Diagnostic Procedures Handbook

including

Key Word Index

2nd Edition

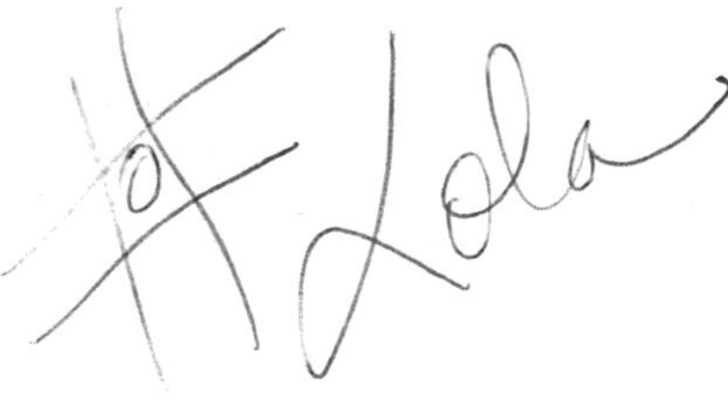

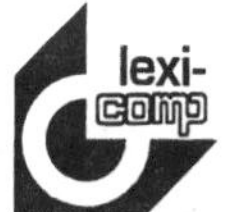

Diagnostic Procedures Handbook

including

Key Word Index

2nd Edition

Franklin A. Michota Jr, MD
Editor
Head, Section of Hospital
and Preoperative Medicine
Department of General Internal Medicine
Cleveland Clinic Foundation
Cleveland, Ohio

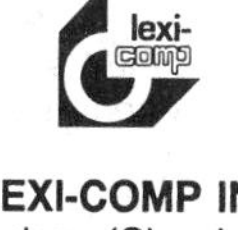

LEXI-COMP INC
Hudson (Cleveland)

CREDITS

Franklin A. Michota Jr, MD
Editor
Head, Section of Hospital
and Preoperative Medicine
Department of General Internal Medicine
Cleveland Clinic Foundation
Cleveland, Ohio

Franklin A. Michota Jr, MD, graduated from The Ohio State University and did his postgraduate work at The Cleveland Clinic Foundation in Cleveland, Ohio. He is a former Chief Medical Resident, and has been a Hospitalist in the Department of General Internal Medicine at the Cleveland Clinic Foundation for the last 4 years. Dr Michota has extensive clinical experience in both acute and subacute inpatient settings. He is currently the Section Chief for Hospital and Preoperative Medicine at the Cleveland Clinic, and serves as an Associate Program Director for the Internal Medicine Residency Program. Dr Michota also has appointments at Ohio State University and Penn State Medical College as an Assistant Professor of Medicine. He has published and presented nationally on the topics of Preoperative Evaluation, Venous Thrombosis, and Hospital Medicine.

This manual was produced using the Pathfinder™ Program — a complete publishing service of Lexi-Comp Inc.

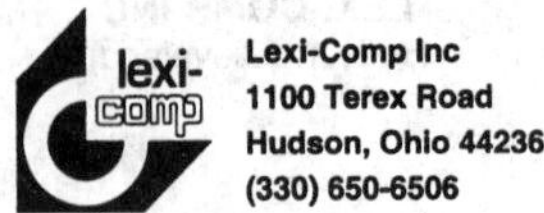

Lexi-Comp Inc
1100 Terex Road
Hudson, Ohio 44236
(330) 650-6506

ISBN 0-916589-73-0

TABLE OF CONTENTS

AUTHORS

Nitamar Abdala, MD
Professor of Radiology
Federal University of São Paulo
São Paulo, Brazil
Magnetic Resonance Imaging

Natalie G. Correia, DO
Associate Director
Internal Medicine Residency Program
Department of General Internal Medicine
Cleveland Clinic Foundation
Cleveland, Ohio
Neurology

Carlos M. Isada, MD
Department of Infectious Disease
Cleveland Clinic Foundation
Cleveland, Ohio
General Internal Medicine

Kevin McCarthy, RCPT
Assistant Technical Director
Pulmonary Function Lab
Cleveland Clinic Foundation
Cleveland, Ohio
Pulmonary Medicine and Critical Care

Peter Mazzone, MD
Fellow
Department of Pulmonary Medicine
Cleveland Clinic Foundation
Cleveland, Ohio
Pulmonary Medicine and Critical Care

Franklin A. Michota Jr, MD
Head, Section of Hospital and Preoperative Medicine
Associate Director
Internal Medicine Residency Program
Department of General Internal Medicine
Cleveland Clinic Foundation
Cleveland, Ohio
General Internal Medicine
Invasive Radiology
Pulmonary Medicine and Critical Care
Ultrasound
Urology

James K. O'Donnell, MD
Director
Department of Nuclear Medicine
Marymount Hospital
Cleveland, Ohio
Nuclear Medicine

Peter B. O'Donovan, MD
Head, Section of Chest Imaging
Department of Diagnostic Radiology
Cleveland Clinic Foundation
Cleveland, Ohio
Computed Tomography
General Radiology

Janus Ong, MD
Fellow
Department of Gastroenterology
Cleveland Clinic Foundation
Cleveland, Ohio
Gastroenterology

Laura Palcisko, RN
Department of General Internal Medicine
Cleveland Clinic Foundation
Cleveland, Ohio
Women's Health

Curtis M. Rimmermann, MD, FACC
Head, Section of Clinical Cardiology
Associate Director
Internal Medicine Residency Program
Department of Cardiology
Cleveland Clinic Foundation
Cleveland, Ohio
Cardiology

Holly Thacker, MD
Head, Section of Women's Health
Department of General Internal Medicine
Cleveland Clinic Foundation
Cleveland, Ohio
Women's Health

CONTRIBUTING AUTHORS TO WOMEN'S HEALTH

Linda Bradley, MD
Department of Obstetrics/Gynecology
Cleveland Clinic Foundation
Cleveland, Ohio

Chad Deal, MD
Department of Rheumatology
Cleveland Clinic Foundation
Cleveland, Ohio

Susan Kalucis, CNP
Department of General Internal Medicine
Cleveland Clinic Foundation
Cleveland, Ohio

AUTHORS *(Continued)*

Mark E. Mayer, MD
Department of General Internal Medicine
Cleveland Clinic Foundation
Cleveland, Ohio

Elisa Ross, MD
Department of Obstetrics/Gynecology
Cleveland Clinic Foundation
Cleveland, Ohio

Holly J. Smedira, MD
Department of General Surgery
Cleveland Clinic Foundation
Cleveland, Ohio

Kristine Zanotti, MD
Department of Obstetrics/Gynecology
Cleveland Clinic Foundation
Cleveland, Ohio

EDITORIAL ADVISORY PANEL

Judith A. Aberg, MD
Director of HIV Services
Washington University School of Medicine
St. Louis, Missouri

Lora L. Armstrong, PharmD, BCPS
Clinical Pharmacist
Caremark Rx, Inc
Northbrook, Illinois

Verna L. Baughman, MD
Associate Professor
Anesthesiology
University of Illinois
Chicago, Illinois

Judith L. Beizer, PharmD, FASCP
Acting Chair and Associate Clinical Professor
Department of Clinical Pharmacy Practice
St John's University College of Pharmacy and Allied Health Professions
Jamaica, New York

Mark F. Bonfiglio, BS, PharmD
Director of Pharmacotherapy Resources
Lexi-Comp, Inc
Hudson, Ohio

Linda R. Bressler, PharmD, BCOP
Department of Pharmacy Practice
University of Illinois College of Pharmacy
Chicago, Illinois

Marcelline Burns, PhD
Research Psychologist
Director, Southern California Research Institute
Los Angeles, California

Harold L. Crossley, DDS, PhD
Associate Professor
Pharmacology
Dental School
University of Maryland at Baltimore
Baltimore, Maryland

Francesca E. Cunningham, PharmD
Program Director for Pharmacoepidemiologic Research
Veterans Affairs
PBM/SHG
Associate Professor
Pharmacy Practice/Anesthesiology
University of Illinois
Chicago, Illinois

Wayne R. DeMott, MD
Pathologists Chartered
Overland Park, Kansas

EDITORIAL ADVISORY PANEL *(Continued)*

Polly E. Kintzel, PharmD, BCPS, BCOP
Clinical Pharmacy Specialist
Bone Marrow Transplantation
Detroit Medical Center
Harper Hospital
Detroit, Michigan

Donna M. Kraus, PharmD
Associate Professor of Pharmacy Practice
Departments of Pharmacy Practice and Pediatrics
Pediatric Clinical Pharmacist
University of Illinois at Chicago
Chicago, Illinois

Charles Lacy, PharmD, FCSHP
Coordinator of Clinical Services
Director, Drug Information Services
Cedars-Sinai Health System
Los Angeles, California

Brenda R. Lance, RN, MSN
Nurse Coordinator
Ritzman Infusion Services
Akron, Ohio

Leonard L. Lance, RPh, BSPharm
Clinical Pharmacist
Lexi-Comp Inc
Hudson, Ohio

Jerrold B. Leikin, MD
Associate Director
Emergency Services
Rush Presbyterian-St Luke's Medical Center
Chicago, Illinois

Timothy F. Meiller, DDS, PhD
Professor
Department of Oral Medicine and Diagnostic Sciences
Baltimore College of Dental Surgery
Professor of Oncology
Greenebaum Cancer Center
University of Maryland at Baltimore
Baltimore, Maryland

Eugene S. Olsowka, MD, PhD
Pathologist
Institute of Pathology PC
Saginaw, Michigan

Thomas E. Page, MA
Drug Recognition Expert and Instructor
Pasadena, CA

Frank P. Paloucek, PharmD
Clinical Associate Professor
University of Illinois
Chicago, Illinois

Christopher J. Papasian, PhD
Director of Diagnostic Microbiology and Immunology Laboratories
Truman Medical Center
Kansas City, Missouri

EDITORIAL ADVISORY PANEL *(Continued)*

FOREWORD

Supporting the difficult-to-achieve national goal of providing the best and most cost-effective medical care dictates that today's medical practitioners take into account a significant array of factors when selecting the appropriate diagnostic procedure for their patients. The dynamics of medical technology, everchanging and expanding regulatory or reimbursement requirements, and the increasing medical awareness on the part of patients are just a few of the important considerations that are likely to affect a practitioner's ultimate approach to use of a diagnostic procedure.

This *Diagnostic Procedure Handbook with Key Word Index (DPH),* which details 309 common and less common procedures, is offered as a handy comprehensive yet concise quick reference for practitioners and other healthcare professionals at all levels of experience or training. The authors, as practicing physicians, have attempted to provide up-to-date information with emphasis on consensus interpretations and practical considerations concerning the diagnostic procedures described in their specialty section.

All procedures covered in this reference are logically structured, with specifications of the procedure presented in a functional and consistent format that allows rapid review of an area of specific interest. Salient points of information pertinent to each major aspect of the procedure are provided: procedure name, abstract, patient care/scheduling, method, specimen (when appropriate), interpretation, footnotes, and references. To be useful, the information contained within a book must be quickly accessible to the user. Therefore, heavy emphasis also has been placed on providing comprehensive indexing and extensive cross-referencing within procedure sections as well as in the Key Word Index and the Alphabetical Index. The arrangement of two major sections, Internal Medicine and Diagnostic Radiology, facilitates access to related procedures or ready review of a specific diagnostic discipline.

The concept for this handbook evolved from the widely used *Laboratory Test Handbook*. The availability of state-of-the-art computer driven typesetting, data base management, and indexing systems (which are Lexi-Comp's specialty) contribute substantially to the ease with which this handbook can be used by the reader.

We hope that this handbook will prove to be not only a valued quick reference but that it will also serve as a useful base to help broaden the user's general knowledge of the many diagnostic tools available today.

ACKNOWLEDGMENTS

The *Diagnostic Procedures Handbook* exists in its present form as the result of the concerted efforts of the following individuals: Robert D. Kerscher, publisher and president of Lexi-Comp Inc; Lynn D. Coppinger, managing editor; Barbara F. Kerscher, production manager; Mark F. Bonfiglio, BS, PharmD, director pharmacotherapy resources; Leonard L. Lance, RPh, BSPharm, pharmacist; Elizabeth Tomsik, PharmD, pharmacotherapy specialist; Joni L. Stahura, BD, PharmD, pharmacotherapy specialist; Matthew Fuller, PharmD, clinical pharmacy specialist, psychiatrist; David C. Marcus, director of information systems; Tracey J. Reinecke, graphic designer.

Special acknowledgment goes out to all Lexi-Comp staff members for their contributions to this handbook.

HOW TO USE THIS HANDBOOK

The *Diagnostic Procedure Handbook with Key Word Index (DPH)* is divided into two primary sections: 1) Internal Medicine and 2) Diagnostic Radiology. Major diagnostic disciplines in each section and the related procedures within the specified discipline are listed alphabetically.

Listed under **Internal Medicine** are:

- **Cardiology**
- **Gastroenterology**
- **General Internal Medicine**
- **Neurology**
- **Pulmonary Medicine and Critical Care**
- **Urology**
- **Women's Health**

Listed under **Diagnostic Radiology** are:

- **Computed Tomography**
- **General Radiology**
- **Invasive Radiology**
- **Magnetic Resonance Imaging**
- **Nuclear Medicine**
- **Ultrasound**

Sections and the procedures within are arranged alphabetically and are cross-referenced with synonyms referring the user to the preferred (appropriate) procedure name.

Each procedure is presented in a consistent format. Information relevant to the given procedure includes:

Name	Specific procedure name
Related information	Cross-reference to other pertinent drug information found elsewhere in this handbook
Synonyms	Other names or accepted abbreviations for the procedure
Applies to	Procedures which are not exact synonyms but have similar instructions or require similar consideration
Replaces	An outdated procedure that has been replaced by a newer procedure
Procedure commonly includes	An abstract of what the procedure includes
Indications	Current use of the procedure
Contraindications	Inappropriate use of the procedure
Patient preparation	Patient care considerations prior to performance of the diagnostic procedure or collection of a specimen

HOW TO USE THIS HANDBOOK *(Continued)*

Aftercare	Patient care considerations following performance of the procedure or specimen collection
Turnaround time	Amount of time needed to obtain results of the procedure
Special instructions	Logistical (scheduling, timing, etc) aspects necessary to appropriately accomplish the procedure or obtain a specimen
Complications	Associated side effects that may occur
Equipment	Specific instruments, tools, supplies required to perform the procedure
Technique	Instructions as to how the procedure is performed
Data acquired	What data can be expected one the procedure is complete
Specimen	Specific specimen required, when appropriate
Volume	Amount of specimen required to perform the procedure, if appropriate
Minimum volume	Minimum amount of specimen required to perform the procedure, if appropriate
Container	Appropriate container into which the specimen is to be drawn, stored, or transported
Collection	Specific information regarding the collection of the specimen
Storage instructions	Indications for storage and/or transport to maintain specimen at optimum condition for testing
Causes for rejection	Circumstances which may invalidate the specimen or procedure
Normal findings	Normal values expected for the procedure
Limitations	Circumstances which may limit the effectiveness of the procedure
Additional information	Information which may contribute to interpretation or utilization of the procedure
Footnotes	Specific literature quotations, specific points of information, or opinions.
References	Selected general documentation from current literature

Acronyms and Abbreviations Glossary

This glossary is a useful listing of acronyms and abbreviations commonly associated with diagnostic procedures. The glossary is not offered as an exhaustive authoritative list, but more as a guide to assist in interpreting frequently used terminology.

Key Word Index

The Key Word Index is not intended in any way to suggest patterns of physicians' orders, nor is it complete. Rather, it is the intent of the authors and editors to make the information easier to find and utilize in order to support better patient care.

The Key Word Index provides a reference to the procedure name based on a diagnostic property, disease entity, organ system, or syndrome for which the procedure is useful. It lists descriptions of specific procedures. Some may support possible clinical diagnoses or rule out other diagnostic possibilities.

Each procedure relevant to the indexed diagnosis is listed and weighted. Two symbols (••) indicate that the procedure is diagnostic, that is, it documents the diagnosis if the expected result is found. A single symbol (•) indicates a procedure frequently used in the diagnosis or management of the particular disease. The other listed procedures are useful on a selective basis with consideration of clinical factors and specific aspects of the case.

Diagnoses with *International Classification of Disease—Clinical Modification* (ICD-9-CM) codes are indicated within the [ ] symbol.

Alphabetical Index

The most expedient method for locating a certain procedure is the alphabetical index in the last section of the handbook. Procedure names and synonyms are listed alphabetically and the page number on which the procedure description may be found is given.

INTERNAL MEDICINE

CARDIOLOGY

- ♦ **Ablation** *see* Electrophysiology Catheter Ablation *on page 31*
- ♦ **Adult Cardiac Catheterization** *see* Cardiac Catheterization, Adult *on page 21*
- ♦ **Ambulatory Electrocardiography** *see* Holter Monitorization *on page 35*
- ♦ **Ambulatory Holter Electrocardiography** *see* Holter Monitorization *on page 35*

Arterial Cannulation

Related Information

Arterial Blood Gases *on page 191*
Pulse Oximetry *on page 245*
Swan-Ganz Catheterization *on page 258*

Synonyms Arterial Catheterization; Arterial Line Placement; Direct Arterial Pressure Monitoring

Procedure Commonly Includes Insertion of an indwelling catheter directly into the arterial circulation for continuous blood pressure (BP) monitoring.

Indications

May be divided into four categories:

- hemodynamic monitoring of the unstable patient (acutely hypotensive or hypertensive) including those on vasopressor or vasodilator agents
- multiple sampling of arterial blood, particularly in the mechanically ventilated patient
- determination of cardiac output (less common)
- administration of local intra-arterial chemotherapy (less common)

Contraindications Poor collateral circulation around the artery to be cannulated constitutes a relative contraindication. Thrombus formation at the catheter site is common and can result in distal extremity ischemia if collaterals are inadequate. Also, coagulopathies, systemic anticoagulation (eg, heparin), and interventional thrombolysis are considered contraindications and reversal may be required.

Patient Preparation The risks and benefits of the procedure are explained. After the site of cannulation is selected by the physician, the area is prepared using povidone-iodine scrub for a minimum of 30 seconds. A sterile technique should be maintained.

Aftercare Meticulous care is required to avoid line-related infections. Recommendations by the Centers for Disease Control include:[1]

- handwashing prior to any manipulation of the system
- applying topical antiseptics to the insertion site immediately after catheter is placed
- covering the site with sterile dressing
- recording date of catheter insertion and each dressing change
- daily inspection of catheter site
- replacing sterile dressing every 48-72 hours with new antibiotic ointment
- flushing of line using normal saline in a closed flush system
- changing flush solution every 24 hours
- changing arterial line site every 4 days or less
- removing catheter promptly at the first sign of infection

Complications Estimates of significant complications range from 15% to 40%. Thrombosis is the most frequent complication. Incidence of thrombosis increases if:

- the catheter is left in place more that 3-4 days
- a large diameter catheter is used

(Continued)

Arterial Cannulation *(Continued)*

- multiple puncture attempts are required
- hypotension, decreased cardiac output, atherosclerosis, or hypothermia are present
- prolonged pressure is required to control bleeding after catheter removal; thrombosis rate under optimal conditions is approximately 5% to 8%; symptomatic occlusion requiring surgery is much less (<1%).

Infectious complications are also frequent, with the catheter serving as either a primary or secondary site of bacteremia. Factors predisposing to infection include prolonged (more than 4 days) catheter insertion, the use of cutdown for insertion, local inflammation, and infection from a secondary source. Other complications include hemorrhage or hematoma formation, pseudoaneurysms, vasovagal reactions, and local skin necrosis. Distal embolization of small clots or air may occur if improper line-flush technique is used.

Equipment Varies somewhat depending on artery selected. A 19- or 20-gauge teflon catheter-over-needle is used in most instances. 16 cm catheters are used for femoral and axillary sites, shorter (1¼" to 2") catheters are used for radial, brachial, and dorsalis pedis sites. If the Seldinger technique is used, a flexible guidewire is also needed. Other equipment includes sterile gloves, hair covers, povidone-iodine, 1% lidocaine without epinephrine, and 3-0 or 4-0 silk suture and suture equipment.

Technique The radial artery is generally considered the site of choice; alternate sites include femoral, axillary, brachial and dorsalis pedis arteries. For radial artery cannulation, the presence of collateral flow must first be established using the modified Allen test. Following this, the wrist is dorsiflexed 60° and using a sterile technique 1% lidocaine is used to infiltrate overlying skin. Catheter-over-needle is inserted at a 30° angle to skin and advanced until arterial blood is seen in the needle hub. The needle is held fixed while the surrounding catheter is advanced into the artery. The needle is removed and the catheter hub is attached to the connecting tubing. After suturing the catheter in place, a wrist board may be used to stabilize the neutral wrist position. The Seldinger technique may be used for larger arteries. Here, the artery is located with a simple 20-gauge needle. Once arterial blood is returned, a flexible guidewire is passed through the needle; the needle is removed and the teflon catheter is threaded over the guidewire into the artery.

Data Acquired Graphic waveform of arterial pressure, with pressure on the vertical axis (mm Hg) and time on the horizontal axis

Normal Findings A typical arterial pressure tracing for a normal individual is depicted in Figure A on the following page.

The peak of each waveform represents the systolic blood pressure and the trough represents the diastolic blood pressure (in mm Hg). Normal values for blood pressure obtained by arterial cannulation are slightly higher than those obtained by routine sphygmomanometry, ranging from 5-20 mm Hg higher. This is due to a combination of physiologic and technical factors, reviewed elsewhere.[2] If indirect pressure readings (ie, cuff pressures) are greater than arterial line readings, instrument error is likely. The entire system (tubing, calibration, seals, catheter, etc) should be carefully inspected; the transmitted arterial waveforms may also appear "damped," further suggesting technical error. A normal "square wave" response is also shown in Figure A. This waveform is seen whenever the tubing system is flushed. Most monitoring systems are equipped with a "flush valve" which can be opened and closed rapidly (routinely performed by nursing staff). A rapid-velocity stream flows through the tubing, removing bubbles and debris. The resulting waveform is by nature artifactual, but abnormalities in its configuration suggest underlying technical problems. See Figure B. on page 20.

In normal individuals, peak systolic blood pressures vary somewhat with respiration, a finding difficult to appreciate with bedside sphygmomanometry, but easily observed with direct arterial blood pressure monitoring. When a healthy person inspires, there is a transient fall in blood pressure. On the blood pressure monitoring screen, this appears as a "dip" in the pressure tracings, which returns to baseline during expiration. The maximum drop in systolic blood pressure (pulsus paradoxus) should not exceed 8-10 mm Hg. Values

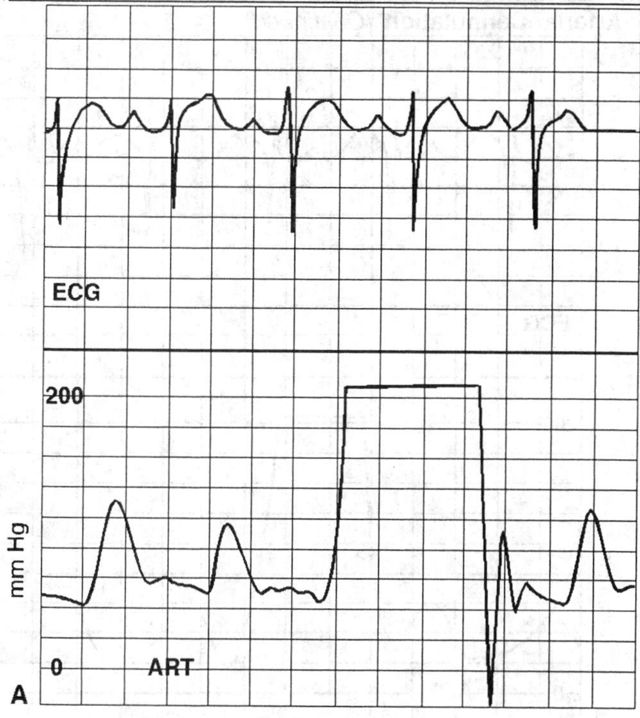

Normal arterial pressure tracing (lower panel) with simultaneous electrocardiogram (upper). Marker indicates start of square wave. Reproduced with permission from *Textbook of Advanced Cardiac Life Support*, American Heart Association, 1987.

less than this are physiologic and should not be confused with cardiac tamponade.

Critical Values Cutoff values for hypertension, as defined in textbooks, are the same for blood pressure obtained by arterial cannulation and routine sphygmomanometry. A "hypertensive urgency" is characterized by marked elevations in diastolic (and sometimes systolic) blood pressure, accompanied by retinal hemorrhages, exudates, and papilledema. End-organ damage is likely within several days if blood pressure is not adequately controlled. In a "hypertensive emergency" (malignant hypertension), the retinal findings described are present along with such alarming features as acute renal failure, seizures, blurred vision, mental status deterioration, stroke, and congestive heart failure. End-organ damage is already apparent. Although both hypertensive urgencies and emergencies show marked blood pressure elevations (eg, diastolic blood pressure >120-140 mm Hg), there are no precise cutoff values. These syndromes should not be arbitrarily diagnosed or excluded on the basis of arterial line blood pressure readings alone; they are complex clinical diagnoses. Similarly, no black-and-white cutoff values exist for defining hypotension. Most physicians would consider a systolic blood pressure in the 70-80 mm Hg range abnormal if the individual was previously healthy. However, systolic blood pressures in the 80-90 mm Hg range are not unheard of in the patient with end stage cardiac disease or on multiple vasodilatory agents. Conversely, a "normal" systolic blood pressure of 110 mm Hg may indicate significant hypotension in the dialysis patient whose baseline is 200 mm Hg. A drop in systolic blood pressure during inspiration >10 mm Hg is significant. (Continued)

Arterial Cannulation *(Continued)*

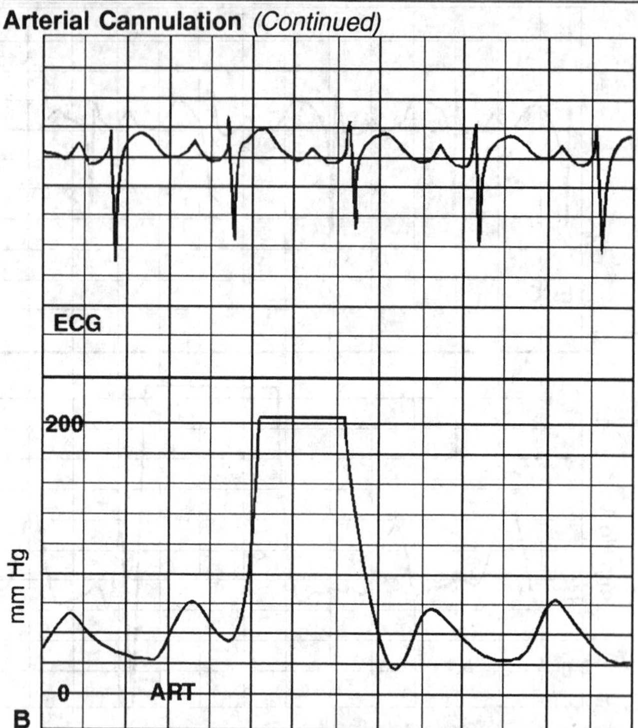

Damped arterial pressure tracing (lower panel) with simultaneous normal electrocardiogram (upper). Configuration of square wave is also damped, suggesting technical error. Reproduced with permission from *Textbook of Advanced Cardiac Life Support*, American Heart Association, 1987.

This increased paradoxical pulse may be seen in cardiac tamponade, severe asthma, pulmonary embolism, and other conditions. Arterial cannulation is useful in monitoring the patient with cardiac tamponade, but is seldom used to make the diagnosis. Disparity in blood pressure readings between direct and indirect measurements >20 mm Hg may occur in shock states. This is due to reflex peripheral vasoconstriction (increased systemic vascular resistance). Korotkoff sounds may be barely audible when direct measurement of central arterial pressures are low-normal. Large discrepancies may also be seen in patients with severe peripheral atherosclerosis (arteriosclerosis obliterans), where systolic pressure drops off dramatically distal to a luminal occlusion. It should be emphasized that inaccuracies may occur in **both** direct and indirect systems. Clinical importance should be placed on the trends in blood pressure values, regardless of the system used.

Limitations Accuracy is limited by errors introduced by the equipment, which transforms mechanical energy (pulse) into electrical energy (tracing). Factors such as the natural frequency of the transducer, clamping, and compliance may cause artifact. Other sources of error include improper leveling of equipment, improper assembly, and air in the tubing.

Additional Information Arterial cannulation is generally considered a procedure of low technical difficulty. The true difficulty lies in avoidance of thrombosis and infection and careful patient selection.

Footnotes

1. Center for Disease Control Working Group Guidelines for Prevention of Intravascular Infections, "Guidelines for the Prevention and Control of Nosocomial Infection," U.S. Department of Health and Human Services, Public Health Service, 1981.
2. American Heart Association, *Textbook of Advanced Cardiac Life Support*, 1987.

References

Mandel MA and Dauchot PJ, "Radial-Artery Cannulation in 1000 Patients: Precautions and Complications," *J Hand Surg*, 1977, 2:482-5.

Pearson ML, Hierholzer WJ, Garner JS, et al, "Guidelines for Prevention of Intravascular Device-Related Infections: Hospital Infection Control Practices Advisory Committee," *Am J Infect Control*, 1996, 24(4):267-77.

Venus B, Mathru M, Smith RA, et al, "Direct Versus Indirect Blood Pressure Measurements in Critically Ill Patients," *Heart Lung*, 1985, 14(3):228-31.

♦ **Arterial Catheterization** *see* Arterial Cannulation *on page 17*

♦ **Arterial Line Placement** *see* Arterial Cannulation *on page 17*

Cardiac Catheterization, Adult

Related Information

Pericardiocentesis *on page 39*

Swan-Ganz Catheterization *on page 258*

Synonyms Adult Cardiac Catheterization; Cineangiocardiography; Coronary Arteriography; Left Heart Catheterization; Right and Left Heart Catheterization; Right Heart Catheterization

Applies to HIS Bundle Electrograms

Procedure Commonly Includes

Left heart catheterization: In the fasting state the right femoral area is topically anesthetized including the subcutaneous tissue. After adequate anesthesia, using a guidewire, a preformed coronary artery catheter is advanced under x-ray guidance to the right and left coronary ostia respectively. Dye is injected into the coronary ostia to delineate the coronary artery anatomy and assess for coronary artery stenoses. In addition, a separate catheter called a pigtail catheter is introduced retrograde across the aortic valve into the left ventricular cavity and a left ventriculogram is obtained. The left ventriculogram helps delineate global and regional left ventricular systolic function and assess for the presence of mitral insufficiency.

Right heart catheterization: The femoral vein is accessed and under fluoroscopic guidance a catheter is advanced via the inferior vena cava to the right atrium, right ventricle, and main pulmonary artery. The subclavian vein and internal jugular vein may also be used for central venous access. Intracardiac pressure recordings, oxygen saturation levels, and cardiac output measurements are frequently obtained.

Indications

- evaluate patients being considered for coronary bypass surgery
- evaluate patients to determine whether angina is the result of aortic stenosis or coronary artery disease
- determine if bypass grafts are patent
- evaluate patients in whom surgical repair is being considered (ie, left ventricular aneurysm, perforated interventricular septum, mitral insufficiency)
- definitive determination of the presence of coronary artery disease
- evaluate structural, valvular, and vascular abnormalities
- measurement of intracardiac pressures, cardiac output, and oxygen saturation

Contraindications

Left heart catheterization

- severe congestive heart failure
- advanced renal insufficiency
- severe peripheral vascular disease
- history of cholesterol embolization

Right heart catheterization

- tricuspid valve prosthesis
- right-sided intracardiac mass

Patient Preparation Patients scheduled for a left heart catheterization must have a written and properly identified consultation from a cardiologist recorded

(Continued)

Cardiac Catheterization, Adult *(Continued)*

in the chart prior to the procedure. The consultant's note should state indications for the procedure and evaluation of risk to the patient.

Left heart catheterization: CBC, BUN, creatinine, chest x-ray, and electrocardiogram should be recorded in the chart the day before the test. A serum potassium should also be ordered the day before the test on all patients receiving diuretics; if the Judkin's technique will be used, shave the patient's iliofemoral areas the day before the procedure; two units of blood may be on call in the Blood Bank. The requesting physician may need to obtain a signed procedure permit for the invasive diagnostic test. Patients younger than 18 years of age must have a parent or legal guardian sign the permit. Patients receiving digitalis should be given their usual dose the morning of the catheterization. A sedative such as midazolam should be given on call from the Cardiac Catheterization Laboratory. For AM patients, omit breakfast on the day of the test. For PM patients, juice and coffee may be given at breakfast time. The patient's weight is obtained on the day of the procedure and recorded in the chart. All patients are sent to the laboratory on a stretcher wearing a hospital gown and regular slippers.

Aftercare Right heart catheterization (including HIS bundle electrograms): Remove dressing after 4 hours. Check for hematoma or bleeding at catheter insertion site twice in 1 hour. If a cutdown was performed, remove the sutures in 5-7 days.

Left heart catheterization (including coronary angiograms): Check the patient's heart rate, blood pressure, arterial puncture site, and distal pulses four times at 15-minute intervals, then four times at 30-minute intervals, then four times at 1-hour intervals. If the femoral approach has been used, enforce absolute bedrest for 6 hours.

Turnaround Time Preliminary reports will be recorded in the chart on the day of the procedure. Final reports will be sent to the chart approximately 72 hours after the procedure.

References

"ACC/AHA Guidelines for Cardiac Catheterization and Cardiac Catheterization Laboratories. American College of Cardiology/American Heart Association Ad Hoc Task Force on Cardiac Catheterization," *J Am Coll Cardiol*, 1991, 18(5):1149-82.

♦ **Cardiogram** *see* Electrocardiography *on page 30*

Cardiopulmonary Stress Test

Related Information

Cardiac Catheterization, Adult *on page 21*

Synonyms ETT; Exercise Tolerance Test; Graded Exercise Test; Metabolic Stress Test

Indications

- determine the presence and severity of exercise-induced myocardial ischemia
- evaluate the potential for exercise-induced rhythm disturbances
- evaluate the hemodynamic responses to activity
- evaluate the effect of medical or interventional therapy
- prescribe appropriate activity guidelines
- evaluate patient's exercise/work tolerance
- evaluate the impact of cardiac rehabilitation intervention
- assess the functional significance of valvular heart disease
- evaluate oxygen and carbon dioxide consumption

Contraindications

- acute MI
- severe symptomatic valvular heart disease
- uncontrolled ventricular arrhythmias
- uncontrolled supraventricular arrhythmias compromising cardiac function
- unstable or rest angina
- uncompensated congestive heart failure
- suspected or known dissecting aortic aneurysm
- thrombophlebitis
- left ventricular outflow tract (LVOT) obstruction with resting symptoms

- clinically significant acute pericarditis or myocarditis
- symptomatic complete heart block
- mobile intracardiac thrombus with peripheral embolization
- significant psychiatric disturbance
- neuromuscular complications that prevent or severely limit ambulation

Patient Preparation The patient is examined and assessed for exercise candidacy by a physician. Test procedure, risks, and benefits are explained to the patient and informed consent is obtained. All clothes above the waist are removed. Female patients may wear a loose-fitting hospital gown that offers easy access to electrodes and lead wires. The skin at electrode sites is vigorously prepared to remove dirt and oils. Electrodes and lead wires are secured to minimize motion artifact. Resting, supine, and standing 12-lead EKGs are recorded and compared to previous EKGs to identify changes. A 30-second posthyperventilation EKG is often recorded prior to exercise to identify ventilatory-induced changes in the ST segments. The patient receives instruction and demonstration regarding walking on the treadmill. The patient is encouraged to walk upright, take long steps, and rely on the treadmill bar only for balance and not for support. After a brief trial period when the patient is adapted to treadmill ambulation, the protocol is initiated.

Aftercare The patient is monitored until hemodynamically stable and blood pressure and pulse values return to a near-baseline level. Patients should check with laboratory personnel before leaving the area.

Special Instructions Outpatients are by appointment only. Inpatients are scheduled as soon as possible (usually within 24 hours of request). Patients are instructed not to eat or drink for 3-4 hours before the test and are also instructed to bring or wear clothes suitable for exercise. Patients are variably requested to discontinue medication as instructed by their personal physicians. Other medications should be taken as prescribed unless instructed differently. The procedure, risks, and benefits should be explained by the physician and the receipt of patient consent should be documented prior to beginning the test.

Equipment Motor driven treadmill, multichannel electrocardiograph with real-time monitor display and printer; sphygmomanometer; cardiac emergency equipment (defibrillator, oxygen, suction, I.V. kits and fluid, emergency drugs, airway management equipment). A nose clip and computerized equipment are used to measure both oxygen and carbon dioxide consumption.

Technique The skin at the electrode sites is vigorously prepared with alcohol and mild abrasion to remove superficial layers of skin. Electrodes are attached to the chest wall. Baseline, pretest 12-lead electrocardiograms are recorded in the supine and standing positions and compared to previous standard 12-lead EKGs for new changes. Post 30-second hyperventilation electrocardiograms are often performed to identify ventilatory-induced electrocardiogram changes. The test procedure is explained to the patient and informed consent is obtained. The patient during testing wears a nose clip and breathes through a nonrebreathing valve that separates expired air from room air. The technician verbally instructs and demonstrates proper treadmill walking technique. The test is performed with a technician and at least one other qualified professional present. The physician is available in the testing area. An appropriate exercise protocol is selected based on the clinical questions asked, the patient's medical status, and the predicted exercise ability of the patient. Every 2-3 minutes the speed and/or grade of the treadmill are increased to yield an increment of ½-2 METS increase per stage. At least one channel (V_5) and preferably three channels of the electrocardiogram are continuously monitored on a real-time visual display monitor. Twelve-lead electrocardiograms and blood pressures are recorded at least once at every stage (usually within the last 30 seconds of each stage). Heart rate, ST segments, arrhythmias, symptoms, and subjective patient responses are also continuously monitored. The test is terminated when the patient achieves a subjective maximal effort, significant ischemic changes are observed, significant rhythm disturbances are observed, hemodynamic status is compromised, the patient requests to stop the test, the equipment fails, or a predetermined endpoint is achieved. During the test, measurements of expired gas are obtained including oxygen tension, carbon dioxide tension, and air flow. In addition,

(Continued)

Cardiopulmonary Stress Test *(Continued)*

ventilatory measurements are also obtained including respiratory rate, minute ventilation, and tidal volume. Both oxygen and carbon dioxide tension are sampled by utilizing a mixed chamber. Oxygen and carbon dioxide consumption can be calculated from ventilatory volumes and also by utilizing differences between expired and inspired gas analysis. These measurements are equivalent to total body oxygen consumption and carbon dioxide production. Noninvasive measurement of oxygen saturation can be obtained by using oximetry. At the conclusion of the exercise test, the treadmill speed and grade are lowered to a baseline level and the patient is encouraged to ambulate as tolerated to avoid venous pooling and a vasovagal response. Patients should ambulate for 3-5 minutes or until the heart rate and blood pressure plateau. Patients are then observed in the sitting or supine position. Patients unable to ambulate after the test should be immediately placed in the prone position and monitored. During recovery, the EKG is continuously monitored and recorded, along with blood pressure and symptoms every minute, until the patient is hemodynamically stable and has returned to a near pretest level.

Data Acquired 12-lead EKG, heart rate, arrhythmias, ST segment values, blood pressure, symptoms, patient subjective responses (eg, rating of perceived exertion, angina scale, dyspnea scale), oxygen tension, carbon dioxide tension, air flow, ventilatory measurements, oxygen and carbon dioxide consumption

Normal Findings Shortening of the PR and QT intervals and J point depression may occur. Less than 1 mm upsloping ST segment depression 60-80 msec after the J point as compared to resting measures. A linear increase in heart rate with activity >85% predicted maximal heart rate (if not on a chronotropic medication, most commonly a beta blocker). A continuous increase of 7-12 mm Hg in systolic blood pressure per MET achieved to a peak systolic blood pressure <220 mm Hg. A fall, no change, or >20 mm Hg increase in diastolic blood pressure to a peak <120 mm Hg. Occasional ventricular or supraventricular ectopy that does not significantly increase with activity. Test termination because of leg or general fatigue and appropriate shortness of breath. Nausea and dizziness early in recovery are not uncommon.

Critical Values 1 mm or more upright, horizontal, or downsloping ST segment depression; 60-80 msec beyond the J point as compared to rest without any confounding medication; metabolic or baseline electrocardiogram abnormalities. Horizontal or downsloping ST segment depression carries a greater probability of significant coronary artery disease compared to rapid recovering upsloping depression. Greater than or equal to 1 mm ST segment elevation of the J point in leads without significant Q waves. Greater than 10 mm Hg fall in systolic blood pressure with increasing workloads recorded on two separate readings at least 30 seconds apart (especially if associated with symptoms of exercise intolerance). An increase of the systolic blood pressure >250 mm Hg, increasing ventricular ectopy to >30% of all complexes, and the onset of complete left or right bundle branch block. The onset of second or third degree heart block, lightheadedness or cyanosis, ataxia, confusion, or nausea during activity.

Limitations

- ST segments cannot be accurately interpreted if patient has left bundle branch block, left ventricular hypertrophy with secondary ST-T changes, the Wolff-Parkinson-White syndrome, digitalis administration, ventricular pacing, electrolyte abnormalities, or baseline ST-T wave abnormalities.
- Sudden intense activity can cause false-positive ST segment depression.
- Medications such as beta blockers, calcium blockers, vasodilators, and afterload reducing agents may reduce myocardial oxygen demand and ameliorate ischemia during activity.
- The early termination of the test by the patient or investigator limits predictive ability.
- Exercise stress testing has an average sensitivity of 60% to 70% and specificity of 80% to 90% for the detection of flow-limiting coronary artery disease.
- The less severe the disease the lower the sensitivity.

- Orthopedic complications and the lack of patient motivation both limit the predictive ability of the test if peak myocardial oxygen demand is not achieved.
- Women yield a higher false-positive rate than men.

References

McKelvie RS and Jones NL, "Cardiopulmonary Exercise Testing," *Clin Chest Med*, 1989, 10(2):277-91.

Wasserman K, Hanson JE, Su DY, et al, *Principles of Exercise Testing and Interpretation*, Philadelphia, PA: Lea and Febiger, 1987.

♦ **Cineangiocardiography** *see* Cardiac Catheterization, Adult *on page 21*

Color Doppler

Synonyms Color Flow Doppler; Color Flow Mapping

Procedure Commonly Includes Color Doppler echocardiography integrates the structural information provided by 2-D echocardiography with pulsed Doppler color-coded flow maps that depict the direction, velocity, and turbulence of blood flow through the cardiac chambers and great vessels. A true noninvasive color Doppler assessment is now part of each complete transthoracic echocardiogram examination.

Indications Color Doppler complements two-dimensional echocardiography and conventional Doppler techniques by providing color flow maps that improve the spatial characterization of flow disturbances. It is proven to be of most value in the detection and specifically the quantitation of regurgitant lesions. The gradation of aortic, mitral, tricuspid, and pulmonic insufficiency can now be assessed with the help of color Doppler. The localization and direction of regurgitant jets, via color Doppler display, has provided useful insight regarding the etiology of regurgitant lesions. Color Doppler can also assist in the evaluation of stenotic lesions by providing a clear visual display of jet directions from which continuous wave Doppler velocities can be measured. It also aids in determining the size of valve orifices. Additionally, the diagnosis of intracardiac shunts in congenital heart disease has been greatly enhanced by color Doppler echocardiography. Increased color Doppler flow velocities also assist in determining the level of left ventricular outflow obstruction in the presence of hypertrophic obstructive cardiomyopathy.

Contraindications There are no contraindications for a color Doppler examination. Like all other forms of cardiac ultrasound technically poor studies may be obtained in patients with chronic lung disease or obesity. The registration of color Doppler decreases in the far field and flow abnormalities may not be obvious in areas distant to the transducer.

Patient Preparation No special patient preparation is required. Fasting is not necessary. No special time of day is preferred.

Technique The color Doppler study is performed simultaneously with the 2-D echocardiogram. After obtaining the initial echocardiographic views and optimizing the settings, the color Doppler is activated to survey the flow pattern through the cardiac chambers and great vessels. The operator next focuses on specific flow abnormalities of interest. The long axis left parasternal view is most useful to evaluate flow through the mitral valve into the left ventricle and out of the left ventricle through the left ventricular outflow tract and aortic valve. Mitral insufficiency and aortic insufficiency can be evaluated from this view. The left parasternal short axis view at the base of the heart best depicts antegrade flow through the tricuspid valve into the right ventricle and through the pulmonic valve to the pulmonary artery. The apical 4-chamber view permits study of flow through the tricuspid and mitral valves into the right ventricle and left ventricle respectively. This view also permits evaluation and quantification of mitral and tricuspid regurgitation. The apical 5-chamber view permits the study of flow through the left ventricular outflow tract. It also permits evaluation and quantification of aortic and mitral insufficiency. The subcostal view permits study of the right ventricle and left ventricular inflow patterns through the tricuspid and mitral valves. It also permits determination of the presence and severity of mitral and tricuspid insufficiency. The suprasternal view provides an opportunity to study flow in the ascending aorta, aortic arch, and descending aorta. Conditions such as aortic stenosis and coarctation of the aorta can often be best studied from this region.

(Continued)

Color Doppler *(Continued)*

Normal Findings A good understanding of normal and abnormal cardiac physiology is needed to adequately interpret color Doppler echocardiography. It is also important to recognize that mild degrees of valvular incompetence, especially tricuspid and mitral, are frequently present in normal subjects. When significant insufficiency is present, this must be evaluated from different orthogonal planes to best obtain a volumetric estimation of the regurgitant jet. A detailed description of the size, direction, and number of jets helps in assessing the severity and etiology of the regurgitant lesion. Similar detailed analysis should be made in intracardiac shunt lesions so that the precise anatomic site and size can be determined. The direction of color flow, including right-to-left, left-to-right, or bidirectional, should be described. In patients with stenotic lesions, color flow can further elucidate the site of obstruction and aid in the precise determination of orifice areas. The degree of flow disturbance is also related to the severity of the stenosis.

References

Otto C, *The Practice of Clinical Echocardiography*, Philadelphia, PA: WB Saunders Co, 1997.

♦ **Color Flow Doppler** *see* Color Doppler *on page 25*

♦ **Color Flow Imaging** *see* Transesophageal Echocardiography *on page 42*

♦ **Color Flow Mapping** *see* Color Doppler *on page 25*

♦ **Continuous Wave Doppler** *see* Transesophageal Echocardiography *on page 42*

♦ **Coronary Arteriography** *see* Cardiac Catheterization, Adult *on page 21*

♦ **Cross-Sectional Echocardiography** *see* Two-Dimensional Echocardiography *on page 46*

♦ **2-D Echo** *see* Two-Dimensional Echocardiography *on page 46*

♦ **Direct Arterial Pressure Monitoring** *see* Arterial Cannulation *on page 17*

Dobutamine Echocardiography

Synonyms Stress Echocardiography

Indications

- determine the presence and severity of exercise-induced myocardial ischemia
- evaluate the potential for exercise-induced rhythm disturbances
- evaluate the hemodynamic responses to activity
- evaluate the effect of medical or interventional therapy
- prescribe appropriate activity guidelines
- evaluate patient's exercise/work tolerance
- evaluate the impact of cardiac rehabilitation intervention
- assess the functional significance of valvular heart disease
- evaluate for myocardial viability

Contraindications

- acute MI
- severe symptomatic valvular heart disease
- uncontrolled ventricular arrhythmias
- uncontrolled supraventricular arrhythmias compromising cardiac function
- unstable or rest angina
- uncompensated congestive heart failure
- suspected or known dissecting aortic aneurysm
- thrombophlebitis
- recent embolism
- symptomatic left ventricular outflow tract (LVOT) obstruction
- clinically significant acute pericarditis or myocarditis
- mobile intracardiac thrombus
- significant psychiatric disturbance

Patient Preparation The patient is examined and assessed for dobutamine echocardiogram candidacy by a physician. The test procedure, risks, and benefits are explained to the patient and informed consent is obtained. All clothes above the waist are removed. The skin at the electrode site is prepared with alcohol to remove dirt and oils. Electrodes are attached to the chest wall. A supine 12-lead electrocardiogram is recorded and compared to previous electrocardiograms to identify changes. The patient receives test instructions and expectations during the protocol.

Aftercare The patient is monitored until hemodynamically stable and blood pressure and pulse values return to a near baseline level. The patient should check out with laboratory personnel when leaving the area.

Special Instructions Outpatients are by appointment only. Inpatients are scheduled as soon as possible (usually within 24 hours of request). Patients are instructed not to eat or drink for 3-4 hours before the test and are also instructed to bring or wear clothes suitable for exercise. Patients are variably requested to discontinue medication as instructed by their personal physicians. Other medications should be taken as prescribed unless instructed differently. The procedure, risks, and benefits should be explained by the physician and the receipt of patient consent should be documented prior to beginning the test.

Equipment Multichannel electrocardiograph with real-time monitor display and printer, sphygmomanometer, cardiac emergency equipment (defibrillator, oxygen, suction, I.V. kits and fluid, emergency drugs, airway management equipment), echocardiogram machine and computerized digitalization equipment for echocardiogram images

Technique The patient is brought to the Echocardiogram Laboratory in a prescheduled 4-hour fasting state. The patient may take medications as instructed by his/her individual physician prior to the test. Atrioventricular nodal suppressing medication such as beta blockers and calcium blockers which may blunt heart rate are typically held prior to the test. The skin at the electrode sites is prepared with alcohol and mild abrasion to remove superficial skin layers of skin. Electrodes are attached to the chest wall. Pretest 12-lead electrocardiograms are recorded in the supine position and compared to previous standard 12-lead electrocardiograms for new changes. The test procedure is explained to the patient and informed consent is obtained. A peripheral intravenous line is placed. A complete resting echocardiogram is obtained including computer digitized images of the left ventricle fully assessing regional wall motion. All cardiac valves, chamber dimensions, and the ascending aorta are fully evaluated and imaged. Once a baseline echocardiogram has been obtained, in the presence of a cardiac sonographer and supervising physician, the dobutamine infusion is begun. Dobutamine is begun at a dose of 5 μg/kg/minute with 3-minute stages increasing to 10 μg/kg/minute, 20 μg/kg/minute, 30 μg/kg/minute to a maximal dose of 40 μg/kg/minute. An electrocardiogram is obtained at each stage as is continuous blood pressure and pulse rate assessment. If 85% of the age-predicted maximum heart rate is not obtained by 40 μg/kg/minute, atropine in 0.25 mg aliquots is given intravenously to a total dose of 2 mg. Atropine is contraindicated in the presence of glaucoma or significantly symptomatic prostatic hypertrophy. During each dobutamine stage, further echocardiogram images are obtained and selected images are digitized for post-test analysis and comparison. At the conclusion of the test, after all echocardiogram images are obtained and a maximal heart rate has been achieved, the dobutamine infusion is stopped. The patient is observed in the recovery period until the heart rate returns to the pretest level and the blood pressure has also returned to baseline. The intravenous line is disconnected, and the patient leaves the Echocardiogram Laboratory under his/her own power.

Data Acquired 12-lead electrocardiogram, heart rate, arrhythmias, ST segment values, blood pressure, symptoms, patient's subjective responses, a full resting and dobutamine echocardiogram

Normal Findings Shortening of the PR and QT intervals and J point depression may occur. Less than 1 mm upsloping ST segment depression 60-80 msec after the J point as compared to resting measures. A linear increase in heart rate with dobutamine infusion >85% of the predicted maximum heart rate if not on a chronotropic medication such as a beta blocker. Occasional ventricular supraventricular ectopy which does not significantly increase with dobutamine infusion. A symmetric decrease in end-systolic dimensions and increase in endocardial thickening with dobutamine infusion as observed by (Continued)

Dobutamine Echocardiography *(Continued)*

echocardiography. The regional wall motion response and endocardial thickening extent should be equivalent in all myocardial segments. Test termination secondary to maximal predicted heart rate attained, significant dysrhythmia and/or significant hypertensive/hypotensive response to dobutamine infusion.

Critical Values Significant nonsustained ventricular tachycardia, sustained atrial arrhythmias, a hypertensive response >220 mm Hg, a hypotensive response >20 mm Hg less than the starting baseline blood pressure, angina pectoris, and an abnormal echocardiogram response to dobutamine infusion

Limitations

- patients with difficult echocardiogram windows where visualization of the left ventricle is limited
- failure to achieve a maximum predicted heart rate and therefore a nondiagnostic test
- premature test termination secondary to angina, significant arrhythmia, or abnormal blood pressure response
- glaucoma and/or symptomatic benign prostatic hypertrophy precluding atropine administration

References

Poldermans D, Fioretti PM, Boersma E, et al, "Safety of Dobutamine-Atropine Stress Echocardiography in Patients With Suspected or Proven Coronary Artery Disease," *Am J Cardiol*, 1994, 73(7):456-9.

Sawada SG, Seger DS, Ryan T, et al, "Echocardiographic Detection of Coronary Artery Disease During Dobutamine Infusion," *Circulation*, 1991, 83(5):1605-14.

♦ **Doppler Echo** *see* Doppler Echocardiography *on page 28*

Doppler Echocardiography

Related Information

Pericardiocentesis *on page 39*

Synonyms Doppler Echo; Doppler Ultrasound

Procedure Commonly Includes The clinical application of Doppler echocardiography is based on the Doppler shift principle. Sound waves increase or decrease their frequency as the object that produces or reflects the Doppler signal transmits or moves away from a given point. A transducer that acts as a transmitter and receiver is placed on the chest wall as the ultrasound waves are sent parallel to cardiac flow. The red cells reflect these waves and alter the frequency of the ultrasound wave proportionately to their velocity. By knowing the velocity of ultrasound through cardiac tissue, the frequency of the transmitted and received sound waves, and the angle of incidence, it is possible to calculate the velocity of blood flow. Volume measurements can be calculated by measuring the diameter or area of a given vessel or chamber and multiplying this by the Doppler-derived velocity. Pressure gradients can be measured by Doppler echocardiography using the simplified Bernoulli's equation:

$P = 4V^2$ where P is the pressure gradient and V is the Doppler-derived velocity

Doppler echocardiography can be used as a stand alone technique with a Piddof transducer or it can be image guided by 2-D echocardiography. Doppler can be pulsed wave or continuous wave depending upon the transducer sending and receiving ultrasound waves intermittently or continuously. The pulsed wave Doppler has the advantage of permitting the precise location of the Doppler flow (range resolution) but is limited to the maximal flow velocity, usually 1-1.5 m/second. Continuous wave Doppler does not possess a high spatial resolution but can detect high velocities of flow as seen in stenotic or regurgitant lesions. In most situations, both forms of Doppler ultrasound are required; the pulsed wave form to determine the origin and extent of the flow disturbance and continuous wave Doppler to detect the maximal velocities present.

Indications Doppler echocardiography complements 2-D echocardiography by providing hemodynamic information not available through conventional echocardiography. The most common application of Doppler echocardiography includes evaluation of stenotic and regurgitant valve lesions and the study of intracardiac shunts. Continuous wave Doppler echocardiography permits precise measurement of gradients in aortic stenosis and, when combined with 2-D echo, permits calculation of the aortic valve area. In mitral stenosis, it permits the measurement of the transmitral gradient. Through the use of the pressure half-time calculation, it allows for estimation of the mitral valve area. Pulsed wave Doppler permits not only the diagnosis but an approximate quantification of aortic and mitral insufficiency. Other applications of Doppler echocardiography include cardiac output calculations and intracardiac pressure measurements such as right ventricular and pulmonary artery systolic pressure.

Contraindications There are no contraindications to Doppler echocardiography. Similar to 2-D echocardiography, technical difficulties may exist in patients with chronic lung disease or obesity. The utmost care must be used to obtain the best spectral display in every patient. This frequently requires the use of multiple transducer locations to best evaluate the flow disturbance.

Patient Preparation No special patient preparation is required. Fasting is not necessary. No special time of the day is preferred.

Special Instructions A complete Doppler study takes approximately 20 minutes. If a patient is scheduled for a full Doppler and two-dimensional echocardiogram examination, 45 minutes of scheduled time will be necessary. A note in the chart or requisition form detailing the reason for the Doppler study request will greatly help the Echocardiography Laboratory personnel to provide a goal-directed study. Other useful information includes age, weight, and height.

Technique Most patients will have a Doppler study in conjunction with a 2-D echocardiogram. Initial patient interaction is similar in both cases. After the 2-D echocardiogram is completed, a Doppler study can then be performed to address specific unanswered questions. Routinely, a Doppler study will include a flow interrogation of the aortic valve from the cardiac apex, right parasternal window, and suprasternal window. The mitral and tricuspid valves can be best interrogated from the left parasternal window and from the cardiac apex. The pulmonic valve is best interrogated from the left parasternal window. Recordings at all these levels are made on a video cassette recorder and selected images are digitized for cine-loop playback. All necessary measurements are made from the video recordings through built-in computer measurement packages.

Normal Findings Adequate interpretation of Doppler echocardiograms requires a comprehensive understanding of cardiovascular physiology and hemodynamics, knowledge of the normal Doppler flow patterns, plus a working understanding of the normal range of velocities through the cardiac valves and chambers. Distinct abnormalities have been characterized by Doppler echocardiography in most cardiac disorders. See table.

Peak Doppler Velocities (m/sec)

	Children	Adults
Mitral flow	1.0 (0.8-1.2)	0.9 (0.4-1.3)
Tricuspid flow	0.6 (0.5-0.8)	0.5 (0.3-0.7)
Pulmonary artery	0.9 (0.7-1.1)	0.75 (0.6-0.9)
Left ventricle	1.0 (0.7-1.2)	0.9 (0.7-1.1)
Aorta	1.5 (1.2-1.8)	1.35 (1.0-1.7)

Reproduced with permission from Hatle L and Angelson B, *Doppler Ultrasound in Cardiology: Physical Principles and Clinical Applications,* 2nd ed, Philadelphia, PA: Lee & Febiger, 1985.

References

Otto C, *The Practice of Clinical Echocardiography,* Philadelphia, PA: WB Saunders Co, 1997.

♦ **Doppler Ultrasound** *see* Doppler Echocardiography *on page 28*

♦ **Dynamic Electrocardiography** *see* Holter Monitorization *on page 35*

♦ **ECG** *see* Electrocardiography *on page 30*

♦ **EKG** *see* Electrocardiography *on page 30*

♦ **EKG, 2-Step Test** *see* Electrocardiogram, Adult, Exercise EKG Test *on page 30*

Electrocardiogram, Adult, Exercise EKG Test

Synonyms Exercise Stress Test; Multistage Exercise Electrocardiographics Test; TMET; Treadmill Exercise Test

Replaces EKG, 2-Step Test

Procedure Commonly Includes The skin is prepared and electrodes are attached. A set of three control electrocardiograms are obtained (resting, standing, and post 1-minute hyperventilation). The patient is instructed and shown by an exercise physiologist or supervising physician how to walk on the treadmill. The test is performed with a qualified professional present. A 12-lead electrocardiogram is obtained each minute during exercise. Every 2-3 minutes the speed and incline of the treadmill are increased to reach a predetermined age predicted maximum heart rate. Once exercise is terminated, the patient lies down and an EKG is recorded every minute for 5 minutes or until ischemic changes have returned to normal and/or heart rate has returned to normal.

Indications

- determine the presence of exercise-induced myocardial ischemia
- evaluate exercise tolerance
- evaluate the blood pressure response to exercise
- evaluate the presence of an exercise-induced arrhythmia
- evaluate the results of medical and surgical therapy
- evaluate symptoms of dyspnea

Contraindications

- inability to walk on treadmill
- unstable angina
- severe hypertension
- fever/sepsis
- presence of left bundle branch block and/or resting ST-T changes precludes the electrocardiogram diagnosis of myocardial ischemia

Patient Preparation Instruct the patient not to eat or drink anything except water after midnight if the appointment is in the morning. Patients to be tested in the afternoon should have nothing to eat or drink after a light breakfast - coffee or juice and toast - at least 4 hours before the test. When clinically feasible, it is preferred that the patient be off digitalis at the time of testing; 3 days for digoxin and 10-14 days for long-acting preparations. Patients need tennis shoes and shorts or pants. Loose clothing is suggested.

Aftercare The patient may need a wheelchair to return to his/her room, if performed as an inpatient. The patient should rest following the test.

Equipment Treadmill

Turnaround Time Final report is given within 2 work days after the test.

Limitations Patients must be able to walk safely at a high rate of speed and with an incline in order to perform the test.

Additional Information The test is supervised by a physician who may terminate the test at his or her discretion.

References

Pina IL, Balady GJ, Hanson P, et al, "Guidelines for Clinical Exercise Testing Laboratories. A Statement for Health Care Professionals From the Committee on Exercise and Rehabilitation, American Heart Association," *Circulation*, 1995, 91(3):912-21.

Electrocardiography

Synonyms Cardiogram; ECG; EKG

Procedure Commonly Includes The electrocardiogram is widely applied in patients with suspected or known heart disease and serves as a baseline reference for most other cardiology tests. Although the single-lead electrocardiogram is used as a reference for most cardiology diagnostic procedures, the electrocardiogram in the present context will be the 12-lead recording.

Indications In patients without known heart disease, the electrocardiogram is used as a screening test for occult coronary artery disease, cardiac arrhythmias, cardiomyopathies, and chamber hypertrophy/enlargement. The electrocardiogram is used as a baseline for future reference to evaluate a patient preoperatively. The electrocardiogram may also provide useful insight for the presence of metabolic alterations such as hypercalcemia, hypocalcemia, hyperkalemia, and hypokalemia. In patients with known heart disease, the electrocardiogram serves as a noninvasive marker for disease severity and progression. It is invaluable for the evaluation of patients with acute chest pain and acute myocardial injury. Most patients with myocardial, valvular, and congenital heart disease will eventually demonstrate electrocardiogram abnormalities. This test is warranted in these situations for both diagnostic and management purposes.

Patient Preparation No special patient preparation is needed. Patients do not need to fast before the electrocardiogram is obtained. No special time of day is preferable.

Special Instructions Inpatients will often have a bedside electrocardiogram performed. Outpatients will travel to the Electrocardiogram Laboratory. Patients can be scheduled for a routine electrocardiogram within 24 hours of the request or a stat electrocardiogram immediately. The reason for the request should be noted in the chart or on the requisition form. Additional information of interest includes the patient's age, sex, race, as well as any current cardiac medications. Situations that require special lead placement should be noted. These include the use of back leads if a posterior myocardial infarction is suspected and the use of right precordial leads if a right ventricular myocardial infarction is suspected. If the patient has a rhythm disturbance, a rhythm strip may be requested.

Technique A brief description of the procedure is provided to the patient. With the patient in a supine and relaxed position the wrists and ankles are prepared for the extremity electrocardiogram leads. The precordium is prepared and marked for the precordial leads and the self-adhesive electrodes are placed. The patient's data is entered. After making sure the calibration settings are appropriate recording of the 12 leads is accomplished. This can be done by selecting lead by lead, or with the newer electrocardiogram recorders by simultaneous recordings of 3-6 leads. The recordings are usually made at a paper speed of 25 mm/second. A copy is left in the chart and another copy is printed in the Electrocardiogram Laboratory for interpretation.

Normal Findings Proper interpretation of electrocardiograms is essential for all physicians and especially for those who take care of patients with potential heart problems. Interpretation of the normal electrocardiogram and its variants needs to be emphasized at all levels of medical training, and continued interpretation and education is required if a person is to maintain proficiency in electrocardiogram interpretation. Distinct abnormalities exist on the electrocardiogram in the presence of chamber dilatation or hypertrophy, in the presence of acute or remote myocardial infarction, pericarditis, ventricular aneurysms, and conduction abnormalities.

References

Chou TC, *Electrocardiography in Clinical Practice*, Philadelphia, PA: WB Saunders Co, 1991.

Grauer K and Curry RW Jr, *Clinical Electrocardiography: A Primary Care Approach*, Oradell, NJ: Medical Economics Books, 1987.

Electrophysiology Catheter Ablation

Synonyms Ablation; EPS Ablation

Procedure Commonly Includes Invasive cardiac electrophysiologic studies are utilized to evaluate patients with complex arrhythmias and conduction abnormalities. Electrode catheters are introduced percutaneously via peripheral veins and are directed to cardiac chambers with the aid of fluoroscopy for recording intracardiac electrocardiograms. In patients with symptomatic cardiac dysrhythmias of atrial, atrioventricular and ventricular origin, catheter-guided ablation at the time of electrophysiology study is a curable technique now available.

Indications

- determine symptomatic and recurrent atrial dysrhythmias such as atrial tachycardia, atrial fibrillation, and atrial fibrillation with Wolff-Parkinson-White syndrome
- determine symptomatic atrioventricular nodal re-entrant tachycardia
- determine symptomatic junctional tachycardia
- determine symptomatic sinus node re-entrant tachycardia
- determine symptomatic atrioventricular macro re-entrant tachycardia

(Continued)

Electrophysiology Catheter Ablation *(Continued)*

- determine symptomatic Wolff-Parkinson-White syndrome
- determine ventricular tachycardia

Contraindications There are no absolute contraindications for electrophysiologic study but as with all invasive procedures a careful risk-to-benefit analysis should be obtained before proceeding with the procedure. A relative contraindication includes patients with advanced coronary artery disease where arrhythmia induction may induce significant myocardial ischemia.

Patient Preparation The procedure generally lasts from 2-6 hours. Electrophysiologic studies are performed in the postabsorptive state and are carried out with light sedation, however, in the presence of arrhythmia induction requiring defibrillation, greater amounts of sedation may be administered. Sufficient time is allowed for elimination of antiarrhythmic medications which may alter the electrical system of the heart, roughly the duration of five half-lives of a given drug. There is no need to discontinue other cardiac medications indicated for nonarrhythmic problems. For the introduction of catheters, the femoral area is scrubbed and shaved prior to the patient arriving in the Electrophysiology Laboratory.

Technique On arrival to the laboratory, the patient is greeted and given a detailed explanation of the procedure and is placed on the electrophysiology table where he/she is draped and prepared for the study. At the completion of the study, gentle pressure is applied to the site of catheter insertion with patients permitted to ambulate after 4-6 hours of bedrest. The ablation procedure is similar to a baseline electrophysiologic study with the addition of a special ablation catheter which is carefully placed via intracardiac electrode mapping. Small bursts of carefully delivered radiofrequency energy transpires and an attempt of arrhythmia reinduction is made. In the absence of arrhythmia reinduction, a successful ablation procedure is concluded. During the procedure, continuous arterial blood pressure and electrocardiogram rhythm strips are obtained. All catheters are advanced under fluoroscopic guidance. Depending on the site of electrophysiologic ablation, catheters may also be placed on the left side of the heart. Not infrequently, the transeptal approach is used to place catheters within the left-sided cardiac chambers.

References

Kay GN, Epstein AE, Dailey SM, et al, "Role of Radiofrequency Ablation in the Management of Supraventricular Arrhythmias: Experience in 760 Consecutive Patients," *J Cardiovasc Electrophysiol*, 1993, 4(4):371-89.

Weber H and Schmitz L, "Catheter Technique for Closed-Chest Ablation of an Accessory Pathway," *N Engl J Med*, 1983, 308(11):653-4.

Electrophysiology Studies

Synonyms EPS; HIS Bundle Recordings; Invasive Cardiac Electrophysiologic Studies; Programmed Electrical Stimulation

Procedure Commonly Includes Invasive cardiac and electrophysiologic studies are utilized to evaluate patients with complex arrhythmias and conduction abnormalities. Electrode catheters are introduced percutaneously via peripheral veins and are guided to cardiac chambers with the aid of fluoroscopy for intracardiac electrocardiogram recordings.

Indications Electrophysiologic studies are performed for diagnostic and therapeutic purposes. The most common diagnostic indications for EPS include:

- evaluating patients with sinus node dysfunction through the measurement of sinus node recovery time
- evaluating atrioventricular conduction to identify the level of the conduction abnormality and to better determine candidates for permanent pacing
- the differential diagnosis of wide QRS complex tachycardia
- the differential diagnosis and mechanism of supraventricular tachycardia
- diagnosing and managing patients with ventricular tachycardia
- evaluating and managing survivors of sudden cardiac death

The most common therapeutic uses of EPS include:

- pharmacologic control of tachycardia where tachycardia is induced and an intravenous therapeutic agent is administered, arrhythmia reinduction is attempted and the response is evaluated

- selecting patients for nonpharmacologic controlled tachycardias such as electrophysiology-guided ablation therapy, antitachycardia pacemakers, and implantable cardiac defibrillators

Contraindications There are no absolute contraindications for electrophysiologic study. As with all invasive procedures, a careful risk-to-benefit analysis should be obtained before proceeding with the study. A relative contraindication includes patients with advanced coronary artery disease where arrhythmia induction may induce significant myocardial ischemia.

Patient Preparation The procedure takes from 2-4 hours. Electrophysiologic studies are performed in the postabsorptive state and are usually carried out without sedation, although in apprehensive patients mild sedation is advisable. Sufficient time is allowed for the elimination of drugs that alter the electrical system of the heart, roughly the duration of five half-lives. For the introduction of catheters, the femoral area is aseptically scrubbed and shaved prior to the patient arriving in the Electrophysiology Laboratory.

Aftercare On completion of the electrophysiology study, gentle pressure is applied to the catheter insertion area with patients permitted to ambulate 4-6 hours after bedrest.

Technique On arrival to the laboratory the patient is greeted and given a detailed explanation of the procedure. The patient is then placed on the electrophysiology table where he/she is draped and prepared for the study. Routinely, at least three surface electrocardiogram leads are recorded as a reference. A temporary pacemaker is placed under local anesthesia and with fluoroscopic guidance at least three catheters are advanced to the appropriate right-sided cardiac chambers. Usually these will include a catheter in the right atrium and/or coronary sinus, one catheter across the tricuspid valve near the bundle of HIS, and another catheter in the right ventricle. A multichannel recorder with precise intracardiac interval measurement capabilities is used to record and interpret the electrophysiology data. Well-placed catheters with appropriate amplification and filtering provide diagnostic recordings in most patients.

Normal Findings Appropriate interpretation of electrophysiology studies requires knowledge of the electrode site and specific electrophysiology study protocol used, as well as a precise understanding of the electrophysiology properties of the heart in health and disease. Measurement of electrophysiology intervals obtained from intracardiac recordings at the level of the coronary sinus, atrioventricular node, HIS bundle, and right ventricle are usually obtained. These include the A-V, atrial-HIS, and HIS-ventricular intervals. Abnormalities of these intervals suggest the presence of different types of atrioventricular conduction abnormalities. By these means, it is possible to diagnose malfunction of the sinus node, to characterize intra-atrial, atrioventricular nodal, HIS bundle system and intramyocardial conduction, and to determine the presence, location, and electrophysiology properties of accessory pathways when present. The site and form of initiation and termination of supraventricular and ventricular tachycardias can also be characterized by electrophysiology study.

References

Zipes DP, DiMarco JP, Gillette PC, et al, "Guidelines for Clinical Intracardiac Electrophysiological and Catheter Ablation Procedures. A Report of the American College of Cardiology/American Heart Association Task Force on Practice Guidelines (Committee on Clinical Intracardiac Electrophysiologic and Catheter Ablation Procedures), Developed in Collaboration With the North American Society of Pacing Electrophysiology," *J Am Coll Cardiol*, 1995, 26(2):555-73.

Endomyocardial Biopsy

Synonyms Heart Biopsy; Right Ventricular Endomyocardial Biopsy

Procedure Commonly Includes The skin is prepared with an aseptic solution. A #8 French arterial introducer is placed percutaneously, most typically in the right internal jugular vein. A sterile biopsy forceps is then advanced under fluoroscopic guidance to the right ventricle and endomyocardial samples are obtained from the right ventricular and interventricular septal walls.

Indications

- evaluate cardiac histology in cardiac transplant patients to monitor for recipient cardiac rejection
- evaluate patients for suspected myocardiopathies or myocarditis

(Continued)

Endomyocardial Biopsy *(Continued)*

Since right-sided intracardiac pressures are measured during the procedure, a Swan-Ganz catheter for evaluation of hemodynamics is also obtained.

Contraindications

- mechanical tricuspid valve
- tricuspid valve endocarditis
- tricuspid valve thrombus
- right internal jugular and/or superior vena caval deep venous thrombosis

Turnaround Time A report of the immediate procedure is written on the chart at the time of cardiac biopsy. Results are usually available from the Pathology Department within 48 hours of arrival of the specimen.

Causes for Rejection If the patient is found to have significantly elevated right ventricular and pulmonary artery blood pressure, the test may be cancelled.

References

Billingham ME, "Endomyocardial Biopsy Diagnosis of Acute Rejection in Cardiac Allografts," *Prog Cardiovasc Dis*, 1990, 33(1):11-8.

♦ **EPS** *see* Electrophysiology Studies *on page 32*

♦ **EPS Ablation** *see* Electrophysiology Catheter Ablation *on page 31*

Ergonovine Provocation Test

Synonyms Provocation Test, Ergonovine

Procedure Commonly Includes This test is performed on patients with angina pectoris for the evaluation of suspected coronary artery vasospasm. Ergonovine malleate is an ergoalkaloid which exerts a vasoconstrictor direct effect on vascular smooth muscle. This provides a sensitive and specific test for provoking coronary artery vasospasm. It is administered intravenously in conjunction with coronary artery angiography. It is carefully administered in small incremental doses. Continuous electrocardiogram and blood pressure measurements are obtained.

Indications Evaluate patients for suspected coronary artery vasospasm especially in the absence of significant coronary artery obstructive disease

Contraindications

- hypersensitivity to ergonovine
- advanced coronary artery obstructive disease
- typical angina pectoris not felt to represent coronary artery vasospasm

Patient Preparation The patient undergoes a standard left heart catheterization. After the coronary artery anatomy is well delineated ergonovine is administered intravenously in doses ranging from 0.05-0.40 mg. Repeat coronary angiography is obtained during the administration of ergonovine to evaluate the coronary arteries for ergonovine-induced vasospasm. Intracoronary nitroglycerin can be administered to reverse the ergonovine-induced vasospasm. A normal response of the coronary arteries to high-dose ergonovine infusion is diffuse coronary vasoconstriction. In true coronary vasospasm, severe focal spasm transpires in the presence of ergonovine administration, unlike the nonspecific diffuse coronary artery vasospasm seen with higher-dose ergonovine infusion.

Aftercare The patient is monitored for the presence of chest discomfort, electrocardiogram changes, and blood pressure changes. Once all vital signs have returned to baseline and no symptoms of angina are present, the patient is discharged from the Cardiac Catheterization Laboratory.

Complications Prolonged coronary artery vasospasm resulting in acute myocardial injury, prolonged angina pectoris, cardiac dysrhythmias

References

Kimball BP, LiPreti V, and Aldridge HE, "Quantitative Arteriographic Responses to Ergonovine Provocation in Subjects With Atypical Chest Pain," *Am J Cardiol*, 1989, 64(12):778-82.

♦ **Esophageal Echo** *see* Transesophageal Echocardiography *on page 42*

♦ **ETT** *see* Cardiopulmonary Stress Test *on page 22*

♦ **Exercise Stress Test** *see* Electrocardiogram, Adult, Exercise EKG Test *on page 30*

♦ **Exercise Tolerance Test** *see* Cardiopulmonary Stress Test *on page 22*

♦ **Graded Exercise Test** *see* Cardiopulmonary Stress Test *on page 22*

♦ **Heart Biopsy** *see* Endomyocardial Biopsy *on page 33*
♦ **HIS Bundle Electrograms** *see* Cardiac Catheterization, Adult *on page 21*
♦ **HIS Bundle Recordings** *see* Electrophysiology Studies *on page 32*
♦ **Holter Electrocardiogram** *see* Holter Monitorization *on page 35*

Holter Monitorization

Synonyms Ambulatory Electrocardiography; Ambulatory Holter Electrocardiography; Dynamic Electrocardiography; Holter Electrocardiogram

Procedure Commonly Includes Holter monitorization is a method for recording an electrocardiogram from an ambulatory subject for extended periods of time. Holter monitoring has emerged as a sensitive and specific means of detecting and evaluating supraventricular and ventricular arrhythmias. The conventional Holter recording obtains electrocardiogram data comparable to leads V_{1-5} on a standard 12-lead electrocardiogram. The electrical signal is recorded onto a cassette magnetic tape. The usual recording time on Holter monitorization is 24 hours, but new recorders allow for up to 5 days of continued monitorization. Using a light portable tape recorder, prolonged recordings can be made while the patient engages in usual daily activities and records these activities as well as suspect correlative symptoms in a diary.

Indications

- assessment of symptoms that may be arrhythmia related
- assessment of R:R interval characteristics
- assessment of risk in patients with or without arrhythmia
- assessment of antiarrhythmic therapy efficacy
- assessment of pacemaker function
- detection of myocardial ischemia

Patient Preparation To maximize the usefulness of ambulatory electrocardiography, the following information should be provided: general patient information, reason for performing the test, medications, and the presence and type of a pacemaker. On scheduling the Holter monitorization, the request should specify if the monitorization should be continuous, intermittent, patient-activated, or event recording. Routine Holter monitorization is continuous. No specified patient preparation is required. Patients are instructed to perform normal daily activities and to record these activities as well as any symptoms in a diary.

Technique When the patient arrives at the Holter Monitor Laboratory, he/she is greeted by the Holter Laboratory personnel and a detailed explanation of the procedure is given. Any previous history of an allergic reaction to tape or electrode gel is obtained. The chest is prepared and the electrodes are firmly put in place. The electrodes are looped and securely taped to minimize movement and artifact. The operation of the recorder and event marker is explained to the patient and information on how to complete the diary is provided. The patient is given instructions on how to continue normal daily activities. Instructions on how to turn off the instrument, how to change the batteries, and how to disconnect the monitor are provided.

Additional Information Interpretation of Holter monitorization is done with the aid of an analysis system which includes a playback deck for cassette tapes and a screen for operator system interaction. Modern scanners have analog-to-digital converter and electronic memories for the EKG to be memorized and played back providing real-time EKG strip documentation. The scanner provides information regarding duration of taping, amount of time deleted from analysis because of artifact, maximal and minimal heart rate, number of ventricular and supraventricular complexes, and number of nonsustained and sustained arrhythmia episodes, if present. The Holter technician will select potential abnormal areas of interest for further analysis and interpretation. Most recorders have dual channel electrocardiogram monitorization to facilitate arrhythmic and ST segment displacement interpretation. Some systems provide "full disclosure" capability in which each complex during the recording is plotted on a compressed time and voltage scale. This is particularly helpful to detect the sequence of premature ventricular complexes and episodes of ventricular tachycardia. Since the patient keeps a diary of activities, symptoms, and time of medication, the scanner can

(Continued)

Holter Monitorization *(Continued)*

determine the time of arrhythmia occurrence and possibly correlate symptoms with the presence or absence of rhythm abnormalities.

References

DiMarco JP and Philbrick JT, "Use of Ambulatory Electrocardiographic (Holter) Monitoring," *Ann Intern Med*, 1990, 113(1):53-68.

Knoebel SB, Crawford MH, Dunn MI, et al, "Guidelines for Ambulatory Electrocardiography. A Report of the American College of Cardiology/American Heart Association Task Force on Assessment of Diagnostic and Therapeutic Cardiovascular Procedures (Subcommittee on Ambulatory Electrocardiography)," *Circulation*, 1989, 79(1):206-15.

Sheffield LT, Berson A, Bragg-Remschel D, et al, "Recommendations for Standards of Instrumentation and Practice in the Use of Ambulatory Electrocardiography. The Task Force of the Committee on Electrocardiography and Cardiac Electrophysiology of the Council on Clinical Cardiology," *Circulation*, 1985, 71(3):626A-36A.

Intravascular Coronary Ultrasound

Synonyms IVUS; Vascular Coronary Ultrasound

Indications

- characterize coronary artery stenosis severity, location, and length
- clarify an indeterminate coronary angiogram for the presence of significant coronary artery obstructive disease
- classify coronary atheromata as either soft and lipid-laden vs fibrotic and calcified
- assess for the presence and severity of cardiac transplant coronary artery disease
- guide preintervention device selection such as sizing of an angioplasty balloon and/or stent

Contraindications

- severe peripheral vascular disease
- bleeding diatheses where arterial puncture may be high risk
- severe congestive heart failure
- advanced renal insufficiency
- history of cholesterol embolization

Patient Preparation Patients scheduled for an intravascular ultrasound are prepared similarly as if scheduled for a left heart catheterization. Indications for the procedure are reviewed with the patient as are the risks, benefits, and alternatives. A complete blood count, BUN, creatinine, chest x-ray, and electrocardiogram should be recorded in the chart the day before the test. A serum potassium should also be ordered before the test. Both femoral areas are shaved and aseptically prepared. A sedative is given on call to the Cardiac Catheterization Laboratory. The patient is in a fasting state.

Aftercare After the left heart catheterization (including coronary angiograms and intravascular ultrasound) check heart rate, blood pressure, arterial puncture site, and distal pulses four times at 15-minute intervals, then four times at 30-minute intervals, then four times at 1-hour intervals. Presuming the femoral approach has been used, absolute bedrest for 6 hours is advised.

Technique This procedure is most commonly performed via the right femoral artery approach. The patient is brought to the Cardiac Catheterization Laboratory and informed of the procedure and its risks. After informed consent is obtained, an intravenous line is started and mild sedatives may be administered. The right femoral artery is palpated and the femoral area is shaved and sterilely prepared with an aseptic solution. After proper draping of the femoral area, a local anesthetic is administered topically. After topical anesthesia is achieved, a deeper anesthetic is administered. Once a thorough anesthesia of the femoral area is complete, a small needle is introduced into the femoral artery. This is exchanged for a guidewire whose position is confirmed by fluoroscopic guidance. Over the guidewire a #8 French introducing catheter is threaded and the guidewire is removed. The catheter position is confirmed by achieving an arterial blood return and flushed with a heparinized saline solution. Under fluoroscopic guidance a #8 French coronary artery guiding catheter is advanced to the coronary artery under evaluation. Through the guiding catheter, the vessel of interest is subselectively cannulated using a steerable angioplasty guidewire. The imaging ultrasound catheter is then advanced and retracted over the wire to examine the coronary artery vessel in real time, recording ultrasound images on video tape for subsequent quantitative or qualitative analysis. Some ultrasound imaging catheters have a motorized pullback system which permits retraction of the ultrasound catheter at a constant speed. This permits a cross-sectional assessment of the coronary arteries and a more quantitative assessment of coronary artery lesion severity by calculating a measurement of cross-sectional lumen area and stenosis severity. It also permits assessment of stenosis severity at bifurcation sites, ostial locations, and also a more accurate measurement of eccentric stenoses.

Turnaround Time Preliminary reports are available on-line during the procedure. Quantitative measurements often occur after the procedure via detailed off-line analysis.

References

Hodgson JM, Reddy KG, Suneja R, et al, "Intracoronary Ultrasound Imaging: Correlation of Plaque Morphology With Angiography, Clinical Syndrome, and Procedural Results in Patients Undergoing Coronary Angioplasty," *J Am Coll Cardiol*, 1993, 21(1):35-44.

Nissen SE and Gurley JC, "Quantitative Assessment of Coronary Dimensions, Lumen Shape and Wall Morphology by Intravascular Ultrasound," *Intravascular Ultrasound*, Tobis JM and Yock PG, eds, New York, NY: Churchill Livingstone, 1992, 71-83.

♦ **Invasive Cardiac Electrophysiologic Studies** *see* Electrophysiology Studies *on page 32*

♦ **IVUS** *see* Intravascular Coronary Ultrasound *on page 36*

♦ **Left Heart Catheterization** *see* Cardiac Catheterization, Adult *on page 21*

♦ **Metabolic Stress Test** *see* Cardiopulmonary Stress Test *on page 22*

♦ **M-Mode Echo** *see* M-Mode Echocardiography *on page 37*

M-Mode Echocardiography

Related Information

Transesophageal Echocardiography *on page 42*
Two-Dimensional Echocardiography *on page 46*

Synonyms M-Mode Echo; Unidimensional Echo

Procedure Commonly Includes M-mode echocardiography, the first form of cardiac ultrasound used in clinical practice, takes its name from the motion of the cardiac structures that were possible to visualize when this diagnostic method was introduced. M-mode echocardiography provides an "ice pick" view of the heart with a very high temporal and unidimensional space resolution, so that it provides an excellent method to measure chamber dimensions and to time cardiac events. It is used as an adjunct to two-dimensional echocardiography.

Indications

The most common indications for this test include:

- wall thickness measurement of the interventricular septum, posterior left ventricular wall, and right ventricular free wall
- measurement of end-diastolic and end-systolic left ventricular internal dimensions
- percent of fractional shortening (difference between end-diastolic and end-systolic dimensions divided by end-diastolic dimension)
- measurement of right ventricular dimension
- measurement of the anteroposterior diameter of the ascending aorta and left atrium

Contraindications There are no contraindications for M-mode echocardiography but patients with chronic obstructive lung disease or marked obesity may have tests of poor diagnostic quality.

Patient Preparation No special patient preparation is required. Fasting is not necessary. The procedure can be done at any time. In scheduling patients that will have multiple cardiac diagnostic procedures, it will be best to order the echocardiogram before Holter monitoring since the multiple electrodes placed on the chest for this procedure may interfere with performance of the echocardiogram. Also, if a patient is to have a stress test on the same day, enough time (2-3 hours) should be allowed after the exercise test to perform the echocardiogram under basal conditions.

Special Instructions In most cases, the M-mode echocardiogram is performed as part of a more complete cardiac ultrasound study that includes

(Continued)

M-Mode Echocardiography *(Continued)*

either 2-D echocardiography and/or Doppler echocardiography. The test that provides the most information should be requested, although sometimes this decision is left to personnel in the Echo Laboratory. A complete cardiac ultrasound study takes anywhere from 30-60 minutes, the "M-mode" part of it takes approximately 5-10 minutes. To optimize the diagnostic yield of the echocardiogram, a note relating the reason for the request should be made in the patient's chart or on a requisition form. Other useful information includes the patient's age, weight, and height.

Technique A patient arriving at the Echo Laboratory is greeted by laboratory personnel. He/she is asked about any previous experience with the procedure and is given a brief description of the test. The patient is asked to undress from the waist up and is provided a gown to be worn with the opening in the front. Three electrodes for EKG monitorization are placed on the chest and the patient is asked to lie in the left lateral decubitus position. Currently, most M-mode echocardiograms are obtained by using a 2-D echocardiographic probe and selecting M-mode information. Briefly, the transducer is placed at the left parasternal border, the long axis view is selected, and the M-mode line is moved from the left ventricle to the mitral valve and finally to the aorta and left atrium. Recordings at these levels are registered in a strip chart recorder, a video recorder, or a page printer. These recordings become part of the report and of the Echo Laboratory file.

Normal Findings Adequate interpretation of M-mode echocardiography requires knowledge of the normal values of the dimensions of the cardiac chambers and great arteries (see table), and an understanding of the normal motion of the valves and different walls of the cardiac system. Distinct abnormalities can be characterized by M-mode echocardiography for many cardiovascular disorders. See table.

Normal M-Mode Echocardiographic Values

	Mean (cm)	Range (cm)
RVD	1.7	0.9-2.6
LVIDD	4.7	3.5-5.7
PLVWT	0.9	0.6-1.1
IVSWT	0.9	0.6-1.1
LA	2.9	1.9-4.0
AO	2.7	2.0-3.7
FS	36%	34%-44%

RVD = Right ventricular dimension

LVIDD = Left ventricular internal dimension in diastole

PLVWT = Posterior left ventricular wall thickness

IVSWT = Interventricular wall thickness

LA = Left atrium

AO = Aorta

FS = Fractional shortening

Reproduced with permission from Feigenbaum H, *Echocardiography,* 4th ed, Philadelphia, PA: Lea & Febiger, 1986.

References

Sahn DJ, DeMaria A, Kisslo J, et al, "Recommendations Regarding Quantitation in M-Mode Echocardiography: Results of a Survey of Echocardiographic Measurements," *Circulation,* 1978, 58(6):1072-83.

♦ **Multistage Exercise Electrocardiographics Test** *see* Electrocardiogram, Adult, Exercise EKG Test *on page 30*

Pacemaker Check

Synonyms Pacemaker Follow-up; Pacer Check

Procedure Commonly Includes Pacemaker checks are part of the routine follow-up of all patients with permanent pacemakers. These routine assessments are designed to anticipate pacemaker generator failure, to find its cause, and to provide appropriate and timely preventive measures. Pacemakers have become more sophisticated as has the required follow-up. Although some routine check-ups can be made in the physician's office with the aid of an EKG alone, most medical centers implanting a large volume and variety of pacemakers have an electronic surveillance center with transtelephonic transmission. These devices underscore and analyze the pacemaker wave form and carry out a full programming assessment.

Indications All patients with permanent pacemakers qualify as candidates for routine pacemaker follow-up. The frequency and depth of the check-up depends on the type of pacemaker, the time elapsed since implantation, and the underlying cardiac rhythm disorder.

Patient Preparation No special patient care or preparation is required for the routine pacemaker check. It is essential to instruct the patient to bring to the visit all pertinent pacemaker implantation information regarding the pacemaker. This is usually provided by the pacemaker manufacturing company in the form of a personalized card with the type and serial number of the device as well as the date of implantation. Laboratories typically maintain patient specific information on record for each patient.

Technique A comprehensive pacemaker check should include an initial clinical evaluation including a history, physical exam, chest x-ray, and a 12-lead electrocardiogram with a rhythm strip. Additionally, and at intervals mandated by the type and length of device implantation, a detailed analysis of the pacemaker wave form should be performed, including analysis of the precise pacemaker rate, amplitude, duration, and contour of the impulse. Proof of appropriate pacing by analyzing a rhythm strip with the pacer in the asynchronous mode should transpire. In programmable pacemakers, a full programming routine should be carried out at appropriate intervals. A highly successful extension of the pacemaker check center has been developed for the use of transtelephonic monitoring. This has permitted many of the pacemaker check functions routinely carried out in the hospital or physician's office to be performed via the telephone from the patient's home. Transtelephonic monitoring has facilitated follow-up of distant patients and has increased the frequency of evaluation without the logistical problems of patient transport.

References

Goldschlager N, Ludoner P, and Creamer C, "Follow-up of the Paced Outpatient," *Clinical Cardiac Pacing*, Ellenbogen KA, Kay GN, and Wilkoff BL, eds, Philadelphia, PA: WB Saunders Co, 1995, 780-808.

♦ **Pacemaker Follow-up** *see* Pacemaker Check *on page 39*
♦ **Pacer Check** *see* Pacemaker Check *on page 39*
♦ **Pericardial Drainage** *see* Pericardiocentesis *on page 39*

Pericardiocentesis

Synonyms Pericardial Drainage

Indications

- cardiac tamponade
- pericardial effusion of unknown etiology for primary diagnostic purposes
- palliative removal of pericardial fluid in patients with advanced malignant disease

Contraindications

- known bleeding diathesis
- therapeutic anticoagulation medications concurrently administered
- very small pericardial effusions where a significant chance of complications exists
- constrictive pericarditis where the pericardium is adherent to the cardiac surface

Patient Preparation For the elective procedure, the patient arrives in the laboratory in the fasting state. After an adequate and thorough explanation of the procedure, the skin is aseptically prepared. Electrocardiogram wires are

(Continued)

Pericardiocentesis *(Continued)*

placed in locations outside of the operative field. Intravenous sedatives may be administered depending on the individual situation. Once the procedure is completed, the pericardial fluid is removed. When the patient is judged to be hemodynamically stable, alert, and responsive, he/she is released from the Pericardiocentesis Laboratory and returned to the hospital bed.

Aftercare The patient is monitored until hemodynamically stable. The operative site is closely monitored for evidence of bleeding or drainage around the catheter and the site is sterilely dressed with bandages.

Equipment The Cardiac Catheterization Laboratory most commonly is utilized, along with fluoroscopy, pericardiocentesis kit including anesthetics, syringes with needles, dilator, exchange wire, and pericardiocentesis catheter

Technique The skin is aseptically prepared over the anterior chest wall and draped with sterile towels. The patient is fully informed regarding the indications and risks of the procedure and informed consent is obtained. Twelve lead electrocardiogram electrodes are applied and continuous electrocardiogram rhythm strip monitoring is obtained during the procedure. A pulse oximeter is also applied and a continuous readout of oxygen saturation is rendered. A pneumatic blood pressure cuff monitors blood pressure every 3 minutes during the procedure. The patient is awake and alert for the procedure but may receive intravenous sedating medications during periods of extreme anxiety. A predetermined location on the anterior chest wall is infiltrated with a topical anesthetic. Once the topical anesthetic has taken effect, deeper tissues are infiltrated. The superficial needle is exchanged for a longer needle and during the anesthetic administration of the deeper tissues an initial attempt at accessing the pericardial space is made with continuous negative pressure on the syringe. If the pericardial space is entered, the depth of access is noted as is the angle of approach. Once the skin and subcutaneous tissues are adequately anesthetized, a syringe with a higher gauge and longer needle is again passed through a similar access channel and directed to enter the pericardial space. Once a free flow of pericardial fluid is obtained, the syringe is removed and a small wire is carefully passed through the entry needle into the pericardial space. X-ray fluoroscopy is utilized to confirm the presence of the wire within the pericardium. Once confirmation of the wire in the pericardium is obtained, the needle is removed with the wire remaining. A scalpel is used to slightly increase the size of the portal of entry at the base of the skin and a rubber dilator is introduced over the wire to dilate the channel. A larger catheter is then passed over the wire and the wire is removed through the catheter. A syringe is attached to the larger catheter and a free flow of pericardial fluid should transpire. With large pericardial fluid accumulations, commonly, a vacuum bottle or bag is attached to the pericardial catheter to assist with more prompt drainage. In emergency situations during hemodynamic compromise and suspected cardiac tamponade, this procedure frequently transpires in a similar fashion but without fluoroscopic guidance. Once all the pericardial fluid is drained, the catheter is removed at a point determined by the supervising physician.

Specimen Pericardial fluid is routinely sent for Gram stain, culture, cell count and differential, pH, LDH, and total protein values. In addition, cytology is routinely performed.

References

Heierli B, Anderes U, and Follath F, "Diagnosis and Therapy of Cardiac Tamponade. An Analysis of 50 Patients," *Schweiz Med Wochenschr*, 1981, 111(21):735-41.

Krikorian JG and Hancock EW, "Pericardiocentesis," *Am J Med*, 1978, 65(5):808-14.

Morgan CD, Marshall SA, and Ross JR, "Catheter Drainage of the Pericardium: Its Safety and Efficacy," *Can J Surg*, 1989, 32(5):331-4.

♦ **Programmed Electrical Stimulation** *see* Electrophysiology Studies *on page 32*

♦ **Provocation Test, Ergonovine** *see* Ergonovine Provocation Test *on page 34*

♦ **Pulsed Doppler** *see* Transesophageal Echocardiography *on page 42*

♦ **Right and Left Heart Catheterization** *see* Cardiac Catheterization, Adult *on page 21*

♦ **Right Heart Catheterization** *see* Cardiac Catheterization, Adult *on page 21*

♦ **Right Ventricular Endomyocardial Biopsy** *see* Endomyocardial Biopsy *on page 33*

♦ **Stress Echocardiography** *see* Dobutamine Echocardiography *on page 26*

♦ **Stress Echocardiography** *see* Treadmill Exercise Echocardiography *on page 43*

♦ **TEE** *see* Transesophageal Echocardiography *on page 42*

Thallium Stress Testing

Procedure Commonly Includes Thallous chloride (^{201}TH) is a radiopharmaceutical injected at peak exercise. Images are traditionally obtained immediately after exercise and at redistribution, typically 3-4 hours after exercise cessation. Resting images are compared to the stress images, specifically assessing for flow heterogeneity, which may suggest flow-limiting coronary artery disease and myocardial ischemia.

Indications

- determine the presence and severity of exercise-induced myocardial ischemia.
- evaluate the potential for exercise-induced cardiac rhythm disturbances
- evaluate the hemodynamic responses to activity
- evaluate the effect of medical or interventional therapy
- prescribe appropriate activity guidelines
- evaluate patient's exercise/work tolerance
- evaluate the impact of cardiac rehabilitation intervention
- evaluate patients for suspected false-positive electrocardiogram stress tests prior to proceeding with cardiac catheterization
- evaluate for peri-infarction myocardial ischemia

Contraindications

- acute myocardial infarction
- severe symptomatic valvular heart disease
- uncontrolled ventricular arrhythmias
- uncontrolled supraventricular arrhythmias compromising cardiac function
- unstable or rest angina
- uncompensated congestive heart failure
- suspected or known dissecting aortic aneurysm
- thrombophlebitis
- recent pulmonary or systemic embolism
- severe symptomatic left ventricular outflow tract obstruction
- clinically significant acute pericarditis and/or myocarditis
- complete heart block
- mobile intracardiac thrombus
- significant psychiatric disturbance

Patient Preparation The patient is instructed to eat 4 hours prior to the test and not to eat, smoke, or drink until the test is completed. The patient is also instructed to wear clothes suitable for exercise, preferably tennis shoes and shorts.

Special Instructions By appointment only. Must be scheduled 24 hours in advance. The physician in charge of the stress test should be present in a supervisory role. Patients on a cardiac medication will be instructed accordingly. Consent forms routinely inform patients of the benefits and risks.

Technique The skin is prepared. Electrodes are attached to the chest. The patient is instructed to properly walk on the treadmill. The patient is also hyperventilated (deep fast breathing for 30 seconds) to evaluate for electrocardiogram ST segment and T-wave lability.

A thallium stress test is similar to a treadmill stress test except the patient is intravenously administered thallium, approximately 45 seconds before the cessation of exercise. An inpatient's intravenous lines are started in the patient's room. Outpatient intravenous lines are started in the heart station by a technician. Once the thallium is administered and exercise is stopped, the patient is placed under a gamma camera for thallium cardiac imaging.

Turnaround Time 24-48 hours

(Continued)

Thallium Stress Testing *(Continued)*

References

Verani MS, "Pharmacologic Stress Myocardial Perfusion Imaging," *Curr Probl Cardiol*, 1993, 18(8):481-525.

Tilt Table Evaluation

Synonyms Tilt Table Test

Procedure Commonly Includes Evaluation of patients with suspected vasovagal syncope. The patient is maintained in the head-up position for a brief period to provoke syncope, bradycardia, or hypotension. The upright position leads to blood pooling with a reduction in central venous pressure and blood pressure.

Indications

- determine suspected vasodepressor syncope
- determine syncope of unknown origin not felt related to a cardiac dysrhythmia

Patient Preparation The patient should be fasting.

Technique The patient is brought to the Tilt Table Testing Laboratory in the fasting state. The patient is situated on the tilt table with straps loosely applied to prevent the patient from losing balance. An intravenous peripheral line is placed. A continuous 12-lead electrocardiogram rhythm strip is obtained. In addition, an automatic inflating sphygmomanometer is also placed. Intravenous isoproterenol is variably administered depending on the initial patient response to position changes.

References

Grubb BP, Temesy-Armos P, Hahn H, et al, "Utility of Upright Tilt-Table Testing in the Evaluation and Management of Syncope of Unknown Origin," *Am J Med*, 1991, 90(1):6-10.

♦ **Tilt Table Test** *see* Tilt Table Evaluation *on page 42*

♦ **TMET** *see* Electrocardiogram, Adult, Exercise EKG Test *on page 30*

Transesophageal Echocardiography

Related Information

M-Mode Echocardiography *on page 37*
Two-Dimensional Echocardiography *on page 46*

Synonyms Esophageal Echo; TEE

Applies to Color Flow Imaging; Continuous Wave Doppler; Pulsed Doppler

Procedure Commonly Includes Transesophageal echocardiography (TEE) has been developed to solve one of the imaging limitations of transthoracic echocardiography. Suboptimal image quality is seen in some patients in whom bony structures, as well as increased lung interface, degrade image resolution. By placing an echo transducer at the tip of a gastroscope and advancing it into the esophagus, the heart can be imaged posteriorly without lung or chest cage interference. The closer proximity to the heart allows for utilization of higher frequency transducers which provide high resolution images. Transesophageal echocardiography has provided a new window through which the heart can be examined with far greater detail than was once thought possible. The mild inconvenience of having to pass a transesophageal probe has been far outweighed by the enhanced images obtained. Presently, transesophageal echocardiography includes M-mode echocardiography, two-dimensional echocardiography, pulsed Doppler, continuous wave Doppler, and color flow imaging.

Indications Transesophageal echocardiography is currently being used intraoperatively to monitor cardiac function during cardiac and noncardiac surgery, in intensive care units to follow and evaluate critically ill patients, and in the study of ambulatory patients to better evaluate cardiovascular disorders. Transesophageal echocardiography has been found most useful in the evaluation of prosthetic valve dysfunction, particularly mitral valve prostheses in the quantification and diagnostic characterization of native mitral valve insufficiency, in the evaluation of left atrial thrombosis and masses, in the evaluation of bacterial endocarditis and its complications, and in the evaluation of intracardiac shunts.

Contraindications Transesophageal echocardiography is contraindicated in patients with esophageal obstructions or in nonintubated patients with respiratory failure.

Patient Preparation The patient should fast 6-8 hours prior to the test to minimize the risk of aspiration.

Special Instructions An intravenous line is placed to administer pretest sedating medications such as midazolam and meperidine. Most patients will be able to resume a full activity level after the procedure. Outpatients are advised to have a companion drive them back home to minimize risks from sedation and analgesics.

Technique A patient arriving at the Echocardiography Laboratory is greeted by laboratory personnel. A fasting period of 6-8 hours is confirmed, the reasons indicated for the test are reviewed, vital signs are obtained, symptomatic status is determined, history of allergies is determined, and a detailed explanation of the procedure is provided. The patient is asked to undress from the waist up and is provided a gown to be worn with the opening in the front. Electrocardiographic and blood pressure monitorization is made throughout the procedure. The laboratory is prepared for cardiopulmonary resuscitation in the rare event that it is necessary. The supervising physician performs a cardiopulmonary examination prior to the procedure. An aerosolized local anesthetic is administered to the back of the throat and a rapid-acting hypnotic and analgesic are given intravenously. The patient is then placed in the left lateral decubitus position and the esophageal probe is passed. A dental suction set minimizes the flow of saliva out of the mouth and nasal cannula oxygen with continuous finger tip oximetry is in place. The patient stays awake and comfortable throughout the procedure, in most cases. A systematic and complete study should be performed in each patient. Additionally, the area of specific concern should be evaluated in further detail. A complete study will include 2-D imaging and color flow Doppler study of all cardiac chambers, valves, and great vessels. The study is initiated with the probe placed most distally, which provides a short axis view of the left ventricle. As the probe is removed a view equivalent to an apical four chamber is obtained. This allows for the best view of the mitral and tricuspid valves. Further removal of the probe allows for visualization of the outflow tract of the left ventricle and aortic valve, the left atrial appendage, interatrial septum, and pulmonary veins. Finally, with further removal of the probe the aortic arch is visualized. The color Doppler is used to evaluate normal and abnormal flow patterns. A continuous video recording is obtained throughout the study for later study and analysis. After completion of the study, the transesophageal probe is removed and the patient is kept under observation until regaining a prestudy status.

Normal Findings Transesophageal echocardiography has provided a new window to the heart. The operator must recognize and become familiar with the different orientations of cardiac structures and tomographic planes, as seen from a new perspective. The current omniplane transesophageal echo probes permit a full 0° to 180° cardiac evaluation combined with retroflexion/anteflexion and lateral/medial probe tip mobility.

References

Seward JB, Khandheria BK, Oh JK, et al, "Transesophageal Echocardiography: Technique, Anatomic Correlations, Implementation, and Clinical Applications," *Mayo Clin Proc*, 1988, 63(7):649-80.

Treadmill Exercise Echocardiography

Synonyms Stress Echocardiography

Indications

- determine the presence and severity of exercise-induced myocardial ischemia
- evaluate the potential for exercise-induced rhythm disturbances
- evaluate the hemodynamic responses to activity
- evaluate the effect of medical or interventional therapy
- prescribe appropriate activity guidelines
- evaluate patient's exercise/work tolerance
- evaluate the impact of cardiac rehabilitation intervention
- assess the functional significance of valvular heart disease

(Continued)

Treadmill Exercise Echocardiography *(Continued)*

Contraindications

- acute MI
- severe symptomatic valvular heart disease
- uncontrolled ventricular arrhythmias
- uncontrolled supraventricular arrhythmias compromising cardiac function
- unstable or rest angina
- uncompensated congestive heart failure
- suspected or known dissecting aortic aneurysm
- thrombophlebitis
- recent embolism
- left ventricular outflow tract (LVOT) obstruction
- clinically significant acute pericarditis or myocarditis
- complete heart block
- mobile intracardiac thrombus
- significant psychiatric disturbance
- neuromuscular complications that prevent or severely limit ambulation

Patient Preparation The patient is examined and assessed for exercise candidacy by a physician. Test procedure, risks, and benefits are explained to the patient and informed consent is obtained. All clothes above the waist are removed. Female patients may wear a loose-fitting hospital gown that offers easy access to electrodes and lead wires. The skin at the electrode sites is prepared to remove dirt and oils. Electrodes and lead wires are secured to minimize motion artifact. Resting, supine and standing 12-lead EKGs are recorded and compared to previous EKGs to identify changes. A 30-second posthyperventilation EKG is often recorded prior to exercise to identify ventilatory-induced changes in the ST segments. The patient receives instruction and demonstration regarding walking on the treadmill. The patient is encouraged to walk upright, take long steps and rely on the treadmill bar only for balance and not for support. After a brief trial period when the patient is adapted to treadmill ambulation the protocol is initiated.

Aftercare The patient is monitored until hemodynamically stable and blood pressure and pulse values return to a near-baseline level. Patients should check out with laboratory personnel when leaving the area.

Special Instructions Outpatients are by appointment only. Inpatients are scheduled as soon as possible (usually within 24 hours of request). Patients are instructed not to eat or drink for 3-4 hours before the test and are also instructed to bring or wear clothes suitable for exercise. Patients are variably requested to discontinue medication as instructed by their personal physicians. Other medications should be taken as prescribed unless instructed differently. The procedure, risks, and benefits should be explained by the physician, and the receipt of patient consent should be documented prior to beginning the test.

Equipment Motor-driven treadmill, multichannel electrocardiograph with real-time monitor display and printer; sphygmomanometer; cardiac emergency equipment (defibrillator, oxygen, suction, I.V. kits and fluid, emergency drugs, airway management equipment). A computerized digitizer and an echocardiogram machine is also necessary.

Technique The patient is brought to the Echocardiography Laboratory in a prescheduled 4-hour fasting state. The skin at the electrode sites is prepared with alcohol and mild abrasion to remove superficial layers of skin. Electrodes are attached to the chest wall. Pretest 12-lead electrocardiograms are recorded in the supine and standing positions and compared to previous standard 12-lead EKGs for new changes. Post 30-second hyperventilation electrocardiograms are often performed to identify ventilatory-induced electrocardiogram changes. The test procedure is explained to the patient and informed consent is obtained. The technician verbally instructs and demonstrates for the patient proper treadmill walking technique. The test is performed with a technician and at least one other qualified professional present. A physician is available in the testing area. An appropriate exercise protocol is selected based on the clinical questions asked, the patient's medical status, and the predicted exercise ability of the patient. Every 2-3 minutes the speed and/or grade of the treadmill are increased to yield an increment of 1/2-2 METS increase per stage. At least one channel (V_5) and preferably three channels of the electrocardiogram are continuously monitored on a real-time visual display monitor. Twelve-lead electrocardiograms and blood pressures are recorded at least once at every stage, usually within the last 30 seconds of each stage. Heart rate, ST segments, arrhythmias, symptoms, and subjective patient responses are also continuously monitored. The test is terminated when the patient achieves a subjective maximal effort, significant ischemic changes are observed, significant rhythm disturbances are observed, hemodynamic status is compromised, the patient requests to stop the test, the equipment fails, and/or a predetermined end-point is achieved. At the conclusion of the exercise test, the treadmill speed and gradient are lowered to a base level and the patient is encouraged to ambulate as tolerated to avoid venous pooling and a vasovagal response. Patients ambulate for 3-5 minutes or until the heart rate and blood pressure plateau. Patients are then observed in a sitting or supine position. If patients cannot ambulate after the test or ambulation is contraindicated, patients should be immediately placed in the prone position and monitored. During recovery, the EKG is continuously monitored and recorded along with the blood pressure and symptoms every minute until the patient is hemodynamically stable and has returned to a near pretest level. A complete resting echocardiogram including color and spectral Doppler is obtained at rest. Immediately after exercise the patient is guided to the padded echo bed. Computer digitized images are obtained with videotape back-up. Both the digitized images and videotape are carefully reviewed for inducible myocardial ischemia and an exercise-induced decrement in regional left ventricular myocardial thickening, indicative of inducible myocardial ischemia.

Data Acquired 12-lead EKG, heart rate, arrhythmias, ST segment values, blood pressure, symptoms, patient subjective responses (eg, rating of perceived exertion, angina scale, dyspnea scale), left ventricular systolic function, regional wall motion, assessment of the pericardial space, assessment of the cardiac valves and the ascending aorta

Normal Findings Shortening of the PR and QT intervals and J point depression may occur. Less than 1 mm upsloping ST segment depression 60-80 msec after the J point as compared to resting measures. A linear increase in heart rate with activity >85% predicted maximal heart rate (if not on a chronotropic medication, most commonly a beta blocker). A continuous increase of 7-12 mm Hg in systolic blood pressure per MET achieved to a peak systolic blood pressure <220 mm Hg. A fall, no change, or >20 mm Hg increase in diastolic blood pressure to a peak <120 mm Hg. Occasional ventricular or supraventricular ectopy that does not significantly increase with activity. Test termination because of leg or general fatigue and appropriate shortness of breath. Nausea and dizziness early in recovery are not uncommon. On echocardiography, the left ventricular cavity should symmetrically reduce in end-systolic size/dimension. There should be a uniform response of the left ventricle in a hypercontractile manner in all segments without evidence of regional myocardial dysfunction.

Critical Values 1 mm or more upright, horizontal or downsloping ST segment depression, 60-80 msec beyond the J point as compared to rest without any confounding medication, metabolic or baseline electrocardiogram abnormalities. Horizontal or downsloping ST segment depression carries a greater probability of significant coronary artery disease than rapid recovering upsloping depression. A ≥1 mm ST segment elevation of the J point in leads without significant Q waves. A >10 mm Hg fall in systolic blood pressure with increasing workloads recorded on two separate readings at least 30 seconds apart (especially if associated with symptoms of exercise intolerance). An increase of the systolic blood pressure >250 mm Hg, increasing ventricular ectopy to >30% of all complexes and the onset of complete left or right bundle branch block. The onset of second- or third-degree heart block, lightheadedness or cyanosis, ataxia, confusion, or nausea during activity. Left ventricular cavity enlargement on echocardiography, failure to reduce the left ventricular end-systolic volumes or exercise-induced regional left ventricular systolic dysfunction.

(Continued)

Treadmill Exercise Echocardiography *(Continued)*

Limitations

- ST segments cannot be accurately interpreted if the patient has left bundle branch block, left ventricular hypertrophy with secondary ST-T changes, the Wolff-Parkinson-White syndrome, digitalis administration, ventricular pacing, electrolyte abnormalities, or baseline ST-T-wave abnormalities.
- Sudden intense activity can cause false-positive ST segment depression.
- Medications such as beta blockers, calcium blockers, vasodilators, and afterload reducing agents may reduce myocardial oxygen demand and ameliorate ischemia during activity.
- The early termination of the test by the patient or investigator limits predictive ability.
- Exercise stress testing has an average sensitivity of 60% to 70% and sensitivity of 80% to 90% for the detection of flow-limiting coronary artery disease.
- The addition of an echocardiogram to an exercise stress test raises the sensitivity to approximately 90% and the specificity to approximately 90%.
- The less severe the disease the lower sensitivity.
- Orthopedic complications and the lack of patient motivation both limit the predictive ability of the test if peak myocardial oxygen demand is not achieved.
- Women yield a higher false-positive rate than men.

References

Marwick TH, "How to Perform Stress Echocardiography: Practical Aspects," *Stress Echocardiography: Its Role in the Diagnosis and Evaluation of Coronary Artery Disease*, Marwick TH, ed, Boston, MA: Kluwer Academic Publishers, 1994.

Sawada SG, Ryan T, Conley MJ, et al, "Prognostic Value of a Normal Exercise Echocardiogram," *Am Heart J*, 1990, 120(1):49-55.

♦ **Treadmill Exercise Test** *see* Electrocardiogram, Adult, Exercise EKG Test *on page 30*

Two-Dimensional Echocardiography

Related Information

M-Mode Echocardiography *on page 37*

Transesophageal Echocardiography *on page 42*

Synonyms Cross-Sectional Echocardiography; 2-D Echo

Procedure Commonly Includes Two-dimensional echocardiography is the most common cardiac ultrasound technique in use today. It provides real-time high resolution tomographic images of the heart and great vessels. It is the preferred noninvasive imaging technique for a wide spectrum of cardiovascular disorders.

Indications Two-dimensional echocardiography provides information for the diagnosis and management of patients with congenital, pericardial, myocardial, and valvular heart disease. It provides accurate information regarding chamber size and ventricular function. The high resolution and clear anatomic detail provided by 2-D echo makes this technique ideally suited for the analysis of common and complex congenital heart disease. It permits the diagnosis and classification of intra-atrial and interventricular septal defects as well as atrioventricular canal defects. The diagnosis of pulmonic stenosis, bicuspid aortic valve, Tetralogy of Fallot, transposition of the great arteries, and Ebstein's anomaly is greatly enhanced by the use of 2-D echocardiography. Two-dimensional echocardiography allows for the diagnosis and sizing of pericardial effusions and can be used as a guide to performing pericardiocentesis. The diagnosis and characterization of left ventricular dilatation and dysfunction has been greatly aided by 2-D echo; it permits differentiation between congestive, restrictive, and obstructive cardiomyopathies. The left ventricular ejection fraction obtained by 2-D echo correlates well with that obtained by angiography and nuclear ventriculography. Two-dimensional echocardiography is firmly established as an ideal imaging technique to evaluate patients with valvular heart disease. In mitral stenosis, it not only provides an accurate diagnosis, but it allows for gradation of severity, pliability, and presence of calcification, and aids in determining the timing for surgery. In patients with mitral insufficiency, it provides accurate assessment of the pathologic and physiologic processes responsible for the cause of regurgitation. In patients with aortic valve disease, two-dimensional echocardiography permits establishment and quantification of the diagnosis. It may also allow for the determination of the etiology. Two-dimensional echocardiography has been most useful in the evaluation of intracardiac tumors, clots, and vegetations.

Contraindications There are no contraindications for 2-D echocardiography. As with M-mode echocardiography, patients with chronic obstructive pulmonary disease or obesity may have tests of poor diagnostic quality. An advantage of 2-D echo over M-mode echo is the possibility of performing studies from the apical and subcostal windows which may provide improved cardiac visualization and greater diagnostic information.

Patient Preparation No special patient preparation is required. Fasting is not necessary. Optimally, the patient should be able to rest supine and in the left lateral decubitus position comfortably. The procedure can be done at any time.

Special Instructions A 2-D echocardiogram takes approximately 45 minutes to perform. Most laboratories allow 1 hour per test to allow for patient preparation and chart handling. To optimize the diagnostic yield of the echocardiogram, a note listing the indication for the study should be made in the patient's chart or on a requisition form. Other useful accompanying information includes the patient's age, weight, and height.

Technique A patient arriving at the Echocardiogram Laboratory is greeted by laboratory personnel. He/she is asked about any prior experience with the procedure and is given a brief description of the test. The patient is asked to undress from the waist up and is provided a gown to be worn with the opening in the front. Three electrodes for EKG monitorization are placed on the chest and the patient is asked to lie in the left lateral decubitus position. A complete 2-D echocardiogram includes multiple tomographic views from the left parasternal area, the cardiac apex, the subcostal region, and the suprasternal fossa. Recordings at all these levels are made on a video cassette recorder and selected frames are registered for the final report. All necessary measurements are made either from still frames during the study or afterwards off line from the video tape.

Normal Findings Adequate interpretation of 2-D echocardiography requires knowledge of the normal cardiac chamber dimensions, great artery dimensions, and blood flow velocity through the respective cardiac valves. In addition, a thorough understanding of the normal motion of the cardiac valves, global and regional left ventricular systolic function is most important. Distinct abnormalities can be characterized by 2-D echocardiography for most cardiovascular disorders. See table.

Two-Dimensional Echocardiography

	Male	Female
Left ventricle end diastolic volume	130±27 (73-201) mL	92±19 (53-146) mL
Left atrial volume	50 mL	36 mL
Left ventricular mass	135 g	99 g

Reproduced with permission from Schiller NB, "Cardiology," *Echocardiography and Doppler in Clinical Cardiology,* Chapter 41, Parmley WW and Chartarjee K, eds, Philadelphia, PA: JB Lippincott Co, 1987.

References

Otto C, *The Practice of Clinical Echocardiography,* Philadelphia, PA: WB Saunders Co, 1997.

♦ **Unidimensional Echo** *see* M-Mode Echocardiography *on page 37*

♦ **Vascular Coronary Ultrasound** *see* Intravascular Coronary Ultrasound *on page 36*

GASTROENTEROLOGY

♦ **Abdominal Paracentesis** *see* Paracentesis *on page 86*
♦ **Acid Infusion Test** *see* Bernstein Test *on page 54*
♦ **Acid Perfusion Test for Esophagitis** *see* Bernstein Test *on page 54*
♦ **Ambulatory pH Monitoring** *see* pH Study, 12- to 24-Hour *on page 92*
♦ **Anal Rectal Motility** *see* Anorectal Manometry *on page 49*

Anorectal Manometry

Synonyms Anal Rectal Motility; ARM; Balloon Manometry for Fecal Incontinence; Rectosphincteric Manometry

Procedure Commonly Includes Direct measurement of pressures in the anal canal, including the internal and external anal sphincters, along with assessment of rectal sensation and reflexes. This is performed by using either a manometry probe or a 3-balloon apparatus with external pressure transducers. It is most useful in the evaluation of suspected Hirschsprung disease and difficult cases of fecal incontinence.

Indications Only carefully selected patients should undergo anorectal manometry (ARM). Certainly, not every patient presenting with fecal incontinence warrants invasive testing. The procedure is indicated when:

- evaluating cases of suspected Hirschsprung disease, in both children and adults; particularly useful in patients with megacolon of unknown etiology or adults with possible "short-segment" Hirschsprung disease
- evaluating difficult cases of fecal incontinence, especially if one of the following is suspected: surgical trauma to anal sphincters or nerve structures; invasive perianal disease compromising regional nerve or muscle; impaired motor function and/or sensory innervation involving one or both anal sphincters from systemic disease (eg, scleroderma, polymyositis, etc); impaired sensation of rectal distention, as in diabetes mellitus
- assessing fecal continence mechanisms following surgery for defecation disorders (surgery for imperforate anus, Hirschsprung disease, etc)

In addition to diagnostic indications, ARM has an important therapeutic role in the treatment of fecal incontinence with biofeedback.[1] Retraining the external anal sphincter in patients with weak voluntary contractions has been successful; biofeedback data is based on continuous external sphincter pressure readings.

Contraindications

- uncooperative patient
- confused or comatose patient; ARM usually requires the patient to voluntarily squeeze and relax muscles controlling continence
- active lower GI bleeding
- history of allergy to rubber or latex products

Patient Preparation The details of the procedure are discussed with the patient and consent is obtained. Patient should understand that the procedure involves inflation of a balloon in the rectum. In many centers, cleansing of the rectal vault is performed routinely, using saline or Fleet® enemas, sometimes also cathartics. Some specialists do not request any bowel prep unless hard stool is expected. Sedatives should not be automatically given, but instead should be reserved for the very young (and extremely anxious) patient.

Aftercare No specific postprocedure restrictions are necessary. Patient may resume previous level of activity.

(Continued)

Anorectal Manometry *(Continued)*

Complications ARM is a very safe procedure. To date, only one major complication has been reported, that of systemic anaphylaxis.[2] This was presumed to be an IgE-mediated hypersensitivity reaction to the latex manometry balloon, as it came in contact with the rectal mucosa.

Equipment Two different systems for performing ARM are popular, and equipment for each is different. (The First International Symposium on ARM reported a wide variety of commercial devices in common use, the majority deemed acceptable[3]). In the first system, "perfusion manometry," a small diameter (0.7-2 mm) manometry probe is utilized, resembling an esophageal manometry catheter. In some models, there is a large inflatable rectal balloon at the distal tip. This probe is a soft plastic catheter with radially arranged ports (sensing orifices) and uses a standard water perfusion system. Other acceptable devices include stiff, hollow metal catheters and dacron-woven catheters with microtip sensors. Attached to the manometry catheter is a pressure transducer for each sensing orifice. Results are recorded on a multichannel polygraph machine. The second system is a nonperfused or "balloon manometry" system. Here, three balloons are aligned in series on a hollow metal cylinder. The largest balloon (50 mL capacity) is the "rectal balloon," and is attached to the end of the cylinder. After proper placement, it will be located in the upper anal canal. The middle balloon is doughnut-shaped and will be positioned in the anal ampulla, surrounded by the internal (and part of the external) anal sphincter. The external balloon will lie at the anal verge, within the external anal sphincter. Each balloon is connected to its own pressure transducer, which in turn transmits to the multichannel recorder. The large rectal balloon may be inflated or deflated by means of an air-filled syringe.

Technique The procedure is performed only by an experienced GI specialist in a fully equipped procedure room.

Perfusion manometry technique: With patient in supine position (or left lateral), a standard digital examination is carried out and anal wink reflex tested. Manometry probe is advanced per rectum approximately 10 cm (in the adult), then slowly withdrawn using station pull-through technique. Pressures are continuously observed and the area of high pressure corresponding to the anal sphincters is located. (This may require several repetitions to ensure reproducibility of results.) This so-called "basal anal pressure" is recorded with the patient relaxed. The patient is then asked to perform a maximal sphincter squeeze, and again, highest pressures are recorded. This is termed the "maximal squeeze pressure". Following this, the manometry catheter is reinserted as before and the 50 mL rectal balloon inflated slowly. Patient reports the first conscious sensation of rectal fullness and the volume of the rectal balloon is recorded at that time. In addition, response of the anal sphincters to rectal distention may be measured with some devices.

Balloon manometry technique: If the 3-balloon apparatus is used, it is inserted per rectum following a digital rectal exam. This device is advanced approximately 8 cm or until the distal (external) balloon is just inside the anal verge and can barely be visualized. Both the middle and external balloons are then inflated and pressure tracings noted. The large internal rectal balloon is inflated with up to 50 mL air. Patient reports the first sensation of rectal fullness. A "threshold value" of rectal sensation is obtained by deflating the balloon slowly and noting the smallest volume sensed. Following this, the large rectal balloon is reinflated and simultaneous pressures recorded from the middle balloon (reflecting internal and external sphincter in upper anal canal) and external balloon (reflecting external sphincter in anal verge).

Additional pressure tracings reflecting the external sphincter may be obtained during cough, anal pinprick, and other maneuvers.

Data Acquired

With perfusion manometry:

- basal pressure of sphincter zone (mm Hg)
- maximal squeeze pressure with maximum voluntary sphincter contraction
- squeeze increment (maximal squeeze pressure minus basal pressure)
- rectal sensation and threshold if rectal balloon is used

With balloon manometry:

- rectal sensation and rectal distention sensory threshold
- urge to defecate following rectal distention
- response of internal sphincter to rectal distention
- response of external sphincter to rectal distention
- estimation of rectal compliance

A compliance curve may be generated if the pressure within the large rectal balloon is plotted against its volume over a range of values.

Normal Findings Testing information is reported by an experienced GI specialist. For basal and squeeze pressures, a wide range of normal values has been reported due to the variety of manometric devices in use. Thus, normal ranges for men and women must be defined by each individual laboratory. Representative normal values of basal anal squeeze and canal pressures are summarized in a recent American Gastroenterological Association position paper on anorectal testing techniques.[4] The normal response to rectal distention (simulated by the inflated rectal balloon) is reflex relaxation of the internal sphincter. This is the "rectoanal inhibitory reflex" under autonomic nervous system control. This occurs within seconds of rectal distention (14-25 mL in balloon[4]) and a 30-40 mm Hg drop in sphincter pressure is seen. This is measured by the middle balloon of the 3-balloon system. Simultaneously, there is contraction of the external anal sphincter, the "rectoanal contraction response". This response to rectal distention is felt to be a learned phenomenon and not a reflex per se. When the large rectal balloon is slowly inflated, most normal individuals can consciously sense distention with approximately 10 mL air. Rectal compliance curves generated from pressure-volume measurements are compared against the norm for an individual laboratory.

Critical Values Test is considered positive (abnormal) if a measured variable or reflex response consistently falls outside the established normal range.

Additional Information In certain disease states, ARM abnormalities may be pathognomonic. In Hirschsprung disease, for example, rectal distention may lead to paradoxical internal sphincter contraction, rather than relaxation. Aganglionosis invariably involves the internal sphincter, and due to involvement of the intramural plexus, the rectoanal inhibitory reflex is abolished. Accuracy is high enough to obviate the need for deep muscle biopsy in some cases. In the adult with short segment Hirschsprung disease, ARM may be the only practical means of establishing the diagnosis. Although ARM is rarely diagnostic of a specific disease in patients with fecal incontinence, important information regarding sphincter failure may be obtained. Abnormally low basal pressures (with normal squeeze pressures) indicate isolated internal anal sphincter dysfunction. Abnormally low squeeze pressures (with normal basal pressures) are characteristic of isolated external sphincter dysfunction. Systemic involvement of neuromuscular disease may at times be confirmed by ARM in patients with fecal incontinence. In scleroderma, for instance, incontinence may be due to selective involvement of the smooth muscle in the internal sphincter. Striated muscle characteristically is spared. There is loss of the rectoanal inhibitory reflex, but external sphincter contraction remains intact. In polydermatomyositis, only striated muscle is involved. External sphincter contraction is impaired but the rectoanal inhibitory reflex is normal. It should be noted that a number of underlying systemic diseases may also cause fecal incontinence and isolated external sphincter dysfunction, including myotonic dystrophy, hyperthyroidism, myasthenia gravis, and perhaps diabetes mellitus. Abnormal sensory threshold for rectal distention suggests a lesion in sensory neural pathways. This has been demonstrated in some diabetics with fecal incontinence where the required distending volume of the rectal balloon is >10 than normal controls. Decreased rectal compliance is the etiology of fecal incontinence in a limited number of diseases. These include radiation proctitis, inflammatory bowel disease with rectal involvement, rectal ischemia, and (possibly) fecal impaction.

Anorectal Biofeedback: Biofeedback is the process by which information is provided to a patient with anorectal disorder about physiologic functions to gain control over these functions. It is indicated in patients with either spastic pelvic floor syndrome or anismus or fecal incontinence. For patients with anismus, the patient can learn to defecate without contracting the pelvic floor (Continued)

Anorectal Manometry *(Continued)*

(either external anal sphincter and/or puborectalis muscle) by comparing his manometric and EMG recordings to that of a normal person's tracing. On the other hand, a patient with fecal incontinence is trained to contract the external sphincter in response to various thresholds of rectal distention. This is again accomplished with the patient observing his own manometric tracings and comparing these to normal tracings. Several sessions are usually required for training and home biofeedback training is available.

Footnotes

1. Marzuk PM, "Biofeedback for Gastrointestinal Disorders: A Review of the Literature," *Ann Intern Med*, 1985, 103(2):240-4.
2. Sondheimer JM, Pearlman DS, and Bailey WC, "Systemic Anaphylaxis During Rectal Manometry With a Latex Balloon," *Am J Gastroenterol*, 1989, 84(8):975-7.
3. Mishalany H, Suzuki H, and Yokoyama J, "Report of the First International Symposium of Anorectal Manometry," *J Pediatr Surg*, 1989, 24(4):356-9.
4. Diamant NE, Kamm MA, Wald A, et al, "American Gastroenterological Association Medical Position Paper on Anorectal Testing Techniques," *Gastroenterology*, 1999, 116:732-60.

References

Griner PF, Black ER, and Panzer RJ, "Laboratory Testing in Gastroenterology," *Bockus Gastroenterology*, 5th ed, Chapter 13, Haubrich WS, Schaffner F, and Berk JE, eds, Philadelphia, PA: WB Saunders Co, 1995, 157-72.

Stendal C, "Anorectal Manometry," *Practical Guide to Gastrointestinal Function Testing*, Oxford, England, Blackwell Science, 1997, 213-24.

Wald A, Caruana BJ, Freimanis MG, et al, "Contributions of Evacuation Proctography and Anorectal Manometry to Evaluation of Adults With Constipation and Defecatory Difficulty," *Dig Dis Sci*, 1990, 35(4):481-7.

Anoscopy

Related Information

Colonoscopy *on page 59*

Flexible Fiberoptic Sigmoidoscopy *on page 76*

Synonyms Proctoscopy

Procedure Commonly Includes Direct examination of the lower rectal mucosa and anal canal. The device used, the anoscope, is a rigid metal or plastic instrument 5-8 cm in length. In general, this procedure is useful in the diagnosis of diseases of the distal anal canal.

Indications

Common indications include:

- rectal bleeding
- evaluation of the perianal mass discovered on digital rectal examination (eg, hematoma, carcinoma, thrombosed hemorrhoids)
- suspected cases of proctitis; procedure allows visually-directed cultures to be obtained (eg, herpes simplex virus, *Neisseria gonorrhoeae*)
- evaluation of rectal pain, including anal fissures, perianal abscesses, fistulas, hematoma
- diagnosis of internal hemorrhoids

Therapeutic procedures which may be performed along with routine anoscopy include:

- collection of specimens for microbiological staining and culture
- direct dilation
- removal of foreign bodies
- biopsy of suspicious lesions, ulcers, or masses
- removal of polyps, single or multiple
- coagulation of bleeding mucosal lesions
- treatment of hemorrhoids by injection or banding

Contraindications There are few absolute contraindications for diagnostic anoscopy. Anoscopy should not be performed if patient refuses to consent or if severe rectal pain is present. In the latter case, if diagnostic anoscopy is considered crucial (ie, perianal abscess), a formal examination under anesthesia may be warranted. If an uncorrectable coagulopathy is present, biopsy should be avoided.

Patient Preparation An individual patient's candidacy for this procedure is determined by a medical history and physical, including a digital rectal exam. One of the advantages of anoscopy is its convenience. It may be performed in a physician's office on short notice and without bowel preparation. The details of the procedure are explained to the patient and consent is obtained. Often, there is a certain amount of anxiety and embarrassment on the part of the patient. The medical staff can do much to alleviate this problem with some simple reassurance and courtesy.

Aftercare If no therapeutic procedures have been performed (such as biopsy or fulguration), no specific aftercare is required. The patient may be discharged directly to home in many cases. Since sedatives are not administered routinely, patients are allowed to drive postprocedure. If the procedure is lengthy or complicated, the physician may want to observe the patient for a variable period of time.

Complications In skilled hands, anoscopy is a safe procedure. Severe complications are unusual. Potential problems include local pain, hemorrhage, and bowel perforation. If a biopsy is performed, the risk of bleeding will increase, depending on the nature of the lesion.

Equipment The anoscope is a rigid metal or plastic tube. The diameter of the device is about 2 cm and the length is 5-8 cm. A wide variety of models are available. Some models require external illumination but others have a built-in fiberoptic light source.

Technique In the majority of cases, sedatives or anesthetics are not required. Procedure may be performed in an endoscopy suite or a well-lit physician's office. The patient is appropriately positioned on an examination table according to physician preference (eg, left lateral decubitus). With the instrument's obturator (introducer) in place, the anoscope is lubricated and then advanced gently through the anal canal, angled posteriorly towards the umbilicus. Once fully inserted, the introducer is removed. The lumen of the canal is inspected for abnormalities.

Normal Findings The normal rectal mucosa appears pink with visible submucosal vessels. A preliminary report is completed in the patient's chart immediately by endoscopist.

Critical Values A variety of local and systemic diseases can cause rectal pathology. The anoscopist usually addresses the following aspects of the examination:

- type of instrument used
- depth of visualization (eg, 10 cm)
- appearance of the mucosa
- presence of blood or pus
- anal fissures, tumors, polyps
- presence of proctitis, vesicles
- hemorrhoids
- foreign bodies
- therapeutic procedures performed
- complications

Additional Information Proctoscopy is safe and very convenient. It may be performed in a physician's office, and unlike colonoscopy, without a special bowel prep. In addition, proctoscopy is not limited to the gastroenterologist. Physicians in primary care fields may perform routine cases with safety and accuracy after proper training. Some experts feel that the anoscope provides optimal visualization of the distal rectum, superior to flexible sigmoidoscopy and colonoscopy. As such, it is the procedure of choice for evaluating anal diseases.

References

Kelly SM, Sanowski RA, Foutch PG, et al, "A Prospective Comparison of Anoscopy and Fiberendoscopy in Detecting Anal Lesions," *J Clin Gastroenterol*, 1986, 8(6):658-60.

Wexner SD, Jagleman DG, and Johansen OB, "Anoscopy and Perirectal Disorders," *Gastrointestinal Endoscopy*, CD-ROM, 2nd ed, Chapter 89, MV Sivak, ed, Philadelphia, PA: WB Saunders Co, 1999.

♦ **ARM** *see* Anorectal Manometry *on page 49*

♦ **Ascites Fluid Tap** *see* Paracentesis *on page 86*

♦ **Bacterial Overgrowth Testing** *see* Breath Hydrogen Analysis *on page 57*

♦ **Balloon Manometry for Fecal Incontinence** *see* Anorectal Manometry *on page 49*

♦ **BAO (Basal Acid Output)** *see* Gastric Acid Analysis *on page 78*

♦ **Basal Acid Output** *see* Gastric Acid Analysis *on page 78*

♦ **Basal Serum Gastrin Determination** *see* I.V. Secretin Gastrin Levels *on page 81*

Bernstein Test

Related Information

Esophageal Motility Study *on page 68*
Standard Acid Reflux Test *on page 99*

Synonyms Acid Infusion Test; Acid Perfusion Test for Esophagitis

Procedure Commonly Includes Infusion of acid (0.1 N HCl) into the distal esophagus to determine if a patient's complaints of chest pain originate in the esophagus. Both acid and a saline control are alternately infused through a nasogastric (NG) tube, without the patient being aware of the identity of the solution. Any subjective symptoms of chest or abdominal discomfort are recorded.

Indications

- determine if symptoms in an individual patient are caused by esophageal disease, most commonly gastroesophageal (GE) reflux disease
- help objectively discriminate between angina pectoris and esophageal disease in the patient with atypical chest pain

Contraindications

- confused or agitated patient; the Bernstein test requires accurate verbal descriptions of symptoms by the patient during acid infusion
- active upper GI bleeding
- nausea and vomiting at test time
- possibly, severe coronary artery disease (CAD)

Patient Preparation Technique and risks of the procedure are explained and consent is obtained. Requisition from referring physician should specify whether Bernstein test is to be performed alone or in conjunction with formal esophageal manometry testing. The patient should be NPO for at least 8 hours before testing and preferably overnight. Avoid antacids and H_2 blockers prior to procedures (check with the GI Laboratory if there are questions regarding medications).

Aftercare If no complications have occurred, patient may be dismissed from GI procedure room. No particular postprocedure restrictions are required, with activity *ad libitum* as tolerated. Usually, the patient is given 30 mL antacid before leaving. If test is positive, inform the patient that he/she will be contacted by the referring physician for specific antireflux instructions.

Complications This procedure is considered quite safe. Minor complications include nausea, vagal reactions, and pyrosis, all usually transient. Mellow et al[1] reported that in patients with documented coronary artery disease (CAD), acid infusion with resultant chest pain was associated with transient myocardial ischemia.

Equipment In GI procedure room: nasogastric tube, connecting tubing, 3-way stopcock, solutions of normal saline and 0.1 N HCl, and lubricant. Commonly, this procedure is done in conjunction with esophageal manometry, in which case the manometer replaces the NG tube.

Technique The procedure is usually performed by a GI specialist. However, if manometry is not desired, the Bernstein test may be safely carried out by a general physician. In the original description of this procedure by Bernstein, patients were positioned in an upright, seated fashion throughout. More recently, however, this has become a matter of preference and many GI specialists opt for the supine position. Following this, the NG tube is lubricated and advanced through the nares 30-35 cm by convention, placing the tip in the distal esophagus. Separate bottles of 0.1 N HCl and saline solution are connected to the NG tube through the 3-way stopcock and clear tubing. Initially, the stopcock is set such that the saline solution is infused first through the NG tube, at a rate of 100-120 drops/minute for 5-15 minutes. The patient is instructed to describe any symptoms in detail, whether or not it is typical of the chief complaint. After this control period, the stopcock is turned so that the infusing solution is changed from saline to 0.1 N HCl without the patient's knowledge. The acid infusion is continued until symptoms appear or until 30 minutes have elapsed. As a general rule, symptoms of pyrosis or abdominal pain should be persistent as long as acid is infusing and worsening in severity over several minutes. "Twinges" or other transient sensations should be recorded but are probably insignificant. If clearly persistent symptoms of retrosternal burning are described, the infusing solution is changed back to saline (again, unknown to patient). Saline is continued for at least 5 minutes. Note whether or not symptoms are alleviated; if so, restart acid infusion and record patient reaction. Alternatively, some clinicians give 30 mL antacid after the initial episode of acid-induced chest pain, foregoing the traditional saline "washout". Patient describes degree of pain relief with antacids, if any. Test is then continued with saline or acid as before.

Data Acquired Presence or absence of symptoms with each infusion, along with duration of symptoms. Nature of symptoms is documented carefully. Reproduction of patient's symptoms is more important than simple presence of a symptom such as heartburn or a new complaint.

Normal Findings No symptoms during either saline or acid infusion

Critical Values A positive test is defined as reproduction of the original chest pain or symptom with infusion of acid, but not saline. This should occur consistently with each separate acid infusion. As an aside, some clinicians through the years have asserted that disappearance of symptoms after cessation of acid infusion (or after administration of antacids) is also a requisite for a positive test. This criterion was not a part of the Bernstein test, as originally described. Winnan et al prospectively investigated this issue and found that a significant number of patients with documented GE reflux experienced persistent chest pain following acid infusion, not relieved by antacids or a replacement saline infusion.[2] They concluded that this clinical adage is probably incorrect and need not be used to define a positive test.

An "inconclusive" test is defined as either:

- chest pain with both saline and acid infusions equally or
- development of a new pain, different from the original chief complaint

Additional Information The Bernstein test has gained clinical acceptance as a rapid and inexpensive means of diagnosing gastroesophageal reflux disease. In cases of atypical chest pain, a positive result may be quite useful in identifying a sensitive lower esophagus as an origin of symptoms. Richter et al (1982) reviewed the literature relating a positive Bernstein test with gastroesophageal reflux and found a sensitivity of 79% and specificity of 82%. Some authors believe that specificity is increased if the patient experiences symptoms within 7 minutes of acid infusion. However, false-negative tests have been documented in nearly all clinical series. Some experts feel that the Bernstein test may be falsely positive in patients with gastritis, further compromising test specificity.[3] This procedure does not objectively measure acid reflux, nor does it diagnose esophagitis. Despite these limitations, this procedure may still be useful, especially when performed in combination with esophageal manometric studies. This appears to be its most accepted role in recent years, especially with the advent of highly elaborate tests for reflux esophagitis.

Footnotes

1. Mellow MH, Simpson AG, Watt L, et al, " Esophageal Acid Perfusion in Coronary Artery Disease: Induction of Myocardial Ischemia," *Gastroenterology*, 1983, 85(2):306-12.
2. Winnan GR, Meyer CT, and McCallum RW, "Interpretation of the Bernstein Test: A Reappraisal of Criteria," *Ann Intern Med*, 1982, 96(3):320-2.
3. De Moraes-Filho JP, "Lack of Specificity of the Acid Perfusion Test in Duodenal Ulcer Patients," *Am J Dig Dis*, 1974, 19(9):785-90.

References

Kahrilas PJ, "Gastroesophageal Reflux Disease and Its Complications," *Gastrointestinal and Liver Disease: Pathophysiology, Diagnosis, and Management*, 6th ed, Chapter 33, Feldman M, Scharschmidt BF, and Sleisenger MH, eds, Philadelphia, PA: WB Saunders Co, 1998, 498-517.

Orlando RC, "Reflux Esophagitis," *Textbook of Gastroenterology*, 3rd ed, Yamada T, Alpers DH, Laine L, eds, Philadelphia, PA: Lippincott Williams & Wilkins, 1999, 1235-63.

Sandler RS, "Bernstein (Acid Perfusion) Test", *Manual of Gastroenterologic Procedures*, 3rd ed, Drossman DA, ed, New York, NY: Raven Press, 1993, 56-60.

Biliary Drainage

Synonyms Biliary Drainage With Cholecystokinin; CCK Test; Duodenal Aspirate; Duodenal Drainage; Gallbladder Stimulation; Transduodenal Drainage With CCK

(Continued)

Biliary Drainage *(Continued)*

Applies to Endoscopic Biliary Drainage; Standard Duodenal Intubation Method of Biliary Drainage

Replaces Biliary Drainage With Magnesium Sulfate

Procedure Commonly Includes Light microscopic and polarized scope examination of "B" bile for cholesterol and calcium bilirubinate crystals

Indications Evaluate by light and polarized microscopy the "B" bile obtained from patients with persistent symptoms of biliary colic who have had negative or inconclusive oral cholecystograms and biliary ultrasound, or who are allergic to radiographic dye. Cholelithiasis or acalculous cholecystitis are suggested by the presence of cholesterol or calcium bilirubinate crystals, by the absence of "B" bile, or by the reproduction of symptoms upon injection of cholecystokinin (CCK). Such supportive evidence of gallbladder disease suggests that symptomatic relief is likely to occur with cholecystectomy.

Contraindications Blocked common bile duct may yield little fluid return during CCK stimulation test and an absence of crystals. Tumor or gallstones may also be the cause of such obstruction.

Patient Preparation Obtain a signed procedure permit for "Biliary Drainage." The patient should have nothing by mouth after the evening meal on the day before the test. Start an I.V. of normal saline. If using the endoscopic method, give 5-10 mg Valium® (no atropine). Anesthetize posterior pharynx with 5% Cetacaine® spray prior to duodenal intubation or endoscopy.

Special Instructions Requisition must state name of test. Procedure is approved by consultation with gastroenterology staff.

Technique Under fluoroscopy, a Dreiling-type, radiopaque, double-lumen tube is intubated. The distal lumen is placed just beyond the papilla of vater in the duodenum, thereby placing the proximal lumen in the gastric antrum. Suction is applied to the gastric lumen and continued throughout the procedure. Cholecystokinin (CCK) is administered by I.V. at the dose of 0.1 mL/kg body weight. Suction is then applied to the duodenal lumen. Three types of bile should be recognized and collected separately. Therefore, the specimen trap should be changed upon recognition of each type of bile. The first bile obtained, "A" bile, is clear and comes from the common bile duct. The second or "B" bile is dark green and comes from the gallbladder. The third or "C" bile is yellow and originates from the biliary radicals. It is the "B" bile that is sent for microscopic analysis. If a satisfactory amount of "B" bile has not been obtained within 15 minutes of CCK injection, the dose should be doubled and repeated. If using an endoscope, the method of collection is basically the same except that the duodenal aspirate is obtained through a suction catheter that is inserted through the biopsy channel.[1]

Data Acquired Presence or absence of cholesterol and calcium bilirubinate crystals; presence or absence of "B" bile; total volume of drainage; patient response.

Turnaround Time 24-48 hours

Specimen 20-25 mL dark "B" bile

Container Any clean plastic container with lid. A Daval mucous specimen trap has been suggested.

Sampling Time 30 minutes - usually begins 10-15 minutes after CCK injection

Causes for Rejection Patient not fasting, administration of peristalsis inhibiting medication (if any questions regarding medications, call the department)

Normal Findings No cholesterol or calcium bilirubinate crystals seen. "B" bile present at least 15-20 mL. Symptoms not reproduced by CCK injection.

Critical Values Test is considered "suspicious" when 1-10 crystals of either calcium bilirubinate or cholesterol are found per slide. Test is considered "positive" when more than 10 crystals of calcium bilirubinate or cholesterol are spotted per slide. No "B" bile obtained even after repeat CCK injection. Symptoms reproduced by CCK injection.

Limitations Reproduction of symptoms alone is only subjective evidence of gallbladder pathology especially since CCK physiologically produces abdominal discomfort and the urge to defecate. However, the CCK test alone has gained popularity in some of the recent literature.[2,3] Liver or pancreatic diseases may cause failure to produce "B" bile and therefore produce a false-positive. A false-positive may also be obtained due to formation of calcium bilirubinate crystals in the presence of pancreatic and liver diseases as well as hemolytic anemias. There is also evidence that cholesterol crystals may be produced physiologically in the fasting state.[4] A false-positive may also be obtained if "false bilirubin" is interpreted as true crystals. These structures are yellow and somewhat amorphous with a pH <4.5 as opposed to the more alkalotic discrete burgundy to brick-red granules of calcium bilirubinate.[1]

Additional Information It is advised to use the cholecystokinin (CCK) stimulation test when other tests to detect gallbladder disease are unsuccessful. This would include an inconclusive finding on a radiology oral cholecystogram test, or when a patient is allergic to the iodine substance contained in most contrast media. Stains and cultures of duodenal aspirates are useful in limited situations. If *Giardia lamblia* or *Strongyloides stercoralis* are suspected, but fecal exams remain negative, stains of duodenal aspirates may prove helpful. Cultures have been proven helpful in typhoid or *Salmonella* carriers.

Footnotes

1. Foss DC and Laing RR, "Detection of Gallbladder Disease in Patients With Normal Oral Cholycystograms," *Am J Dig Dis*, 1977, 22(8):685-9.
2. Sykes D, "The Use of Cholecystokinin in Diagnosing Biliary Pain," *Ann R Coll Surg Engl*, 1982, 64(2):114-6.
3. Lennard TW, Farndon JR, and Taylor RM, "Acalculous Biliary Pain, Diagnosis and Selection for Cholecystectomy Using the Cholecystokinin Test for Pain Reproduction," *Br J Surg*, 1984, 71(5):368-70.
4. Northfield TC and Hoffman AF, "Biliary Lipid Secretion in Gallstone Patients," *Lancet*, 1973, 1:747-8.

References

Burnstein MJ, Vassal KP, and Strasberg SM, "Results of Combined Biliary Drainage and Cholectystokinen Cholecystography in 81 Patients With Normal Oral Cholecystograms," *Ann Surg*, 1982, 196(6):627-32.

♦ **Biliary Drainage With Cholecystokinin** *see* Biliary Drainage *on page 55*

♦ **Biliary Drainage With Magnesium Sulfate** *see* Biliary Drainage *on page 55*

♦ **Blind Liver Biopsy** *see* Liver Biopsy *on page 82*

♦ **Breath Analysis** *see* Breath Hydrogen Analysis *on page 57*

Breath Hydrogen Analysis

Synonyms Breath Analysis; Breath Test; Hydrogen Breath Test; Hydrogen Exhalation Test

Applies to Bacterial Overgrowth Testing; Carbohydrate Malabsorption Tests; Measurement of Intestinal Transit Time

Replaces Carbon-14 Glycine Cholate Test for Bacterial Overgrowth; Carbon-14 Lactose Breath Test; Carbon-14 Stool Excretion; Intestinal Biopsy (for Disaccharidase Deficiency); Intestinal Intubation for Culture; Intestinal Perfusion and Lactose Barium Radiography; Lactose (Sucrose and d-Xylose) Tolerance Test; Stool pH Test; Tests for Fecal Reducing Substances

Procedure Commonly Includes Carbohydrate intolerance: The patient ingests lactose or other carbohydrate feeding. This is followed by collection of samples of expired air. The H_2 content of the expired air is then determined by gas chromatography. Above average H_2 content is considered a positive test.

Measurement of intestinal transit time: The patient ingests a carbohydrate feeding which is followed by a collection of a series of samples of expired air. The H_2 content of each air sample is determined by gas chromatography. The time period between the ingestion of the carbohydrate meal and the first measured increase in expired H_2 is considered to be the small intestinal transit time.

Bacterial overgrowth: The patient ingests a carbohydrate feeding which is followed by a collection of a series of samples of expired air. The H_2 content of each air sample is determined by gas chromatography. The test is considered positive if two distinct H_2 peaks are detected. The first peak corresponds to carbohydrate fermentation by bacteria in the small bowel, and the second to fermentation in the colon (an abnormal finding). Fasting breath H_2 is also usually elevated in this condition.

Indications

- Diagnose carbohydrate malabsorption - lactose, sucrose, DW xylose[1]

(Continued)

Breath Hydrogen Analysis *(Continued)*

- diagnose bacterial overgrowth - H_2 breath test is useful in conjunction with carbon-14 glycolate test
- diagnose motility disorders, such as irritable bowel and postgastrectomy syndromes by measurement of intestinal transit time

Contraindications

- patient unable to drink liquids
- active diarrhea may decrease response
- severe pulmonary disease

Patient Preparation NPO for at least 6-8 hours (preferably overnight) and during test (except for carbohydrate feeding). No smoking 15 minutes prior to test. No antibiotics 7 days prior to test. No grain cereals or foods 12 hours prior to test. Carbohydrate feeding: infants 2 g/kg low fiber, adults 20 g/kg low fiber. Lactulose is the best feeding for bacterial overgrowth testing as it traverses the entire bowel unabsorbed.

Turnaround Time 3-7 days

Container Haldane-Priestly tube for adults; for infants, Rahn-Otis end tidal sampler, nasal prongs, or postnasal catheter connected to bags fitted with 1-way stopcocks. Gas is then transported via an oiled syringe to a Vacutainer®.

Sampling Time Up to 6 hours if interval sampling is used. Interval sampling is usually done every 30 minutes for 2-4 hours.

Collection Usually involves Haldane-Priestly tube into which the patient exhales with nose clamped

Storage Instructions Vacutainer® for up to 3 weeks

Normal Findings For lactose intolerance: if measured in rate of excretion, H_2 >0.5 mL/minute (nL <0.3); if measured as end tidal volume, H_2 >24 ppm or 20 ppm greater than fasting (nL <10). For intestinal overgrowth: two distinct H_2 peaks correspond to carbohydrate fermentation in the small bowel and then the colon.[1] For measurement of intestinal transit time: more than 95 minutes is normal.

Limitations If the test is performed during states of active diarrhea, transit time may not be long enough for sufficient fermentation. Significant bowel, pulmonary, or vascular disease may decrease H_2 absorption and secretion. Idiopathic or iatrogenic absence of intestinal flora makes the test worthless. Presence of normal flora that consume H_2 can give falsely low H_2 excretion. The test is useless in newborns prior to intestinal colonization.[2] The presence of acidic colonic milieu common in infants can give a falsely low H_2 excretion.[3] Exercise also lowers H_2 excretion.[4] Smoking and sleep may falsely elevate H_2 excretion.[5]

Additional Information This test is based on the premise that the normal small bowel absorbs ingested carbohydrate, that the normal small bowel is sterile, and that undigested carbohydrate is then fermented by normal colonic flora with H_2 being the product of that fermentation. The predominence of H_2 produced in the colon is expelled rectally and the remainder is absorbed into the colonic circulation. It is then expelled into the pulmonary tree where it can be measured as exhaled H_2.

Footnotes

1. Bond JH and Levitt MD, "Use of Breath H_2 to Quantitate Small Bowel Transit Time Following Partial Gastrectomy," *J Lab Clin Med*, 1977, 90(1):30-6.
2. Barr RG, Hanley J, Patterson DK, et al, "Breath H_2 Excretion in Normal Newborn Infants in Response to Usual Feeding Patterns: Evidence for "Functional Lactase Insufficiency" Beyond the First Month of Life," *J Pediatr*, 1984, 104(4):527-33.
3. "The Influence of Colonic pH on the Hydrogen Breath-Analysis Test," *Nutr Rev*, 1982, 40(6):172-5.
4. Payne DL, Welsh JD, and Claypool PL, "Breath H_2 Response to Carbohydrate Malabsorption After Exercise," *J Lab Clin Med*, 1983, 102(1):147-50.
5. Rosenthal A and Solomons NW, "Time-Course of Cigarette Smoke Contamination of Clinical H_2 Breath-Analysis Tests," *Clin Chem*, 1983, 29(11):1980-1.

References

Caballero B, Solomons NW, and Torún B, "Fecal Reducing Substances and Breath H_2 Excretion as Indicators of Carbohydrate Malabsorption," *J Pediatr Gastroenterol Nutr*, 1983, 2(3):487-90.

Newcomer AD, McGill DB, and Thomas PJ, et al, "Prospective Comparison of Indirect Methods for Detecting Lactase Deficiency," *N Engl J Med*, 1975, 293(24):1232-6.

♦ **Breath Test** *see* Breath Hydrogen Analysis *on page 57*

Aftercare Following procedure, patient is observed in the recovery area. Vital signs are recorded at least once postprocedure. Once sedation has worn off, patient may be discharged from the testing area. Driving is forbidden due to residual effects from sedatives. The patient is instructed to call physician if complications should develop.

Special Instructions Antibiotic prophylaxis for bacterial endocarditis is commonly administered for patients undergoing colonoscopy with prosthetic valves, a past history of endocarditis, rheumatic valvular disease, or other high risk cardiac lesions. Some authors, however, consider this unnecessary because of the low risk of bacteremia. Regimen for high risk patients recommended by the American Heart Association[3] include:

- ampicillin 2 g I.M./I.V. and gentamicin 1.5 mg/kg given I.M./I.V. 30 minutes before and 6 hours after procedure, 1 g ampicillin I.V./I.M. or amoxicillin 1 g orally
- if penicillin allergic, vancomycin and gentamicin can be administered

Complications Major complications include[1,4,5]:

Perforation: estimated at 0.14% to 0.8% with diagnostic colonoscopy and 1% with polypectomy. This may be recognized immediately (intra-abdominal viscera directly visualized) or may be delayed for days. Perforation may be caused by mechanical trauma from the instrument tip, especially if the wall is weakened (from ischemia, diverticula, colitis), the colon is "tacked down" (previous pelvic surgery, tumor, adhesions), or an obstructive lesion is present. Less commonly, perforation may be noninstrumental, secondary to aggressive insufflation with air (serosal tears). Polypectomy-related perforation may result from a direct luminal laceration from a snare loop or hot forceps, or may be from delayed sloughing of necrotic bowel following thermal coagulation. This latter situation may lead to the "postpolypectomy coagulation syndrome" characterized by fever, evidence of peritoneal irritation (rebound tenderness), and leukocytosis. Radiographic evidence of perforation or free air is lacking, and patients recover without surgery. "Free" perforation from a large transmural laceration is less frequent (0.14% to 0.26%) and requires immediate surgery. Lesser degrees of perforation are more difficult to diagnose. If pneumoperitoneum is detected on KUB a Gastrografin™ (water-soluble) enema x-ray needs to be obtained. If leakage is not demonstrated, many cases can be managed conservatively. The profile of the high risk patient has been described previously. However, serious complications have been reported in routine cases.

Hemorrhage: Incidence of serious bleeding from diagnostic colonoscopy without polypectomy is negligible, 0% to 0.5% of cases. Several large series have reported no incidents of this nature. With polypectomy the rate increases to 0.7% to 2.5% and may be immediate or delayed. Repeat colonoscopy may be necessary to coagulate a bleeding pedicle. In rare instances, angiography and surgery have been required.

Respiratory depression: Usually due to oversedation in the patient with chronic lung disease.

Bacteremia: Incidence varies among series from 0% to 5%. Several large studies have reported no positive blood cultures (see Special Instructions).

Miscellaneous complications:

- vasovagal reactions
- explosion of combustible gases in the colon (H_2, methane) when in contact with an electric spark; this may occur with a grossly inadequate bowel prep
- splenic laceration
- transient EKG changes
- dehydration resulting from excessive use of laxatives and enemas for bowel cleansing
- volvulus

Equipment The standard endoscope is 185 cm in length with a diameter of 12-13 mm. An intermediate length instrument of 140 cm is also available and examines up to the ascending colon. Modern colonoscopes, whether fiberoptic or video, provide a brilliant, high-resolution, color view of the mucosa through wide angle optics. Newer instruments contain two channels within the

(Continued)

Colonoscopy *(Continued)*

endoscope which can accommodate two accessories at the same time, such as a snare wire and forceps. Air for insufflation and a water jet may also be introduced through these channels. The multidirectional tip is controlled at the endoscopist's end by two wheels, for either up-down or right-left deflection. The instrument head is connected to a variety of auxiliary devices via a separate cable, such as a suction box, an external cold light source, and water feed tank.

Technique The procedure is performed by a qualified gastroenterologist in a properly equipped procedure room. At times, colonoscopy may be performed in an ICU, emergency room, or hospital bed using portable equipment. Following sedation, the patient is placed in a left lateral decubitus position. A digital rectal examination is performed. After this the lubricated endoscope is inserted per rectum. Initially, a "red-out" is seen in the rectum and insufflation is used as needed to optimally visualize the lumen. The instrument is advanced then only under direct vision. Landmarks are identified including the rectum (highly vascular, bluish vessels), sigmoid (ring-like valves), descending colon (narrow and tubular), transverse colon (triangular folds), hepatic flexure (dark blue hue from the liver), ascending colon (large lumen), ileocecal valve, and terminal ileum. Mucosal surfaces are reinspected as the endoscope is withdrawn. Minor operative procedures are performed as indicated.

Turnaround Time Final pathology report on biopsy specimens is given within 3-5 days. Microbiologic stains, when performed, are available the same day, but cultures may be variably delayed.

Specimen All biopsy specimens and cytologic brushings are sent to the Pathology Laboratory without delay. Any tissue for microbiological culture should be sent in a sterile container without fixative. Specimen collection, fixative, and transportation are usually the responsibility of the endoscopist.

Normal Findings Preliminary and final report on colonoscopic findings are written immediately by the gastroenterologist, and placed in medical chart. Important aspects of the examination frequently commented upon include:

- adequacy of bowel prep
- type of instrument used
- premedications used, antibiotic prophylaxis if given
- most proximal bowel segment examined
- mucosal abnormalities - polyps (size, appearance), pseudopolyps, hemorrhagic areas, ulcers, neoplastic or obstructing lesions, diverticula, friable areas, lipomas, telangiectasia, spasm, competence of ileocecal valve
- operative procedures performed during colonoscopy
- complications
- recommendations

Limitations This is a relatively expensive procedure in comparison with the barium enema and other related endoscopic studies (eg, EGD, proctoscopy, sigmoidoscopy). The quality of the study, and thus its interpretation, is highly dependent on the skill and experience of the endoscopist. It is also considered more technically difficult than upper endoscopy. Suboptimal studies are not uncommon and often are a result of inadequate bowel preparation.

Footnotes

1. Rankin GB and Sivak MV, "Indications, Contraindications, and Complications of Colonoscopy," *Gastrointestinal Endoscopy*, CD-ROM, 2nd ed, Chapter 80, MV Sivak, ed, Philadelphia, PA: WB Saunders Co, 1999.
2. Waye JD and Williams CB, "Colonoscopy and Flexible Sigmoidoscopy," *Textbook of Gastroenterology*, 3rd ed, Yamada T, Alpers DH, Laine L, et al, eds, Philadelphia, PA: Lippincott Williams & Wilkins, 1999, 2701-17.
3. Dajani AS, Taubert KA, Wilson W, et al, "Prevention of Bacterial Endocarditis. Recommendations by the American Heart Association," *JAMA*, 1997, 277(22):1794-801.
4. MacRae FA, Tan KG, and Williams CB, "Towards Safer Colonoscopy: A Report on the Complications of 5000 Diagnostic or Therapeutic Colonoscopies," *Gut*, 1983, 24(5):376-83.
5. Geenen JE, Schmitt WG, and Hoogan WJ, "Complications of Colonoscopy," *Gastrointest Endosc*, 1974, 66:812.

References

"Appropriate Use of Gastrointestinal Endoscopy," American Society for Gastrointestinal Endoscopy, Standards of Practice Committee, Manchester, MA, 1997.

Overholt BF, "Colonoscopy: A Review," *Gastroenterology*, 1975, 68(5 Pt 1):1308-20.
Ransohoff DF, Lang CA, and Kuo HS, "Colonoscopic Surveillance After Polypectomy: Considerations of Cost-Effectiveness," *Ann Intern Med*, 1991, 114(3):177-82.
Rex DK, Lehman GA, Hawes RH, et al, "Screening Colonoscopy in Asymptomatic Average-Risk Persons With Negative Fecal Occult Blood Tests," *Gastroenterology*, 1991, 100(1):64-7.
Sakai Y, "Technique of Colonoscopy," *Gastrointestinal Endoscopy*, CD-ROM, 2nd ed, MV Chapter 80, Sivak, ed, Philadelphia, PA: WB Saunders Co, 1999.
Waye JD, "Colonoscopy and Proctosigmoidoscopy," *Bockus Gastroenterology*, 5th ed, Chapter 25, Haubrich WS, Schaffner F, and Berk JE, eds, Philadelphia, PA: WB Saunders Co, 1995, 316-30

♦ **Duodenal Aspirate** *see* Biliary Drainage *on page 55*
♦ **Duodenal Drainage** *see* Biliary Drainage *on page 55*
♦ **Duodenal Intubation** *see* Small Bowel Biopsy *on page 95*
♦ **Endoscopic Biliary Drainage** *see* Biliary Drainage *on page 55*
♦ **Endoscopic Retrograde Cannulation of Ampulla of Vater** *see* Endoscopic Retrograde Cholangiopancreatography *on page 63*
♦ **Endoscopic Retrograde Cannulation of Pancreas** *see* Endoscopic Retrograde Cholangiopancreatography *on page 63*
♦ **Endoscopic Retrograde Cannulation of Papilla of Vater** *see* Endoscopic Retrograde Cholangiopancreatography *on page 63*

Endoscopic Retrograde Cholangiopancreatography

Related Information

Esophagogastroduodenoscopy (EGD) *on page 72*
Sphincter of Oddi Manometry *on page 97*

Synonyms Endoscopic Retrograde Cannulation of Ampulla of Vater; Endoscopic Retrograde Cannulation of Pancreas; Endoscopic Retrograde Cannulation of Papilla of Vater; ERCP

Applies to Percutaneous Transhepatic Cholangiogram (PTC)

Procedure Commonly Includes Endoscopic visualization of the duodenum and papilla of vater, followed by radiologic assessment of the pancreatic duct and biliary tree. Procedure is performed on a conscious, but sedated patient. A specialized fiberoptic endoscope is introduced by mouth and advanced through the upper GI tract until the second portion of the duodenum is reached. Under direct visualization, the papilla of vater is located and inspected. A small catheter is then advanced through the papilla of vater and into the pancreatic and biliary duct systems, all under fluoroscopic guidance. Contrast material is injected through the catheter, outlining the pancreatic duct (pancreatogram) and biliary ducts (cholangiogram). Forceps biopsies or cytologic brushings of the periampullary region and ducts may be taken. Endoscopically-guided therapeutic procedures are also possible, including endoscopic sphincterotomy and dissolution of stones. ERCP is a safe, nonsurgical means of assessing the anatomy of the ductal system and is successful in 80% to 90% of attempts.

Indications ERCP has emerged as a widely accepted, standard technique for diagnosing a variety of pancreaticobiliary tract disorders. However, several noninvasive radiologic procedures are also effective in diagnosing these disorders, including percutaneous transhepatic cholangiography (PTC), CT scan of the abdomen, ultrasound of the abdomen, and the radionuclide liver-spleen scan. These imaging techniques should be considered complementary (not competitive) with ERCP. The precise sequencing of studies must be individualized in each case, but generally the high-risk procedures (ERCP, PTC) are reserved for last. With these considerations in mind, the American Society for Gastroenterology Endoscopy (1997) published suggested guidelines for ERCP as follows:[1]

- evaluation of the jaundiced patient in whom biliary obstruction is suspected (if therapeutic ERCP maneuvers can be performed during the procedure)
- evaluation of the nonjaundiced patient whose clinical, biochemical, or imaging data suggests pancreatic or biliary tract disease
- evaluation of the patient with signs or symptoms compatible with pancreatic cancer, when prior imaging studies (eg, CT scan, MRI, or ultrasound) are normal or equivocal

(Continued)

Endoscopic Retrograde Cholangiopancreatography *(Continued)*

- evaluation of pancreatitis of unknown etiology
- preoperative evaluation of a known pancreatic pseudocyst, known chronic pancreatitis, or pancreatic trauma prior to surgical repair or endoscopic therapy
- endoscopic sphincterotomy
  - choledocholithiasis
  - papillary stenosis or sphincter of Oddi dysfunction causing significant disability
  - facilitate placement of biliary stent or balloon dilatation of biliary stricture-sump syndrome
  - choledochocoele involving major papilla
  - ampullary carcinoma in patients who are not candidates for surgery
  - facilitate access to the pancreatic duct
- placement of stents across benign or malignant strictures, fistulas, postoperative bile leak, or in high-risk patients with large unremovable common duct stones
- balloon dilation of ductal strictures
- placement of nasobiliary drains for prevention of or treatment of acute cholangitis or infusion of chemical agents for common duct stone dissolution
- decompression of an obstructed common bile duct or postoperative bile leak
- pseudocyst drainage in appropriate cases
- tissue sampling from pancreatic and bile ducts
- therapy of disorders of the pancreatic duct

ERCP is generally not indicated in:[1,2]

- evaluation of abdominal pain of obscure origin in the absence of objective findings which suggest biliary or pancreatic disease
- evaluation of suspected gallbladder disease without evidence of bile duct disease
- further evaluation of proven pancreatic malignancy unless management will be altered

Contraindications

- patient refusal or poor cooperation
- recent attack of acute pancreatitis, within the past several weeks; one exception is the patient with known choledocholithiasis who will be undergoing endoscopic sphincterotomy or surgery
- recent myocardial infarction
- inadequate surgical back-up
- history of contrast dye anaphylaxis
- poor surgical candidacy; in general, patients should be able to tolerate laparotomy if complications arise
- severe cardiopulmonary background disease
- overlying residual barium in the GI tract from recent abdominal CT scan, lower GI series, etc

Patient Preparation Technique and potential complications of the procedure are discussed with the patient. Informed consent is obtained for ERCP, including likely therapeutic interventions. Formal consultation with gastroenterology staff is required prior to approval and scheduling. The patient is informed that although ERCP is an outpatient procedure, overnight hospitalization may become necessary, especially in difficult and prolonged cases. On the day prior to the procedure, inpatient candidates are routinely seen by the endoscopist (or his representative) to briefly examine the patient, review details of the case, write orders, and answer remaining patient questions. The patient is made NPO after midnight (or at least 8 hours prior to study). Daily oral medications are permitted the morning of ERCP with physician approval. Exceptions include antacids and Carafate® which may interfere with visualization of the mucosa. Aspirin products and nonsteroidal agents must be discontinued well in advance (at least 5 days for aspirin), especially if biopsy or sphincterotomy/papillotomy is anticipated. For hospital inpatients, dentures are removed and patient is transported to endoscopy suite on cart, accompanied by medical chart and relevant x-rays. For outpatients, procedure is the same except that transportation home must be arranged in advance. Once patient is in the procedure room, baseline vital signs are recorded and an intravenous line started. Antibiotic prophylaxis may be given at this time (see Special Instructions). Premedications are routinely given, including parenteral meperidine, and midazolam or diazepam. A topical anesthetic agent such as Cetacaine® spray is applied to the pharynx.

Aftercare The patient is placed at strict bedrest and observed carefully in the recovery area. Vital signs are monitored frequently and physician contacted if any complications arise. If the patient has tolerated the procedure well, he/she may be discharged from the testing area once sedatives have worn off. The patient is made NPO until gag reflux has returned, then clear liquids for 24 hours. Any patient undergoing a complex therapeutic procedure should be observed overnight in the hospital. If a "same day" outpatient procedure is performed, the patient must have ready access to the hospital emergency room should complications develop.

Special Instructions Prior to ERCP, if bile duct obstruction is suspected, antibiotic coverage is usually indicated. If high grade bile duct or pancreatic duct obstruction is confirmed during ERCP, antibiotics should be continued (or begun). Individuals at risk for infective endocarditis are often given antibiotic prophylaxis prior to ERCP, particularly if a therapeutic maneuver such as sphincterotomy is planned. High-risk cardiac lesions include rheumatic valvular disease, prosthetic valves, and prior endocarditis. However, ERCP is considered a relatively low-risk procedure for the development of endocarditis, in comparison with invasive dental procedures and genitourinary tract instrumentation. Some authorities feel that prophylactic antibiotics are not warranted.

Complications In the hands of a skilled endoscopist, diagnostic ERCP is associated with a 3% incidence of morbidity and 0.2% mortality, based on nationwide statistics.[3] Complication rate is considerably higher with an inexperienced endoscopist. If endoscopic sphincterotomy or papillotomy is performed, overall morbidity rate increases to 8% and mortality 1% to 1.5%. Emergent surgical repair is necessary in 2%; it should be noted that these figures are superior to those documented for elective surgical exploration of the common bile duct.

Complications of ERCP may be classified as follows.

- Painless hyperamylasemia: May occur in ≤75% of cases with sometimes striking elevations of serum and urine amylase levels. This is not accompanied by abdominal pain, nausea, or other stigmata of pancreatitis and is clinically inconsequential. Within 4 days, amylase decreases to normal without treatment.
- Acute pancreatitis: Develops in 0.7% to 7.4% of cases and represents a small fraction of patients with elevated amylase levels. Pathogenesis is unclear. Implicated factors include the type of contrast used, the rate and volume of injection, the underlying condition of the pancreas, and the experience of the endoscopist. Management is the same as for gallstone or alcoholic pancreatitis.
- Sepsis: A rare complication but associated with a high mortality. The incidence of bacteremia has been variously estimated at 0% to 14%. Both cholangitis (incidence of 0.65% to 0.8%) and pancreatic sepsis (0.3% incidence) have been reported. The former is almost exclusively associated with ductal obstruction. Biliary stasis predisposes patients to infection of bile fluid, and gram-negative bacteria probably remain dormant behind the obstruction until ERCP. Pancreatic sepsis appears more likely if a pseudocyst is present. Injection of nonsterile contrast into the pseudocyst may lead to abscess if drainage is sluggish. Some authorities consider the presence of pseudocyst a contraindication to ERCP but others feel the statistical risk is unproven.

(Continued)

Endoscopic Retrograde Cholangiopancreatography *(Continued)*

- Complications of upper endoscopy: Nonspecific complications common with upper gastrointestinal endoscopy (EGD) (see listing) include esophageal perforation, hypoxia, adverse drug reactions, and arrhythmias. Drug toxicity may play a more significant role with ERCP due to lengthier procedure time requiring multiple drug administrations.
- Instrumental injury: Uncommon with diagnostic ERCP alone unless anatomy is surgically distorted. Common therapeutic injuries are hemorrhage, laceration, and perforation.

Equipment The duodenoscope used for ERCP is similar to the fiberoptic or video endoscope used for EGD with several modifications. The viewing lens and light window at the instrument tip are arranged for side viewing. Within the duodenoscope is a channel which can accommodate a polyethylene contrast-filled catheter, which can be advanced past the tip of the instrument. This separate catheter is used for cannulating the papilla of vater. Other devices may be passed through the endoscope, including biopsy forceps, electrocautery devices, sphincterotome, cytology brush, etc.

Technique ERCP is performed with the patient on an x-ray table with radiologic equipment and fluoroscopy at hand. Following premedication, the patient is placed in the left lateral decubitus position. The duodenoscope is passed by mouth through the anesthetized pharynx and into the esophagus, stomach, and duodenum. A rapid visual examination of these segments may be made. Once the instrument has reached the second (descending) portion of the duodenum, the ampulla of vater is located, often on the medial wall. The periampullary region is carefully inspected. Often glucagon is given (0.2 mL doses) to decrease duodenal motility and facilitate visualization. The inner catheter (containing contrast dye) is then advanced from the lateral port of the endoscope and guided into the orifice. Once the ampulla has been engaged, the catheter is advanced several millimeters into the duct and a small volume of contrast injected. The dye filling pattern is observed under fluoroscopy ("the test shot") to determine orientation. In this manner, the pancreatic duct and the bile duct may be selectively cannulated and imaged separately with contrast. Fluoroscopy is used as needed to assure proper catheter orientation. Formal spot radiographs are taken of contrast-filled ducts for the permanent record. At times, x-ray table adjustments and patient repositioning may be necessary, particularly if the gallbladder is imaged. Delayed films are also obtained following removal of the duodenoscope since contrast material normally remains in the ductal system for minutes. In addition, suspicious periampullary or ductal lesions may be biopsied and cytologic brush samples obtained. "Blind" biopsies of the ducts and/or pancreas may be taken at physician discretion. A variety of therapeutic procedures, mentioned earlier, may be performed.

Turnaround Time Final report on biopsy and cytology specimen histology is given within 2-3 days (or longer in some cases).

Specimen Biopsy specimens and cytologic brushings are placed in appropriate containers and fixatives and sent to the Pathology Laboratory without delay. Tissue for Gram stain and culture is placed in a sterile jar without fixative and hand carried to the Microbiology Laboratory. Details of specimen collection, fixative, and transportation are handled by the gastroenterology team.

Normal Findings Preliminary written report and final report on endoscopic and radiologic findings is immediately completed by gastroenterology staff. A "normal cholangiogram" implies a normal radiographic appearance of the following structures: common bile duct (CBD), common hepatic duct, left and right hepatic duct (and subdivisions), cystic duct, and gallbladder. Maximum diameter of the normal CBD is approximately 9 mm (range 4-9 mm) providing the gallbladder is present. If the patient has had prior cholecystectomy, diameters may be somewhat increased. The CBD normally will have a tapered appearance at its distal end, the so-called "vaterian segment" where it is surrounded by the papilla and sphincter of Oddi. A "normal pancreatogram" implies a smooth, patent main pancreatic duct which gradually tapers from the body (diameter 3.4 mm) to the tail (1.7 mm). With optimal filling of the pancreatic duct, approximately 15-30 secondary branches will be outlined with contrast. These are straight in appearance and of fine caliber. There is variability in the anatomy of the pancreatic ducts. For example, the duct of Santorini is present in 80% of normal individuals and its communication with the duodenum or main pancreatic duct is variable.

Critical Values In formulating the diagnostic impression, information is obtained from three sources: direct visual examination, radiologic imaging, and biopsy specimens. Endoscopic examination of the papilla of vater may reveal a mucosal mass if carcinoma of the pancreatic head is present. Other malignancies may involve this region including ampullary carcinoma, cholangiocarcinoma, and rarely duodenal cancers. The endoscopic appearance of the papilla may be highly suggestive in other disease states, such as papilla "bulging" (possible impacted stone), edema, erythema, and patency (recently passed stone), visible purulent drainage (suppurative cholangitis), bright red blood through the orifice (hemobilia). Radiologic abnormalities in the cholangiogram may be specific and diagnostic. Certainly, retained stones in the common bile duct are easily recognized by discrete filling defects. Other deviations include biliary strictures, irregular filling defects or mass lesions beyond endoscopic visualization (carcinoma), ductal dilatation (obstruction of any cause), irregular intrahepatic ducts with strictures and ectasia (sclerosing cholangitis), and cystic duct narrowing with cholelithiasis (acute cholecystitis). The pancreatogram may reveal congenital abnormalities (such as pancreas divisum), small pancreatic pseudocysts (not seen on CT scan), and pancreatic duct calculi. The radiologic appearance of carcinoma of the pancreas includes:[4]

- single, irregular abrupt stricture of the pancreatic duct
- gradual occlusion of the main duct
- alterations in the side branches near the tumor such as fragmentation and cystic destruction
- displacement of Wirsung duct
- pooled contrast material in an irregular manner (within necrotic tumor)
- strictured CBD and pancreatic duct ("double duct" sign)

The radiologic appearance of chronic pancreatitis may closely resemble pancreatic cancer. However, the main pancreatic duct in chronic pancreatitis is classically irregular, tortuous, and with **multiple** stenoses - the "chain of lakes" appearance. Single smooth stenosis is also more consistent with chronic pancreatitis. The yield of biopsy in pancreatic cancer is >90% in most large series. Nearly all pancreatic malignancies are ductal carcinomas; thus even small lesions are likely to cause stenosis or occlusion of the main pancreatic duct. In cases where tumor invades the pancreatic duct region or ampulla without entering the lumen, cytology specimens of pancreatic juice may be diagnostic.

Limitations ERCP is relatively expensive and hazardous in comparison with other endoscopic procedures. Results are highly operator dependent, as demonstrated in large series. For both physician and patient, there may be nontrivial radiation exposure if fluoroscopy time is prolonged. This procedure is technically difficult, particularly in patients who have had a Billroth II gastrectomy and gastrojejunostomy.

Footnotes

1. American Society for Gastrointestinal Endoscopy, Standards for Practice Committee, *Appropriate Use of Gastrointestinal Endoscopy*, Manchester, MA: American Society for Gastrointestinal Endoscopy, 1997.
2. Pasricha PJ, "Gastrointestinal Endoscopy," *Cecil Textbook of Medicine*, 21st ed, Chapter 122, Goldman L, and Bennett JC, eds, Philadelphia, PA: WB Saunders Co, 2000, 649-53.
3. Shahmir M and Schuman BM, "Complications of Fiberoptic Endoscopy," *Gastrointest Endosc*, 1980, 26(3):86-91.
4. Cello JP, "Pancreatic Cancer," *Gastrointestinal and Liver Disease: Pathophysiology, Diagnosis, and Management*, 6th ed, Chapter 39, Feldman M, Scharschmidt BF, and Sleisenger MH, eds, Philadelphia, PA: WB Saunders Co, 1998, 604-19.

References

Bilbao MK, Dotter CT, Lee TG, et al, "Complications of ERCP: A Study of 10,000 Cases," *Gastroenterology*, 1976, 70(3):314-20.

(Continued)

Endoscopic Retrograde Cholangiopancreatography *(Continued)*

Cotton PB and Williams CB, "ERCP-Diagnostic Technique," *Practical Gastrointestinal Endoscopy*, 4th ed, Cambridge, MA: Blackwell Science, 1996.

Sivak MV Jr and Sullivan BH Jr, "Endoscopic Retrograde Pancreatography: Analysis of the Normal Pancreatogram," *Am J Dig Dis*, 1976, 21(3):263-9.

Stewart ET, Vennes JA, and Geenen JE, eds, *Atlas of Endoscopic Retrograde Cholangiopancreatography*, St Louis, MO: CV Mosby Co, 1977.

Venu RP, Geenen JE, Toouli J, et al, "Endoscopic Retrograde Cholangiopancreatography. Diagnosis of Cholelithiasis in Patients With Normal Gallbladder X-ray and Ultrasound Studies," *JAMA*, 1983, 249(6):758-61.

♦ **Endoscopic Retrograde Cholangiopancreatography (ERCP) With Pressure Measurement of Sphincter of Oddi** *see* Sphincter of Oddi Manometry *on page 97*

♦ **ERCP** *see* Endoscopic Retrograde Cholangiopancreatography *on page 63*

♦ **Esophageal Manometric Study** *see* Esophageal Motility Study *on page 68*

♦ **Esophageal Manometry** *see* Esophageal Motility Study *on page 68*

Esophageal Motility Study

Related Information

Bernstein Test *on page 54*
Standard Acid Reflux Test *on page 99*

Synonyms Esophageal Manometric Study; Esophageal Manometry

Procedure Commonly Includes Passage of a multilumen manometry catheter into the esophagus and stomach. This device is connected to at least three separate pressure transducers and is capable of sensing squeeze pressures at different sites within the esophageal lumen. Quantitative data is obtained regarding the amplitude (mm Hg) and duration (seconds) of contractions of the upper esophageal sphincter (UES), lower esophageal sphincter (LES), and several sites within the esophageal body. A number of distinct esophageal motility disorders may be diagnosed. Provocative agents may also be employed to induce manometric abnormalities in patients with chest pain of obscure etiology. This procedure has become widely used and is considered the standard of diagnosis for most motor diseases of the esophagus.

Indications Evaluate the patient with suspected primary esophageal motor dysfunction. This includes (but is not limited to) the following:

- primary achalasia
- diffuse esophageal spasm
- chronic idiopathic intestinal pseudo-obstruction (manometry may aid in the initial diagnosis of this entity)
- nutcracker esophagus
- idiopathic LES incompetence

Evaluate the patient with suspected secondary esophageal motility disorder due to systemic disease, including:

- scleroderma
- polydermatomyositis
- systemic lupus erythematosus
- amyloidosis
- Chagas disease
- primary skeletal muscle disease (eg, myotonia dystrophica)
- multiple sclerosis, amyotrophic lateral sclerosis

Evaluate the patient with chest pain of unclear etiology, in order to determine whether symptoms are of an esophageal origin. This usually follows a negative cardiac work-up.

Assess the competence of the LES, in difficult cases of reflux esophagitis, where the diagnosis is still in doubt or where standard medical therapy has failed.

Evaluate the success of various surgical procedures on the esophagus, such as esophageal dilatation, LES myotomy in achalasia, and antireflux surgery.

Ensure proper placement of pH probes (used to diagnose acid reflux) by accurately locating the LES.

Contraindications Few contraindications exist for this procedure. In general, the patient should be alert, able to swallow on command, and capable of verbalizing symptoms. This is particularly true if provocative studies to elicit chest pain are planned. Manometry should not be performed on a patient with tenuous cardiopulmonary status in whom vagal stimulation is hazardous.

Patient Preparation Technique and goals of the procedure are discussed with the patient and informed consent is obtained. No antacids, nitrates, calcium channel blockers, analgesics, promotility agents, sedatives, or anticholinergic agents are permitted for 24 hours prior to procedure (if possible). If study is scheduled for the AM, the patient is made NPO after midnight. If the patient is scheduled for the PM, the patient is made NPO for 8 hours beforehand. Patient is sent to procedure room with medical record. No premedications are given prior to manometry and sedatives are not permitted.

Aftercare There are no specific restrictions postprocedure. The previous level of activity may be resumed if no complications have arisen.

Special Instructions Requisition from ordering physician should state if additional studies, such as pH probe testing, acid perfusion (Bernstein) testing, or pharmacologic provocation, are desired. Otherwise, decision will be left to the discretion of the operator.

Complications Esophageal manometry is considered a safe procedure with little morbidity. Potential complications are those common to any nasogastric (NG) intubation, such as gagging, epistaxis, vasovagal reactions, etc. More serious adverse reactions may result from medications given for provocative testing. In particular, ergonovine is used in some centers to provoke esophageal contraction and spasm. This agent is also used to induce coronary artery spasm during cardiac catheterization in patients with possible variant (Prinzmetal) angina. Thus, there are potential cardiac complications if ergonovine is used. Other agents have come into favor recently, such as edrophonium, which have little cardiac effects. Abdominal cramps and nausea of a transient nature have been reported with edrophonium.

Equipment The manometry probe is a polyvinyl catheter with multiple lumens (from 3-8). Each lumen has a separate orifice. Probe diameter ranges from 1.1-5 mm, depending on the model. There are usually three or more side holes spaced approximately 5 cm apart which act as pressure sensors. Each catheter lumen is independently perfused with water from a multichannel pneumohydraulic infusion device (with low compliances). A separate pressure transducer is also attached to each lumen and pressures are recorded on a multichannel polygraph. A swallowing sensor is also used in some centers.

Technique The procedure is performed in a fully-equipped GI Laboratory. Patient assumes a supine position and a swallowing sensor is placed around patient's neck. The catheter assembly is calibrated and pressures rechecked with a sphygmomanometer. The device is introduced via the nares using standard nasogastric intubation technique (alternatively, per mouth) and advanced until all sensing orifices are recording gastric (cardia) pressures. The station pull-through technique is commonly used. With the recorder on, the catheter is slowly withdrawn until the proximal channel is within the LES. Resting LES tone is measured first. Patient is given water via a 50 mL syringe and is asked to swallow and the relaxation response of LES is noted. The catheter is then pulled out slowly at 0.5 cm increments until the most distal orifice is sensing the LES (all channels having passed through the LES). The catheter is taped into position and patient performs a series of wet swallows (5 mL H_2O) over several minutes. Information is obtained regarding the LES, peristalsis, and esophageal body contractions. The catheter is then withdrawn approximately 3 cm and retaped, so that all sensing orifices are within the esophageal body. Wet swallows are repeated and contractions recorded. Next, pull-through is continued until the proximal orifice is surrounded by the UES; perfusion is stopped in this channel to prevent aspiration. Catheter is withdrawn until the proximal orifice is within the pharynx, the middle is in the UES, and the distal in the upper esophageal body. Ten dry swallows are

(Continued)

Esophageal Motility Study *(Continued)*

performed. This concludes the standard procedure. When indicated, provocative testing is carried out once standard manometry is completed. The catheter is repositioned and edrophonium is injected (10 mg I.V. usually) or a placebo. Again, patient performs wet swallows and esophageal contractions are recorded at different catheter positions. Subjective complaints of chest pain are carefully recorded and correlated temporally with any new manometric findings. The acid perfusion (Bernstein) test may also be performed at this time.

Normal Findings Preliminary written report on manometric findings and provocation testing is completed immediately by gastroenterology staff and placed in medical chart. This includes both selected numerical data and an overall diagnostic interpretation. Normal values are established for each individual testing center, and are dependent to some degree on the equipment system selected. An example of a normal motility and provocation study as reported by one laboratory is shown in the table.

Esophageal Motility Study

Esophageal manometry	
1. Catheter (lumen)	4
2. LES	
Location (cm from nares)	38
Resting pressure (mm Hg)	27
Mean pressure (mm Hg)	15
Relaxation	Complete
3. Esophageal body	
Peristalsis	Normal
Amplitude, mean (mm Hg)	124
Amplitude, peak (mm Hg)	224
Duration, mean (sec)	3.5
Duration, max (sec)	5
4. UES	
Location (cm from nares)	16
Resting pressure (mm Hg)	33
Relaxation	Normal
Coordination with hypopharynx	Normal
Diagnosis: normal motility study	
Edrophonium provocation (1 mg IU)	No chest pain
Bernstein test	Negative

Critical Values A wide variety of esophageal contraction abnormalities is possible. However, several "classic" patterns of manometric readings have been described, and may be diagnostic for a particular motor disorder. Selected patterns are shown in the following figure.

As shown, a normal control subject experiences a short duration wave in the upper esophagus following a wet swallow. (In general, the upper esophagus is composed of striated muscle, and the middle and lower portions contain smooth muscle.) The wave progresses down the esophagus in a characteristic, timed fashion, that is, a peristaltic wave. The LES appropriately relaxes to accommodate the anticipated food bolus. In achalasia, however, the initial striated muscle contraction following a swallow may be normal but smooth muscle contractions (mid and lower esophagus) are of low amplitude and prolonged duration. Characteristically, the LES maintains a high basal pressure and fails to relax after a swallow. In a condition known as diffuse esophageal spasm, there is an increase in the baseline pressure in the mid and lower esophagus after a swallow. In addition to this, multiple repetitive high amplitude (short duration) contractions are seen in smooth muscle. These are "aperistaltic" contractions (ie, not coordinated with the initial skeletal muscle

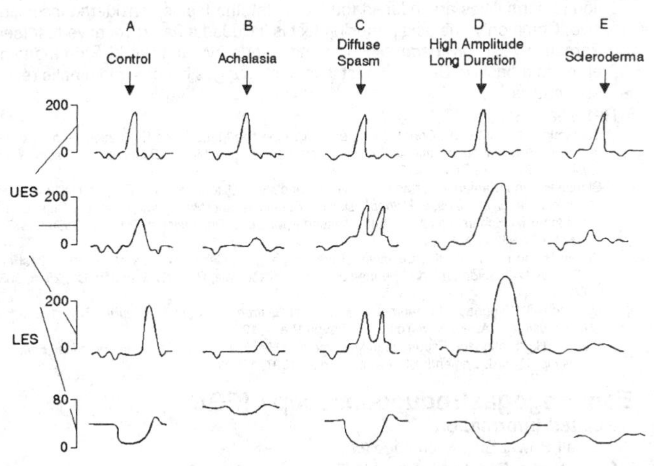

contraction). LES pressures may be normal or high and relaxation is variable. The "nutcracker esophagus" is characterized by smooth muscle contractions of very high amplitude and long duration. Peristalsis is maintained, although propagation may be slowed. LES tone and relaxation are relatively normal. In scleroderma, a unique pattern is seen. Upper esophageal contraction is normal but all smooth muscle contractions are markedly diminished in amplitude or even absent. Unlike achalasia, the LES pressure is low. In polymyositis, (not shown) there is potential involvement of any striated muscle, including the pharynx and UES. Decreased amplitude contractions may be seen in the pharynx along with hypotension in the UES, but smooth muscle contractions remain normal. Milder variants of the idealized patterns in the figure may be seen. Also, mixtures of these contraction abnormalities are possible. In patients with chest pain of obscure etiology, esophageal manometry is often considered to rule out an unspecified motor disorder. If a patient experiences typical chest pain symptoms during the course of a standard examination, and a classic motility disorder is recorded during the same time interval, an esophageal origin of symptoms is likely. Appropriate treatment of the motility disorder should be initiated. However, if typical chest discomfort occurs during standard manometry but pressure tracings are normal, then motility dysfunction is less likely as the cause of symptoms. It is not, however, entirely excluded. Conversely, if manometry is clearly abnormal but the patient denies any chest discomfort, the test is inconclusive. Some clinicians elect to treat the underlying motor disorder empirically. This is based on data which shows that the majority of patients who experience chest pain secondary to an esophageal motor disorder display continuous manometric abnormalities but only intermittent symptoms. In addition, ≤80% of patients with such continuous contraction abnormalities have reported significant chest discomfort. The proper management of this group is still evolving. Various pharmacologic agents have been used to induce abnormal contractions in selected patients with chest pain of obscure origin. This may be attempted in difficult cases where barium enema, upper endoscopy, and standard manometry are nondiagnostic. A cholinergic agonist, edrophonium chloride, is popular because of its specificity and favorable safety profile. If when following injection of edrophonium there are symptoms of typical chest pain and manometric (Continued)

Esophageal Motility Study *(Continued)*

abnormalities, the test is considered positive. If either chest pain or contraction abnormalities are induced (but not both), the test is considered inconclusive. Commonly, the acid perfusion test is included as a provocative test (see Bernstein Test *on page 54*). The finding of a hypotensive LES on manometry and a positive Bernstein test is strongly suggestive of symptomatic reflux esophagitis.

References

Benjamin SB, Richter JE, Cordova CM, et al, "Prospective Manometric Evaluation With Pharmacologic Provocation of Patients With Suspected Esophageal Motility Dysfunction," *Gastroenterology*, 1983, 84(5 Pt 1):893-901.

Clouse RE and Diamant NE, "Motor Physiology and Motor Disorders of the Esophagus," *Gastrointestinal and Liver Disease: Pathophysiology, Diagnosis, and Management*, 6th ed, Chapter 32, Feldman M, Scharschmidt BF, and Sleisenger MH, eds, Philadelphia, PA: WB Saunders Co, 1998, 467-97.

Cohen S and Parkman HP, "Diseases of the Esophagus," *Cecil Textbook of Medicine*, 21st ed, Chapter 124, Goldman L and Bennett JC, eds, Philadelphia, PA: WB Saunders Co, 2000, 658-68.

Orlando RC, "Esophageal Manometry," *Manual of Gastroenterologic Procedures*, 3rd ed, Chapter 4, Drossman DA, ed, New York, NY: Raven Press, 1993, 36-49.

Stendal C, "Stationary Esophageal Manometry," *Practical Guide to Gastrointestinal Function Testing*, Oxford, England: Blackwell Science, 1997, 156-80.

Esophagogastroduodenoscopy (EGD)

Related Information

Small Bowel Biopsy *on page 95*

Synonyms Esophagoscopy (if Esophagus Alone Studied); Peroral Endoscopy; UGI Endoscopy; Upper Endoscopy; Upper Gastrointestinal Endoscopy

Procedure Commonly Includes Direct visual examination of the upper gastrointestinal tract by means of a flexible fiberoptic endoscope. Typically, the procedure is carried out on an awake, but sedated, patient either in a specially equipped endoscopy suite or at the bedside in an intensive care unit. The endoscope is advanced (by mouth) through the oropharynx, esophagus, stomach, and duodenum. Important anatomic landmarks are identified and mucosal surfaces are examined for suspicious lesions such as ulcers, erosions, polyps, strictures, malignancies, varices, bleeding sites, etc. Biopsy specimens are easily obtained, and may be sent for histopathology, cytology, and/or microbiological culture. Other minor operative procedures may be performed utilizing the standard endoscope, including polypectomy, cytologic brushings, sclerotherapy or banding of esophageal varices, extraction of foreign bodies, electrocautery of bleeding sites, and sonographic examination of abnormal lesions.

Indications The precise indications for esophagogastroduodenoscopy (EGD) are still evolving and physician discretion still plays a major role.[1,2] Practice patterns amongst physicians vary considerably. Controversy exists regarding the use of EGD as a first-line diagnostic procedure for suspected upper GI disease. Some clinicians have virtually abandoned the standard upper GI barium swallow in favor of endoscopy. This approach addresses the problem of the false-negative upper GI series but is quite expensive and not without risk. In each case, a number of factors must be individually weighed, such as the risk of complications, cost of the procedure (versus upper GI series), expected diagnostic benefits, and probability of a normal (negative) examination. Diagnostic indications may be grouped as follows.

High yield indications:[1,2,3]

- acute upper GI bleeding, to establish the exact location of hemorrhage prior to endoscopic cautery, surgery, etc
- dysphagia, especially if esophageal strictures or ulcerations are seen on a previous upper GI series. Note that EGD may still be indicated if the barium swallow is normal but clinical suspicion of esophageal disease remains high
- dyspepsia, if refractory to standard medical antireflux therapy. EGD is also indicated whenever a surgical antireflux procedure is planned.
- odynophagia, when inflammation or infection is clinically suspected, especially if esophagitis from *Candida*, cytomegalovirus, or herpes simplex virus is likely

- surveillance endoscopy for known premalignant conditions, such as Barrett esophagus, lye-induced strictures, Plummer-Vinson syndrome and familial adenomatous polyposis
- abnormalities seen on upper GI series which require visual confirmation and tissue biopsy (eg, polyps, gastric ulcers, redundant gastric folds, strictures)
- suspected gastric outlet obstruction and persistent nausea and vomiting
- screening for esophageal varices in patients with cirrhosis who are candidates for primary prophylactic treatment against variceal bleeding.

Lower yield indications (procedure not always appropriate):

- atypical chest pain
- abdominal pain of unknown etiology
- routine, uncomplicated cases of gastroesophageal reflux
- uncomplicated cases of duodenal ulcer demonstrated by upper GI series

Therapeutic indications for EGD are numerous and include:

- sclerotherapy of bleeding esophageal varices
- management of upper GI bleeding using electrocautery, photocoagulation, etc
- laser ablation of esophageal cancer
- endoscopic placement of esophageal stents
- placement of permanent feeding tubes under endoscopic guidance (PEG tubes)
- dilatation of esophageal strictures
- polypectomy
- dissolution of bezoars

Contraindications

- acute myocardial infarction
- hypoxemia with respiratory distress
- hypotension and shock, regardless of etiology
- massive upper GI bleeding with hypotension where emergency surgery is clearly appropriate (EGD may needlessly delay surgery and visualization is often obscured by copious amounts of blood.)
- uncontrolled hypertension
- patient refusal

Relative contraindications (high-risk situations) include:

- noncorrectable coagulopathy
- recent myocardial infarction (within weeks)
- severe coronary artery disease
- recent upper GI tract surgery where anastomotic sites may still be "fresh"
- active peritonitis
- subluxation or instability of the cervical spine
- perforated viscus

Patient Preparation Technique and risks of the procedure are explained to the patient and informed consent is obtained. In some medical centers, formal consultation with gastroenterology staff is mandatory before obtaining an EGD. In other institutions, the procedure is arranged directly with the endoscopy scheduling desk by the primary physician. EGD may be performed on either inpatients or outpatients. Customarily, inpatients are examined briefly by the endoscopist (or his representative) the day prior to EGD in order to review details of the case, write orders, and answer patient questions. It should be emphasized that patients frequently experience apprehension and fear regarding choking on the endoscope. Careful and thoughtful reassurances from the medical team may be quite effective in allaying these anxieties. The patient is kept strictly NPO for 6 hours prior to EGD. If a morning procedure is planned, patient is NPO after midnight. If EGD is scheduled for later in the afternoon, some centers allow a light breakfast that morning. Daily medications are permitted with small sips of water. Medicines which potentially interfere with visualization of the mucosa, such as antacids or Carafate®, should be discontinued beforehand. If a tissue biopsy is anticipated, aspirin products, and nonsteroidal agents are discontinued well in advance (at least 5 days for aspirin). If gastric outlet obstruction is clinically suspected, nasogastric suction is performed prior to EGD in order to remove retained luminal contents. This also applies to the patient with known or suspected impairment

(Continued)

Esophagogastroduodenoscopy (EGD) *(Continued)*

of gastric motility. For inpatients, dentures are removed and patient is transported to endoscopy suite on a cart, along with medical chart and relevant x-rays. For outpatients, arrangements for driver transportation home must be made in advance by the patient, since driving is not permitted after the procedure. Once patient is in the procedure room, baseline vital signs are obtained (pulse, blood pressure, etc). Intravenous sedation is routinely given, commonly diazepam (or another short-acting benzodiazepine) and meperidine several minutes prior to examination. A topical anesthetic agent such as Cetacaine® spray (benzocaine and tetracaine hydrochloride) is often applied to the pharynx.

Aftercare Immediately postprocedure the patient is observed in the recovery area. Vital signs are usually recorded at least once, and prn in the "high-risk" patient. If no complications have occurred and sedation has worn off, the patient may be discharged from the testing area. A normal diet may be resumed once gag reflex has returned. Driving is not allowed due to residual sedative effects.

Complications Morbidity and mortality of upper endoscopy is relatively low, but should not be overlooked. Statistics compiled from several large clinical series suggest an incidence of adverse outcomes of 0.1% to 0.2%. Death has been reported between 0.14-0.65/1000 endoscopies. Major complications, as described by Shamir and Schuman, are as follows.[4]

- Perforation of esophagus or stomach: Up to 0.1% of all EGDs (some large centers report no cases of perforation). The upper esophagus above the cricopharynx appears most vulnerable. Other risk factors are esophageal cancer, strictures, or cervical osteophytes.
- Bleeding: Considered rare even after biopsies, at 0.3/1000 cases. In most cases, bleeding is not due to a coagulation defect, rather it results from biopsy of friable tissue.
- Cardiopulmonary complications: Significant cardiac arrhythmias are distinctly unusual. If a Holter monitor is placed, transient rhythm disturbances such as sinus tachycardia, premature ventricular contractions (PVCs), premature atrial contractions (PACs), and rarely ischemic changes may be recorded in <22% of cases. Few adverse clinical outcomes have been reported.

Other complications include the following.

- Pulmonary aspiration has been estimated at 0.8/1000 cases, but carries a mortality rate of 10%. Prout demonstrated that some degree of aspiration occurs in as many as 25% of cases, using iodinated oil as a marker. No cases of clinical pneumonia developed.[5]
- Toxicity of premedications: Minor complications are fairly common but usually inconsequential. Diazepam or midazolam may cause a local phlebitis and meperidine may induce transient nausea. More importantly, the patient with severe COPD or liver cirrhosis may experience respiratory depression from this combination. In one series from England, 0.67 out of 1000 EGDs were followed by respiratory arrest requiring mechanical ventilation.[6]
- Infection: Prospective studies have shown a bacteremia rate of 3% to 8% (positive blood cultures). Some centers routinely use antibiotic prophylaxis in patients with valvular heart disease, although the risk of endocarditis is probably extremely low.[7]
- Miscellaneous: Parotid swelling, abdominal pain from air insufflation, transient megacolon, transient fever with pulmonary infiltrates (following sclerotherapy of varices).

Equipment The fiberoptic or video endoscope has replaced the rigid endoscope as the instrument of choice. The video endoscope has also largely supplanted the fiberendoscope because of ease of use, less musculoskeletal and eye strain, and the avoidance of getting splashed by body fluids. This device has a length of approximately 1 meter and diameter of 9.5-12.5 mm. Within the instrument shaft are several separate channels designed for passage of optional devices such as biopsy forceps, polyp snare, cytology brush, cautery or laser device, and suction. Air may also be introduced for insufflation of the stomach. For clearing of debris from the viewing area, a jet stream of water from a separate reservoir can be flushed through one channel. At the head or handle of the endoscope are two control devices ("wheels") which maneuver the instrument tip as it is advanced, an up-down angle wheel (deflection of almost 180°) and a right-left angle wheel (deflection of 100°). A side-viewing upper endoscope is also available if close investigation of certain "blind areas" is needed, such as the duodenal bulb and the medial wall of the second portion of the duodenum.

Technique Performed only by an experienced gastroenterologist in a properly equipped endoscopy suite. At times, it may be necessary to carry out this procedure in an emergency room or ICU bed. Following sedation, patient is placed in the left lateral decubitus position (although successful intubation is possible in other positions). A hollow mouthpiece is inserted to protect the patient's teeth and facilitate instrument passage. The endoscope is slowly advanced orally and is "swallowed" by the patient. Once past the cricopharyngeal region, the instrument is guided only under direct visualization. An important landmark is the Z-line at the gastroesophageal junction, approximately 40 cm from the teeth. The tip is then advanced into the cardia, with gentle insufflation of air. The various portions of the stomach are inspected - cardia, fundus, greater and lesser curvature, and antrum. Following this, the tip is then passed through the pylorus, into the duodenal bulb, and sometimes as far as the descending portion of the duodenum. Mucosal surfaces are reinspected as the instrument is withdrawn. Biopsies, cytologic brushings, polypectomy, cauterization of bleeding lesions, etc, are performed as indicated. Sclerotherapy or banding of esophageal varices is not considered part of the routine EGD. This is a separate therapeutic procedure requiring additional equipment and somewhat more involved patient preparation.

Turnaround Time Final report on biopsy specimen histopathology is given within 3-5 days. Gram stain and KOH prep are known immediately (within minutes if necessary) but culture results may require several days (or more than 1 week if viral culture requested).

Specimen All biopsy specimens and cytologic brushings are sent to the Pathology Laboratory without delay in appropriate containers and fixatives. Tissue for Gram stain, KOH prep, and culture should be sent in sterile containers without fixative to the Microbiology Laboratory. The details of proper specimen collection, fixation, and transportation are usually supervised by the gastroenterology team.

Normal Findings No upper GI tract pathology encountered. Preliminary or final written report on endoscopic findings is completed immediately by gastroenterology staff and placed in medical chart before the patient is discharged from the endoscopy suite. In general, the endoscopist comments in detail on all findings, normal and abnormal, and concludes with an overall clinical impression.

Critical Values No grading schemes or numerical "cutoffs" per se. Subjective interpretation of visual findings by an experienced gastroenterologist constitutes the data base. Important aspects of the endoscopic examination frequently commented upon include:

- location of the Z-line
- presence or absence of hiatal hernia
- appearance of mucosal surfaces, with attention to ulcerations, erosions, strictures, masses, streaks, polyps, Barrett-type epithelium, redundant tissue, etc
- location and appearance of bleeding site(s) or varices
- abnormalities in tone (spasm) of the lower esophageal sphincter or pylorus
- miscellaneous abnormalities
- operative procedure(s) performed during endoscopy
- complications
- technical adequacy of the study

In some centers, instant photographs of suspicious lesions are taken during endoscopy and included in the medical chart. Endoscopic examinations are recorded on real-time videotape for later review by the referring physician and endoscopist.

(Continued)

Esophagogastroduodenoscopy (EGD) *(Continued)*

Limitations Quality of study and its interpretation are highly dependent on the expertise of the endoscopist. Recognition of subtle abnormalities and visualization of all portions of the upper GI tract require a high degree of clinical competence. A variety of technical factors may lead to a suboptimal study. Endoscopists refer to "blind spots" - regions difficult to visualize in most cases - which include the superior aspect of the duodenal bulb, portions of the fundus, and the lesser curvature below the incisura. Active uncontrolled bleeding, retained blood in the stomach, and retained food or antacids may also lead to an inadequate study. EGD should not be used for the diagnosis of esophageal motility disorders. The procedure of choice for this entity is esophageal manometry. Similarly, EGD is not a first-line test for the diagnosis of reflux esophagitis (although characteristic histologic changes may be found on mucosal biopsy).

Additional Information Other procedures carried out during an upper gastrointestinal endoscopy include placement of percutaneous endoscopic gastrostomy (PEG) tubes in patients who are unable to feed orally. Percutaneous endoscopic jejunostomy tubes can also be placed in selected patients. Removal of polyps may also be performed. Endoscopic ultrasound probes may be attached to allow examination of suspicious lesions and adjacent structures. This technology is currently being actively investigated and indications for the procedure are being defined at the present time.

Footnotes

1. Gibb SP, Laney JS, and Tarshis AM, "Use of Fiberoptic Endoscopy in Diagnosis and Therapy of Upper Gastrointestinal Disorders," *Med Clin North Am*, 1986, 70(6):1307-24.
2. Grossman MB, "Gastrointestinal Endoscopy," *Clin Symp*, 1980, 32(3):2-36.
3. Cooper GS and Blades EW, "Indications, Contraindications, and Complications of Upper Gastrointestinal Endoscopy," *Gastrointest Endosc*, CD-ROM, 2nd ed, Chapter 37, MV Sivak, ed, Philadelphia, PA: WB Saunders Co, 1999.
4. Shahmir M and Schuman BM, "Complications of Fiberoptic Endoscopy," *Gastrointest Endosc*, 1980, 26(3):86-91.
5. Prout BI and Metreweli C, "Pulmonary Aspiration After Fiberendoscopy of the Upper Gastrointestinal Tract," *Br Med J [Clin Res]*, 1972, 4:269-71.
6. Schiller KFR, Cotton PB, and Salmon PR, "The Hazards of Digestive Fiberendoscopy: A Survey of British Experience," *Gut*, 1972, 13:1027.
7. Dajani AS, Taubert KA, Wilson W, et al, "Prevention of Bacterial Endocarditis. Recommendations by the American Heart Association," *JAMA*, 1997, 277(22):1794-801.

References

Botet JF and Lightdale C, "Endoscopic Sonography of the Upper Gastrointestinal Tract," *AJR Am J Roentgenol*, 1991, 156(1):63-8.

Kahn KL, Kosecoff J, Chassin MR, et al, "The Use and Misuse of Upper Gastrointestinal Endoscopy," *Ann Intern Med*, 1988, 109(8):664-70.

Morrissey JF and Reichelderfer M, "Gastrointestinal Endoscopy (1)," *N Engl J Med*, 1991, 325(16):1142-9.

Schuman BM, "Upper Gastrointestinal Endoscopy," *Bockus Gastroenterology*, 5th ed, Chapter 23, Haubrich WS, Schaffner F, and Berk JE, eds, Philadelphia, PA: WB Saunders Co, 1995, 295-309.

Young HS, and Keefe EB, "Complications of Gastrointestinal Endoscopy," *Gastrointestinal and Liver Disease: Pathophysiology, Diagnosis, and Management*, 6th ed, Chapter 19, Feldman M, Scharschmidt BF, and Sleisenger MH, eds, Philadelphia, PA: WB Saunders Co, 1998, 301-8.

♦ **Esophagoscopy (if Esophagus Alone Studied)** *see* Esophagogastroduodenoscopy (EGD) *on page 72*

♦ **Esophagus Acid Reflux Test With Intraluminal pH Electrode for Detection of Reflux** *see* Standard Acid Reflux Test *on page 99*

♦ **Esophagus Acid Reflux Test With Intraluminal pH Electrode (Prolonged Recording)** *see* pH Study, 12- to 24-Hour *on page 92*

Flexible Fiberoptic Sigmoidoscopy

Related Information

Anoscopy *on page 52*
Colonoscopy *on page 59*

Synonyms Flexible Proctosigmoidoscopy; Sigmoidoscopy, Flexible

Procedure Commonly Includes Direct examination of the rectum, sigmoid colon, and proximal portions of the colon (≤60 cm) by means of a flexible fiberoptic endoscope. Flexible sigmoidoscopy is readily performed in a physician's office with minimal bowel preparation. In comparison with other endoscopic procedures, flexible sigmoidoscopy allows visualization of more proximal colonic segments than either anoscopy or rigid proctosigmoidoscopy, but is more limited than colonoscopy.

Indications Although the precise indications are still being debated, common uses include:

- screening of healthy, asymptomatic adults for colorectal cancer[1]
- evaluation of the patient with suspected lower gastrointestinal pathology in combination with a barium enema study (by itself, the barium radiographs may be insensitive in the distal colon)
- management of lower gastrointestinal bleeding; in selected patients this procedure can detect bleeding polyps, fissures, etc
- evaluation of the patient with suspected inflammatory disease of the colon, such as inflammatory bowel disease, infectious colitis, sigmoid diverticulitis, and others

More controversial indications include:

- temporary decompression of sigmoid volvulus (recurrence of the volvulus is common without prompt surgery)
- cancer surveillance in patients who have undergone surgical resection of a sigmoid colon neoplasia (to rule out recurrence at the anastomosis)

Contraindications Few absolute contraindications exist for this procedure; however, the procedure should best be avoided in the following high-risk situations:

- severe diverticulitis
- acute peritonitis
- toxic megacolon
- severe underlying cardiac or pulmonary disease
- uncorrectable coagulopathy
- acute intestinal perforation
- massive GI bleeding

In addition, flexible sigmoidoscopy should not be performed in situations where colonoscopy is indicated (see Colonoscopy *on page 59*). This includes polypectomy which should be performed by colonoscopy.

Patient Preparation Details of the procedure are discussed with the patient, including goals, technique, and risks. Informed consent is obtained. A number of preparative bowel regimens have been proposed. One popular and effective regimen is administration of a single phosphosoda (Fleet®) enema several minutes before sigmoidoscopy. This results in an adequate bowel prep in nearly 90% of patients. Other bowel regimens include: two phosphosoda enemas immediately prior to procedure, and oral laxative followed by a single enema. These alternative regimens are also effective. In the majority of cases, premedications such as sedatives, narcotics, or anesthetics are not necessary. (Occasionally, a patient may benefit from a short-acting benzodiazepine.)

Aftercare In general, patients may resume their prior level of activity after sigmoidoscopy. Since sedatives are not administered, in most cases, patients may drive home postprocedure.

Special Instructions Due to the risk of bacteremia during sigmoidoscopy, antibiotics may be useful for prevention of bacterial endocarditis in patients with high-risk heart disease. Patients who are at risk for endocarditis include those with prosthetic heart valves, rheumatic valvular disease, previous history of endocarditis, and others. Such patients may benefit from antibiotic prophylaxis, although the risk of endocarditis is low. According to the American Society for Gastrointestinal Endoscopy in 1995,[2] antibiotic prophylaxis is **not** recommended on a routine basis for patients without such heart lesions.

Complications Flexible sigmoidoscopy is a safe procedure in skilled hands. Complications that have been reported in the literature include local pain, bleeding, bacteremia, cardiac arrhythmias, and bowel perforation. The incidence of perforation is quite low, estimated at 0.1% of cases.[3]

Technique The patient is placed in the left lateral decubitus position on an examination table. Digital rectal examination is performed first. Some physicians routinely perform anoscopy prior to flexible sigmoidoscopy, since the former allows superior visualization of the rectum and anal canal (see Anoscopy *on page 52*). Following this, the sigmoidoscope is lubricated and

(Continued)

Flexible Fiberoptic Sigmoidoscopy *(Continued)*

gently inserted into the rectum. The instrument is then advanced under direct visualization. The physician can direct the tip of the scope using handheld controls and guide the shaft of the instrument with torque. Only a minimal amount of insufflation of the bowel is necessary (unlike colonoscopy). The flexible sigmoidoscope is advanced to its full length, either 35 or 60 cm depending on the model. Areas of pathology are noted. Invasive procedures can be performed as needed, such as biopsy, fulguration, stool sampling, etc. As the instrument is withdrawn, all areas of the intestinal mucosa are inspected again. The rectum is well visualized during withdrawal by retroflexing the sigmoidoscope tip 180° in the final 10 cm.

Turnaround Time Final report on biopsy specimens is usually given within 3-5 days. Microbiologic stains, when performed, are often available the same day but bacterial and viral cultures require more time.

Specimen All biopsy specimens and cytologic brushings are sent to the Pathology Laboratory promptly. Any tissue or stool samples for microbiological culture should be sent in sterile containers **without** fixative.

Normal Findings Preliminary and final report on sigmoidoscopic findings are immediately completed by the physician and charted. Important aspects of the examination often commented on include:

- indications for procedure
- type of instrument used
- adequacy of bowel prep
- depth of visualization (eg, 35 cm, 60 cm)
- appearance of the mucosa
- abnormalities such as polyps (size, appearance), pseudopolyps, fissures, neoplasms, ulcers, friable regions, blood, pus, diverticula, and others
- therapeutic procedures performed
- sites of biopsies
- sites of cultures
- complications
- recommendations

Additional Information The flexible sigmoidoscope is now routinely used in the surveillance of neoplasia-polyps in the asymptomatic patient. The procedure is well-tolerated and safe. It is estimated that about 55% of colon cancers and adenomas are within the theoretic reach of the 60 cm instrument. In reality, most but not all such lesions are detected during sigmoidoscopy. The sensitivity of the 60 cm instrument is about 85% (within its 60 cm range). The 35 cm scope is more comfortable and less expensive than its larger counterpart. Of course, the yield of this instrument is somewhat less, with only 40% of malignant or premalignant colonic lesions within its theoretic range.

Footnotes

1. Achkar EA, "Flexible Sigmoidoscopy," *Gastrointestinal Endoscopy*, CD-ROM, 2nd ed, Chapter 91, MV Sivak, ed, Philadelphia, PA: WB Saunders Co, 1999.
2. "Antibiotic Prophylaxis in Gastrointestinal Endoscopy." American Society for Gastrointestinal Endoscopy. *Gastrointest Endosc*, 1995, 42:630-5.
3. Marks G and Borenstein BD, "Complications of Flexible Fiberoptic Sigmoidoscopy. A Conceptual Approach," *Surg Endosc*, 1987, 1:59-62.

References

"Flexible Sigmoidoscopy." American Society for Gastrointestinal Endoscopy, *Gastrointest Endosc*, 1998, 48(6):695-6.

Hocutt JE Jr, Jaffe R, Owens GM, et al, "Flexible Fiberoptic Sigmoidoscopy," *Am Fam Physician*, 1982, 26(5):133-41.

Rex DK and Lewis BS, *Flexible Sigmoidoscopy*, Cambridge, MA: Blackwell Science, 1996.

♦ **Flexible Proctosigmoidoscopy** *see* Flexible Fiberoptic Sigmoidoscopy *on page 76*

♦ **Full Colonoscopy** *see* Colonoscopy *on page 59*

♦ **Gallbladder Stimulation** *see* Biliary Drainage *on page 55*

Gastric Acid Analysis

Applies to BAO (Basal Acid Output); Basal Acid Output; Gastric Acid pH Measurement; Gastric Intubation; MAO (Maximal Acid Output), Gastric Acid Titration; Maximal Acid Output; PAO (Peak Acid Output); Peak Acid Output

Procedure Commonly Includes Intubation of the stomach and suction collection of gastric contents for basal acid output determination. This is followed by pentagastrin injection and continued collection of gastric contents for peak and maximal acid output determination. Following collection, gastric contents undergo pH, acid concentration, and volume measurements.

Indications

Evaluate patients with recurrent ulcer disease after surgery for peptic ulcer disease

- rule out acid hypersecretion
- assess completeness of vagotomy (sham feeding - see Additional Information)

Evaluate patients with an elevated fasting gastrin level

- physiologic response (ie, hypochlorhydria in atrophic gastritis)
- pathologic response (ie, Zollinger-Ellison syndrome, antral G-cell hyperplasia)

Evaluate adequacy of proton-pump inhibitor dosage in patients with Zollinger-Ellison syndrome

Contraindications This test is contraindicated in patients with gastric outlet obstruction, recent upper gastrointestinal bleeding, obstruction to passage of NG tube from nasopharynx to stomach (ie, Zenker's diverticulum, esophageal stricture, etc), and upper respiratory tract infection.

Patient Preparation Discontinue all medications that may influence gastric secretion at least 24 hours before testing (ie, H_2-blockers, antihistamines, cholinergics, anticholinergics, tranquilizers, antidepressants, and carbonic anhydrase inhibitors). Proton pump inhibitors need to be discontinued 1 week before testing and H_2-blockers used instead for symptoms. Patient needs to be NPO after midnight. Procedure is explained to patients and informed consent obtained.

Aftercare Remove NG tube. Resume preprocedure medications.

Equipment 14-18 French NG tube, 60 mL syringe, pentagastrin 6 µg/kg for parenteral injection, eight fluid collection containers, and acid titrating equipment (pH meter, graduated burette, small beakers, and 0.1 N NaOH)

Technique The test is performed in the seated position. Insert NG tube and advance tip to the most dependent portion of the stomach. Confirm fluoroscopically or by the Water Recovery Test. (Infuse 20-50 cc of water into NG and aspirate using a syringe; placement is adequate if recovery is >90%.)

Specimen Gastric aspirate

Collection After a 30-minute washout period, gastric juice is collected by machine suction or manual suction. For BAO (basal acid output), collect gastric secretions for the first hour in four 15-minute samples. After the first hour, pentagastrin is injected subcutaneously. In the postinjection hour, again collect four 15-minute samples for the PAO (peak acid output). Calculate BAO, PAO, and MAO by titration of an aliquot of each of the eight samples with 0.1 N NaOH. Acid content in each of the eight 15-minute collections is calculated by multiplying the mL of NaOH needed for titration to pH 7.0 in aliquot and then using the formula [(mmol H^t in each 15-minute collection = mmol H^t) in aliquot x (volume of 15-minute collection/volume of aliquot)]. BAO in mmol H^t/hour, is the sum of the acid content of the first four 15-minute collections. PAO in mmol H^t/hour is the sum of the two highest acid outputs among the four postpentagastrin injection collections multiplied by 2. MAO in mmol H^t/hour is the sum of the acid content of the four 15-minute collections following pentagastrin injection.

Causes for Rejection Failure to fast or abstain from medications as under preparation. Procedure should not be performed if significant amounts of gastric contents are obtained on insertion of NG tube.

Normal Findings Normal values for BAO and MAO are 2.5 mmol H^t/hour and 25 mmol H^t/hour respectively for males and 1.5 mmol H^t/hour and 15 mmol H^t/hour respectively for females. Normal values for PAO are 35 mmol H^t/hour and 25 mmol H^t/hour respectively for males and females. Values for patients with duodenal ulcer are about twice those of normals and those for patients with gastric ulcers they are generally lower than normal. For Zollinger-Ellison syndrome patients, BAO and MAO are 40 mmol H^t/hour and 65 mmol H^t/hour respectively.

(Continued)

Gastric Acid Analysis *(Continued)*

Limitations The test is rarely helpful in the prediction of the likelihood of recurrence of ulcer disease after surgery, in the evaluation of dyspepsia, in the routine evaluation of patients with peptic ulcer disease, and in the distinction between malignant and benign gastric ulcers.

Additional Information The Hollander test was used to test adequacy of vagotomy. This test is based on the premise that insulin-induced hypoglycemia stimulates the vagus nerve which in turn induces gastric acid secretion. However, because of severe adverse reactions to the Hollander test such as myocardial ischemia, seizures, or in some cases, death, this test has been largely replaced by the sham feeding test.[1] In the sham feeding test, a patient is allowed to see, smell, taste, and chew an appetizing meal. Food is not swallowed to avoid the gastric phase of acid secretion. Gastric contents are collected and acid content (sham acid output - SAO) is calculated as described above. A SAO/PAO <0.1 is abnormal in healthy adults; therefore, a ratio of >0.1 after ulcer surgery signifies an intact vagus innervation to the stomach.

Footnotes

1. Chey WD and Chey WY, "Tests of Gastric and Exocrine Pancreatic Function and Absorption," *Textbook of Gastroenterology*, 3rd ed, Yamada T, Alpers DH, Laine L, et al, eds, Philadelphia, PA: Lippincott Williams & Wilkins, 1999, 2924-37.

References

Feldman M, "Gastric Secretion: Normal and Abnormal," *Gastrointestinal and Liver Disease: Pathophysiology, Diagnosis, and Management*, 6th ed, Chapter 38, Feldman M, Scharschmidt BF, and Sleisenger MH, eds, Philadelphia, PA: WB Saunders Co, 1998, 587-603.

Klein KB, "Gastric Secretory Testing," *Manual of Gastroenterologic Procedures*, 3rd ed, Drossman DA, ed, New York, NY: Raven Press, 1993, 61-7.

♦ **Gastric Acid pH Measurement** *see* Gastric Acid Analysis *on page 78*

♦ **Gastric Intubation** *see* Gastric Acid Analysis *on page 78*

♦ **Gastric Intubation** *see* I.V. Secretin Gastrin Levels *on page 81*

Helicobacter pylori Breath Test

Synonyms ^{13}C and ^{14}C Urea Breath Test

Procedure Commonly Includes Measurement of the ability of the urease enzyme of *Helicobacter pylori* to hydrolyze urea subsequently releasing labeled CO_2

Indications Diagnose *Helicobacter pylori* infection in a patient with peptic ulcer disease; assess *Helicobacter pylori* eradication after treatment in patients with peptic ulcer disease

Patient Preparation NPO for at least 4 hours. No antibiotics or bismuth compounds should be taken for about 4 weeks before the test. Proton pump inhibitors should be discontinued 2 weeks prior to the test as these may lead to false-negative tests.

Technique The patient ingests labeled urea in the liquid form for ^{13}C and in tablet form for ^{14}C. ^{13}C is not radioactive and is safe to be used in children and women of childbearing age. ^{14}C subjects the patient to a small dose of radioactivity. Presence of *Helicobacter pylori* in the stomach allows the labeled urea to be split by the bacterial urease releasing labeled CO_2. This CO_2 is then absorbed into the bloodstream and released in exhaled air. The exhaled air is collected and labeled CO_2 measured by mass spectrometry for ^{13}C and by scintillation counter for ^{14}C. Ingestion of labeled urea followed by collection of breath samples for analysis. Breath analysis for labeled CO_2 is performed by scintillation for ^{14}C and mass spectrometry for ^{13}C.

Sampling Time Expired air: <10 minutes for ^{14}C and 30 minutes for ^{13}C. It is longer for ^{13}C because urea presented in liquid form may be hydrolyzed by oral organisms which may account for an early peak in labeled CO_2. Because of background ^{13}C concentration, a baseline breath sample needs to be collected to which the 30-minute sample is compared.

Normal Findings Labeled CO_2 in exhaled air of <5% for ^{13}C and <200 dpm for ^{14}C

Additional Information In addition to being nonradioactive, ^{13}C labeled urea has the advantage of being easy to perform and of being safe to perform repeatedly. ^{14}C, on the other hand, has the advantage of a shorter sampling time and of not requiring a test meal. It is radioactive and this limits its use in children and women of childbearing age. The sensitivity and specificity of urea breath tests are 90% to 97% and 95% to 96% respectively.

References

Del Valle J, Cohen H, Laine L, et al, "Acid Peptic Disorders," *Textbook of Gastroenterology*, 3rd ed, Yamada T, Alpers DH, et al, eds, Philadelphia, PA: Lippincott Williams & Wilkins, 1999, 1370-444.

Peterson WL and Graham DY, "*Helicobacter Pylori*," *Gastrointestinal and Liver Disease: Pathophysiology, Diagnosis, and Management*, 6th ed, Chapter 39, Feldman M, Scharschmidt BF, and Sleisenger MH, eds, Philadelphia, PA: WB Saunders Co, 1998, 604-19.

Savarino V, Vigneri S, and Celle G, "The ^{13}C Urea Breath Test in the Diagnosis of *Helicobacter pylori* infection," *Gut*, 1999, 45(S1):118-22.

♦ **Hydrogen Breath Test** *see* Breath Hydrogen Analysis *on page 57*

♦ **Hydrogen Exhalation Test** *see* Breath Hydrogen Analysis *on page 57*

♦ **Intestinal Biopsy (for Disaccharidase Deficiency)** *see* Breath Hydrogen Analysis *on page 57*

♦ **Intestinal Intubation for Culture** *see* Breath Hydrogen Analysis *on page 57*

♦ **Intestinal Perfusion and Lactose Barium Radiography** *see* Breath Hydrogen Analysis *on page 57*

♦ **Intravenous Secretin Injection Test** *see* I.V. Secretin Gastrin Levels *on page 81*

I.V. Secretin Gastrin Levels

Synonyms Intravenous Secretin Injection Test

Applies to Basal Serum Gastrin Determination; Gastric Intubation; Secretin Stimulated Serum Gastrin Determination; Serum Radioimmunoassay for Gastrin

Procedure Commonly Includes I.V. injection of secretin and blood sampling at specific intervals for serum gastrin. A basal specimen is drawn and then, 2, 5, 10, 15, 20, 25, and 30 minutes after injection. Radioimmunoassay is used to measure serum for gastrin.

Indications Rule out gastrinoma (Zollinger-Ellison syndrome) in patients with appropriate symptoms (recurrent peptic ulcer unresponsive to appropriate medical or surgical therapy, diarrhea or steatorrhea, multiple endocrine neoplasia (MEN) type I symptomatology) who have gastric acid hypersecretion and a fasting hypergastrinemia that is ≤1000 pg/mL (≥1000 pg/mL with acid secretion and appropriate symptoms is diagnostic of Zollinger-Ellison syndrome). This test, if negative, may suggest a diagnosis of G-cell hyperplasia if the appropriate symptomatology is present (see Additional Information).

Contraindications Allergic to secretin

Patient Preparation NPO after midnight. If on an H_2-blocker, stop 24-48 hours before test. If on a proton pump inhibitor, change to H_2-blocker 7 days before test and stop H_2-blocker 24-48 hours before test.

Technique The secretin test for Zollinger-Ellison syndrome is possible because of an unknown mechanism by which there is a paradoxical increase in serum gastrin following secretin injection. In the normal patient and in the patient with G-cell hyperplasia, the gastrin response is decreased. In the patient with duodenal ulcer, there may be no change, a decrease, or a slight increase in serum gastrin.

Turnaround Time 48 hours

Specimen Blood

Sampling Time 35 minutes

Collection Basal serum gastrin is drawn at 5 minutes preceding and then immediately before secretin injection.[1] Pure porcine GIH secretin 2 units/kg is injected over 30 seconds. Serum gastrin is drawn at 2, 5, 10, 15, 20, 25, and 30 minutes after injection.

Normal Findings ≤200 pg/mL increase in serum gastrin

Limitations Five percent false-negative (often seen in the presence of hypocalcemia[2])

Additional Information Elevated serum fasting gastrins may be elevated ≥1000 pg/mL in pernicious anemia, achlorhydria, hypochlorhydria, chronic gastritis, gastric cancer, rheumatoid arthritis, vitiligo, and diabetes mellitus. (Continued)

I.V. Secretin Gastrin Levels *(Continued)*

However, most of the patients with these maladies are not acid hypersecretory or do not have refractory peptic ulcer disease. After Zollinger-Ellison has been excluded by the secretion test, a meal stimulated gastrin test may be performed. If it causes excess gastrin release, a diagnosis of G-cell hyperfunction is likely. A combined secretion calcium test has been devised which may be a more potent stimulant to gastrin secretion.[3] Following diagnosis of Zollinger-Ellison, an abnormal CT is the most helpful means of locating the potentially malignant gastrinoma.

Footnotes

1. Weisiger R, "Zollinger Ellison Syndrome and Other Hypersecretory States," *Sleisenger & Fordtrans Gastrointestinal and Liver Diseases: Review and Assessment*, 6th ed, Chapter 41, Feldman M, Scharschmidt BF, and Sleisenger MH, eds, Philadelphia, PA: WB Saunders Co, 1998, 679-95.
2. Jansen JB and Lamers CB, "Effect of Changes in Serum Calcium on Secretin-Stimulated Serum Gastrin in Patients With Zollinger-Ellison Syndrome," *Gastroenterology*, 1982, 83(1 Pt 2):173-8.
3. Romanus ME, Neal JA, Dilley WG, et al, "Comparison of Four Provocative Tests for the Diagnosis of Gastrinoma," *Ann Surg*, 1983, 197(5):608-17.

References

McGuigan JE and Wolfe MM, "Secretin Injection Test in the Diagnosis of Gastrinoma," *Gastroenterology*, 1980, 79(6):1324-31.

Wurzelmann JI and Sandler RS, "Secretin Injection Test for Diagnosis of Gastrinoma," *Manual of Gastroenterologic Procedures*, 3rd ed, Drossman DA, ed, New York, NY: Raven Press, 1993, 86-8.

♦ **Lactose (Sucrose and d-Xylose) Tolerance Test** *see* Breath Hydrogen Analysis *on page 57*

♦ **Laparoscopy** *see* Peritoneoscopy *on page 88*

♦ **Laparotomy in Selected Cases** *see* Peritoneoscopy *on page 88*

Liver Biopsy

Related Information

Peritoneoscopy *on page 88*

Synonyms Blind Liver Biopsy; Needle Biopsy of the Liver; Percutaneous Liver Biopsy

Applies to Percutaneous Needle Aspiration Biopsy Under Fluoroscopic, CT, or Ultrasound Guidance; Transjugular Needle Biopsy of the Liver

Procedure Commonly Includes Percutaneous biopsy of liver parenchyma in a "blind" fashion (ie, not under radiologic guidance). This is carried out at the bedside under local anesthesia. A specialized, thin-bore needle is advanced between the ribs overlying the region of hepatic dullness. Several 2 cm cores of deep liver tissue are excised. Fresh specimens may be sent for gross pathologic inspection, routine light microscopy, special stains for liver storage diseases, transmission and immune electron microscopy, immunohistochemistry (using monoclonal antibodies), DNA hybridization studies, and microbiologic culture. Liver biopsy is a valuable and time-honored means of diagnosing diffuse liver parenchymal disease as well as disseminated focal disease.

Indications Candidates for liver biopsy must be carefully selected. This procedure, by nature, is invasive and histologic findings may often be reported as "consistent with" a particular disease (without being pathognomonic) or simply "nondiagnostic". In most cases, noninvasive imaging studies such as CT scan or ultrasound are now obtained first. With these considerations in mind, indications for liver biopsy include:

- suspected cases of liver cirrhosis, in order to confirm the diagnosis pathologically; establish etiology if possible (alcohol, alpha$_1$-antitrypsin deficiency, primary biliary cirrhosis, Wilson disease, hemochromatosis, etc); assess and stage level of activity; assess complications
- chronic hepatitis, with or without cirrhosis, to assess activity and stage of disease for prognosis and for consideration for treatment
- suspected liver disease in the known alcoholic patient, to confirm alcoholic liver disease, exclude alternative causes of liver disease (which may be present in ≤20% of cases), stage and assess disease activity
- diagnosis of hematoma or metastatic neoplasms

- suspected multisystem disease with liver involvement, where traditional diagnostic techniques have not been fruitful (eg, sarcoidosis, amyloidosis, tuberculosis, glycogen storage disease)
- staging of lymphoma
- unexplained hepatomegaly
- cholestasis of unknown etiology, where prior studies for biliary obstruction are negative
- persistently elevated liver enzyme tests
- selected cases of fever of unknown origin
- selected cases of hepatitis of unknown etiology, in order to differentiate viral from drug-induced etiologies (not always possible) or to assess complications, such as cholestasis
- evaluation of response to treatment
- in liver transplant recipients, to evaluate the status of the liver after transplantation

Liver biopsy is less useful in:

- acute hepatitis A or B infection, unless the diagnosis is in question
- extrahepatic biliary obstruction, where percutaneous transhepatic cholangiography and ERCP are considered first-line procedures
- fluid-filled liver cysts detected on ultrasound or CT scan, probably more amenable to guided thin needle aspiration first

Contraindications

- impaired hemostasis, accepted as prothrombin time more than 3 seconds over control, or INR ≥1.5, PTT more than 20 seconds over control, thrombocytopenia (platelets ≤75,000), and markedly prolonged bleeding time (≥10 minutes)
- severe anemia (Hgb ≤9.5 g/dL)
- local infection near needle entry site, such as right-sided pleural effusion or empyema, right lower lobe pneumonia, local cellulitis, infected ascites or peritonitis
- tense ascites (low yield technically, risk of leakage)
- high-grade extrahepatic biliary obstruction with jaundice (increased risk of bile peritonitis)
- septic cholangitis
- possible hemangioma
- possible echinococcal (hydatid) cyst
- lack of compatible blood for transfusion
- uncooperative patient

Patient Preparation Procedures and risks of the procedure are explained and consent is obtained. Formal consultation with gastroenterology staff is usually required. All aspirin products and nonsteroidal anti-inflammatory agents must be discontinued at least 5 days beforehand. If taking oral anticoagulants (Coumadin®), hospitalization is required to convert to heparin therapy before biopsy. Patient is to have a light breakfast 2-3 hours before the biopsy in order to facilitate gallbladder emptying and thereby decreasing the risk of puncturing it during a "blind" procedure. Some prefer patients to be NPO after midnight the evening prior, especially if conscious sedation will be used. Daily medications may be taken on the day of procedure pending physician approval. Screening laboratory studies ordered 24-48 hours in advance commonly include CBC, PT/PTT, BUN, bleeding time, and type and crossmatch for possible transfusion. Electrolytes and liver function tests are optional. If pneumonia or pleural effusion is suspected on examination, PA and lateral chest x-ray are obtained. Premedication with meperidine and/or diazepam may be administered at physician discretion. This is not routine in some centers due to possible toxicity.

Aftercare Liver biopsies are generally outpatient procedures at the present time, provided the following criteria are met.

- Patient must live within 30 minutes of the hospital or should stay in a temporary lodging within 30 minutes of the hospital.
- Patient must stay with a companion who will provide care and transportation to the hospital if necessary.
- Patient should have no serious comorbid conditions.

(Continued)

Liver Biopsy *(Continued)*

- Patient should be watched in the hospital for 4-6 hours after biopsy with no complications occurring during that time.

For the first 2 hours, patient is positioned on his right side. After 4-6 hours, patient may be allowed to sit up. Vitals (blood pressure, pulse) are checked every 15-30 minutes for 2 hours, every 30 minutes for the next 2 hours, and then every hour for 2 hours. Physician should be immediately notified if hypotension, tachycardia, fever, or uncontrolled pain occurs. Acetaminophen or meperidine may be given for pain control.

Special Instructions In the appropriate high-risk patient, antibiotic prophylaxis for infective endocarditis may be considered. Little data exists regarding the risk of bacteremia, however, much less endocarditis.

Complications Based on several large series, serious morbidity has been estimated at 0.1% to 0.2%. Fatality rates have ranged from 0% to 0.17%, both figures being derived from studies involving >20,000 biopsies each. The following are the more commonly seen complications.

- Pain - the most common adverse event, noted in ≤50% of cases. Usually it is confined to the right shoulder, probably referred pain from diaphragmatic pleura. Analgesia is required in approximately 20% of patients with acetaminophen sufficient in most cases. Meperidine may be used if pain does not resolve with acetaminophen. Symptoms resolve in 1-2 days.
- Hemorrhage - minor episodes are common. Self-limited oozing from the puncture site may persist for approximately 1 minute, but with loss of only 5-10 mL blood. Significant hemorrhage is less frequent but is the most common cause of death from liver biopsy. Several series have estimated an incidence of approximately 0.2%, but Sherlock (1984) reported 40 patients out of 6379 required transfusion for intraperitoneal bleeding.[1] She felt these statistics may even underestimate the incidence since those with severe coagulopathies were excluded. Bleeding usually results from a tear of a distended portal or hepatic vein. Specific sites include the abdominal cavity (hemoperitoneum), liver capsule (capsular hematoma), liver parenchyma (intrahepatic hematoma), or biliary tree (hemobilia). Postulated risk factors are coagulopathy, amyloid liver, hepatocellular injury, hemangioma, and vascularized tumor. However, bleeding may be massive when no risk factors are present. Not all episodes require surgery. In one study, 4 out of 7532 patients needed surgical intervention while 12 others with severe hemorrhage were transfused and observed.
- Bile leakage with peritonitis - associated with severe obstruction of the larger bile ducts. This is felt to result from laceration of a small, distended duct or from puncture of the gallbladder. With the widespread use of noninvasive imaging, the size of the bile ducts is known prebiopsy and the complication rate has declined.
- Laceration of internal organs and viscera - right kidney, gallbladder, colon, pancreas, and others
- Others: right-sided pneumothorax, arteriovenous fistula - 5.4% of all biopsies, drug toxicity

Equipment Several biopsy needles are available.

- Menghini needle - 1.9 mm diameter steel shaft with sharpened beveled tip and syringe; specimen is obtained using suction/aspiration into a 10 mL syringe. Requires only 1 second within the liver ("1-second technique") and patient need not hold his breath. Disadvantages are small samples and fragmentation of biopsy specimens.
- "Tru-cut" needle - disposable 2.05 mm diameter needle designed to cut out cores of tissue. Specimens are less fragmented, even in the cirrhotic liver, and thus a high success rate. However, dwell time in liver is longer (5-10 seconds), patient must cooperate more, and several steps are necessary.
- Vim-Silverman needle - sheath with inner cutting blade (similar to a "punch" biopsy). Tru-cut needle is a modernized Vim-Silverman.

Disposable needles that have spring loading and triggering mechanisms are now becoming popular.

Technique Patient lies supine in bed with right hand behind his head. Liver margins are estimated by percussion. If the location of the liver cannot be ascertained, an ultrasound should be performed first. Two approaches are popular, transthoracic (intercostal) or subcostal (anterior). With the former, biopsy site is identified along the midaxillary line in the center of hepatic dullness, usually the eighth or ninth intercostal space. This approach avoids other abdominal organs but always penetrates the pleura. With the subcostal approach, the biopsy site lies below the bottom rib anteriorly, and is used when a liver mass is easily palpable below the right costal margin. The risk of visceral laceration is higher and this approach is infrequently used; fine needle aspiration under CT guidance has become more popular. A wide area is prepped and draped in sterile fashion. The skin is anesthetized with 1% lidocaine, then deeper structures are infiltrated - subcutaneous tissue, intercostal muscles, and diaphragm. Some operators make a small superficial incision with a No. 11 blade at the needle entry site to facilitate needle insertion. Techniques differ with the type of biopsy needle selected. In general, the biopsy needle is advanced as far as the diaphragm (depth estimated by a finder needle). If a Menghini needle is used, suction is applied to the syringe, and the needle is pushed rapidly through the pleura and into the liver parenchyma. A 2.5 cm core of liver is aspirated and needle withdrawn, all within 1 second. If other needles are used, patient may need to hold his breath at the end of expiration to decrease the risk of pneumothorax.

Specimen At least one liver core, ≥2 cm in length. Initial specimen processing and transportation is handled by the gastroenterology team. A typical protocol would be as follows.

- Tissue fixation - for light microscopy, specimen is routinely fixed in a 10% buffered formula within 1 minute. For transmission electron microscopy, 1 mm cubes of specimen are fixed immediately in glutaraldehyde with further processing in the Pathology Laboratory.
- Routine tissue stains including, H & E - general liver histology stain; reticulin stain - for connective tissue, especially cirrhosis, fibrosis, bridging necrosis; trichrome - fibrosis; iron stain - useful for hemosiderosis, hemochromatosis, bile pigments; diastase PAS stain - useful for alpha$_1$-antitrypsin globules, bile ducts, iron; orcein - for hepatitis B surface antigen (if present, fine granular brown material stains in hepatocytes); also for copper-binding protein in Wilson disease
- Cytologic preparation - fluid from aspirating syringe may be smeared on clean microscope slide, fixed, and sent to the Cytology Laboratory.
- Microbiological culture - specimen sent without fixative in sterile container. Special stains (AFB, KOH, etc) and cultures (tuberculosis, viral, *Brucella*, parasites, fungi) as needed.
- Optional special stains (ie, congo red for amyloidosis, immunohistochemistry)

Footnotes

1. Sherlock S, Dick R, and van Leeuwen DJ, "Liver Biopsy Today. The Royal Free Hospital Experience," *J Hepatol*, 1984, 1(1):75-85.

References

Friedman LS, Martin P, and Munoz SJ, "Liver Function Tests and the Objective Evaluation of the Patient With Liver Disease," *Hepatology: A Textbook of Liver Disease*, 3rd ed, Chapter 28, Zakim D and Boyer TD, eds, Philadelphia, PA: WB Saunders Co, 1996, 791-833.

Reddy KR and Jeffers LJ, "Evaluation of the Liver. B. Liver Biopsy and Laparoscopy," *Schiff's Diseases of the Liver*, 8th ed, Chapter 7, Schiff ER, Sorrell MF, and Maddrey WC, eds, Philadelphia, PA: Lippincott Williams & Wilkins, 1999, 245-66.

Schaffner F and Thung SN, "Liver Biopsy," *Bockus Gastroenterology*, 5th ed, Chapter 97, Haubrich WS, Schaffner F, and Berk JE, eds, Philadelphia, PA: WB Saunders Co, 1995.

Sherlock S and Dooley J, "Biopsy of the Liver," *Diseases of the Liver and Biliary System*, 10th ed, Chapter 3, Oxford, England: Blackwell Scientific Publications, 1997,33-42.

Van Ness MM and Diehl AM, "Is Liver Biopsy Useful in the Evaluation of Patients With Chronically Elevated Liver Enzymes?" *Ann Intern Med*, 1989, 111(6):473-8.

♦ **Long-Interval Distal Esophageal pH Monitoring** *see* pH Study, 12- to 24-Hour *on page 92*

♦ **Lower Endoscopy** *see* Colonoscopy *on page 59*

♦ **Lundh Test** *see* Secretin Test for Exocrine Pancreatic Function *on page 94*

♦ **MAO (Maximal Acid Output), Gastric Acid Titration** *see* Gastric Acid Analysis *on page 78*

♦ **Maximal Acid Output** *see* Gastric Acid Analysis *on page 78*

♦ **Measurement of Intestinal Transit Time** *see* Breath Hydrogen Analysis *on page 57*

♦ **Needle Biopsy of the Liver** *see* Liver Biopsy *on page 82*

♦ **Open Small Bowel Biopsy, Laparotomy** *see* Small Bowel Biopsy *on page 95*

♦ **Pancreatic Function Test** *see* Secretin Test for Exocrine Pancreatic Function *on page 94*

♦ **PAO (Peak Acid Output)** *see* Gastric Acid Analysis *on page 78*

Paracentesis

Synonyms Abdominal Paracentesis; Ascites Fluid Tap

Procedure Commonly Includes At the bedside, physician introduces a needle into the peritoneal space of a patient with free ascites, and samples the fluid for diagnostic and/or therapeutic purposes.

Indications Diagnostic indications include:

- patients with new onset of ascites
- ascites fluid of unknown etiology
- patients with clinically suspected ascites fluid infections (abdominal pain, unexplained fever, leukocytosis, declining mental status)

Therapeutic paracentesis is indicated when ascites fluid has accumulated enough to cause respiratory compromise, abdominal pain, or worsening of existing inguinal or umbilical hernias. Paracentesis should not be performed to diagnose the presence of ascites fluid. This should be known prior to the procedure (by physical examination or radiological imaging).

Contraindications Severe coagulopathy not correctable by vitamin K, fresh frozen plasma, etc; inability of physician to demonstrate ascites fluid on physical examination; lack of patient cooperation. Recent literature suggests the following factors are **not** contraindications for paracentesis: morbid obesity, low grade coagulopathy, multiple abdominal surgical scars, and bacteremia.[1]

Patient Preparation Technique and risks of the procedure are explained. Premedications (eg, sedatives or narcotics) are not routinely required. Laboratory requisitions are completed in advance to avoid delay in fluid processing later. Prothrombin and partial thromboplastin times prior to paracentesis are ordered at physician discretion (some elect to transfuse fresh frozen plasma immediately prior to procedure if PT/PTT are prolonged).

Aftercare No special limitations exist for the patient postprocedure. If large amounts of ascites are removed (several liters), frequent blood pressure measurements are needed to monitor possible hypotension. Patients may ambulate postprocedure if vital signs remain stable. Occasionally, ascites fluid may leak persistently from the puncture site. In this instance, the patient should remain supine with the site angled directly upwards, until the leak stops spontaneously. On rare occasions, the paracentesis site may need to be sutured to stop the leak.

Special Instructions In clinical practice, paracentesis is at times performed on patients with significant hepatic encephalopathy. Additional personnel may be required for conferring with family members and for proper patient positioning during the procedure.

Complications The medical literature is divided on the incidence of complications from paracentesis. Earlier literature was more negative and tended to emphasize the possible complications, based on retrospective analysis.[2,3] Some authors suggested that paracentesis itself was the cause of many cases of ascites fluid infection.[4] A prospective study concluded that paracentesis is a safe procedure, carrying <1% risk of major complications and <1% risk of minor complications.[1] No deaths or bowel perforations were seen in 229 consecutive attempts. The most feared complication is needle perforation of an abdominal viscus or solid organ such as liver or spleen. Others include intraperitoneal hemorrhage from laceration of an umbilical vein, scrotal or penile edema, abdominal wall hematoma, and contamination of ascites by nonsterile technique. Hypotension can be seen when large amounts of ascites (>1500 mL) are removed rapidly.

Equipment Sterile gloves, drapes (optional), and adequate local anesthesia (26-gauge subcutaneous needle, 2% lidocaine). In clinical practice, various needles and angiocatheters are used. A 22-gauge, 1.5" metal needle with a plastic catheter is recommended. Recently, longer (3.25") 15-gauge or 17-gauge metal needles with multiple holes specifically made for paracentesis have become available. If a thick panniculus is encountered, a 3" to 5" 22-gauge needle may be substituted. Also required are a sterile 50 mL syringe and, if large volumes of ascites are to be removed, 4-6 or more sterile 1 L vacuum bottles with connecting tubing.

Technique Patient empties bladder prior to procedure. Physician confirms the presence of ascites by physical examination with patient in a semirecumbent position. Preferred site of entry is in the midline, inferior to the umbilicus. If a midline scar is present from prior surgery or if percussion is not reliable, an area near the flank is selected. At times, physician may request patient to assume the hand-knees position if small amounts of ascites are present. The entry site is then caudad to the umbilicus. The site is prepped with iodine solution and skin and deeper tissues are infiltrated with lidocaine. The skin is retracted caudally and the 22-gauge needle (attached to syringe) is inserted into the anesthetized area and advanced while aspirating. When ascites fluid returns freely, the needle is held in position and not advanced further (avoiding bowel trauma). Multiple aliquots (50 mL) may be obtained in this manner. For larger volumes, the syringe is removed and connecting tubing is directly attached to the 22-gauge needle to allow drainage into vacuum bottles. Once the desired amount is collected, the needle is withdrawn quickly and the caudal skin retraction is released, allowing the skin to return to its normal position. This causes the entrance and exit needle sites to form a "Z-tract" which minimizes ascites leakage.

Data Acquired Ascites fluid is routinely analyzed for cell count and differential, chemistries including LDH, albumin and protein, Gram stain, bacterial culture, and cytology. Additional tests include special cultures for tuberculosis or fungi, ascites fluid pH, amylase, lipase, glucose, triglycerides, lactate, CEA, and hyaluronic acid.

Specimen When the procedure is performed therapeutically, the maximum volume of ascites that can be removed safely depends on the presence or absence of peripheral edema.[5] Volumes up to 10-12 L may be obtained in patients with peripheral edema without adverse effects.[6] When performed for diagnostic purposes, smaller volumes (50-100 mL) are adequate for routine studies. If malignancy or fastidious infection is suspected, larger volumes (more than 100 mL) will improve laboratory yield for either culture or cytology.

Container Lavender top tube for cell count; red top tube for routine chemistries; aerobic and anaerobic culture media bottles for bacteriology. For cytology, send sterile vacuum bottles with 5000 units of heparin added. If ascites fluid pH is desired, send specimen in anaerobic syringe (gas bubbles removed) on ice to the Acute Care Laboratory.

Collection Some authorities recommend inoculating the bacterial culture media with ascites fluid immediately at bedside.[7] The average concentration of bacteria in ascites fluid is very low, in most cases, of spontaneous peritonitis. In addition, a significant number of organisms may not survive in the time needed for specimen transport and plating in the Microbiology Laboratory. Bedside inoculation of appropriate media (standard blood culture bottles) may improve the chances of obtaining a positive bacterial culture several fold.

Normal Findings Ascites fluid is traditionally categorized as either "exudative" or "transudative" based on laboratory analysis.[8] More recently, the serum ascites albumin gradient (SAAG) has replaced the transudate-exudate classification of ascitic fluid.[9] A SAAG ≥1.1 is considered "high gradient" and is consistent with portal hypertension representing conditions (eg, cirrhosis, cardiac ascites, Budd-Chiari syndrome, veno-occlusive disease). A SAAG <1.1 is considered "low gradient" and is not consistent with portal hypertension representing conditions such as peritoneal carcinomatosis, tuberculous peritonitis, pancreatic ascites, and nephrotic syndrome.

Critical Values The early diagnosis of spontaneous bacterial peritonitis (SBP) prior to bacterial culture results can frequently be made on routine analysis of ascites fluid.[10] Patients with SBP, or other ascites fluid infections, have ascites

(Continued)

Paracentesis *(Continued)*

WBC count >500/mm³ (along with many polymorphonuclear (PMN) cells on the differential >250/mm³). In addition, two other laboratory indices suggestive of SBP are ascites pH <7.35 and ascites lactate <25 ng/dL.[11] The clinical utility of these last two criteria has not been as well established as the standard PMN count. Many physicians will begin empiric antibiotics on the basis of PMN >250/mm³ alone. Gram stain of ascites fluid has low sensitivity for detecting SBP due to the low bacterial concentration, even on a centrifuged sample. Malignant ascites can be expected to have abnormal cytology in >50% of the cases. Indirect evidence of neoplasm include: grossly hemorrhagic fluid (may also be traumatic); ascites CEA >10 ng/mL with adenocarcinoma; ascites hyaluronic acid >0.25 mg/mL with mesothelioma; high ascites triglyceride levels with chronic chylous ascites (>80% of cases are lymphoma); ascites WBC count >500/mm³ with peritoneal carcinomatosis (but PMN count low, <250/mm³), pH <7.35, lactate <25 mg/dL. None of these values are considered diagnostic of malignancy and should be used only as supportive evidence.

Additional Information Paracentesis is a safe procedure when ascites is easily demonstrable on physical examination. When small amounts of ascites are present, a fluid wave may be difficult to demonstrate even when ≤1.5 L ascites are present. CT scan or abdominal ultrasound guided needle aspiration is particularly useful in these cases. Patients with ascites from cirrhosis may develop SBP and yet have minimal evidence of infection; some patients may be completely asymptomatic.[12] A low threshold for performing paracentesis is recommended in this setting, despite the low-grade coagulopathy that frequently is seen.

Footnotes

1. Runyon BA, "Paracentesis of Ascitic Fluid: A Safe Procedure," *Arch Intern Med*, 1986, 146:2259-61.
2. Liebowitz HR, "Hazards of Abdominal Paracentesis in the Cirrhotic Patient," *N Y State J Med*, 1962, 62:1822-6, 1997-2004, 2223-9.
3. Mallory A and Schaefer JW, "Complications of Diagnostic Paracentesis in Patients With Liver Disease," *JAMA*, 1978, 239(7):628-30.
4. Conn HO, "Bacterial Peritonitis: Spontaneous or Paracentric?" *Gastroenterology*, 1979, 77(5):1145-6.
5. Rocco VK and Ware AJ, "Cirrhotic Ascites: Pathophysiology, Diagnosis, and Management," *Ann Intern Med*, 1986, 105(4):573-85.
6. Korula J, "Ascites: Pathogenesis, Characteristics, Complications, and Treatment," *Liver and Biliary Diseases*, 2nd ed, Kaplowitz N, ed, Baltimore, MD: Wiliams & Wilkins, 1996, 589-602.
7. Runyon BA, Umland ET, and Merlin T, "Inoculation of Blood Culture Bottles With Ascitic Fluid; Improved Detection of Spontaneous Bacterial Peritonitis," *Arch Intern Med*, 1987, 147(1):73-5.
8. Runyon BA, "Ascites and Spontaneous Bacterial Peritonitis," *Gastrointestinal and Liver Disease: Pathophysiology, Diagnosis, and Management*, 6th ed, Chapter 78, Feldman M, Scharschmidt BF, and Sleisenger MH, eds, Philadelphia, PA: WB Saunders Co, 1998, 1310-33.
9. Pare P, Talbot J, and Hoefs JC, "Serum Ascites Albumin Concentration Gradient: A Physiologic Approach to the Differential Diagnosis of Ascites," *Gastroenterology*, 1983, 85(2):240-4.
10. Hoefs JC and Runyon BA, "Spontaneous Bacterial Peritonitis," *Dis Mon*, 1985, 31(9):1-48.
11. Yang CY, Liaw YF, Chu CM, et al, "White Count, pH, and Lactate in Ascites in the Diagnosis of Spontaneous Bacterial Peritonitis," *Hepatology*, 1985, 5(1):85-90.
12. Pinzello G, Simonetti RG, and Craxi A, "Spontaneous Bacterial Peritonitis: A Prospective Investigation in Predominantly Nonalcoholic Cirrhotic Patients," *Hepatology*, 1983, 3(4):545-9.

♦ **Peak Acid Output** *see* Gastric Acid Analysis *on page 78*

♦ **Percutaneous Liver Biopsy** *see* Liver Biopsy *on page 82*

♦ **Percutaneous Needle Aspiration Biopsy Under Fluoroscopic, CT, or Ultrasound Guidance** *see* Liver Biopsy *on page 82*

♦ **Percutaneous Transhepatic Cholangiogram (PTC)** *see* Endoscopic Retrograde Cholangiopancreatography *on page 63*

♦ **Peritoneal Endoscopy** *see* Peritoneoscopy *on page 88*

Peritoneoscopy

Related Information

Liver Biopsy *on page 82*

Synonyms Celioscopy; Laparoscopy; Peritoneal Endoscopy

Replaces Laparotomy in Selected Cases

Procedure Commonly Includes Direct visualization of anterior intra-abdominal structures by means of a rigid laparoscope. This is performed in an endoscopy suite under local anesthesia or in an operating room under general anesthesia. The technique involves insertion of a Veress needle into the peritoneal cavity, followed by insufflation with gas (either CO_2 or nitrous oxide). Once this pneumoperitoneum has been created, the laparoscope is advanced into the peritoneal cavity through a small periumbilical incision. The following structures can be readily visualized: omentum, surface of the liver, peritoneum, gallbladder, portions of the spleen, diaphragm, and the serosal surfaces of the small bowel and colon. In female patients, the ovaries, Fallopian tubes, and uterus are also accessible. The areas of pathology are noted and visually-directed biopsies may be obtained.

Indications The more common diagnostic indications include:

- ascites of unknown etiology. In the majority of cases, bedside paracentesis should be performed first. If the ascites fluid is found to be exudative (but otherwise nondiagnostic), peritoneoscopy may be used to rule out occult malignancy, fungal peritonitis, tuberculosis, and other conditions.
- diffuse or focal liver disease of unknown etiology. Direct inspection of the liver combined with a visually-directed liver biopsy can increase diagnostic accuracy. This may be particularly helpful in suspected cases of hepatocellular carcinoma, lymphoma metastatic to liver, granulomatous hepatitis, and tuberculosis. Even when diffuse liver disease is present, as in cirrhosis, laparoscopic liver biopsy and visual inspection of the liver appears to be more sensitive than "blind" liver biopsy.
- suspected peritoneal carcinomatosis
- cancer staging; peritoneoscopy may be used to determine the stage of malignancies such as ovarian cancer and Hodgkin disease when formal surgical laparotomy is contraindicated.

Additional indications for peritoneoscopy include:

- evaluation of chronic abdominal pain syndromes. This procedure may occasionally be useful in diagnosing abdominal adhesions or endometriosis in patients with chronic pain. Some physicians may use laparoscopy as a means of avoiding a formal laparotomy in difficult cases. The precise role and efficacy of peritoneoscopy in this setting is unclear.
- suspected ectopic pregnancy
- suspected pelvic inflammatory disease
- primary or secondary amenorrhea
- fever of unknown origin; in selected cases to rule out lymphoma or granulomatous diseases
- infertility evaluation (eg, diagnosis of tubal defects)
- suspected appendicitis
- emergency evaluation of abdominal trauma

Therapeutic uses for peritoneoscopy include:

- tubal ligation
- pancreatic biopsy by laparoscope through lesser sac
- therapeutic wedge resection of the ovaries in polycystic ovary syndrome
- lysis of adhesions
- removal of foreign bodies (eg, intrauterine device which has perforated into the Cul-de-sac)
- treatment of endometriosis with electrocautery or laser
- laparoscopic cholecystectomy
- laparoscopic colorectal surgery

Contraindications Absolute contraindications to peritoneoscopy include:

- acute peritonitis, particularly when surgical intervention is warranted
- unstable cardiac or pulmonary status
- acute intestinal obstruction; the presence of multiple dilated loops of bowel increases the risk of perforation by the needle or trocar
- uncorrectable, severe coagulopathy
- uncooperative patient

Relative contraindications are as follows:

- presence of abdominal adhesions, usually from multiple abdominal surgeries or severe peritonitis. This increases the risk of bowel perforation. In each case, the risk-benefit ratio should be carefully considered (some authors consider this an absolute contraindication)

(Continued)

Peritoneoscopy *(Continued)*

- presence of an abdominal hernia. On rare occasions, a hernia can become incarcerated during peritoneal insufflation
- infection involving the abdominal wall, such as cellulitis
- history of multiple abdominal surgeries (increased likelihood of dense adhesions)

Patient Preparation Patients who are candidates for peritoneoscopy must be referred to the appropriate specialist in gastroenterology, obstetrics and gynecology, or surgery. A complete medical history and physical is required. The technique, risks, and benefits of the procedure are discussed with the patient and informed consent is obtained. The details of scheduling are usually the responsibility of the subspecialist performing the procedure (such as date, time, operating area, etc). If peritoneoscopy is to be performed under general anesthesia, preoperative medical clearance may be necessary. The following laboratory studies are routinely obtained: complete blood count (including platelet count), electrolytes, prothrombin time (PT), and partial thromboplastin time (PTT). An electrocardiogram and chest x-ray are usually indicated if general anesthesia is planned. NPO (nothing by mouth) for at least 8 hours before procedure. Usually nothing after midnight the day before. Preoperative enemas are not necessary unless the patient complains of fecal impaction. Laxatives should be avoided. Prescription medications normally taken by the patient must be reviewed in advance by the physician, and explicit instructions provided. This is particularly relevant if the patient is on insulin, antiarrhythmic agents, or antianginals. Patient should avoid taking aspirin products or nonsteroidal anti-inflammatory agents for several days before procedure. On the day of the procedure, the patient is shaved and prepped by the medical team. Premedication is usually with Demerol® and a benzodiazepine. The bladder should be emptied prior to the procedure.

Aftercare Following the procedure, the patient is observed in the endoscopy recovery area or postanesthesia care unit. Vital signs are obtained frequently. The length of time for observation depends on the general medical condition of the patient. It is not mandatory to hospitalize patients overnight, unless the procedure was complicated.

Special Instructions NPO after midnight.

Complications Laparoscopy is considered a safe procedure, especially when candidates are carefully selected. Certainly, the presence of a relative contraindication (eg, multiple surgeries in the past) increases the risk. The incidence of death associated with this procedure has been estimated at 1 in 2000, and severe complications in an additional 1 in 500.[1] A wide variety of adverse outcomes have been reported. Most often these appear related to incorrect placement of the needle used to create the pneumoperitoneum, although complications can occur during any phase. These include:

- injury or perforation of bowel, liver, spleen, ovary, gallbladder
- subcutaneous emphysema, pneumomediastinum
- bleeding, especially at biopsy sites or within the abdominal wall
- vasovagal reactions, myocardial infarction
- fever, infection, peritonitis
- pain, especially in the shoulder from diaphragmatic irritation
- aortic rupture

Technique As indicated previously, the procedure may be performed under local anesthesia (with sedation) or under general anesthesia. For most gastroenterologic indications, local anesthesia is preferable. The patient may be required to perform certain simple maneuvers during laparoscopy. The patient is placed supine on a standard operating room table. The table is equipped with stirrups. The buttocks are extended 4" to 5" over the edge of the table, which is tilted in Trendelenburg position for gynecologic procedures. Table may be tilted in any direction as needed to visualize any area of peritoneum required. The site of needle entry is identified and anesthetized. This is often the inferior rim of the umbilicus, although other areas are acceptable. A small skin incision is made and a Veress needle is advanced into the peritoneal cavity. Approximately 2 L of gas is then instilled into the peritoneal cavity (either CO_2 or nitrous oxide). The Veress needle is then removed. The skin incision previously made is enlarged and the laparoscopic trocar and sleeve are inserted. A twisting motion is used until the trocar is within the gas-filled peritoneal cavity. The laparoscope is then inserted through the sleeve and advanced under direct visualization. Additional volumes of gas may be introduced into the abdomen through the sleeve. The various internal structures are observed directly and pathologic areas biopsied as indicated. In some cases, accessory trocars may be required for introduction of instruments for suction, biopsy, fulguration, hemostasis, etc.

Turnaround Time 2-3 days

Specimen Liver biopsy, tumor biopsy, peritoneal biopsy, ovarian wedge biopsy, ascitic or peritoneal fluid aspiration and washing. Specimens for histopathologic examination should be placed in a clean container with appropriate fixative. Samples for microbial culture should be placed in a sterile container (or syringe) without fixative. Cultures for anaerobic organisms should be inoculated into anaerobic media or transported immediately to the Microbiology Laboratory. For cytologic samples, peritoneal fluid samples should be promptly spread on a clean microscope slide and fixed.

Container Clean container with fixative for tissue specimens for histology. Sterile syringes for peritoneal aspirates for culture. Syringes for peritoneal aspirates for cytology. Fluid should be immediately spread on slide and fixed in 95% alcohol.

Sampling Time 1-2 hours

Normal Findings Preliminary report on gross laparoscopic findings written in patient's chart immediately by operating physician. Final typewritten report is attached to chart within several days. Specifically, the laparoscopist usually comments on the following aspects of the case:

- premedications administered
- type of instrument used
- gross appearance of omentum, peritoneal surfaces
- size and appearance of the liver, gallbladder, spleen, diaphragm, small bowel, colon, female reproductive organs, appendix
- presence or absence of ascites
- areas of pathology including malignancy, endometrial implants, adhesions, vascular abnormalities, abscesses, ectopic pregnancies, foreign bodies, as appropriate
- biopsies, brushings, ascites fluid aspirations
- other operative procedures performed
- complications

The laparoscopist also includes an overall clinical impression, based on the clinical history and visualized abnormalities.

Additional Information Despite the safety and efficacy of peritoneoscopy, it is an infrequently performed gastroenterologic procedure. It is, however, well-established in the field of obstetrics and gynecology, due to the accessibility of the female pelvic organs. From a GI standpoint, peritoneoscopy appears of most benefit in evaluating the patient with ascites of unknown etiology, where malignancy or tuberculosis are possibilities. Clinical trials comparing the diagnostic yield of laparoscopy versus laparotomy are lacking. Until such studies are performed for different clinical indications, the selection of laparoscopy will depend in part on physician familiarity and confidence with the procedure.

Footnotes

1. Vilardell F and Marti-Vicente A, "Laparoscopy," *Bockus Gastroenterology*, 5th ed, Chapter 27, Berk JE, Haubrich WS, and Schaffner F, eds, Philadelphia, PA: WB Saunders Co, 1995, 341-48.

References

Lightdale CJ, "Indications, Contraindications, and Complications of Laparoscopy," *Gastroenterologic Endoscopy*, 2nd ed, Chapter 92, Sivak MV Jr, ed, Philadelphia, PA: WB Saunders Co, 1999.

Nord HJ, "Technique of Laparoscopy," *Gastroenterologic Endoscopy*, CD-ROM, 2nd ed, Chapter 93, Sivak MV, ed, Philadelphia, PA: WB Saunders Co, 1999.

Reddy KR and Jeffers LJ, "Liver Biopsy and Laparoscopy," *Schiff's Diseases of the Liver*, 8th ed, Schiff ER, Sorrell MF, and Maddrey WC, eds, Philadelphia, PA: Lippincott-Raven, 1999, 245-66.

♦ **Peroral Endoscopy** *see* Esophagogastroduodenoscopy (EGD) *on page 72*

♦ **Peroral Jejunal Biopsy** *see* Small Bowel Biopsy *on page 95*

pH Study, 12- to 24-Hour

Related Information

Standard Acid Reflux Test *on page 99*

Synonyms Ambulatory pH Monitoring; Esophagus Acid Reflux Test With Intraluminal pH Electrode (Prolonged Recording); Long-Interval Distal Esophageal pH Monitoring

Procedure Commonly Includes Placing a pH probe into the distal esophagus for a 12- to 24-hour period in order to generate a graph depicting continuous pH readings. Information is obtained regarding quantity and pattern of gastroesophageal (GE) reflux events, the correlation with symptoms, and the efficiency of esophageal acid clearance.

Indications

- quantify the number of acid reflux episodes which occur over 12-24 hours under physiologic conditions; particularly useful in patients with suspected reflux esophagitis (based on the history and physical) who have failed empiric therapy, or whose symptoms are atypical
- further evaluate patients with typical symptoms of reflux esophagitis but whose upper endoscopy is normal
- evaluate difficult cases of nocturnal pulmonary aspiration or noncardiac chest pain, particularly to see if subjective complaints correlate temporally with episodes of acid reflux
- monitor, in selected cases, the effectiveness of medical or surgical antireflux therapy

Contraindications

- any condition that prohibits standard nasogastric intubation - nasal obstruction, maxillofacial trauma, basilar skull fracture, severe coagulopathy, etc
- active upper GI bleeding
- refractory nausea and vomiting
- uncooperative patient, especially in terms of diet, compliance, cigarette use, and coffee intake since these factors are carefully regulated during the procedure
- agitated or confused patient, since an accurate record of reflux events must be kept, including time of day and nature of symptoms

Patient Preparation Technique and risks of the procedure are explained in detail and consent is obtained. Patient is instructed to be NPO for at least 4-6 hours before placement of the pH probe. Discontinue H_2-blockers 24 hours prior to procedure. Proton pump inhibitors need to be discontinued 7 days before procedure unless the test is being done to assess failure of medical therapy.

Aftercare Patient may be discharged if no complications have arisen. Activity may be *ad libitum* or as determined by referring physician. No specific post-procedure restrictions are necessary.

Complications This procedure is considered safe and no significant attendant morbidity has been reported. Potential complications are mainly those related to any nasogastric (NG) intubation (eg, nasal trauma, vasovagal reaction, tracheal intubation, etc).

Equipment In GI procedure room: flexible pH electrode, separate glass reference electrode, pH meter with recording device, reference pH solutions, pH software, and a computer. In most cases, an esophageal manometry system with transducer equipment is needed initially. Also required are tape, electrode gel, and a form in which the patient records time of symptoms and daily activities.

Technique The system is calibrated against the reference pH solutions to ensure accuracy. Esophageal manometry is carried out in most cases to locate the exact position of the lower esophageal sphincter (LES). Following this, a pH probe is passed through the nose, using standard nasogastric intubation technique, and is positioned 5 cm above the LES. If a separate reference electrode is available, it is taped to the skin on the chest. Both pH probe and reference electrode are connected to the pH recording device, which is then strapped to the waist or worn on a belt. In some centers, patients are placed on a restricted diet in which the pH of all food and beverage is >5. Smoking is usually not permitted due to potential effects on lower esophageal sphincter tone. Patients are instructed to fully record the time of symptoms, changes in body position (standing, sitting, lying, etc), and time of meals. Patients are also given full instructions on the operation and care of the pH recording device.

Data Acquired Graphic recording strip of intraesophageal pH over a 12- to 24-hour period where the pH is plotted on the vertical axis and time on the horizontal axis. The data from the pH recording device is downloaded into the computer for analysis. Patient submits his log book of all activities for the 12-24 hours of pH monitoring for comparison analysis.

Normal Findings Individual composite reflux score within two standard deviations of the mean score of a reference group, using the criteria of Johnson and DeMeester. Other definitions may be used and are mentioned in the following information. Data is analyzed and final interpretation is provided by a GI specialist. Basic principles of interpretation are as follows. From the 24-hour pH recording, six variables are analyzed:

- percent of total recording time with intraesophageal pH <4
- percent of time in upright position with pH <4
- percent of time in recumbent position with pH <4
- total number of reflux episodes requiring ≥5 minutes to clear
- average number of reflux episodes per hour
- duration of longest period of esophageal acid exposure (single episode)

A "reflux episode" is defined as a fall in pH to ≤4 for at least 5 seconds. Several methods of interpreting the raw data have been proposed. Johnson and DeMeester described a weighted scoring system utilizing these six variables.[1] A total "reflux score" is calculated and this is compared with reflux scores from an asymptomatic control group. If the reflux score calculated for a patient is more than two standard deviations (SD) above the mean score of 15 control volunteers, the degree of reflux is considered "abnormal". This system has come under some criticism because of complexity and length of time required for calculation. Some researchers advocate independent analysis of each of the six variables, without weighing certain variables more heavily. Schlesinger suggests another, more simple grading system based on a prospective study of 64 patients undergoing 24-hour pH monitoring. Discrimination from asymptomatic controls was best achieved by analyzing only two variables - (the number of reflux events requiring ≥5 minutes to clear and total exposure time of the esophagus to acid).

Critical Values Abnormal reflux defined as reflux score more than two standard deviations above reference group. Again, other definitions may be used, based on the interpreting physician's preference.

Additional Information The patient who presents with symptoms consistent with GE reflux disease is commonly encountered in clinical practice. The majority of cases do not require laboratory testing. Those individuals with typical retrosternal burning pain are usually treated empirically for presumed reflux esophagitis. Diagnostic testing is neither indicated nor economically feasible in this large group of patients. Patients who present with atypical symptoms, who have persistent pain despite aggressive medical treatment, or who may have complications of reflux disease (eg, nocturnal asthma, esophageal strictures) are candidates for additional diagnostic testing. However, no single test for reflux esophagitis is clearly superior. In fact, no sequence of testing or combination of tests has been generally agreed upon. The 24-hour pH test was designed to quantitate exposure of the distal esophagus to acid. Initial studies suggested superior sensitivity (88%) and specificity (98%) for this test, but later studies suggested these figures were inflated. Schlesinger, et al demonstrated a 29% false-negative rate in patients with endoscopically proven erosive esophagitis.[2] In the subgroup of patients with typical reflux symptoms but normal endoscopies, a sensitivity of only 21% was reported. Despite these caveats, this procedure is gaining increasing importance and popularity. No other procedure examines patients over a prolonged period or under near-physiologic conditions. It is based, in part, on the rationale that symptomatic GE reflux is not an "all or none" phenomenon, unlike the rationale underlying the standard acid reflux test. An important clinical application of this test is the temporal correlation of subjective symptoms with objective pH measurements. The occurrence of typical symptoms in the absence of

(Continued)

pH Study, 12- to 24-Hour *(Continued)*

pH changes argues strongly against reflux esophagitis as the etiology of symptoms.

Footnotes

1. Johnston LF and DeMeester TR, "Twenty-Four Hour pH Monitoring of the Distal Esophagus. A Quantitative Measure of Gastroesophageal Reflux," *Am J Gastroenterol*, 1974, 62(4):325-32.
2. Schlesinger PK, Donahue PE, Schmid B, et al, "Limitations of 24-Hour Intraesophageal pH Monitoring in the Hospital Setting," *Gastroenterology*, 1985, 89(4):797-804.

References

Bozymski EM and Orlando RC, "Ambulatory Intraesophageal pH Monitoring," *Manual of Gastroenterologic Procedures*, 3rd ed, Drossman DA, ed, New York, NY: Raven Press, 1993, 50-5.

DeMeester TR, Wang C, Wernly JA, et al, "Technique, Indications, and Clinical Use of 24-Hour Esophageal pH Monitoring," *J Thorac Cardiovasc Surg*, 1980, 79(5):656-70.

Johnson LF, "24-Hour pH Monitoring in the Study of Gastroesophageal Reflux," *J Clin Gastroenterol*, 1980, 2(4):387-99.

Mattox HE and Richter JE, "Prolonged Ambulatory Esophageal pH Monitoring in the Evaluation of Gastroesophageal Reflux Disease," *Am J Med*, 1990, 89(3):345-56.

Stendal C, "Anorectal Manometry," *Practical Guide to Gastrointestinal Function Testing*, Oxford, England: Blackwell Science, 1997, 213-24.

♦ **Proctoscopy** *see* Anoscopy *on page 52*

♦ **Rectosphincteric Manometry** *see* Anorectal Manometry *on page 49*

♦ **SART** *see* Standard Acid Reflux Test *on page 99*

♦ **SBB** *see* Small Bowel Biopsy *on page 95*

♦ **Secretin-CCK test** *see* Secretin Test for Exocrine Pancreatic Function *on page 94*

♦ **Secretin-Pancreozymin test** *see* Secretin Test for Exocrine Pancreatic Function *on page 94*

♦ **Secretin Stimulated Pancreatic Amylase and Bicarbonate Determination** *see* Secretin Test for Exocrine Pancreatic Function *on page 94*

♦ **Secretin Stimulated Serum Gastrin Determination** *see* I.V. Secretin Gastrin Levels *on page 81*

Secretin Test for Exocrine Pancreatic Function

Synonyms Pancreatic Function Test

Applies to Lundh Test; Secretin-CCK test; Secretin-Pancreozymin test; Secretin Stimulated Pancreatic Amylase and Bicarbonate Determination

Procedure Commonly Includes Insertion of a Dreiling tube into the duodenum and intravenous injection of secretin. Duodenal aspiration for volume of pancreatic juice and bicarbonate and amylase determination.

Indications Determine pancreatic exocrine function in patients who are suspected to have chronic pancreatitis based on clinical information, especially in a subset who have normal structural evaluation of the pancreas (ie, plain abdominal radiographs, CT scans, ERCP, and EUS)

Contraindications Allergy to secretin; inability to cooperate because the procedure requires placement of a Dreiling tube

Patient Preparation NPO after midnight. The posterior pharynx is anesthetized with 5% Cetacaine® spray prior to duodenal intubation. Use of a short-acting sedative is left to the discretion of the gastroenterologist.

Technique Under fluoroscopy, a Dreiling-type, radiopaque, double-lumen tube is intubated. The distal lumen is placed just beyond the papilla of vater in the duodenum, thereby placing the proximal lumen in the gastric antrum. Both gastric juice and duodenal contents are separately collected by continuous suction. Gastric contents are discarded while duodenal contents are retained for analysis. Care must be taken so as not to contaminate the duodenal aspirate with gastric contents. Confirmation of correct placement of Dreiling tube by fluoroscopy is key. In addition, the pH of uncontaminated duodenal fluid is ≤7.5. Once the tube is in place, collection is begun. After preinjection samples have been collected, secretin (0.3 μg/kg) is then given as an intravenous bolus. Postinjection samples are then collected. CCK may be added to secretin but there is no evidence that this increases the sensitivity and/or specificity of secretin alone. Alternatively, CCK alone is given and in this case, measurements of trypsin and lipase are obtained.

Specimen Duodenal aspirate

Sampling Time 2-2.5 hours

Collection Preinjection samples are collected every 15 minutes for 1 hour for volume determination and determination of bicarbonate and amylase concentration. Postinjection samples are collected every 15 minutes for 1-1.5 hours.

Normal Findings

After secretin injection:

- normal volume: 107-223 mL/hour
- bicarbonate concentration: 92-124 mEq/L
- bicarbonate output: 14-21 mmol/hour
- amylase output: 174-1270 units/hour[1]

When CCK is used with secretin:

- normal volume: 151 mL/hour
- bicarbonate concentration: 70 mmol/L
- bicarbonate output: 11.3 mmol/hour
- amylase output: 131 units (during 30 minutes of CCK)

After CCK:

- normal lipase output: 77-322 K units/hour
- trypsin is 25-54 K units/hour

Limitations Contamination of duodenal contents with gastric juice will produce inaccurate volume measurements and falsely low bicarbonate concentrations. The test is expensive, time-consuming, and requires tube placement in the duodenum.

Additional Information Occasionally, abnormally low volumes are aspirated. In order to assure that this is true volume rather than a technical error, a nonabsorbable marker is infused into the proximal duodenum and quantification of the marker in the collected duodenal aspirate assists in determining adequacy of duodenal aspiration.[2] The Lundh test determines the pancreatic enzyme concentration after a test meal. After ingestion of a standardized 300 mL meal of dried milk, vegetable oil, and dextrose, duodenal contents are aspirated for enzyme determination. Normal values are trypsin ≥7 IU/L and chymotrypsin ≥12.6 IU/L. This test is less sensitive than secretin or CCK tests.

Footnotes

1. Dreiling DA and Hollander F, "Studies in Pancreatic Function II. A Statistical Study of Pancreatic Secretion Following Secretin in Patients With Pancreatic Disease," *Gastroenterology*, 1950, 15:620.
2. Go VLW, Hofmann AF and Summerskill WHJ, "Simultaneous Measurements of Total Pancreatic, Biliary, and Gastric Outputs in Man Using a Perfusion Technique," *Gastroenterology*, 1970, 58:321.

References

Banks PA, "Acute and Chronic Pancreatitis," *Gastrointestinal and Liver Disease: Pathophysiology, Diagnosis, and Management*, 6th ed, Chapter 48, Feldman M, Scharschmidt BF, and Sleisenger MH, eds, Philadelphia, PA: WB Saunders Co, 1998, 809-62.

Chey WD and Chey WY, "Tests of Gastric and Exocrine Pancreatic Function and Absorption," *Textbook of Gastroenterology*, 3rd ed, Yamada T, Alpers DH, Laine L, et al, eds, Philadelphia, PA: Lippincott Williams & Wilkins, 1999, 2924-37.

♦ **Serum Radioimmunoassay for Gastrin** *see* I.V. Secretin Gastrin Levels *on page 81*

♦ **Sigmoidoscopy, Flexible** *see* Flexible Fiberoptic Sigmoidoscopy *on page 76*

Small Bowel Biopsy

Synonyms Peroral Jejunal Biopsy; SBB; Small Intestinal Biopsy

Applies to Duodenal Intubation

Replaces Open Small Bowel Biopsy, Laparotomy

Procedure Commonly Includes Obtaining specimens of small bowel tissue by means of a small bowel intubation with an endoscope. The procedure is performed under the same conditions as an upper endoscopy except that the endoscopes used are longer for intubation of the small intestine. Fresh specimens of small bowel are sent for histologic analysis and/or other specialized studies (microbiologic culture, enzyme assay, immunocytochemistry).

Indications Small bowel biopsy (SBB) is useful in diagnosing diseases of the duodenum and jejunum safely and rapidly. SBB is an invaluable means of diagnosing primary diseases of the small intestine. In certain cases, it may also be used to diagnose systemic diseases which involve the small bowel

(Continued)

Small Bowel Biopsy *(Continued)*

secondarily. The clinical utility of the SBB depends largely on the diagnoses being considered in an individual case.

SBB is definitely useful in the following diseases (histologic abnormalities are distinctive)[1]:

- Whipple disease
- abetalipoproteinemia
- agammaglobulinemia

SBB is probably useful in the following diseases (mucosal lesions are patchy and may be missed):

- giardiasis
- amyloidosis
- small bowel lymphoma
- eosinophilic gastroenteritis
- intestinal lymphangiectasia
- systemic mastocytosis

SBB is possibly useful in the following diseases (histologic abnormalities may be nonspecific):

- celiac sprue (however, a normal biopsy excludes this disease)
- tropical sprue
- vitamin B_{12} as folate deficiency
- scleroderma
- radiation enteritis

In clinical practice, this procedure is most commonly performed to evaluate malabsorption of uncertain etiology, or diarrhea from the small intestine. SBB may also be used to monitor response to therapy, particularly when the clinical improvement is limited.

Contraindications

- tight stricture
- pyloric obstruction
- uncorrectable coagulopathy
- uncooperative or comatose patient
- contraindications as stated for esophagogastroduodenoscopy (EGD)

Patient Preparation Technique and risks of the procedure are explained to the patient and informed consent is obtained. In some medical centers, formal consultation with gastroenterology staff is mandatory before obtaining a SBB. In other institutions, the procedure may be arranged directly by the ordering physician with the gastroenterology procedure laboratory. The patient should be fasting for 6-8 hours prior to SBB. If a morning procedure is planned, patient is NPO after midnight. If SBB is scheduled for later afternoon, some centers allow a light breakfast that morning. Daily medications are permitted with small sips of water. Due to the risk of bleeding, aspirin products and nonsteroidal anti-inflammatory agents should be discontinued well in advance (at least 5 days for aspirin). If a bleeding disorder is suspected, a complete blood count, prothrombin time (PT), and partial thromboplastin time (PTT) should be drawn.

Aftercare Patient should remain NPO until the topical anesthetic has worn off (usually 1-2 hours). If intravenous sedatives were administered during the procedure, patient should not drive for the remainder of the day. Prior to discharge, patient should be carefully instructed to contact a physician if severe abdominal pain occurs or rectal bleeding is seen.

Complications In the great majority of cases, SBB is a safe procedure. The most serious complication is bleeding. In one reported series, only three bleeding episodes occurred after 4200 small bowel biopsies, and none were severe enough to warrant blood transfusion. Other complications include abdominal pain, bacteremia, and aspiration during passage of the tube or capsule.

Technique A topical anesthetic such as Cetacaine® spray is applied to the pharynx. Intravenous sedation is given for the endoscopic procedure. The endoscopy is performed as described above for EGD except that intubation as far into the small bowel is attempted. The entire procedure may be completed in minutes. Fluoroscopy may be used to document the location of the endoscope in the jejunum. Several devices may be used for biopsy. To increase diagnostic yield, multiple biopsies are usually taken. "Blind biopsies" may be obtained in cases where there are no gross abnormalities seen on endoscopy. If a lesion or mucosal abnormality is present, then directed small bowel biopsy can be performed. Duodenal aspiration may be performed to obtain fluid for quantitative culture for bacterial overgrowth.

Specimen Fresh duodenal or jejunal tissue. All biopsy specimens are sent to the Pathology Laboratory without delay in appropriate containers and fixatives. The details of specimen collection, fixation, and transportation are usually supervised by the gastroenterology team.

Normal Findings No abnormalities seen on gross examination or light microscopy. However, a "normal" biopsy may also be a result of sampling error, especially in small bowel diseases which are "patchy." A formal report is issued by pathologist.

Critical Values Abnormalities are as noted by the pathologist. Examples of histologic patterns in specific disease states include:

- Whipple disease - clusters of periodic acid-Schiff (PAS)-positive macrophages in the lamina propria
- abetalipoproteinemia - vacuolated epithelial cells secondary to fat stores
- intestinal lymphoma - characteristic lymphoma cells in lamina propria and submucosa
- eosinophilic enteritis - mucosa invaded by numerous eosinophils, often patchy
- amyloidosis - amyloid fibrils present on Congo red staining
- giardiasis - parasites visibly adhering to the mucosa
- Crohn disease - noncaseating granulomas identified
- celiac sprue - almost complete absence of villi, hypertrophy, and elongation of crypts, infiltration of mononuclear cells

Additional Information Small bowel biopsy is done in adults as well as children if malabsorption is suspected. Usually these patients exhibit symptoms of chronic diarrhea or steatorrhea, weight loss, failure to thrive, as well as hematologic or laboratory evidence of malabsorption (ie, hypoalbuminemia, anemia, electrolyte abnormality, etc).

Footnotes

1. Greenberger NJ and Isselbacher KJ, "Disorders of Absorption," *Harrison's Principles of Internal Medicine*, 11th ed, Chapter 237, Braunwald E, Isselbacher KJ, Petersdorf RG, et al, eds, New York, NY: McGraw-Hill Inc, 1987, 1260-76.

References

Heizer WD, "Mucosal Biopsy of the Duodenum and Small Bowel in Adult Patients and Duodenal Aspiration," *Manual of Gastroenterologic Procedures*, 3rd ed, Chapter 20, Drossman DA, ed, New York, NY: Raven Press, 1993, 145-9.

Lewis BS, "Endoscopy of the Small Intestine," *Gastrointestinal Endoscopy*, CD-ROM, 2nd ed, Chapter 50, MV Sivak, ed, Philadelphia, PA: WB Saunders Co, 1999.

Perera DR, Weinstein WM, and Rubin CE, "Symposium on Pathology of the Gastrointestinal Tract - Part II. Small Intestinal Biopsy," *Hum Pathol*, 1975, 6(2):157-217.

Weinstein WM, "Gastrointestinal Mucosal Biopsy and Cytology," *Bockus Gastroenterology*, 5th ed, Chapter 29, Haubrich WS, Schaffner F, and Berk JE, eds, Philadelphia, PA: WB Saunders Co, 1995, 355-69.

♦ **Small Intestinal Biopsy** *see* Small Bowel Biopsy *on page 95*

Sphincter of Oddi Manometry

Related Information

Endoscopic Retrograde Cholangiopancreatography *on page 63*

Synonyms Endoscopic Retrograde Cholangiopancreatography (ERCP) With Pressure Measurement of Sphincter of Oddi; Sphincter of Oddi Pressure Measurement or Profile

Procedure Commonly Includes Placement of a manometry catheter within the sphincter of Oddi to diagnose abnormalities in motor function. Performed during the course of ERCP as an optional, adjunctive test. Baseline sphincter pressures are measured by means of a water-filled, pressure-sensitive catheter. A continuous graph of sphincter of Oddi pressure (mm Hg) versus time (seconds) is generated. This procedure is useful in evaluating patients with "idiopathic" pancreatitis, and is based on the concept that intermittent biliary obstruction (and pancreatitis) may result from sphincter of Oddi dysfunction.

(Continued)

Sphincter of Oddi Manometry *(Continued)*

Indications This procedure has only recently gained clinical acceptance, and thus applications are still evolving. Sphincter manometry may be indicated in patients with recurrent pancreatitis with normal ERCP examinations. Recent studies suggest that a subgroup of patients with "idiopathic" recurrent pancreatitis (no structural lesions on ERCP) will demonstrate abnormally elevated resting pressures of the sphincter of Oddi.

Contraindications If a formal ERCP is planned in addition to sphincter of Oddi manometry, contraindications include:

- patient refusal or poor cooperation
- recent attack of acute pancreatitis within the past several weeks
- recent myocardial infarction
- inadequate surgical back-up
- history of contrast dye anaphylaxis

Relative contraindications include:

- poor surgical candidacy; in general patients should be able to tolerate laparotomy if complications arise
- ascites
- severe cardiopulmonary background disease
- overlying residual barium in the GI tract from recent abdominal CT scan, lower GI series, etc

Patient Preparation Since this procedure is performed in conjunction with ERCP, the same considerations apply.

Equipment A triple lumen water-perfused manometry catheter with or without aspiration port is commonly used. This catheter contains side-hole orifices for pressure sensing, spaced approximately 2 mm apart. Each catheter lumen is separately perfused with a low compliance hydraulic system.

Technique After completion of the standard ERCP, contrast dye is allowed to drain from the ducts. The manometry catheter is then advanced through the biopsy channel within the endoscope. Under direct visualization, the catheter is introduced into the papilla of vater and advanced into either the common bile duct or pancreatic duct. Baseline ductal pressures are recorded. The catheter is then withdrawn at 2 mm intervals while continuous pressure measurements are being taken. This has been termed the "station pull-through technique". Pressures within the sphincter of Oddi are obtained, including a baseline resting tone and superimposed phasic contractions. Depending on results, a variety of pharmacologic interventions may be attempted, including:

- cholecystokinin-octapeptide (CCK-OP), which abolishes phasic activity of sphincter of Oddi and increases duodenal contractions
- glucagon, which also eliminates sphincter phasic activity
- pentagastrin, which increases both basal and phasic pressures
- bethanechol, which stimulates sphincter phasic activity and others

Normal Findings Preliminary report is written in chart by the gastroenterologist before the patient leaves the procedure area. Final typewritten report of manometry accompanies final ERCP report.

- baseline (resting) sphincter of Oddi pressure: 15-25 mm Hg
- superimposed phasic pressure waves at sphincter of Oddi: 50-200 mm Hg (3-5 cycles/minute)
- pancreatic duct pressure: 10 mm Hg

Critical Values Abnormalities in either resting pressures and/or phasic pressures. Most common abnormality is increased resting pressure ≥30 mm Hg (without pharmacologic provocation).

Limitations

- clinical indications and applications are limited
- technically difficult procedure
- not available in all gastroenterology laboratories

Additional Information Despite the clinician's best efforts, a small number of patients with recurrent bouts of pancreatitis will continually defy diagnosis. In this problematic group, no clues regarding etiology can be found on clinical examination, noninvasive imaging studies, or ERCP. The syndrome is characterized by recurrent abdominal pain, abnormal liver function tests (often despite prior cholecystectomy), hyperamylasemia, and delayed drainage of contrast material from the biliary tree. Through the years, this clinical presentation has been variously called biliary dyskinesia, papillary stenosis, or sphincter of Oddi spasm. More recently, researchers have found that roughly 20% of such patients with "idiopathic" recurrent pancreatitis manifest significant motor abnormalities in the sphincter of Oddi. Dysfunction of this sphincter may be due to either fixed stenosis (from inflammation or fibrosis) or "functional" abnormalities (motor). Sphincter of Oddi manometry has become the standard means of evaluating the latter condition, supplanting previous criteria such as the Nardi test, sphincter of Oddi biopsy, and delayed drainage of contrast material. Studies have shown that some patients with sphincter of Oddi abnormalities may benefit from surgical intervention. Both sphincteroplasty (with septectomy) and endoscopic sphincterotomy have eliminated attacks of pancreatitis in certain patients.

References

Gilbert DA, DiMarino AJ, Jensen DM, et al, " Status Evaluation: Sphincter of Oddi Manometry," *Gastrointest Endosc*, 1992, 38(6):757-9.

Banks PA, "Acute and Chronic Pancreatitis," *Gastrointestinal and Liver Disease: Pathophysiology, Diagnosis, and Management*, 6th ed, Chapter 48, Feldman M, Scharschmidt BF, and Sleisenger MH, eds, Philadelphia, PA: WB Saunders Co, 1998, 809-62.

Bar-Meir S, Geenen JE, Hogan WJ, et al, "Biliary and Pancreatic Duct Pressures Measured by ERCP Manometry in Patients With Suspected Papillary Stenosis," *Dig Dis Sci*, 1979, 24(3):209-13.

Geenen JE, "New Diagnostic and Treatment Modalities Involving Endoscopic Retrograde Cholangiopancreatography and Esophagogastroduodenoscopy," *Scand J Gastroenterol*, 1982, 77(Suppl):93-106.

Moody FG, Calabuig R, Vecchio R, et al, "Stenosis of the Sphincter of Oddi," *Surg Clin North Am*, 1990, 70(6):1341-54.

Toouli J, Roberts-Thomson IC, Dent J, et al, "Sphincter of Oddi Motility Disorders in Patients With Idiopathic Recurrent Pancreatitis," *Br J Surg*, 1985, 72(11):859-63.

Venu RP, Geenen JE, Hogan W, et al, "Idiopathic Recurrent Pancreatitis. An Approach to Diagnosis and Treatment," *Dig Dis Sci*, 1989, 34(1):56-60.

♦ **Sphincter of Oddi Pressure Measurement or Profile** *see* Sphincter of Oddi Manometry *on page 97*

Standard Acid Reflux Test

Related Information

Bernstein Test *on page 54*
Esophageal Motility Study *on page 68*
pH Study, 12- to 24-Hour *on page 92*

Synonyms Esophagus Acid Reflux Test With Intraluminal pH Electrode for Detection of Reflux; SART; Tuttle Test

Procedure Commonly Includes Placement of a pH probe and manometer into the esophagus to objectively demonstrate the presence of gastroesophageal (GE) reflux. With the patient in a supine position, an abrupt fall in esophageal pH at rest, following strain maneuvers, or after exogenous gastric acid loading indicates acid reflux. This serves as a convenient, introductory test for suspected reflux esophagitis.

Indications

- objectively demonstrate the presence of GE reflux under controlled conditions; particularly useful when the diagnosis of reflux esophagitis is still somewhat in doubt
- evaluate cases of noncardiac chest pain, in which acid reflux is a reasonable possibility
- monitor, in selected cases, the effectiveness of antireflux interventions, both surgical and medical

Contraindications SART requires an alert, cooperative subject who, at the minimum, can perform Valsalva maneuvers, Müeller maneuvers, and leg raises. Thus, for the obtunded, agitated, or critically ill patient this test should be deferred. Other contraindications include active upper GI bleeding, nausea and vomiting, and possibly active peptic ulcer disease. In addition, since passage of the probe/manometer via a nasogastric (NG) approach often engenders a vagal response, patients with malignant cardiac arrhythmias or unstable hemodynamics should be tested with caution, if at all.

Patient Preparation Technique and risks of the procedure are explained and consent is obtained. The patient should be kept NPO at least 8 hours prior to (Continued)

Standard Acid Reflux Test *(Continued)*

testing, and preferably overnight. Avoid antacids and H_2 blockers prior to procedure (check with the GI Laboratory if there are questions regarding medications).

Aftercare The patient may be discharged from GI procedure room providing no complications have occurred. Activity may be *ad libitum* as tolerated and no specific postprocedure restrictions are necessary. If patient experiences pyrosis after the acid-loading step of the procedure, give 30-60 mL antacid. If SART is positive, inform patient that he will be contacted by the referring physician for specific antireflux instructions.

Complications SART is considered quite safe and no significant morbidity or mortality has been reported. Minor complications include nausea, eructation, vagal reactions, and transient dyspepsia (if acid load test is positive), with little long-term clinical significance.

Equipment In GI procedure room: pH electrode probe (eg, Beckman glass electrode or MI-506 flexible microelectrodes), pH meter (eg, Beckman Laboratory model), reference electrode, pen recording device, reference pH solutions, esophageal manometry catheter with transducer equipment (see Esophageal Motility Study *on page 68*), and solutions of 0.1 N HCl

Technique Performed by GI specialist in adequately equipped procedure room. Initially, pH meter and probe are calibrated against standard reference pH solutions. Afterwards, the pH probe may be threaded through the lumen of certain manometry catheters, so that the distal tip of the probe protrudes 1 cm. The probe and catheter assembly are advanced into the stomach, using a nasogastric approach. With the patient in a supine position, gastric pH is recorded (expected value ≤4). The probe is then slowly withdrawn, crossing the lower esophageal sphincter (LES); location of LES is verified by pressure tracings from the manometer. By convention, the probe is then fixed into position 5 cm above the LES. Intraesophageal pH is recorded and compared with gastric pH. If no difference in pH is found between stomach and esophagus, free GE reflux is suspected. If such is the case, instruct patient to make frequent swallows. Failure to raise intraesophageal pH ≥6 despite multiple swallows confirms free GE reflux. Procedure may be stopped at this point. If, however, intraesophageal pH is normal on the initial reading (ie, pH ≥6), four types of straining maneuvers are carried out. In the supine position, patient performs Valsalva maneuvers, Müller maneuvers, and leg raises. In the fourth maneuver, the examiner compresses patient's abdomen by hand. Each maneuver is performed twice. Intraesophageal pH is recorded during and immediately after each event. An abrupt fall in luminal pH may indicate GE reflux (see Critical Values). Eructation, wretching, or belching at this stage may require repetition of some maneuvers since each lowers LES tone. If esophageal pH stays >6 despite these straining maneuvers, the acid-loading step may be performed, especially if clinical suspicion of reflux is still high. The probe and catheter are readvanced into the stomach and 200-300 mL 0.1 N hydrochloric acid is infused. The pH probe is then withdrawn and, as before, positioned 5 cm above the LES. Again, patient performs two sets of the four straining maneuvers (Valsalva, Müller, etc), with frequent pH recordings.

Data Acquired Various pH measurements, as described. Subjective complaints of pyrosis may be noted but are not a part of the SART per se.

Normal Findings pH in esophagus remains >6 despite straining maneuvers and acid loading.

Critical Values

- If pH in esophagus equals pH in stomach (and both ≤4) when patient is supine, acid reflux is present, probably "free" reflux. Failure to raise pH with swallowing saliva further confirms free reflux.
- If the criteria for "free" reflux are not met, positive test for GE reflux may also be defined as an abrupt fall in intraesophageal pH ≤4 during or immediately following any **two** straining maneuvers.
- If the first two criteria are not met, a positive test may still be seen if intraesophageal pH falls to 4 during or immediately after two straining maneuvers during the acid-loading step.

Limitations Severe nausea, emesis, inability to pass catheter back to stomach

References

Benz LJ, Hootkin LA, Margulies S, et al, "A Comparison of Clinical Measurements of Gastroesophageal Reflux," *Gastroenterology*, 1972, 62:1-5.

Orlando RC, "pH Probe for Reflux (Turtle Test)," *Manual of Gastroenterologic Procedures*, 2nd ed, Drossman DA, ed, New York, NY: Raven Press, 1987, 51-4.

Tuttle SG, DeHarello A, and Grossman MI, "Esophageal Acid Perfusion Test and a Gastroesophageal Reflux Test in Patients With Esophagitis," *Gastroenterology*, 1960, 38:861-72.

♦ **Standard Duodenal Intubation Method of Biliary Drainage** *see* Biliary Drainage *on page 55*

♦ **Stool pH Test** *see* Breath Hydrogen Analysis *on page 57*

♦ **Tests for Fecal Reducing Substances** *see* Breath Hydrogen Analysis *on page 57*

♦ **Transduodenal Drainage With CCK** *see* Biliary Drainage *on page 55*

♦ **Transjugular Needle Biopsy of the Liver** *see* Liver Biopsy *on page 82*

♦ **Tuttle Test** *see* Standard Acid Reflux Test *on page 99*

♦ **UGI Endoscopy** *see* Esophagogastroduodenoscopy (EGD) *on page 72*

♦ **Upper Endoscopy** *see* Esophagogastroduodenoscopy (EGD) *on page 72*

♦ **Upper Gastrointestinal Endoscopy** *see* Esophagogastroduodenoscopy (EGD) *on page 72*

GENERAL INTERNAL MEDICINE

Allergy Testing, Intracutaneous (Intradermal)

Related Information

Allergy Testing, Percutaneous *on page 106*
Bronchial Challenge Test *on page 202*
Penicillin Allergy Skin Testing *on page 140*

Synonyms Immediate Hypersensitivity Skin Test; Intracutaneous (Intradermal) Allergy Testing

Procedure Commonly Includes Injection of one or more allergenic substances into the skin, including certain inhalants (grasses, molds, trees, weeds), epidermals (animal dander and house dust), ingestants (foods and food additives), and insect venoms. Intradermal testing is an objective, *in vivo* means of evaluating IgE-mediated hypersensitivity.

Indications

- objectively demonstrate the presence of immediate-type hypersensitivity to foreign substances (allergens) suspected from the clinical history; potential test substances include common allergens to which the atopic individual is often sensitive: pollens, grasses, animal dander, as well as individual substances such as antibiotics (prototype penicillin), stinging insect venom, and certain foods
- determine if allergic disease underlies difficult to manage cases of asthma, rhinitis, dermatitis, angioedema-urticaria, or anaphylaxis
- further evaluate "indeterminate" test results obtained on prior skin prick testing (percutaneous allergy testing)
- follow up on negative skin prick tests when the clinical suspicion for a particular allergen remains high
- document immediate hypersensitivity prior to provocative allergy testing or prior to allergy desensitization therapy (immunotherapy)

Contraindications

- recent use of medications known to inhibit the wheal and flare skin response; this includes antihistamines, hydroxyzine, tricyclic antidepressants, and phenothiazines. Newer antihistamines with longer half-lives may interfere with testing for more than 1 week.
- documented anaphylactic reaction on prior skin testing; any foreign substance causing a serious systemic reaction under controlled test conditions should never be retested in the same individual. Unrelated substances are not necessarily contraindicated but should be approved by the physician.
- known hypersensitivity to a stabilizer or diluent found in some commercial allergen preparations; 0.03% human serum albumin is often used as a stabilizer in solutions used for intradermal testing. The patient should be routinely questioned prior to testing regarding egg allergy.

Patient Preparation Requisition should include current medications, including last dose of antihistamines or other drugs which may interfere with testing; contact physician if these medications have been recently used (see Contraindications). Procedure and risks are explained. Once in testing center, the nurse or physician should perform a brief dermatologic exam to ensure adequate areas of normal appearing skin and to identify the rare patient with dermographism.

Aftercare If no procedural complications have occurred, the patient may be discharged from the testing center. Skin sites should be kept clean until well healed. The patient should contact a physician immediately if 6-8 hours later

(Continued)

Allergy Testing, Intracutaneous (Intradermal) *(Continued)*

symptoms of wheezing, lightheadedness, or shortness of breath develop (the unusual case of a "late phase response").

Special Instructions A physician must be immediately available if skin testing is performed by a nurse or other trained personnel. Emergency equipment should be close by in the rare case of anaphylaxis. Materials such as tourniquets, aqueous epinephrine for injection, needles, and syringes should be conveniently available.

Complications Intradermal testing is generally safe, but the possibility of a systemic reaction does exist as with any mode of allergy skin testing. During intradermal testing, inadvertent overpenetration of the needle beyond the dermis may lead to injection of the allergen into the subepidermal capillary bed (and from there, into the systemic circulation). In contrast, with skin prick testing, the allergen is introduced only into the epidermis and penetration into deeper layers is unlikely. In theory, this may lead to less profound adverse reactions. The incidence of systemic reaction with intradermal testing has been estimated between 0.03% and 0.49%, with at least 14 documented fatalities.[1,2] Systemic reactions include generalized urticaria, hypotension, and anaphylaxis. Local complications are generally minor and resolve quickly; these include subcutaneous hemorrhage (clinically negligible), localized pruritus, and nonspecific irritant reactions. The risk of bacterial infection or hepatitis B is diminishingly small if proper technique is followed and needles are not reused between patients. A "late phase response" has been described and is an unusual and unpredictable occurrence. This occurs 6-18 hours after a positive wheal and flare response; test site(s) develop inflammatory edema or induration which resolves in 24 hours without specific treatment.

Equipment Allergens used for intradermal testing are commercially prepared extracts of foreign substances, buffered in saline solution and stabilized with human serum albumin. Commonly tested substances include:

- inhalants such as trees and shrubs (ash, birch, cottonwood poplar, maple, and others), weeds (ragweed, English plantain, cocklebur, sheep sorrel, and others), grasses (Bermuda, bluegrass, fescue), molds and fungi (*Alternaria, Aspergillus, Fusarium, Mucor*)
- epidermals such as house dust, house mites, feathers, cat and dog dander
- ingestants such as foods, food additives, drugs (penicillin)
- injectants such as drugs or stinging insect venom (*Hymenoptera*)

Hundreds of standardized extracts are available, but not all foreign substances are suitable for intradermal testing. Some have not undergone proper biologic standardization in terms of potency, purity, and efficacy, while others cause immediate irritant skin reactions (not IgE-mediated). Also required are 0.5 mL or 1 mL tuberculin syringes, alcohol swabs, sterile gauze, and 26- to 30-gauge needles. A separate needle and syringe is needed for each allergen.

Technique Physician reviews and confirms selection of allergens. The volar aspect of the arm or forearm is the preferred site for testing. Each allergen is individually drawn up into the tuberculin syringe and bubbles are eliminated to avoid nonspecific "splash reactions". The allergen is then injected into the dermis using a 27-gauge needle angled at approximately 45°. The volume of solution injected should be enough to raise a small bleb 2 mm in diameter, usually 0.01-0.02 mL. Larger volumes (more than 0.05 mL) may result in nonimmunologic irritant skin reactions (false-positives). Needle and syringe are discarded. Serial intradermal injections may be made in this fashion but must be adequately spaced (>2 cm apart) to avoid errors in interpretation. A negative and positive skin test control is often included, consisting of saline and histamine, respectively.

Data Acquired Test sites are examined at 15-20 minutes for a wheal and flare reaction. Late phase reactions occurring more than 6 hours later are not recorded because their significance is not known. The largest diameter of the wheal and/or erythema is measured and recorded in millimeters.

Normal Findings No wheal or erythema found at allergen test sites. The histamine control site should be positive and saline control site (if used) should be negative.

Critical Values A wheal >5 mm with accompanying erythema is considered a positive test. This was defined in a position paper from the American College of Physicians.[3] A number of alternative grading schemes are also commonly used in clinical practice. However, the specific criteria applied in these grading schemes vary considerably, and this lack of consistency is a potential source of confusion and error.[4] One such system is as follows:

- 0: wheal and erythema <5 mm
- 1+: wheal 5-10 mm; erythema 11-20 mm
- 2+: wheal; erythema 21-30 mm
- 3+: pseudopods; erythema 31-40 mm
- 4+: wheal >15 mm or pseudopods; erythema >40 mm

Intradermal allergy testing plays an integral role in the evaluation of the patient with suspected allergic disease. Following the history and physical examination, it is considered by some as the initial diagnostic test of choice to objectively confirm the presence of allergic disease. Some individuals have symptomatic IgE-mediated hypersensitivity to multiple common environmental substances (pollens, grass, animal dander, etc), and are termed "atopic". These allergic reactions in atopic individuals represent a type I Gell and Coombs' reaction. That is, an individual exposed to a relevant allergen (one to which he has been previously sensitized) manifests a characteristic series of immunologic events. Mast cells are activated, leading to release of inflammatory mediators such as histamines, leukotrienes, and eosinophil chemotactic factors. This process is mediated by IgE antibodies. Clinical manifestations of this immediate hypersensitivity are variable and include bronchospasm, urticaria, rhinitis, food allergy, and even anaphylaxis. Nonatopic individuals may also develop IgE-mediated hypersensitivity. Often, there is sensitivity to only one substance, such as stinging insect venom. Intradermal testing is useful in documenting IgE-mediated allergy in both atopic and nonatopic individuals. Intradermal testing induces a characteristic inflammatory response in the skin when the proper antigen is reintroduced into a sensitive patient. Mast cells in the skin release histamine, causing increased vascular permeability and dilation of blood vessels. This "wheal and flare" dermal response is seen with IgE-mediated allergy, regardless of whether the patient's main symptoms are located in the airways, skin, nasal mucosa, gastrointestinal tract, etc. Proper interpretation of skin test results requires consideration of the history and physical in each case. Even if technical errors are minimized (see Limitations), test results cannot be interpreted in isolation. A positive test result by itself does not necessarily denote clinical allergy. Strictly speaking, a positive skin response indicates only a state of potential hypersensitivity, a heightened immunologic reactivity towards a particular allergen. Instances of positive skin tests in asymptomatic, nonallergic individuals have been well documented. Symptoms characteristic of allergic disease (rhinorrhea, sneezing, wheezing, etc) may result from:

- true allergic disease with a positively reacting intradermal test
- allergic disease with a negatively reacting skin test (false-negative from technical error)
- allergic disease caused by a substance not tested
- nonimmunologic, non-IgE mediated disease

By itself, the intradermal test does not definitively discriminate between these possibilities and does not prove causality. If a positive skin test occurs in response to an allergen strongly suspected from the history, most clinicians would consider that allergen the likely etiology of symptoms. A negative skin test occurring with a substance not suspected from the history strongly rules out that substance as the cause of allergic symptoms. The relevance of a positive test occurring with an allergen not suspected from the history and physical is problematic and may require repeat testing or further serologic or provocative allergy testing. A negative skin test occurring with an allergen strongly suspected from the history should be repeated carefully with attention

(Continued)

Allergy Testing, Intracutaneous (Intradermal) *(Continued)*

to technical factors; a repeatedly negative result casts doubt on the substance as the cause of symptoms.

Limitations

False-positives may result from the following:

- nonspecific irritant skin reactions interpreted as positive. This is a significant problem with intradermal testing. The volume of test substance introduced with intradermal injection is considerably greater than that used with skin prick testing, making the intradermal test potentially "too sensitive".
- hemorrhage at injection site interpreted as erythema
- dermographism interpreted as a wheal
- allergen contaminating neighboring sites
- test sites too close together
- impurities or contaminants in allergen preparations or the use of nonstandardized test materials
- small wheals (eg, 2 mm) interpreted as positive

False-negatives may result from the following:

- subcutaneous (not intradermal) injection of allergen
- waning allergen potency or improper volume or concentration
- drugs such as H_1 antagonists, hydroxyzine, tricyclic antidepressants, phenothiazines, dopamine
- active skin disease such as atopic dermatitis
- possibly extremes of age

Additional Information Intradermal testing is more expensive and time-consuming than the skin prick test. Both procedures evaluate the presence of IgE-mediated hypersensitivity. Although some physicians screen patients with suspected allergic disease by using intradermal testing exclusively, others begin with the more convenient prick test and follow up on negative or equivocal results with the more sensitive intradermal test. Positive results obtained on the skin prick test generally do not mandate further intradermal testing with the same antigen. Technically, intradermal allergy tests and the tuberculin skin test are performed in a nearly identical manner. However, the latter evaluates type IV cell-mediated immunity (delayed hypersensitivity) rather than type I antibody-mediated immunity (immediate hypersensitivity). This is due to the nature of the host immune response. Individuals exposed to *Mycobacterium tuberculosis* (MTB), for example, characteristically develop type IV cell-mediated immunity rather than IgE-mediated hypersensitivity. The skin response to intradermal injection of MTB antigen usually consists of erythema and induration at 24-48 hours, not an immediate wheal and flare reaction.

Footnotes

1. Bousquet J, Demoly P, and Michel FB, "*In Vivo* Methods for Study of Allergy: Skin Tests, Techniques, and Interpretation," *Allergy, Principles and Practice*, 5th ed, Chapter 32, Middleton E Jr, Reed CE, Ellis EF, et al, eds, St Louis, MO: CV Mosby Co, 1998, 430-39.
2. Nelson HS, "Diagnostic Procedures in Allergy. I. Allergy Skin Testing," *Ann Allergy*, 1983, 51(4):411-8.
3. Terr AI, "Allergic Diseases," *Basic and Clinical Immunology*, 6th ed, Stites DP, Stabo JD, and Wells JV, eds, Norwalk, CT: Appleton and Lange, 1987, 435-56.
4. VanArsdel PP Jr and Larson EB, "Diagnostic Tests for Patients With Suspected Allergic Disease. Utility and Limitations," *Ann Intern Med*, 1989, 110(4):304-12.

Allergy Testing, Percutaneous

Related Information

Allergy Testing, Intracutaneous (Intradermal) *on page 103*
Fungal Skin Testing *on page 122*
Penicillin Allergy Skin Testing *on page 140*

Synonyms Immediate Hypersensitivity Skin Test; Percutaneous Allergy Testing; Prick Test; Puncture Test; Scratch Test; Skin Prick Test

Procedure Commonly Includes Skin testing patients with suspected immediate-type hypersensitivity to one or more environmental substances. The test is performed by placing a drop of allergen(s) on the skin and making a needleprick through the drop(s) and into the underlying epidermis. Puncture sites are examined over the next 20 minutes for a wheal and flare skin response which, if present, indicates antibody-mediated (IgE) hypersensitivity to the test allergen.

Indications

- confirm the presence of immediate-type hypersensitivity to foreign substances (allergens) suspected from the patient's clinical history; in addition to commonly encountered allergens (eg, pollens, animal dander, grasses, molds, house dust) other potential test substances include antibiotics, stinging insect venom, and a variety of foods
- determine whether environmental allergens are playing a role in difficult to manage cases of asthma, urticaria, eczema, or anaphylaxis
- document immediate hypersensitivity prior to more elaborate allergy testing, such as provocation testing (bronchial provocation, oral food provocation) or prior to allergy desensitization therapy (immunotherapy)

Contraindications

- use of antihistamine medications (H_1 antagonists) within 48 hours of skin testing; antihistamines may inhibit the wheal and flare response, potentially causing false-negative results. Newer antihistamines with longer half-lives may interfere with testing for more than 1 week.
- use of hydroxyzine (Atarax®) within 1 week of testing
- documented anaphylactic reaction on prior percutaneous testing; allergens causing systemic reaction under test conditions should never be retested in the same patient. Unrelated substances, however, are not necessarily contraindicated but require physician approval.
- known systemic reaction to stabilizers or diluents contained in some allergen preparations; albumin is sometimes used as a stabilizer in commercial preparations; some testing centers routinely question patients regarding egg allergy

Patient Preparation Requisition should include current medications, including last dose of antihistamines if applicable. Contact physician if there has been recent use of antihistamines or hydroxyzine (see Contraindications). Procedures and risks are explained to the patient beforehand. Once in the testing center, a brief dermatologic exam should be performed to ensure adequate areas of normal appearing skin for test purposes (and to identify the rare case of dermographism).

Aftercare If no adverse reaction has occurred postprocedure, patient is free to leave testing area. Instruct patient to keep the skin puncture sites clean until well healed. The patient should contact a physician immediately if symptoms of dyspnea, wheezing, lightheadedness, severe pruritus, etc develop later that day (the rare case of "late phase response").

Special Instructions Prior to testing, patient ideally should undergo a complete medical history and physical, with attention to allergy-related signs and symptoms. This allows a more directed and rational selection of antigens to be tested. Although skin testing may be performed by nurses or other trained personnel, a physician must be immediately available at all times to treat the rare case of anaphylaxis. Emergency equipment should be conveniently located and should include tourniquets, aqueous epinephrine, syringes, etc.

Complications The most common complication is a mild pruritus localized to positive test sites, usually resolving overnight. The incidence of significant bleeding or superficial skin infection is diminishingly low. However, as with other types of allergy skin testing, the possibility of systemic reaction exists. The exact incidence is unclear, but is felt to be rare and only at a case report level. It is generally regarded as safer than the closely related intradermal allergy test (estimated incidence of systemic reaction in the latter is >0.03%). Reported complications include generalized urticaria and anaphylaxis.

Equipment Allergens used for prick testing are commercially prepared liquid extracts of a wide variety of foreign substances, numbering in the hundreds. It should be noted that some commercial allergens have not undergone biologic standardization for potency and purity. In addition, other allergen extracts are known to cause nonimmunologic irritant skin reactions which cannot be interpreted (codeine, radiographic contrast dye). Thus, not all foreign substances are suitable for skin testing. Commonly used allergen extracts include:
(Continued)

Allergy Testing, Percutaneous *(Continued)*

- trees (cottonwood, poplar, ash, birch, maple, oak, elm, hickory, pecan, and others)
- weeds (including ragweed, English plantain, sorrel-dock, pigweed)
- grasses (Timothy, Johnson, Bermuda, fescue, bluegrass)
- molds or fungi (*Alternaria, Fusarium, Hormodendrum, Aspergillus, Mucor*); hypersensitivity to *Aspergillus fumigatus* is often tested in patients with suspected allergic bronchopulmonary aspergillosis (ABPA)
- epidermals (house dust, house mites, feathers, cat and dog dander).

Standardized extracts are also available for foods, antibiotics, and insect venoms. Most prick test allergens are stabilized in 50% glycerol to prevent spontaneous degradation (human serum albumin is more often used as a stabilizer with intradermal testing). A supply of 27-gauge disposable hypodermic needles is also required, one needle for each allergen. Various automatic lancet devices and reusable solid needles are being promoted as alternatives to the hollow needle (possibly with some cost savings), but these devices remain optional.

Technique The physician reviews and confirms selection of allergens to be tested. Preferred test areas are the back or volar aspect of the forearm. A drop of each allergen is individually placed in a predetermined location on the skin. Usually less than 30 allergens are tested in one session and drops are placed in parallel rows approximately 2 cm apart. A 27-gauge needle is then passed through the drop at a 20° angle and the epidermis is penetrated with a stabbing motion. The needle tip is lifted slightly to tent the skin upwards, with care taken not to induce bleeding, and the needle is then removed. This constitutes the "prick" or "puncture". Over 30 separate pricks may be made in this fashion in several minutes using a new needle for each allergen. The drop of solution is wiped off 1 minute after needle puncture (some physicians prefer to wait up to 20 minutes). Frequently, a negative and positive skin test control is included in the test battery consisting of glycerol and histamine, respectively. Minor variations in the overall techniques may be necessary if optional devices (such as the Morrow Brown needle) are used. Important differences exist between the prick test (described previously) and the technically similar "scratch test". In the scratch test a superficial linear abrasion is made in the epidermis (instead of a "prick") and a drop of allergen is placed on the scratch. Multiple scratches are often required. This technique has fallen out of favor due to a high incidence of nonimmunologic irritant reactions, patient discomfort, scar formation, and poor reproducibility.

Data Acquired Test sites are examined for a wheal and erythema reaction, maximal at 15-20 minutes. Late phase reactions (6-8 hours) are not recorded routinely since their significance is unclear. Largest diameter of the wheal and/or erythema is measured and recorded in millimeters. Alternatively, the shape of wheal and flare may be permanently recorded by placing transparent paper directly onto the patient's back and outlining the skin reaction with a pen. Advanced techniques using ultrasound or Doppler flowmetry of the skin reaction are still primarily research tools.

Normal Findings No wheal or erythema at test sites except for histamine control

Critical Values A wheal <5 mm in transverse diameter is of questionable significance. A wheal >5 mm with accompanying erythema constitutes a positive test, as defined in a position paper issued by the American College of Physicians.[1] In clinical practice, grading systems are often employed, but grading criteria lack uniformity. One example is as follows:

- negative: no reaction
- 1+: no wheal, erythema <20 mm
- 2+: no wheal, erythema >20 mm
- 3+: definite wheal and erythema
- 4+: pseudopods, wheal and erythema

In this system, grades 2+ through 4+ are considered positive. The evaluation of the patient with suspected allergic disease is based on the history, physical examination, and allergy skin tests. Some individuals suffer from antibody (IgE) - mediated sensitivity to multiple commonly encountered substances, such as pollens, grass, and animal dander. These symptomatic individuals are termed "atopic" and represent approximately 10% of the population in the United States. Nonatopic individuals may also develop IgE-mediated allergy, as in the case of acquired hypersensitivity to insect venom. Percutaneous allergy testing is an *in vivo* method of identifying afflicted individuals in both these groups and identifying the most likely causative agents. Allergic reactions of the immediate hypersensitivity variety represent type I Gell and Coombs' reactions. Exposure to a relevant allergen (true antigen) leads to mast cell activation with release of mediators of inflammation such as histamine, leukotrienes, and eosinophil chemotactic factors. This process is mediated by IgE antibodies. A wide spectrum of symptoms may be seen in association with allergic disease and ranges from rhinitis, dermatitis, and asthma to urticaria-angioedema and anaphylaxis.

It should be noted that each of these conditions may also be caused by nonallergic mechanisms without direct involvement of the host immune system. Percutaneous allergy testing may be useful in this setting, as in differentiating allergic from nonallergic asthma. When a sensitized individual is re-exposed to antigen by means of the prick test, the skin undergoes characteristic inflammatory changes. Mast cells in the skin release histamine causing increased vascular permeability and vasodilatation. This dermal response, the wheal and flare, is uniformly seen in patients with IgE-mediated disease regardless of the location of the patient's presenting symptoms: nasal mucosa, skin, airways, or gastrointestinal tract. Prick testing has been critically evaluated in the medical literature and found to have acceptable sensitivity, specificity, and reliability for clinical practice. The challenge in prick testing lies not in its technical aspects but in the interpretation of a positive or negative result. A number of potential false-positive and false-negative results may complicate interpretation (see Limitations). Yet, even if these usually procedural errors are eliminated, correct interpretation requires consideration of the clinical history and physical along with skin test results. A positive test by itself indicates only a state of potential hypersensitivity, a heightened immunologic reactivity towards a particular allergen. In a study involving scratch testing of college students, 17% of asymptomatic subjects had one or more positive skin tests, indicating that immunologic sensitivity may exist in the absence of symptoms.[2] There is no guarantee that a positive reacting allergen is the cause of a patient's symptoms (rhinorrhea, bronchospasm, etc). Symptoms of allergic disease may be caused by:

- a positive reacting test material (true positive)
- a negative reacting test material (false-negative)
- a foreign substance not tested
- nonimmunologic, non-IgE-mediated disease

By itself, the prick test does not prove causality. If a positive skin test occurs with an allergen strongly suspected from the history, most clinicians consider this presumptive evidence of causality. Similarly, a negative test occurring with a test substance of low suspicion effectively rules out that substance as the cause of a patient's symptoms. The clinical relevance of a positive test occurring with an allergen not suspected from clinical presentation is very problematic and may require repeat testing or further serologic or provocative testing. A negative skin test occurring with an allergen strongly suspected from the history may require follow-up with the somewhat more sensitive intradermal allergy test.

Limitations False-positives: nonspecific irritant reactions; dermographism interpreted as a wheal; hemorrhage at prick site interpreted as erythema; allergen spread from one site to another when the same needle is reused; small wheals (eg, 2 mm) interpreted as significant; impurities or contaminants in allergen preparations; test sites improperly spaced; inappropriate allergen concentrations

False-negatives: waning potency of allergens; inadequate concentration of allergen; technical errors in epidermal puncture; drugs such as H_1 antagonists, hydroxyzine, tricyclic antidepressants, phenothiazines, dopamine; skin diseases such as atopic dermatitis; possibly extremes of age

(Continued)

Allergy Testing, Percutaneous *(Continued)*

Additional Information Some allergists test for immediate hypersensitivity exclusively with the prick test, while others use intradermal testing instead. The prick test is simpler, faster, safer, and possibly less painful to the patient than intradermal testing. However, there is a higher rate of false-negatives and sensitivity is somewhat less. A common compromise is to begin evaluation of the allergic individual with the prick test and follow up indeterminate reactions or negative reactions of strongly suspected allergens with the intradermal test.

Footnotes

1. "Allergy Testing." American College of Physicians, *Ann Intern Med*, 1989, 110(4):317-20.
2. Hagy GW and Settipane GA, "Prognosis of Positive Allergy Skin Tests in an Asymptomatic Population: A Three Year Follow-up of College Students," *J Allergy Clin Immunol*, 1971, 48(4):200-11.

References

Council on Scientific Affairs, "*In Vivo* Diagnostic Testing and Immunotherapy for Allergy: Report 1, Part II, of the Allergy Panel," *JAMA*, 1987, 258(11):1505-8.

Demoly P, Michel F, and Bousquet J, "*In Vivo* Methods for Study of Allergy: Skin Tests, Techniques, and Interpretation," *Allergy: Principles and Practice*, 5th ed, Middleton E Jr, Reed CE, Ellis E, et al, eds, St Louis, MO: CV Mosby Co, 1998, 430-4.

Van Arsdel PP Jr and Larson EB, "Diagnostic Tests for Patients With Suspected Allergic Disease. Utility and Limitations," *Ann Intern Med*, 1989, 110(4):304-12.

♦ **Anergy Control Panel** *see* Anergy Skin Test Battery *on page 110*

Anergy Skin Test Battery

Related Information

Fungal Skin Testing *on page 122*
Tuberculin Skin Testing, Intracutaneous *on page 144*

Synonyms Anergy Control Panel; Anergy Skin Testing; Delayed Reaction Intracutaneous Tests; Skin Test Battery

Procedure Commonly Includes Intradermal injection of several common antigenic substances to which a cell-mediated immune response would be expected. Anergy skin testing utilizes recall antigens such as *Candida*, mumps, *Trichophyton*, and other substances as a way of evaluating cell-mediated, delayed-type hypersensitivity (DTH) responses *in vivo*. Most of the general population has had contact or infection with one or more of the skin test antigens, and would be expected to have a cutaneous reaction when re-exposed to a "recall antigen." Skin injection sites are examined at 48-72 hours. The development of local induration to one or more antigens indicates adequate delayed hypersensitivity response and implies relatively competent T-cell function. Failure to respond to all of the skin test antigens is termed cutaneous anergy and can be seen in a variety of medical conditions and at the extremes of age.

Indications

- assess the cellular immune system, especially in patients with suspected immunodeficiency syndromes (inherited or acquired). Often this procedure is performed as part of an initial assessment of the immune system in patients with recurrent infections, involuntary weight loss, or other symptoms to suggest a defect in the cell-mediated immune system.
- serve as "control" skin tests when given in conjunction with a tuberculin skin test (PPD test). In the past, the assumption has been that persons who react adequately to anergy skin testing have intact DTH responses and a negative PPD skin test result in an individual could be safely interpreted as a true negative (ie, no infection with *M. tuberculosis*). Similarly, a person who had inadequate DTH responses and failed to respond to the skin test antigens would also fail to respond to PPD skin testing, even if infected with *M. tuberculosis*. Anergy skin testing was particularly important in the HIV-infected person given the high rates of both tuberculosis and cutaneous anergy, and anergy skin testing has been routinely used to help interpret PPD skin test results. However, recent guidelines from the Centers for Disease Control and Prevention (CDC,1998) no longer recommend routine anergy skin testing in conjunction with PPD testing for screening for tuberculosis in persons with HIV (see Additional Information). Physicians may decide to administer anergy tests along with

the PPD on a case-by-case basis, but the usefulness of the anergy test is probably limited.

- provide prognostic information in persons infected with HIV; recent data suggest that anergy skin testing may provide additional information about disease progression and death in persons with HIV, independent of $CD4^+$ cell counts. Some researchers have also reported that anergy skin testing may provide prognostic information in other situations such as sepsis, cancer, and postoperative complications.

Contraindications

- history of hypersensitivity reaction to any of the antigens included in the skin battery
- history of hypersensitivity to eggs or egg products, or to stabilizer or diluent used in commercial antigen preparations. For example, commercially available mumps skin test antigen is derived from virus incubated in chicken embryo and preserved in thimerosal (a mercury derivative). **The mumps skin test antigen is contraindicated in persons with a history of hypersensitivity to eggs or egg products.**
- history of hypersensitivity to **thimerosal** (or mercury products)
- the safety and efficacy of some of the antigens has not been demonstrated in pregnancy and should be avoided unless clearly needed. The safety of the mumps antigen in children has not been established. The safety and efficacy of the mumps antigen in young adults who have been immunized with the mumps vaccine is unknown.

The use of corticosteroids is not necessarily a contraindication for anergy skin testing, although individuals are likely to be anergic. However, some studies suggest that anergy skin testing may still be accurate if performed up to 1 week after starting corticosteroids.

Patient Preparation Due to the risk of anaphylactic reaction associated with any type of allergy skin testing including anergy skin testing, epinephrine injection (1:1000) should be immediately available. Procedure and risks are explained to the patient. No specific skin preparation is necessary. However, those patients with generalized skin disease, such as psoriasis, should be examined beforehand to ensure that there are suitable areas of normal appearing skin. Although testing need not be performed by a physician, one should be immediately available in the event of a systemic reaction.

Aftercare If no adverse reaction has occurred within 30 minutes, patient may be discharged from the testing center. Test sites should be kept reasonably clean for 72 hours. No restrictions on bathing are necessary. The patient should contact a physician if severe local reactions develop, extensive erythema beyond the test site occurs, or if fever, dyspnea, or lightheadedness develops.

Special Instructions Requisition should include a list of all current medications, with attention to corticosteroids or other immunosuppressive agents.

Equipment As of this writing (January 2000) only mumps and *Candida* skin test antigens have been approved by the U.S. Food and Drug Administration (FDA). Mumps skin test antigen has been approved for some years prior to the more recent approval of the *Candida* skin test antigen. A number of other antigens have been used for anergy skin testing, most of which are allergenic extracts usually employed in allergy testing. Allergens such as tetanus toxoid and *Trichophyton* are frequently included in the skin test battery because exposure to these substances in the general population is expected and most individuals should have a positive DTH response. However, limited information is available regarding the sensitivity and specificity of the various skin test antigens used together.

The optimal choice of antigens and the total number employed has yet to be determined. Most test centers use less than five antigens in their routine battery, but considerable variation exists. Different preparation, dilutions, and dosages are used for even the more commonly used antigens. In one literature review, more than 30 different antigens were found to be in routine use at major centers. Palmer, et al discovered that 90% of 750 hospitalized patients reacted to one or more of the following: mumps, *Candida*, *Trichophyton*, and tuberculin.[1] Increasing the total number of antigens improved the rate of skin reactions by only 1%. A typical anergy battery might include *Candida*,

(Continued)

Anergy Skin Test Battery *(Continued)*

measles, *Trichophyton*, and mumps. The CDC feels that the number of antigens used is influenced by the purpose of the anergy testing in an individual. If the main issue is to avoid misdiagnosing anergic persons as nonanergic, then two antigens are sufficient. If the issue is to avoid misdiagnosing immunocompetent persons as anergic, then multiple antigens might be indicated.

Other equipment necessary includes disposable plastic tuberculin syringes, along with 26- or 27-gauge short (1/4" to 1/2") needles, alcohol pads, and gauze pads.

Technique An alternative technique, Multitest CMI®, has been in use for several years. This multiple-puncture device is FDA approved and includes seven standardized antigens and one diluent which are injected simultaneously into the dermis. Antigens included are tetanus toxoid, diphtheria toxoid, streptococcal antigen, *Proteus*, tuberculin, *Candida*, and *Trichophyton*. This device obviates the need for separate syringes, needles, and antigens. The use of the Multitest CMI® may prove to be limited by factors such as availability and cost.

Mantoux method: All of the antigens must be injected **intradermally**. A subcutaneous injection may lead to no reaction. Antigens are injected separately. Antigens are individually drawn up into tuberculin syringes immediately prior to testing. The volar aspects of the arms or forearms are the preferred test sites. Only normal appearing skin should be used. Sites are prepared with alcohol swabs. Using a 26- or 27-gauge needle, each antigen is injected intradermally at a 45° angle, bevel down. A small bleb approximately 2-3 mm in diameter should be raised; usually an injected volume of 0.05 mL is sufficient. Care should be taken to avoid deeper subcutaneous injections. Each antigen is separately planted in this fashion with adequate spacing between injection sites (>2 cm).

Multipuncture method: Antigens are placed simultaneous by means of the Multitest® CMI device. Seven antigens and one glycerol control are standardized with respect to selection and concentration and are preloaded onto this disposable plastic device. A different antigen coats each of seven multiple puncture heads, which are spaced approximately 2 cm apart, in two parallel rows of four. The skin over the forearm is held taut. The device is then oriented per manufacturer's instructions ("T" bar towards the head) and applied to the skin with a rocking motion. Each head must sufficiently puncture the skin. Regardless of technique, all test sites should be examined immediately and at 24, 48, and 72 hours. Date and time of injection must be recorded. The precise location, identity, and concentration of each antigen should be recorded, most often in a pictorial format or standardized table. It may be helpful to circle and label each antigen with a waterproof pen directly onto the skin, but this must not replace formal notations in the medical chart.

Data Acquired The transverse diameter of induration at each test site should be carefully measured by both inspection and palpation. Results are recorded in millimeters at the appropriate 24-hour intervals. Areas of erythema are also measured but play a minor role in most grading schemes.

Normal Findings Normal individuals should demonstrate a positive skin reaction to one or more test antigens.

Critical Values A positive skin test is usually defined as the presence of induration and accompanying erythema ≥5 mm in transverse diameter at an injection site at 24, 48, or 72 hours. Immediate skin reactions (ie, within minutes) are due to mechanisms other than cellular immunity and do not define a positive test. When the Multitest® CMI system is used, induration ≥2 mm in transverse diameter is considered significant. This disparity in definition between the intradermal and multiple puncture technique results from a variety of technical factors including volume of antigen introduced, depth of skin penetration, etc.

A state of anergy is defined as an inability to mount an appropriate delayed hypersensitivity response. In clinical practice this is manifested as a complete absence of reactivity to a skin test battery of at least four to five antigens. Some authorities require repetition of the test battery at least once before labeling a patient "anergic". Normal individuals are expected to develop a positive skin test in response to at least one antigen, barring technical error. Anergy may be present as a generalized defect in T-cell function, as in sarcoidosis, AIDS, or tuberculosis, or as a specific defect in cellular immunity, as in mucocutaneous candidiasis where T-cell response to *Candida* is selectively deficient. There are numerous causes of anergy and these may be categorized as follows:

- infections: bacterial, tuberculosis, disseminated fungal infections, viral (influenza, mumps, mononucleosis, hepatitis, and others), parasitic
- congenital: cell-mediated deficiency (DiGeorge syndrome), combined cellular and humoral deficiency (Nezelof's, Wiskott-Aldrich syndrome, etc)
- acquired/iatrogenic: neoplasms (solid tumors, lymphomas, leukemias), medications (corticosteroids, antineoplastic agents, methotrexate, and others), AIDS
- rheumatic diseases: rheumatoid arthritis, lupus, Behçet disease
- miscellaneous: uremia, diabetes mellitus, inflammatory bowel disease, sarcoidosis, extremes of age, malnutrition

Limitations "Traditional" skin test battery limitations, mentioned previously, include variation in selection and total number of antigens used as well as a lack of standardization of antigen potency. However, some practitioners consider the inability to select and interchange antigens in the Multitest® CMI system a major drawback.

False-positive reactions may occur when:

- an immediate wheal and flare is interpreted as delayed hypersensitivity
- intradermal bleeding is interpreted as erythema
- dermographism is present

False-negative reactions may be caused by:

- lack of antigen potency
- subcutaneous injection
- inadequate dose or concentration
- incomplete skin puncture by the Multitest® device
- attenuated skin response, as in atopic dermatitis

Additional Information The most common use of the anergy skin test has been in conjunction with the PPD skin test. In 1991, the CDC recommended routine anergy testing in HIV-infected persons who were undergoing PPD testing for assessment of latent tuberculosis. HIV-infected persons who were at risk for tuberculosis but were PPD negative and anergic were considered candidates for isoniazid preventive therapy. Since then, a number of studies have shown significant difficulties in interpreting the anergy battery for HIV-infected persons, and challenged the recommendation for isoniazid treatment for PPD negative/anergic persons. In 1998, the CDC issued revised guidelines which do not recommend the routine use of anergy testing when screening for tuberculosis in HIV-infected persons in the U.S.

This change in recommendation for HIV-infected persons is based in part on the following observations.

- There remains considerable variability in the methodology of anergy skin testing
- Persons with active tuberculosis may demonstrate selective nonreactivity to PPD (ie, adequate DTH on anergy testing but PPD negative). Thus, reactivity to one or more skin test antigens in a person with a negative PPD test placed simultaneously does not prove a lack of infection from *M. tuberculosis*.
- Persons may have a positive PPD test but do not respond to other skin test antigens. This was demonstrated mainly in areas of the world where tuberculin reactivity was high, but has also been reported in populations where tuberculin skin reactivity was low.
- The results of anergy skin tests can be inconsistent and unpredictable in an HIV-infected individual when repeated over time.
- There is no definite association between anergy and the risk of developing active TB in persons with HIV. Several studies have shown such a relationship but others have not.
- Empiric isoniazid treatment of HIV-infected persons who are anergic and PPD negative does not appear to reduce the rate of active tuberculosis.

(Continued)

Anergy Skin Test Battery *(Continued)*

The CDC states that anergy testing in HIV-infected persons may be useful in individual situations but the individual patient's risk of exposure to tuberculosis and possibility of infection with TB should be taken into account.

Footnotes

1. Palmer D and Reed W, "Delayed Hypersensitivity Skin Testing: I. Response in a Hospitalized Population," *J Infect Dis*, 1973, 130:132-7.

References

Blatt SP, Hendrix CW, Butzin CA, et al, "Delayed-Type Hypersensitivity Skin Testing Predicts Progression to AIDS in HIV-Infected Patients," *Ann Intern Med*, 1993, 119(3):177-84.

Centers for Disease Control and Prevention, "Anergy Skin Testing and Preventive Therapy for HIV-Infected Persons: Revised Recommendations," *MMWR Morb Mortal Wkly Rep*, 1998, 46(No. RR-15).

Huebner RE, Schein MF, Hall CA, et al, "Delayed-Type Hypersensitivity Anergy in Human Immunodeficiency Virus-Infected Persons Screened for Infection With *Mycobacterium tuberculosis*," *Clin Infect Dis*, 1994, 19(1):26-32.

Wright PW, Crutcher JE, and Holiday DB, "Selection of Skin Test Antigens to Evaluate PPD Anergy," *J Fam Pract*, 1995, 41(1):59-64.

♦ **Anergy Skin Testing** *see* Anergy Skin Test Battery *on page 110*

Arthrocentesis

Related Information

Ingestion Challenge Test *on page 125*

Synonyms Closed Joint Aspiration; Joint Tap

Procedure Commonly Includes Passing a needle into a joint space and aspirating synovial fluid for diagnostic analysis

Indications

Diagnostic indications include:

- joint effusions of unknown etiology
- arthritis of unclear etiology
- all cases of suspected infectious arthritis (bacterial, fungal, tuberculous)
- confirmation of a diagnosis strongly suspected on clinical grounds, such as suspected gout in patients with podagra
- monitoring synovial fluid response to antibiotic therapy in established cases of septic arthritis

Therapeutic indications include:

- decompression of a tense, painful joint effusion
- evacuation of pus in bacterial arthritis (repeated closed drainage)
- removal of inflammatory cells and crystals in selected cases of gout or pseudogout
- intra-articular injection of corticosteroids

Contraindications

- local infection along the proposed needle entrance tract (eg, overlying cellulitis, periarticular infection)
- uncooperative patient, especially if unable to keep the joint immobile throughout procedure
- difficult to identify boney landmarks
- a poorly accessible joint space, as in hip aspiration in the obese patient
- inability to demonstrate a joint effusion on physical examination, except when septic arthritis is strongly suspected (and effusions may be barely detectable)

In addition, some authors consider bacteremia (documented or suspected) a contraindication to arthrocentesis based on the theoretical concern of seeding a sterile joint when the entering needle ruptures surrounding capillaries. No data is available to support or refute this. Clinical judgment must be individualized in each case. If infectious arthritis is suspected, arthrocentesis should be promptly performed even with documented bacteremia. However, more elective indications for the procedure, such as corticosteroid injection, should be deferred, at physician's discretion.

Patient Preparation Procedure and risks are explained and consent is obtained. No intravenous pain medications or sedatives are required.

Aftercare Determined by results of procedure, as outlined by physician. May range from joint immobilization with passive range of motion, as in septic arthritis, to full weight-bearing, as in effusions secondary to osteoarthritis. No specific joint positioning postprocedure has been demonstrated to reduce complications.

Complications Arthrocentesis is a generally safe procedure, especially when performed on a large, easily accessible joint such as the knee. Potential complications include:

- iatrogenic joint space infection (if properly performed, incidence has been estimated at 1 in 15,000 cases)
- hemorrhage or hematoma formation (usually when alternative approaches are used and blood vessels are ruptured on the flexor surface of the joint)
- local pain caused by needle trauma to the periosteum
- injury to cartilage, particularly problematic due to slow repair rate
- tendon rupture
- nerve palsies

Equipment Alcohol swabs, povidone-iodine prep solution, sterile gloves and towels, gauze, and forceps. Local anesthesia with ethyl chloride vinyl spray and/or lidocaine 1% with appropriate syringes and subcutaneous needles. If the joint to be aspirated is large, use 18- or 20-gauge 1.5" needle on a 20 mL syringe (additional syringes should be available). If joint is small or effusion minimal, use 20- or 22-gauge 1.5" needle on 3 mL syringe. In this latter case, additional tubes for fluid collection will not be needed. Otherwise, use three sterile tubes for collection, the first one with either EDTA additive or a small amount of heparin. If gonococcal arthritis is suspected, obtain chocolate (Thayer-Martin) media. Glass slides and polarized microscope are necessary if crystalline arthropathy is suspected.

Technique Procedure should be performed by an experienced physician only. The following description details the technique of knee arthrocentesis, a joint commonly aspirated by the generalist. Presence of effusion is confirmed on physical examination. If the effusion appears small, an elastic wrap (or manual pressure) may be placed around the knee to compress mobile fluid into the joint space. The patient is instructed to lie supine and remain relaxed. Ideally, the operator should be seated and the height of patient's bed adjusted accordingly. Physician selects the type of approach: suprapatellar, parapatellar, or infrapatellar. The parapatellar approach is popular and effective with tense effusions. Here, the knee is placed in 20° flexion to relax the quadriceps. The preferred entry site is the midportion of the patella (approximately 2 cm superior to the inferior portion of the patella), preferably the medial aspect. This site is marked by indenting the skin with the retracted end of a ballpoint pen. The skin is prepped with alcohol first, then povidone-iodine. Some clinicians prefer strict aseptic technique (5-minute scrub, masks, gowns, and drapes) whereas others do not use even sterile gloves or drapes. We prefer a middle-ground approach, using sterile gloves and towels but foregoing masks and gowns. The use of local anesthesia also varies amongst practitioners. If the joint is tense, and anatomical landmarks easily palpable, we prefer cutaneous anesthesia with only a spray of ethyl chloride solution. Alternatively, a subcutaneous wheal of lidocaine may be raised in the usual fashion. Injection of lidocaine into deeper structures is not usually required (where it may potentially interfere with culture results because of bacteriostatic properties). Following this, the needle-on-syringe is passed through the marked skin site and advanced slowly while aspirating. A "pop" may be felt as the needle penetrates the capsule. The needle should be directed parallel to the plane of the synovial capsule if the parapatellar approach is used. Once fluid is returned, the needle should not be advanced further in order to avoid cartilage damage. Only mild suction should be used to aspirate so that trauma and hemorrhage do not occur. In general, joint effusions should be drained completely. A blind "search" with the needle (often with vigorous aspiration) is hazardous and should not be attempted. Forceps may be used to stabilize the needle if several syringe changes are required. Once completed, withdraw the needle, apply pressure, and place adhesive tape over puncture site. If persistent pain is encountered during the procedure, trauma to cartilage or periosteum is likely. Do not reflexly anesthetize these deeper tissues with lidocaine; instead, withdraw the needle and redirect it along a new plane. Correct placement of the needle in the joint space is normally painless. In the case of a "dry tap," folds of synovium may be acting as a valve obstructing the needle lumen.

(Continued)

Arthrocentesis *(Continued)*

Reposition the needle slightly, or if there is fluid in the syringe, inject a small amount to clear the needle bevel. This problem can be avoided by using the infrapatellar approach. The technique for suprapatellar and infrapatellar aspiration has been detailed elsewhere. The suprapatellar approach is most useful in tense effusions where the suprapatellar bursa (usually in communication with the joint space) is visibly distended. While easily performed, there is a potential for sinus tract formation especially if the entry site is directly over the bursa, rather than several centimeters away. The infrapatellar approach has a low risk of cartilage damage compared with the parapatellar approach and is useful for patients with marked flexion contractures of the knee. However, clinicians may not be familiar with the technical details of this approach. Similar principles apply to aspiration of joints other than the knee and are referenced.

Data Acquired A wide array of tests on synovial fluid is available. Routine tests on effusions of unknown etiology include cell count, glucose, Gram stain and routine culture, and microscopic examination for crystals (urate, calcium, pyrophosphate dihydrate). Optional tests include viscosity, mucin clot test, uric acid level, and culture for *Neisseria gonorrhoeae*, tuberculosis, etc. Occasionally ordered tests include synovial fluid protein, LDH, cytology, rheumatoid factor, and complement.

Specimen Synovial fluid

Container For small fluid volumes, send capped syringe without needle to laboratory; otherwise, fluid may be carefully transferred to sterile tubes.

Collection

- Tube 1: Gram stain and culture
- Tube 2: mucin clot, if ordered (no heparin)
- Tube 3: (add heparin or EDTA) cell count, chemistries, crystals, additional studies

If gonococcal arthritis is suspected, chocolate (Thayer-Martin) agar should be inoculated, either at the bedside or during initial specimen processing.

Storage Instructions Specimen should be hand carried to the laboratory, preferably by the physician. Delay in processing may spuriously lower synovial fluid glucose levels.

Normal Findings In the absence of disease, synovial fluid usually cannot be aspirated. Normal synovial fluid is clear and viscous. A drop placed between the thumb and forefinger (or two microscope slides) can form a string >2 cm long as the fingers are separated, indicating high viscosity. Similarly, the mucin clot test is performed by adding 1 mL synovial fluid to a 5% solution of acetic acid. Normally, a firm clot forms. Both tests reflect high viscosity of synovial fluid caused by leukocyte hyaluronic acid. Cell count and differential normally reveal <200 WBCs/mm^3 with <25% neutrophils. Chemistries show protein <2 g/dL, uric acid <8 mg/dL, synovial glucose nearly equal to serum glucose, and synovial LDH less than serum LDH. Gram stain and cultures are negative (acellular).

Critical Values Abnormal synovial fluid can be divided into four diagnostic categories. Considerable overlap exists among these categories and correlation with the clinical presentation is required.

Group I synovial fluids are seen commonly in degenerative joint disease (osteoarthritis) and trauma. Fluid is clear or yellow tinged, viscous and mucin clot firm. WBC count is <200/mm^3 with <25% neutrophils (often mononuclears >50%). Chemistries including glucose are normal and microbiologic cultures are negative. This is considered a "noninflammatory" effusion. Some inflammatory conditions may at times cause a group I fluid, such as acute rheumatic fever and systemic lupus erythematosus.

Group II fluids are "inflammatory" in nature. Diseases leading to this category include crystal-induced arthropathies (gout, CPPD or "pseudogout"), rheumatoid arthritis, connective tissue diseases (SLE, polymyositis, etc), ankylosing spondylitis and other seronegative spondyloarthropathies (Reiter's syndrome, psoriatic arthritis), and acute rheumatic fever. Synovial fluid appears opaque and turbid from cellular fragmentation. Viscosity is similar to water and the "string test" yields only short strings. Mucin clot testing results in a friable gel rather than a tight, rope-like clot. WBC counts are elevated, 5000-75,000/mm^3 with >50% neutrophils. Synovial glucose tends to be lower than serum glucose, especially if synovial WBCs are elevated (neutrophils consume glucose). Gram stain and cultures are negative.

Group III effusions are characteristic of septic arthritis. Fluid appears grossly turbid and may be frankly purulent. WBC count as a rule is >50,000/mm^3 and may be >1,000,000/mm^3. Differential shows preponderance of neutrophils (>90%), with the exception of tuberculous arthritis where lymphocytes may comprise 50% of leukocytes. Synovial glucose is characteristically <50% of simultaneous serum glucose and this finding strongly suggests septic arthritis. Glucose values <10 mg/dL have been reported and support classification into group III (rather than group II) in cases where WBC count is moderately elevated. However, sensitivity of low glucose levels in the septic joint is approximately 50%. Gram stain yield in group III effusions varies with the bacteria isolated. In patients with staphylococcal septic arthritis, the Gram stain is diagnostic in 75% of cases, with gram-negative arthritis, 50% of Gram stains are diagnostic, but with gonococcal arthritis, only 25% of Gram stains are positive. In nongonococcal septic arthritis, the bacterial culture is more helpful than the Gram stain, the former being positive in 85% to 95% of cases (provided no recent antibiotic use). However, with gonococcal arthritis, the culture is less sensitive, with only a 25% positive yield.[1]

Group IV synovial effusions are grossly hemorrhagic. Etiologies include systemic abnormalities (eg, excessive heparin anticoagulation, severe thrombocytopenia) and local joint pathology (eg, femur fracture, neuropathic joint).

As mentioned earlier, diagnostic groups are not mutually exclusive. Certain disease entities may fall into more than one diagnostic category. For example, synovial fluid in acute rheumatic fever may appear as either a group I or a group II effusion; neuropathic arthropathy may appear as group I or IV; and lupus-associated effusions as group I or II. In addition, an individual patient may befall more than one pathologic process over the course of time. It has been demonstrated that rheumatoid arthritis (group II effusion) is a predisposing factor for the later development of bacterial arthritis (group III) and both may be present in the same patient. Finally, some diseases may change from one diagnostic category to another over a short time period. For example, septic arthritis in an early stage may present with a low synovial WBC count and normal glucose (group I) and only later on progress to a typical septic arthritis (group III) picture on subsequent arthrocentesis.

Additional Information Arthrocentesis is indispensable for the accurate diagnosis (or exclusion) of septic arthritis and crystal-induced arthropathy and therein lies its greatest utility. Despite the difficulties with the classification scheme described above, synovial fluid findings in both these treatable conditions is often pathognomonic. Practically, the procedure carries a low risk of complications and can be performed in minutes when an accessible joint is involved. The general physician often handles aspirations of the knee, elbow, and first metatarsal phalangeal joint. When septic arthritis is suspected in a less accessible area, such as the sacroiliac joint, aspiration should not be delayed due to a lack of familiarity. Rheumatologic consultation should be obtained promptly.

Footnotes

1. Goldenberg DL and Reed JI, "Bacterial Arthritis," *N Engl J Med*, 1985, 312(12):764-71.

References

Gatter RA, "Arthrocentesis Technique and Intrasynovial Therapy," *Arthritis and Allied Conditions: A Textbook of Rheumatology*, 13th ed, Chapter 38, Koopman WJ, ed, Baltimore, MD: Williams & Wilkins, 1997, 751-60.

♦ **Bone Marrow** *see* Bone Marrow Aspiration and Biopsy *on page 117*

Bone Marrow Aspiration and Biopsy

Applies to Bone Marrow; Bone Marrow Iron Stain; Bone Marrow Sampling; Bone Marrow Trephine Biopsy; Iron Stain

Procedure Commonly Includes Aspiration and/or biopsy of bone marrow (BM) for microscopic analysis. Both procedures are carried out under local (Continued)

Bone Marrow Aspiration and Biopsy *(Continued)*

anesthesia at the patient's bedside. For aspiration, a specialized hollow needle is advanced into the intramedullary cavity (usually iliac crest). Approximately 0.4 mL liquid marrow and bone fragments are aspirated into a syringe, then smeared onto a slide. Frequently, a bone marrow biopsy is performed as a complementary, but separate, procedure (different equipment and site). A specialized biopsy needle (eg, Jamshidi needle) is used to obtain a core of solid cortical bone. This technique preserves the normal marrow architecture of the biopsy sample and allows for formal for histologic analysis.

Indications Bone marrow sampling is indicated in the evaluation of a wide variety of hematologic disorders, usually noted first on the CBC or peripheral smear. It is also useful in the diagnosis of systemic diseases which may potentially involve the marrow, such as infectious or granulomatous processes. Bone marrow aspiration and biopsy should be considered separate procedures, although indications often overlap. Indications for bone marrow **aspiration** include:

- evaluation of severe anemia, especially when etiology is in doubt and reticulocyte count is low
- evaluation of macrocytic anemia, to confirm the presence of megaloblastic anemia or to exclude sideroblastic anemia and normoblastic erythropoiesis
- leukopenia and/or thrombocytopenia, to differentiate excessive consumption from decreased production
- persistent leukocytosis of unknown etiology
- suspected myelodysplastic syndrome
- suspected leukemia, to confirm diagnosis and to classify subtype (FAB categorization)
- suspected immunoglobulin disorders, such as multiple myeloma, for diagnosis and staging
- evaluation of lipid storage diseases
- evaluation of suspected iron storage abnormalities
- acquisition of marrow for chromosomal analysis
- acquisition of tissue for microbiological culture (fungi, bacteria, mycobacteria, parasites)
- evaluation of response to therapy for hematologic malignancies

Bone marrow biopsy preserves the marrow architecture and is useful in evaluating systemic diseases secondarily involving the marrow. Bone marrow **biopsy** indications include:

- evaluation of pancytopenia
- evaluation of possible myelophthisic anemia (bone marrow infiltrated with leukemic cells, metastatic tumor, lymphoma, granulomas, etc)
- diagnosis and staging of solid tumors or lymphoma
- evaluation of selected cases of fever of unknown origin
- diagnosis of systemic amyloidosis when other methods have failed
- suspected cases of myelofibrosis
- evaluation of myeloproliferative syndromes (polycythemia vera, essential thrombocythemia, etc)
- failed bone marrow aspiration attempts (the so-called "dry tap")

Authorities differ on the exact indications for both bone marrow aspiration and biopsy. Some believe that most hematologic abnormalities are adequately evaluated by bone marrow aspiration alone (without biopsy). Bone marrow biopsy should not be routinely performed with aspiration, it is argued, due to the following reasons:

- diagnosis can often be made by aspiration
- significant patient discomfort accompanies biopsy
- there is needless expense and patient risk

Thus, bone marrow biopsy should only be performed if specific indications are present (as listed).

Other experts routinely include a biopsy whenever aspiration is performed. The following reasons are cited.

- Bone marrow biopsy may be diagnostic in cases where aspiration is negative or equivocal.
- It is nearly impossible to predict in advance which aspiration attempts will be technically difficult.
- Bone marrow biopsy actually causes less discomfort than aspiration in some cases.
- Cost-benefit analysis may favor the combined approach. The cost to physician, technologist, and patient may be doubled if patient is forced to undergo a separate bone marrow biopsy at a later date.

Contraindications

- uncooperative patient
- cellulitis, osteomyelitis, or radiation therapy involving the proposed site of needle entry
- severe, noncorrectable coagulopathy
- thoracic aortic aneurysm if a sternal approach is used
- Paget disease involving the iliac bone represents a high risk situation, due to excessive bleeding at trephine biopsy site (but not necessarily a contraindication)

Patient Preparation Technique and risks of the procedure are explained to the patient and consent is obtained. Considerable patient apprehension often accompanies this procedure and requires thorough, step-by-step explanation beforehand. If coagulopathy is known or suspected, a recent CBC and PT/PTT should be drawn. Requisition must state in advance any special studies to be performed on specimen, such as AFB stain, Congo red stain for amyloid, cytogenetics studies, etc. Contact referring physician if any questions arise or contact appropriate laboratories directly. Patients are commonly premedicated with a short-acting benzodiazepine or analgesic such as meperidine.

Aftercare Needle puncture site(s) are covered with a dry sterile dressing. If the bone marrow biopsy is performed from the posterior iliac crest, patient must lie on back for a full 30 minutes before being discharged. In the presence of a low-grade coagulopathy or mild thrombocytopenia, direct pressure should be applied by operator (not patient) to puncture sites until local bleeding ceases. Instruct patient to keep dressings dry. Ideally, puncture sites should be examined approximately 24 hours later by nurse or physician, but this is not always feasible.

Special Instructions This procedure requires at least two operators. The first obtains the aspiration and/or biopsy specimen in a sterile fashion (usually a physician or specialized nurse clinician) and the second immediately examines and prepares the specimen (usually a nurse or technologist from the Hematology Laboratory).

Complications Bone marrow sampling is considered a relatively safe but invasive procedure. Minor complications include local bleeding, hematoma, and discomfort at the needle puncture site. Local infection is rarely seen if proper aftercare is followed. Major complications have been reported with sternal biopsy (Bahir 1963), including fatal puncture of mediastinal structures. Historical reports of fistula formation, osteomyelitis, and profuse bleeding were associated with biopsy of what are now considered nonstandard sites, such as the tibia. Minimal complications are associated with sampling of the iliac crest, the preferred site.

Equipment Commercially assembled trays for aspiration and biopsy are widely available. These prepackaged kits typically contain a bone marrow biopsy needle (usually Jamshidi needle), aspiration needle (usually Illinois needle), various syringes (5 mL, 10 mL, 20 mL), assorted needles (18-gauge, 25-gauge), and 1% lidocaine with epinephrine for local anesthesia. Also included are gauze, sterile gloves, drapes and towels, No 11 scalpel blade, and alcohol and iodine prep. The Jamshidi needle is a large-bore (usually 11-gauge), hollow needle with a tapered tip, thin metal stylet, and wide plastic grip to allow easy needle rotation. The Illinois needle is somewhat smaller, but likewise comes with a stylet and plastic sheath for improved grip. Smaller gauge needles are available for use in the pediatric population.

(Continued)

Bone Marrow Aspiration and Biopsy *(Continued)*

Technique The procedure is performed by experienced operators only. May be carried out at the bedside if adequate lighting is available, otherwise done in a procedure room.

Aspiration: Preferred site is the posterior superior iliac spine (PSIS), alternatively the sternum. The patient is placed on his side or lies prone. Landmarks are identified by palpation - the PSIS primarily, but the anterior superior iliac spine also. A wide circular area (approximately 5" in diameter) overlying the PSIS is prepped with povidone-iodine in the usual sterile fashion. Using the 25-gauge needle and lidocaine, the skin directly over the PSIS is anesthetized. Following this, deeper structures are liberally anesthetized with the 18-gauge needle, including a several centimeter area of the periosteum. A 4 mm long skin incision is made over the PSIS by means of the No 11 scalpel blade, then extended deeper through fatty tissues down to the anesthetized periosteum. The Illinois aspiration needle (with stylet in place) is advanced through this soft tissue incision and firmly into the cortex of the PSIS, using a constant rotary motion of the needle ("drilling"). Once the needle has penetrated approximately 1 cm into the marrow cavity, the stylet is removed and a 10 mL syringe is attached to the open (distal) end of the aspiration needle. At least 4-5 mL marrow is aspirated using firm suction. This volume is adequate for most routine hematologic studies, but larger volumes are usually needed for fungal or tuberculous cultures, cytogenetics, cell markers, etc. This step often causes the most patient discomfort. After aspiration, the syringe is detached and immediately handed over to the technologist in order to prevent the specimen from clotting (aspiration needle is still in the PSIS). The technologist examines the specimen grossly for marrow particles, which may be visible to the naked eye. If present, this signifies that an adequate marrow specimen has likely been obtained; if absent, the aspiration needle is redirected slightly and the previous listed steps repeated. After completion, the needle is removed and direct pressure applied.

Biopsy: May be carried out immediately following aspiration, while patient is still under local anesthesia. Preferred site is again the PSIS; however, unlike bone marrow aspiration, biopsy is never obtained from the sternum. A Jamshidi biopsy needle is passed through the same skin and soft tissue incision used for aspiration (alternatively, a completely new site may be used). However, a separate hole in the PSIS must be made. Once into the cortical bone, the needle is advanced using a pronounced clockwise/counterclockwise rotary motion. The needle is oriented along an imaginary line connecting the PSIS and the anterior superior iliac spine, forcing a slight angle of the needle with respect to the skin. The needle should **not** be advanced perpendicular to the skin; this results in poor quality biopsies (often with mostly cartilage). The stylet is then removed. The "drilling" is continued until the needle is at least 2 cm deep into the cortex. This may be estimated by periodically replacing the stylet into the needle and noting the distance the stylet protrudes. The biopsy core is subsequently "sheared off" by the following maneuvers:

- needle is rotated a full 10 turns clockwise then 10 turns counterclockwise
- needle is withdrawn slightly and redirected at a different angle
- needle is readvanced
- steps 1-3 are repeated (until the core is sheared off). The needle is withdrawn, again using rotary motions so as not to lose the core. The blunt obturator or "push wire" is passed through the sharp tip of the Jamshidi needle and the specimen pushed gently out of the needle base and onto a sterile gauze. The technologist immediately makes imprints of the core then places the specimen in fixative.

The techniques for aspiration and biopsy outlined are generally agreed upon in major textbooks. However, some clinicians strongly believe that bone marrow biopsy should always **precede** aspiration, despite the "textbook" recommendations. They argue that artifacts in the core biopsy may be induced by aspiration.

Specimen The bone marrow aspirate is immediately examined for visible bone spicules. The presence of these small spicules suggests an adequate specimen. Direct smears of the aspirate fluid are prepared by the technologist at the bedside. These smears consist of marrow particles and free marrow cells spread onto coverslips. This technique helps to preserve the cytologic appearance of individual blood cells. Bone marrow biopsy samples are handled differently. In many institutions, touch preparations are made first, before specimen fixation. The marrow specimen is touched gently to a clean glass slide in several places, without smearing. These "touch preps" are allowed to air-dry and subsequently undergo routine staining. This technique also helps preserve cytologic detail. Once the touch preparations are completed, the remainder of the specimen is placed in a fixative such as formalin or Zenker's solution. The specimen is then processed according to individual laboratory protocol (for example, overnight fixation, decalcification, wash steps, dehydration, and serial sectioning). Routine stains are performed on processed specimens. These include hematoxylin and eosin (H & E), Wright-Giemsa stain, and iron stain. Optional studies may be obtained at physician request such as cytogenetic analysis, flow cytometry, electron microscopy, and amyloid stains. The Hematology Laboratory must be notified in advance for these studies. Bone marrow specimens may also be submitted for microbiological analysis. Cultures may be obtained for aerobic and anaerobic bacteria, fungi (eg, *Histoplasma capsulatum*), acid-fast bacilli (eg, *Mycobacterium tuberculosis* or *Mycobacterium avium-intracellulare*), and viruses (cytomegalovirus). Fixatives should **not** be added to specimens submitted for culture. Again, it is important to notify the Microbiology Laboratory in advance for these cultures.

Normal Findings The bone marrow aspirate and biopsy are reviewed by a staff pathologist or hematologist. The preliminary report on the bone marrow aspirate may often be available several hours after the procedure, on request. Normal values for bone marrow cell lines in the adult are as follows:

Granulocytes

- blasts: 0% to 1 %
- promyelocytes: 1% to 5%
- neutrophil myelocytes and metamyelocytes: 7% to 25%
- neutrophil bands and segs: 20% to 60%
- eosinophils: 0% to 3%
- basophils: 0% to 1%
- monocytes: 0% to 2%
- lymphocytes: 5% to 15%
- plasma cells: 0% to 2%

Erythrocytes

- proerythrocytes: 0% to 1%
- early erythrocytes: 1% to 4%
- late erythrocytes: 10% to 20%
- normoblasts: 5% to 10%

The above bone marrow differential cell counts are calculated from the bone marrow aspirate specimen. Other useful data provided by the bone marrow aspirate include:

- myeloid/erythroid ratio (normal ratio 3-4:1)
- total cells counted
- overall cellularity
- erythropoiesis
- granulopoiesis

The bone marrow biopsy provides additional information on marrow architecture (which cannot be obtained from the aspirate). When examining the biopsy specimen, the pathologist may comment on:

- gross description including size of sample
- overall cellularity
- presence of granulomas
- infiltrative marrow processes such as lymphoma, carcinoma, granulomas
- iron stores
- results of special stains

References

Batjer JP, "Preparation of Optimal Bone Marrow Samples," *Lab Med*, 1979, 10:101-6.

Beckstead JH, "The Bone Marrow Biopsy: A Diagnostic Strategy," *Arch Pathol Lab Med*, 1986, 110(3):175-9.

(Continued)

Bone Marrow Aspiration and Biopsy *(Continued)*

Brynes RK, McKenna RW, and Sundberg RD, "Bone Marrow Aspiration and Trephine Biopsy: An Approach to a Thorough Study," *Am J Clin Pathol*, 1978, 70(5):753-9.

Williams WJ and Nelson DA, "Examination of the Marrow," *Hematology*, 5th ed, Chapter 3, Williams WJ, Beutler E, Lichtman MA, et al, eds, New York, NY: McGraw-Hill Book Co, 1995, 15-24.

♦ **Bone Marrow Iron Stain** *see* Bone Marrow Aspiration and Biopsy *on page 117*

♦ **Bone Marrow Sampling** *see* Bone Marrow Aspiration and Biopsy *on page 117*

♦ **Bone Marrow Trephine Biopsy** *see* Bone Marrow Aspiration and Biopsy *on page 117*

♦ **Closed Joint Aspiration** *see* Arthrocentesis *on page 114*

♦ **Closed Kidney (Renal) Biopsy** *see* Kidney Biopsy *on page 126*

♦ **Contact Dermatitis Skin Test** *see* Patch Test *on page 138*

♦ **Delayed Hypersensitivity Fungal Skin Tests** *see* Fungal Skin Testing *on page 122*

♦ **Delayed Reaction Intracutaneous Tests** *see* Anergy Skin Test Battery *on page 110*

♦ **Epicutaneous Patch Test** *see* Patch Test *on page 138*

♦ **Food Allergy Test** *see* Ingestion Challenge Test *on page 125*

Fungal Skin Testing

Related Information

Allergy Testing, Percutaneous *on page 106*
Anergy Skin Test Battery *on page 110*
Tuberculin Skin Testing, Intracutaneous *on page 144*

Synonyms Delayed Hypersensitivity Fungal Skin Tests; Skin Tests for Histoplasmosis, Blastomycosis, Coccidioidomycosis

Procedure Commonly Includes Intradermal injection of fungal antigen(s) to determine if a delayed hypersensitivity reaction is present to a given fungus. Skin test sites are examined at 24, 48, and 72 hours for induration which, if present, implies prior infection with the tested fungus.

Indications Fungal skin testing has been applied for the following reasons:

- as an epidemiologic tool for defining geographic regions of endemic fungal infection
- as a diagnostic aid in individual cases of suspected primary fungal infection (limited usefulness)
- as a prognostic indicator in culture-proven cases of fungal infection (particularly coccidioidomycosis)
- as a component of a comprehensive cutaneous anergy panel, used to assess the integrity of a patient's cell-mediated immune system (T-cell function); this standardized panel is usually comprised of *Candida*, mumps, and *Trichophyton* antigens

Contraindications Prior systemic reaction to fungal skin testing; known immediate hypersensitivity (IgE-mediated) to the specific fungus to be tested; known immediate hypersensitivity to mercury, which is contained in some commercial preparations of *Coccidioides* antigen; the presence of erythema nodosum (high risk for adverse reaction - see following information).

Patient Preparation Procedure and risks are explained to the patient. No specific skin preparation is necessary. However, those patients with generalized skin disorders such as extensive psoriasis should be examined beforehand for suitable areas of normal appearing skin. If immediate hypersensitivity to the fungal antigen is even remotely suspected, a physician should be in attendance.

Aftercare Fifteen to 30 minutes after injections, sites should be examined for adverse reactions ranging from the IgE wheal and flare response to systemic reactions; otherwise, close observation postprocedure is generally not necessary and patients should be instructed to keep test sites clean for 72 hours. No restrictions on bathing or cleaning injection sites are necessary.

Special Instructions Requisition should state the specific fungal antigens to be planted, as well as whether a simultaneous skin anergy panel is desired.

Current medications should also be included in the requisition, with attention to corticosteroids or other immunosuppressive agents.

Complications As with other forms of skin testing, immediate IgE-mediated local reactions are possible, although unusual. Erythema, vesiculation, and skin necrosis may be seen, at times involving large areas. Systemic reactions, including anaphylaxis, have rarely been reported. Patients with infection with *Coccidioides immitis* who manifest erythema nodosum may be at an increased risk of a major systemic reaction after skin testing. However, in the vast majority of cases, fungal skin testing is safe.

Equipment Skin test materials are derived from cultures of the appropriate fungi and most are available commercially in standardized concentrations. Common fungal antigens tested include *Histoplasma capsulatum*, *Coccidioides immitis*, *Blastomyces dermatitidis* (not available commercially), *Candida*, and *Trichophyton*. Disposable plastic or glass tuberculin syringes are required along with 26- or 27-gauge short (¼" to ½") beveled needles.

Technique The volar aspect of the forearm is prepped with alcohol swabs. Skin test material(s) are injected intradermally so that discrete wheals are raised. Generally, 0.1 mL skin test antigen is injected, but more dilute solutions may be used if a severe reaction is anticipated. Subcutaneous injections should be avoided. Multiple fungal antigens may be injected at separate sites using this method. Test sites should be examined at 24, 48, and 72 hours. Date and time of injection should be recorded along with the location of each fungal antigen.

Data Acquired The transverse diameter of induration should be carefully measured by inspection and palpation and results recorded (in millimeters) at 24-hour intervals. Areas of erythema, however, are not as important as induration and are excluded in most grading schemes unless extensive (>10 mm).

Normal Findings No induration or erythema

Critical Values A positive skin test is defined by many authorities as a diameter of induration ≥5 mm.[1] Induration of 0-4 mm is considered negative. Alternatively, a standardized grading scale, which is popular with general delayed-type hypersensitivity skin testing, may be used:[2]

- 0: no reaction
- 1+: erythema >10 mm and/or induration 1-5 mm
- 2+: induration 6-10 mm
- 3+: induration 11-20 mm
- 4+: induration >20 mm

The interpretation of a positive (or negative) skin test is so problematic that the clinical utility of fungal skin testing is significantly limited. A positive reaction indicates only that exposure to the relevant fungus has occurred at some time in the past, whether recent or remote. In addition, fungal infections are endemic in many areas of the United States, where >90% of the local population may be skin test positive following asymptomatic or subclinical infections (eg, histoplasmosis in the Ohio River Valley). Thus, in the individual patient with suspected active fungal infection, a positive skin test adds little new diagnostic information and fails to establish the fungus as the infecting agent.[1] This becomes especially relevant if the patient has ever lived in a known endemic area. In the patient with pulmonary nodules, the importance of a positive test is also unclear. Some authorities consider a positive histoplasmin test in an area of low prevalence as strong evidence for histoplasmosis.[3] Others argue that lung nodules may still be due to bronchogenic carcinoma despite a positive histoplasmin test, and skin testing adds little to clinical decision making. Similarly, a negative skin test presents major problems in interpretation. Lack of reactivity may be seen in the following situations:

- no previous fungal infection
- previous fungal infection in an immunocompromised patient
- acute systemic fungal infection, where skin test positivity is often delayed for 2-4 weeks
- waning skin test reactivity to a given fungus, as occurs in the elderly
- technical errors in antigen placement

Even the documentation of skin test conversion (ie, negative test converting to positive or serial testing) is regarded as only indirect evidence of fungal

(Continued)

Fungal Skin Testing *(Continued)*

exposure in the interim and does not necessarily imply active infection. Regarding the specific fungal antigens, the derivative of *Histoplasma capsulatum* is termed histoplasmin. An older preparation of histoplasmin cross reacted frequently with *Blastomyces* and *Coccidioides* and caused a rise in complement fixation titers to *Histoplasma*. A newer histoplasmin preparation ameliorates, but does not entirely eliminate, these problems. The histoplasmin skin test may cause a spurious increase in *Histoplasma* complement fixation titers. Since the CF serologic test is clinically more useful than the histoplasmin skin test, serologies should be drawn first in suspected cases. Coccidioidomycosis skin testing shares many of the same interpretive difficulties as histoplasmosis testing, such as waning reactivity over time, delay in test positivity during acute fungal infection, and areas of high prevalence. Two preparations of *Coccidioides* antigen are available, the older coccidioidin (derived from the mycelia phase) and Spherulin® (derived from lysed spherules). Spherulin® may have superior sensitivity and has been found to be positive in 30% more cases than coccidioidin. Although testing is not useful in the individual with suspected *Coccidioides* pneumonia, it may provide prognostic information in culture proven cases. In a classic study, patients with disseminated coccidioidomycosis had a higher survival rate if their skin test was positive (75%) compared with those who tested negative (15%).[4] Patients with limited coccidioidomycosis almost always develop a positive test; failure to do so may predict impending disseminated disease.[5]

In one recent study,[6] serial fungal skin testing was useful in identifying individuals with nonmeningeal coccidioidomycosis who were at high risk for relapse following a course of antifungal therapy. Patients with persistently negative coccidioidin skin tests (administered at the time of the initial diagnosis and repeated serially prior to completion of antifungal therapy) were more likely to relapse than those who had serial positive tests. The clinical utility of this observation is not clear[7] and serial skin tests are not performed routinely during the treatment of coccidioidomycosis.

Use of the coccidioidin preparation may cause false-positive histoplasmosis serologic tests, but neither Spherulin® nor coccidioidin interferes with serologic tests for coccidioidomycosis. Coccidioidal skin tests are generally positive before coccidioidal serologic tests; some clinicians use this fact to justify skin testing in acute cases (despite its limited diagnostic utility).

Skin tests for blastomycosis are presently of questionable value due to poor sensitivity and specificity, even in the study of epidemics. Fungal antigens derived from *Candida albicans* and *Trichophyton* are primarily used only for anergy testing because of the high prevalence of positive skin tests in the general population. (See Anergy Skin Test Battery *on page 9999*).

Additional Information Fungal skin testing is a form of delayed hypersensitivity skin testing and as such is an assessment of cell-mediated immunity. Delayed hypersensitivity is a clinical phenomenon based on the reaction of the skin to intradermal injection of an antigen. It is a common form of immune protection against a wide range of infectious agents, including fungi. Following initial exposure to a fungus, a population of transformed T-lymphocytes is created, the so-called memory cells. When fungal antigen is introduced intradermally at a later date, these sensitized T cells are activated and initiate a cascade involving lymphokines, neutrophils, and macrophages. Clinically, this is manifested by the delayed formation of significant skin induration. Delayed hypersensitivity fungal skin testing should be differentiated from immediate hypersensitivity skin testing. The former is primarily T-cell mediated and the latter is mediated by IgE mechanisms. Skin testing for common allergies to molds or fungi is carried out using the percutaneous allergy testing method (see Allergy Testing, Percutaneous *on page 106*) and is IgE-mediated. Similarly, skin tests for immediate hypersensitivity to *Aspergillus fumigatus* also use this method. This is commonly obtained in the evaluation of patients with suspected allergic bronchopulmonary aspergillosis.

Footnotes

1. Davies SF and Sarosi GA, "Role of Serodiagnostic Tests and Skin Tests in the Diagnosis of Fungal Disease," *Clin Chest Med*, 1987, 8(1):135-46.
2. Bates SE, Suen JY, and Tranum BL, "Immunological Skin Testing and Interpretation. A Plea for Uniformity," *Cancer*, 1979, 43(6):2306-14.
3. Ahmed AR and Blose DA, "Delayed-Type Hypersensitivity Skin Testing," *Arch Dermatol*, 1983, 119(11):934-45.
4. Smith CE, Whiting EG, Baker ES, et al, "The Use of Coccidioidin," *Am Rev Respir Dis*, 1948, 57:330-60.
5. Drutz D and Catanzaro A, "Coccidioidomycosis. Part I," *Am Rev Respir Dis*, 1978, 117(3):559-85.
6. Oldfield EC, Bone WD, Martin CR, et al, "Prediction of Relapse After Treatment of Coccidioidomycosis," *Clin Infect Dis*, 1997, 25(5):1205-10.
7. Stevens DA, "Adequacy of Therapy for Coccidioidomycosis," *Clin Infect Dis*, 1997, 25(5):1211-2.

♦ **Immediate Hypersensitivity Skin Test** *see* Allergy Testing, Intracutaneous (Intradermal) *on page 103*

♦ **Immediate Hypersensitivity Skin Test** *see* Allergy Testing, Percutaneous *on page 106*

Ingestion Challenge Test

Related Information

Arthrocentesis *on page 114*

Bronchial Challenge Test *on page 202*

Synonyms Food Allergy Test; Oral Provocation Test

Procedure Commonly Includes *In vivo* testing of patients with suspected food allergy. This procedure is useful in evaluating patients with a clinical history consistent with IgE-mediated hypersensitivity to specific foods. Other substances may also be tested, such as food additives (metabisulfites) and certain medications (nonsteroidal anti-inflammatory agents). The patient is asked to ingest capsules containing fixed amounts of a specific food (or food additive) and is then observed for the development of allergic symptoms.

Indications Ingestion challenge testing is useful in the following situations:

- clinical history typical for IgE-mediated food allergy but relevant skin prick tests are negative or nondiagnostic
- clinical history of nonspecific "food intolerances" of uncertain significance but skin tests are positive
- prior diagnosis of "food allergy" established by unknown or unproven methods

Formal testing is not required in every case of suspected food allergy; this procedure yields useful clinical information in only a limited number of situations. When the patient's clinical history is compatible with IgE-mediated food allergy and subsequent skin prick tests confirm the diagnosis, formal oral testing is probably unnecessary. Under these circumstances many clinicians would simply instruct the patient to avoid the food (or food additive) in question. If the results of this are equivocal, then ingestion challenge testing may be indicated.

Contraindications

- documented anaphylactic reaction in the past to food substance in question (eg, anaphylaxis from prior skin testing)
- inadequate medical supervision or resuscitation equipment

Patient Preparation In general, a patient with suspected food allergy should undergo a careful history and physical examination before any laboratory testing. Following this, if a formal oral challenge test appears indicated, the purpose, risks, and technique of this procedure should be reviewed with the patient. All foods suspected of causing allergy should be avoided prior to testing in order to simplify test interpretation. Antihistamines should also be discontinued before testing, since H_1 antagonists depress the IgE response. All such medication changes must be reviewed and approved by the physician.

Aftercare Per protocol of the individual testing center. In general, the patient is carefully observed for varying lengths of time after completion of the study, depending on the nature and severity of the allergic reaction. Rarely, complications may develop some hours after discharge from the testing center; patient should be instructed to contact a physician immediately.

(Continued)

Ingestion Challenge Test *(Continued)*

Complications A number of physiologic reactions may occur as a result of a positive test. These "complications" include potentially life-threatening events such as anaphylactic shock, acute asthma, and angioedema. Other complications are less severe and include nausea, diarrhea, rhinitis, and urticaria. These complications are not unique to oral provocation testing, and are shared by other allergy tests which evaluate immediate hypersensitivity.

Equipment Several food preparations are available for oral provocation testing. One such preparation is a gelatin capsule containing 500 mg of a single food substance. These are popular and well tolerated. Placebo capsules may also be necessary if a blinded challenge is planned.

Technique Specific protocols for testing vary. Usually, the patient ingests food capsules at specific time intervals and is carefully observed by a physician for signs of allergy. Placebo capsules are included in single-blinded or double-blinded trials. If no reaction has occurred after 12 capsules, the test is terminated. If a severe allergic reaction is expected based on the clinical history, smaller doses are given at 1-hour intervals.

Normal Findings No adverse reactions after ingestion of multiple food capsules

Critical Values Test is considered positive when typical symptoms of food allergy develop shortly after administration of a specific food capsule, but not after placebo. The validity of such allergic reactions relies on the clinical judgment of the testing physician. Typical symptoms are urticaria, wheezing, angioedema, and rhinitis. Other possible symptoms include nausea, vomiting, diarrhea, and abdominal pain, which may be difficult to interpret.

Additional Information The ingestion challenge test has also been used to evaluate allergy to certain drugs, particularly nonsteroidal anti-inflammatory agents. Often, bronchial provocation is used in conjunction with the oral ingestion of the medication (see Bronchial Challenge Test *on page 202*). In this way, bronchospasm may be objectively documented in response to the oral challenge. Much controversy surrounds the subject of food allergy in general. The medical literature is filled with various testing techniques for food intolerance, but they are often uncontrolled and anecdotal. A position paper, issued by the American College of Physicians[1], addressed the many controversies in allergy testing, including the ingestion challenge test. The information presented in this entry is in keeping with the recommendations of the American College of Physicians.

Footnotes

1. "Allergy Testing." American College of Physicians, *Ann Intern Med*, 1989, 110(4):317-20.

References

Lessof MH, Wraith DG, Merrett TG, et al, "Food Allergy and Intolerance in 100 Patients - Local and Systemic Effects," *Q J Med*, 1980, 49(195):259-71.

Metcalfe DD, "Diagnostic Procedures for Immunologically-Mediated Food Sensitivity," *Nutr Rev*, 1984, 42(3):92-7.

VanArsdel PP Jr and Larson EB, "Diagnostic Tests for Patients With Suspected Allergic Disease. Utility and Limitations," *Ann Intern Med*, 1989, 110(4):304-12.

♦ **Intracutaneous (Intradermal) Allergy Testing** *see* Allergy Testing, Intracutaneous (Intradermal) *on page 103*

♦ **Iron Stain** *see* Bone Marrow Aspiration and Biopsy *on page 117*

♦ **Joint Tap** *see* Arthrocentesis *on page 114*

Kidney Biopsy

Related Information

Ultrasound, Kidney Biopsy *on page 491*

Synonyms Closed Kidney (Renal) Biopsy; Renal Biopsy

Procedure Commonly Includes Biopsy of the renal parenchyma for diagnostic purposes. In most cases, this is performed percutaneously under local anesthesia, either as a "blind" procedure or under ultrasound guidance. Fresh kidney specimens are sent for gross and microscopic analysis, including H & E stain, PAS/PAMS stain, immunofluorescence staining, and in selected cases, scanning electron microscopy. Kidney biopsy is useful in diagnosing primary (intrinsic) renal disease, assessing the nature and severity of renal involvement in various systemic disorders, and (less commonly) establishing the diagnosis of certain systemic diseases (eg, amyloidosis).

Indications The exact indications for performing a renal biopsy are not universally agreed upon and opinions vary widely amongst nephrologists, despite almost four decades of experience. There continues to be lively debate in the medical literature over these indications. Glassock and Massry classify their procedural indications as follows:[1]

"Most useful" indications include:

- idiopathic nephrotic syndrome in the adult (prior to empirical glucocorticoid therapy)
- non-nephrotic range proteinuria (1-2 g/day) of unknown cause accompanied by an abnormal urinary sediment
- proteinuria with glomerular hematuria (ie, urinary tract infections and neoplasms have been excluded)
- acute renal failure of unknown cause, when obstruction has been ruled out the diagnosis of acute tubular necrosis cannot be established clinically, both kidneys are of normal size
- suspected cases of rapidly progressive glomerulonephritis (RPGN) or the acute nephritic syndrome
- suspected cases of active lupus nephritis, characterized by hematuria (>6 RBCs/hpf), proteinuria (>200 mg/day), and elevated serum creatinine
- suspected cases of renal vasculitis, particularly polyarteritis nodosa and Wegener granulomatosis (which often requires aggressive combination therapy)
- evaluation of the renal allotransplant patient with possible graft rejection, acute tubular necrosis (ATN), drug-induced interstitial nephritis, infarction, or recurrence of original disease in the graft

"Possible useful" indications include:

- persistent glomerular hematuria without proteinuria
- proteinuria >1 g/day with normal urinary sediment
- evaluation of suspected inherited glomerular diseases such as Alport's or Fabry disease
- evaluation of the known diabetic with rapid, unexpected deterioration of renal function, sudden development of nephrotic syndrome, or early development of azotemia in the absence of diabetic retinopathy

Renal biopsy is "not useful" in evaluating:

- malignant hypertension
- polycystic kidney disease
- hepatorenal syndrome
- pyelonephritis
- chronic renal failure with shrunken kidneys
- routine cases of diabetic nephropathy
- clinically silent lupus nephritis (controversial)

Proponents of kidney biopsy believe that a definitive histologic diagnosis of a specific renal disease should be made prior to any empirical trial of immunosuppressives (ie, cases of nephrotic syndrome, RPGN, etc). Opponents of early kidney biopsy believe that empirical steroids should be attempted first with careful monitoring of renal function. Usually kidney biopsy is unnecessary whether or not the renal disease is steroid-responsive. This latter opinion is based primarily on group statistical studies and decision analysis theory. Certainly, the details of each individual case must be reviewed prior to decision-making regarding biopsy. The costs and potential complications of the procedure should be weighed against the probability of altering patient management based on the biopsy results.

Contraindications

Absolute contraindications:

- uncorrectable and clinically severe bleeding diathesis
- patient refusal

Relative contraindications:

- severe thrombocytopenia, <50,000/mm^3 (usually correctable by platelet infusion)
- solitary kidney (except with a renal allograft)
- renal artery aneurysm

(Continued)

Kidney Biopsy *(Continued)*

- active pyelonephritis or perinephric abscess
- hydronephrosis
- uncontrolled severe hypertension
- uncorrected volume depletion

A prolonged Ivy bleeding time is commonly seen in patients with renal failure, due in part to platelet dysfunction. This does **not** represent a contraindication to kidney biopsy.[1] At the worst, it should be considered a high risk situation. Experience in several centers has demonstrated the safety of kidney biopsy in this setting. In some centers, however, desmopressin (DDAVP®) is infused prior to biopsy in order to normalize the bleeding time in azotemic patients but this practice has not been widely accepted. Other potentially high risk situations (not contraindications) include:

- moderate thrombocytopenia, 100,000-150,000/mm^3
- moderate hypertension
- BUN >100 mg/dL (considered a contraindication in the 1950s)

Patient Preparation Procedure and risks of the procedure are explained and informed consent is obtained. The patient should understand that kidney biopsy usually requires a 24-hour hospital stay postprocedure. All administrative issues related to the planned hospitalization should be completed in advance. If patient is on antihypertensive medications he/she should be instructed to continue these up to and including the day of admission (unless directed otherwise by physician). Some nephrologists customarily obtain a platelet count, PT, and PTT on the day of the procedure, while others order these tests only when coagulopathy is suspected. As previously mentioned, the Ivy bleeding time has limited clinical utility in this setting and need not be routinely ordered for the azotemic patient. A hematocrit and urinalysis are often obtained as a baseline reference for later comparison with postprocedure values. Except in unusual, high risk situations, it is not necessary to type and crossmatch blood for transfusion. Premedication with a short-acting benzodiazepine may be helpful in the anxious patient. In some centers, I.V. access is routinely established (heparin lock and D_5W at a maintenance rate). Vital signs are recorded beforehand and physician is informed if blood pressure is elevated.

Aftercare Immediately after biopsy is completed, vital signs are obtained. If stable, patient should lie supine in bed for at least 12 hours. Pulse and blood pressure are monitored four times at 15-minute intervals, two times at 30-minute intervals, three times at 1-hour intervals, then every 4 hours until discharge (usual total hospital time is 24 hours). Hematocrits are obtained at 12 and 24 hours after procedure routinely or prn if gross hematuria or hypotension develops. Commonly, all voided urine samples are collected by nursing staff, saved in labeled plastic containers at the bedside, and serially examined for gross and microscopic hematuria. Physician should be contacted if gross hematuria occurs, hematocrit drops significantly, severe pain at biopsy site persists, or blood pressure falls. These may be indicative of an enlarging hematoma. After hospital discharge, patient should avoid heavy lifting, strenuous exercise, and contact sports for 1-2 weeks.

Special Instructions Special handling of the specimen may be necessary when certain diseases are suspected. Standard tissue processing is usually insufficient for analyzing glycogen, uric acid crystals, and other crystal diseases. The Pathology Laboratory should be contacted in advance in these special circumstances.

Complications The precise complication risk for an individual patient is difficult to predict, since this figure is heavily influenced by the skill of the operator and the presence of relative contraindications.

Common complications include:

- microscopic hematuria, present in nearly every case (thus, some authorities do not consider this a complication)
- perirenal hematoma, also very common; usually self-limited and asymptomatic, but may be seen on ultrasound or CT scan
- postbiopsy pain, usually described as a dull ache. More pronounced pain may signify expanding hematoma.

Less common complications:

- aggravation of hypertension
- persistent perirenal bleeding and gross hematuria. Blood transfusion is required in approximately 1 out of 500 biopsies; surgical intervention in 1 out of 1000.[1]
- arteriovenous fistula formation; reported in ≤10% of biopsies, usually asymptomatic but sometimes may cause hematuria
- kidney rupture
- calyceal fissure
- puncture of pancreas, bowel, spleen, liver
- laceration of aorta or renal artery
- death (1:1000 to 1:3000)

In one large series, overall complication rate was estimated at 2.1%, out of 5500 reported biopsies.[2] Complications included expanding hematoma and bleeding requiring blood transfusion or nephrectomy. Mortality was approximately 1 in 1000. In another recent survey, 94 complications were reported from 1000 consecutive biopsies (gross hematuria accounted for 73%).[3] Thus, textbook estimates of complications range from 2% to 10%.

Equipment Kidney biopsy is obtained using either a Travenol Tru-cut needle or a Vim-Silverman needle. The former is a one-piece, disposable apparatus 11.4 cm long (≤15 cm), consisting of a needle with cannula and obturator. The Vim-Silverman needle is also commonly employed and is composed of three separate pieces: obturator, cannula with sharpened end, and two semicircular cutting blades. A 23-gauge finder needle is used by some nephrologists. Various needles and syringes are used for local anesthesia, with some preferring a long needle (6" - 20-gauge) for deep tissue anesthesia. Other standard equipment includes a scalpel blade, lidocaine, sterile drapes, Betadine®, gauze, gowns and masks, specimen containers.

Technique The procedure is performed by an experienced nephrologist. This procedure requires subspecialty training and is outside the realm of the generalist. Briefly, the patient is placed in a prone position with a pad or rolled towel under the abdomen. Either the right or left kidney may be biopsied and individual physician preferences differ. The ideal site is the outer aspect of the lower pole of the selected kidney where there is less risk of vascular puncture. This is located by using either bedside ultrasound or anatomic landmarks (lower portion of the 12th rib and spinous processes of the lumbar vertebrae) and usually lies approximately 2 cm inferior to the 12th rib. Using formal sterile technique (masks, caps, gowns, etc), the desired area is prepped with Betadine® and draped. Skin is anesthetized with lidocaine in the usual manner. A small cutaneous incision is made with the scalpel blade and then carried several centimeters deeper into subcutaneous tissues. Lidocaine is liberally injected along this incision using a long (6") anesthesia needle, infiltrating down to the kidney. (At this point, some physicians opt to use a "finder needle" in order to estimate the depth of the kidney below the skin.) The biopsy needle is then advanced slowly through this incision with the patient holding his breath each time the needle is pushed forward. Once the renal capsule has been penetrated, the patient is asked to breathe normally. If the needle apparatus is in proper position, the distal (visible) end of the needle will move in a pendulous fashion with inspiration and expiration in a characteristic "arc". The patient holds his breath in inspiration and the biopsy core is obtained. Details regarding biopsy trocar manipulation differ for the Vim-Silverman and the Travenol Tru-cut needles. The biopsy needle is withdrawn from the patient and the specimen is removed. In most instances, a second (and sometimes third) pass is made with the biopsy needle, using identical technique, so that several tissue cores are obtained.

Data Acquired Biopsy tissue for laboratory analysis

Specimen Fresh renal parenchymal tissue (not yet placed in fixative). Usually has a somewhat cylindrical appearance and may be up to 2 cm long, although often smaller (ie, 4-8 mm). To date, no one single method of tissue fixation has been devised for light microscopy, electron microscopy (EM), and immunofluorescence (IF) staining. Thus, if only a single biopsy core has been obtained it must be physically sectioned, usually into three portions along the short axis. At the minimum, Pathology Laboratories require 6-12 glomeruli for (Continued)

Kidney Biopsy *(Continued)*

light microscopy, 4-6 glomeruli for IF, and 2-3 for EM. Of course, larger numbers of glomeruli are always preferred so as not to overlook focal renal disease, but technically this is not always possible. Three separate biopsy cores from three separate needle passes is ideal from the pathologist's viewpoint.

Container Sterile jar or Petri dish, sterile towels, or gauze moistened with saline are sometimes used for transport of specimen for frozen sectioning.

Collection For light microscopy, specimen is placed in buffered formalin. Alternative fixatives include Zenker's and Bouin's solutions, among others. Later, the fixed specimen undergoes dehydration prior to being embedded (usually in paraffin), then is sectioned and mounted on slides. Commonly used tissue stains include H & E, PAS, and PAMS (periodic acid-methanamine silver); optional stains include congo red for amyloid. For electron microscopy, the specimen is placed in glutaraldehyde solution. All further specimen processing takes place in a specialized EM Laboratory. For immunofluorescence microscopy, the specimen needs to be immediately frozen then cryosectioned. Subsequently, the specimen is stained for the presence of IgG, IgM, IgA, C3, C1q, and other serum proteins. Either monoclonal antibodies or fluorescent antisera directed against these proteins is used.

Causes for Rejection Initial specimen allowed to dry out before fixing, incorrect fixative, inadequate specimen size, delay in transit time to laboratory (especially for frozen sections)

Normal Findings No abnormalities seen on gross, histologic, IF microscopy, or EM. However, a "normal" biopsy in a patient with clinically suspected renal disease (elevated serum creatinine, active urinary sediment, etc) may be solely a result of sampling error. In other words, some disease processes may be focal (eg, focal segmental glomerulosclerosis), variable (lupus nephritis), or early. A typical biopsy section may sample only 10 glomeruli, out of >1,000,000 glomeruli found in each kidney. Final report is issued by pathologist.

Critical Values The specimen is examined by the pathologist in a step-wise, systematic manner. Any abnormal finding is reported along with pertinent normal structural findings.[4]

Gross examination: specimen size, color, and consistency noted. Proportion of cortex and medulla estimated. Pale areas with surrounding hyperemia may be suggestive of necrosis, infarction, infectious inflammation.

Light microscopy: H & E, PAS, PAMS sections systematically studied. Features such as sample size (number of glomeruli), integrity of renal architecture, and acute vs chronic nephron loss noted. The following structures are examined.

- Glomeruli: Attention paid to important abnormalities such as glomerulosclerosis, crescents, thickened or disrupted glomerular basement membrane (GBM), mesangial expansion
- Renal tubules: Rule out ischemic or toxic tubular damage, tubular atrophy, epithelial abnormalities, inflammatory infiltrates, intraluminal casts and RBCs, etc
- Interstitium: Rule out interstitial fibrosis, extracellular crystals, edema, inflammatory cells (ie, perivascular or peritubular inflammation), granulomas
- Vasculature: Rule out emboli, thrombi, arteriosclerosis, hyaline deposits, necrotizing vasculitis

When present, glomerular disease is conventionally reported as "focal" (some glomeruli diseased but most are normal), "generalized" (only a few glomeruli spared), "segmental" (only a portion of an individual glomerulus effected), "diffuse" (entire glomerulus diseased).

Electron microscopy: Typically, only a few nephrons are scanned in detail. Of the different components of the nephron, EM is most useful in detecting glomerular pathology. Anatomic structures within the glomerulus can be examined with high resolution, including Bowman's capsule, the glomerular basement membrane (GBM), endothelium, and mesangium. Some structural abnormalities can only be demonstrable by EM. In minimal change disease, diffuse foot process effacement is detectable on EM but not light microscopy. Also, immune complex deposition disease may sometimes be evident by EM when light microscopy and IF microscopy are negative or equivocal. Immune complexes typically appear as "election dense deposits" on EM. Of clinical importance, these deposits may be accurately localized to the subendothelium, subepithelium, mesangium, or basement membrane. The location and pattern of these deposits may be diagnostic of specific renal disease. Other pathologic conditions that may be evident on EM are amyloidosis, microangiopathic injury (as in thrombotic thrombocytopenia purpura), and various storage diseases (Gaucher).

Immunofluorescence microscopy: Frozen sections are analyzed for the presence and distribution of serum proteins in kidney tissue, particularly immune complexes, or antibodies to GBM. After "staining" with monoclonal antibodies directed against immunoglobulins and complement, the specimen is studied under a fluorescence microscope. Four staining patterns are common:

- linear deposits along the GBM
- granular deposits in subepithelium, coarse (as in poststreptococcal glomerulonephritis) or fine (as in membranous glomerulonephritis)
- granular subendothelial deposits, coarse or fine
- mesangial deposits

Data acquired separately from histologic inspection, IF microscopy, and EM are integrated to form the final interpretation. As mentioned, a combination of findings may be pathognomonic. For example, Goodpasture syndrome is characterized by linear deposits of specific anti-GBM antibody with C_3 deposition on immunofluorescence, but light microscopy is variable (from nearly normal glomeruli to many crescents) and EM findings are negative for dense deposits. For a discussion of typical biopsy findings in the many primary and secondary renal diseases see Schrier's textbook, *Diseases of the Kidney*.[4]

Limitations When primary (intrinsic) renal disease is present, kidney biopsy is in many instances diagnostic. Exceptions to this include advanced glomerular disease where pathologic findings become nonspecific, technical error, and sampling bias (diseased glomeruli not present on small biopsy sample). Primary glomerular disease is also one cause of rapidly progressive glomerulonephritis (RPGN), a syndrome characterized by extracapillary crescent formation. However, a long list of diseases is associated with crescent formation and this often becomes a nonspecific finding. Unless other clues are present in such cases, the precise nature of the underlying renal disease (whether primary or not) will remain obscure. When the kidney is secondarily involved by systemic disease, biopsy findings are often nondiagnostic. Pathologic changes may be reported as "typical of" or "consistent with" a particular systemic disease, but findings are seldom pathognomonic. For example, biopsy results are usually nonspecific in Wegener granulomatosis, diabetes mellitus, TTP, and multiple myeloma.[5] These multisystem diseases are more easily diagnosed by alternative methods of testing.

Additional Information Kidney biopsy is valuable in diagnosing primary renal disease and in assessing the severity of renal disease in known systemic disorders. In addition, prognostic information and response to medical therapy may be gained from biopsy. Despite the controversy surrounding the exact indications for this procedure, it is often clinically important to define the nature and extent of kidney pathology, in order to guide therapy in a rational manner and predict the natural course of disease. This becomes particularly important in the renal transplant candidate. On occasion, a high risk patient may undergo an open surgical kidney biopsy instead of a closed needle biopsy. The former is performed by a urologist in a formal operative suite and is usually reserved for the patient with a significant coagulopathy which might require direct tamponade of bleeding sites.

Footnotes

1. Glassock RJ and Massry SG, eds, "Renal Biopsy," *Textbook of Nephrology*, 3rd ed, Chapter 93, Baltimore, MD: Williams & Wilkins, 1994, 1739-43.
2. Hlatky MA, "Is Renal Biopsy Necessary in Adults With Nephrotic Syndrome?" *Lancet*, 1982, 2(8310):1264-7.
3. Diaz-Buxo JA and Donadio JV Jr, "Complications of Percutaneous Renal Biopsy: An Analysis of 1000 Consecutive Biopsies," *Clin Nephrol*, 1975, 4(6):223-7.

(Continued)

Kidney Biopsy *(Continued)*

4. Tisher CC and Croker BP, "Indications for and Interpretation of the Renal Biopsy: Evaluation by Light, Electron, and Immunofluorescence Microscopy," *Diseases of the Kidney*, 6th ed, Chapter 15, Schrier RW and Gottschalk CW, eds, Boston, MA/Toronto: Lippincott, 1997, 435-64.
5. Dennis VW, "Investigations of Renal Function," *Cecil Textbook of Medicine*, 18th ed, Chapter 76, Wyngaarden JB and Smith LH, eds, Philadelphia, PA: WB Saunders Co, 1988, 527-8.

References

Andreucci VE, Fuiano G, Stanziale P, et al, "Role of Renal Biopsy in the Diagnosis and Prognosis of Acute Renal Failure," *Kidney Int Suppl*, 1998, 66:S91-5.

Bajema IM, Hagen EC, Hermans J, et al, "Kidney Biopsy as a Predictor for Renal Outcome in ANCA-Associated Necrotizing Glomerulonephritis," *Kidney Int*, 1999, 56(5):1751-8.

Benfield MR, Herrin J, Feld L, et al, "Safety of Kidney Biopsy in Pediatric Transplantation: A Report of the Controlled Clinical Trials in Pediatric Transplantation Trial of Induction Therapy Study Group," *Transplantation*, 1999, 67(4):544-7.

Fuiano G, Mazzo G, Comi N, et al, "Current Indications for Renal Biopsy: A Questionnaire-Based Survey," *Am J Kidney Dis*, 2000, 35(3):448-57.

Gimenez LF, Micali S, Chen RN, et al, "Laparoscopic Renal Biopsy," *Kidney Int*, 1998, 54(2):525-9.

Haas M, Meehan SM, Josephson MA, et al, "Smooth Muscle-Specific Actin Levels in the Urine of Renal Transplant Recipients: Correlation With Cyclosporine or Tacrolimus Nephrotoxicity," *Am J Kidney Dis*, 1999, 34(1):69-84.

Haas M, Spargo BH, Wit EJ, et al, "Etiologies and Outcome of Acute Renal Insufficiency in Older Adults: A Renal Biopsy Study of 259 Cases," *Am J Kidney Dis*, 2000, 35(3):433-47.

Khajehdeni P, Junaid SM, Salinas-Madrigal L, et al, "Percutaneous Renal Biopsy in the 1990s: Safety, Value, and Implications for Early Hospital Discharge," *Am J Kidney Dis*, 1999, 34(1):92-7.

Nass K and O'Neill WC, "Bedside Renal Biopsy: Ultrasound Guidance by the Nephrologist," *Am J Kidney Dis*, 1999, 34(5):955-9.

Nguyen GK and Akin MR, "Fine Needle Aspiration Cytology of the Kidney, Renal Pelvis, and Adrenal," *Clin Lab Med*, 1998, 18(3):429-59.

Oberbauer R, Rohrmoser M, Regele H, et al, "Apoptosis of Tubular Epithelial Cells in Donor Kidney Biopsies Predicts Early Renal Allograft Function," *J Am Soc Nephrol*, 1999, 10(9):2006-13.

Platt JF, Rubin JM, and Ellis JH, "Lupus Nephritis: Predictive Value of Conventional and Doppler US and Comparison With Serologic and Biopsy Parameters," *Radiology*, 1997, 203(1):82-6.

Randhawa PS, Saad RS, Jordan M, et al, "Clinical Significance of Renal Biopsies Showing Concurrent Acute Rejection and Tacrolimus-Associated Tubular Vacuolization," *Transplantation*, 1999, 67(1):85-9.

Rodriguez F, Krayenbuhl JC, Harrison WB, et al, "Renal Biopsy Findings and Follow-up of Renal Function in Rheumatoid Arthritis Patients Treated With Cyclosporin A. An Update From the International Kidney Biopsy Registry," *Arthritis Rheum*, 1996, 39(9):1491-8.

Tan PH, Yadin O, Kleinman KS, et al, "Simultaneous Postinfections Glomerulonephritis and Thrombotic Microangiopathy: A Renal Biopsy Study," *Am J Kidney Dis*, 1998, 31(3):513-20.

Labial Salivary Gland Biopsy

Synonyms Lower Lip Biopsy for Sjögren Syndrome; LSG Biopsy; Minor Salivary Gland Biopsy

Indications

- diagnose Sjögren syndrome: LSG biopsy is useful in selected cases of Sjögren syndrome, especially when the diagnosis remains in doubt. Biopsy is indicated when histologic confirmation of salivary gland involvement is necessary for clinical management. Although a number of diagnostic criteria for Sjögren syndrome have been published from different study groups worldwide, most include a positive LSG biopsy as an important diagnostic test.
- aid in the diagnosis of sarcoidosis: Granulomatous inflammation from lip biopsies are suggestive (but not diagnostic) of sarcoidosis. However, LSG biopsy is seldom necessary in the diagnostic work-up of sarcoidosis; biopsies from commonly involved sites, such as the lung and/or lymph nodes, have a higher yield.

Contraindications

- severe coagulopathy
- systemic anticoagulation
- hypersensitivity to lidocaine or epinephrine
- local infection, mouth ulcers (relative contraindications)

Patient Preparation Procedure and possible complications are discussed in detail with the patient and informed consent is obtained. The details of scheduling (date of procedure, time, location, etc) are handled by the surgical team following a formal evaluation. All aspirin and aspirin-containing products should be discontinued 5-7 days prior to procedure; nonsteroidal anti-inflammatory agents should also be held at least 2-3 days beforehand. Routine patient medications may be taken the morning of surgery. If a bleeding disorder is suspected, obtain a complete blood count, PT, and PTT.

Aftercare As per surgical team recommendations. In general, solid foods are avoided for several hours postprocedure. The patient should be instructed to contact surgeon or primary physician promptly if complications arise. A follow-up visit is usually arranged by the surgical team.

Complications LSG biopsy is considered a very safe procedure. Reported complications include:

- persistent numbness in the lower lip, at the incision site; this may occur if small sensory branches are severed during incision or, less commonly, dissection. This complication has been associated with the use of older surgical techniques, which include the blind "punch biopsy" labial midline biopsies, and others. With newer surgical approaches, where the glands are dissected free of the various vascular and neural structures, the incidence of lip numbness is <1%.
- excessive bleeding at the biopsy site. This is an unusual complication and associated more with earlier surgical techniques.
- torn stitches

Technique As previously mentioned, a variety of surgical techniques may be employed; only recent techniques will be described. The procedure is carried out on an alert patient, seated comfortably in a dental chair. The lower lip is anesthetized using lidocaine with epinephrine, then everted. Only areas of normal mucosa are suitable for biopsy. Daniels (1984) advocates making a single horizontal incision approximately 2 cm long between the midline and commissure. Following this, blunt dissection is carried out to free the salivary glands from the surrounding fascia. This technique allows direct visualization of sensory nerves, which are then easily avoided. At least five glands should be removed; due to their small size, histologic findings (eg, lymphocytic infiltration) may not be present in all glands.

Specimen An adequate specimen consists of 5-10 minor salivary glands. Tissue processing is supervised by the surgical staff. Routine histologic processing is sufficient in most cases. Electron microscopy, microbiologic culture, and cytology are optional and are at the physician's discretion.

Normal Findings General histopathology and degree of glandular inflammation is determined by a pathologist. There is some disagreement in the rheumatologic literature concerning the precise pathologic criteria for Sjögren syndrome. The "focus scoring method" is the most widely accepted method of interpretation and involves semiquantitative grading of salivary gland inflammation. Based on the early work of Chisholm and Mason (1968), more than one focus of lymphocytes/4 mm^2 of minor salivary gland tissue accurately distinguishes Sjögren syndrome from normal controls. A focus of lymphocytes has been defined as an aggregate of 50 or more round cells. Focus score of 0 or 1 is normal. Scattered foci of lymphocytes may still yield a focus score of 0-1 if the number of lymphocytes in a given focus is small (<50 cells), or foci are widely spaced (>4 mm^2 of gland). Background glandular tissue must be normal as well.

Critical Values A focus score >1 is consistent with Sjögren syndrome. In other words, two or more focal aggregates of lymphocytes (>50 cells each) are seen consistently in most glands of the specimen. Biopsies are assigned a Chisholm-Mason score of 0-4. It is important that normal-appearing acini should be visible adjacent to lymphocyte aggregates to avoid confusion with other diseases such as chronic sialadenitis. Salivary gland biopsies which show evidence of duct obstruction or nonspecific injury are excluded from analysis.

Limitations There is still some disagreement over the histologic criteria for Sjögren syndrome by LSG biopsy. For example, a Chisholm-Mason score of 1 is sufficient in some studies to qualify as a positive test, but in others the score must be ≥2. False-positive results have been reported if the biopsy is taken in an area of chronic mucosal inflammation such as lichen planus, repeated trauma, mucocele, etc. The false-positive rate may be as high as 20%. Potential sampling variation may lead to false-negative results since histologic

(Continued)

Labial Salivary Gland Biopsy *(Continued)*

involvement of salivary glands can be patchy. Finally, LSG biopsy establishes the presence of the salivary component of Sjögren syndrome only, not the ocular component.

Additional Information Sjögren syndrome is a common systemic autoimmune disease that may affect 1% of the population. Persons with primary Sjögren syndrome present with xerostomia and xerophthalmia, which result from inflammatory infiltrates involving exocrine glands. Secondary Sjögren syndrome occurs when the abnormalities are associated with another connective tissue disease such as systemic lupus erythematosus or rheumatoid arthritis. Several sets of criteria have been published to diagnose this syndrome, with subtle but important differences[1]. The "California (San Diego)" criteria[2], for example, includes the following:

- subjective symptoms: dry mouth
- ocular component: Schirmer test, Rose-Bengal test, fluorescent test
- oral component: reduced basal and stimulated salivary flow, labial salivary gland biopsy
- serological studies: rheumatoid factor, antinuclear antibody, anti-Ro/SSA, La/SSB

In contrast, the Copenhagen criteria do not require subjective symptoms or serologic tests, and base the diagnosis on objective test abnormalities such as the Schirmer test and LSG biopsy. Greek criteria emphasize subjective symptoms more than the California criteria, and do not include serologic variables. The (revised) European criteria has the most specific subjective symptoms (daily dry mouth >3 months, artificial tear use >3 times per day, daily dry eyes >3 months, recurrent swelling of the salivary glands, and need for liquids for swallowing food)[3]. In general, the various diagnostic criteria worldwide include LSG biopsy as an important (but not sole) variable in the diagnosis of Sjögren syndrome. Some authors believe that LSG biopsy is most useful in patients who meet the San Diego criteria for sicca and positive anti-Ro or anti-La antibody; the biopsy adds little in persons with a clinically obvious diagnosis or in cases where Sjögren syndrome is not reasonably suspected[4].

Footnotes

1. Bell M, Askari A, Bookman A, et al, "Sjögren Syndrome: A Critical Review of Clinical Management," *J Rheumatol*, 1999, 26(9):2051-61.
2. Fox RI, Robinson CA, Curd JG, et al, "Sjögren Syndrome: Proposed Criteria for Classification," *Arthritis Rheum*, 1986, 29(5):577-85.
3. Vitali C, Bombardieri S, Moutsopoulos HM, et al, "Preliminary Criteria for the Classification of Sjögren Syndrome: Results of a Prospective Concerted Action Supported by the European Community," *Arthritis Rheum*, 1993, 36(3):340-7.
4. Lee M, Rutka JA, Slomovic AR, et al, "Establishing Guidelines for the Role of Minor Salivary Gland Biopsy in Clinical Practice for Sjögren Syndrome," *Rheumatology*, 1999, 25(2):247-53.

References

Daniels TE and Fox PC, "Salivary and Oral Components of Sjögren Syndrome," *Rheum Dis Clin North Am*, 1992, 18(3):571-89.

Fox RI, Tornwall J, and Michelson P, "Current Issues in the Diagnosis and Treatment of Sjögren Syndrome," *Curr Opin Rheumatol*, 1999, 11(5):364-71.

♦ **Lower Lip Biopsy for Sjögren Syndrome** *see* Labial Salivary Gland Biopsy *on page 132*

♦ **LSG Biopsy** *see* Labial Salivary Gland Biopsy *on page 132*

♦ **Mantoux Test** *see* Tuberculin Skin Testing, Intracutaneous *on page 144*

♦ **Minor Salivary Gland Biopsy** *see* Labial Salivary Gland Biopsy *on page 132*

♦ **Nailfold Capillaroscopy** *see* Widefield Capillary Microscopy *on page 149*

♦ **Nailfold Capillary Microscopy** *see* Widefield Capillary Microscopy *on page 149*

Nasal Endoscopy

Synonyms Rhinolaryngoscopy; Rhinopharyngoscopy

Procedure Commonly Includes Direct examination of the nasal passages, nasopharynx, oropharynx, and larynx by means of a flexible fiberoptic endoscope. This procedure permits visualization of upper airway structures inaccessible to the conventional otoscope or nasal speculum. Nasal endoscopy is carried out by an allergist or otolaryngologist in an outpatient setting. It is a safe and rapid (10-15 minutes) means of evaluating complicated upper airway and sinus disorders, particularly those refractory to standard medical therapy.

Indications The precise role of nasal endoscopy in clinical practice is still evolving. Although it has been applied to a wide variety of clinical situations, some experts warn against its indiscriminate use. Clearly, not every patient who presents with symptoms referable to the nasopharynx need undergo endoscopy.

General indications for this procedure are:

- upper airway disease of unclear etiology
- chronic or recurrent upper airway disease, despite appropriate therapy

Specific indications for nasal endoscopy include:

- suspected nasal polyposis (or when polyps are seen on speculum exam); to confirm the diagnosis, assess extent of disease, check response to treatment, and screen for recurrence after polypectomy
- chronic or recurrent sinusitis; purulent material may be visualized directly and the source located (sphenoid, maxillary, ethmoid ostia)
- persistent nasal obstruction, not due to septal deviation and not responding to decongestants
- chronic nasal discharge of unknown etiology, especially if unilateral (ie, undiagnosed nonallergic rhinitis)
- anosmia
- recurrent epistaxis or serosanguineous nasal discharge
- persistent hoarseness
- chronic use of steroid nasal sprays for perennial rhinitis, especially after several years of therapy
- suspected cases of adenoidal hypertrophy (eg, young child with sleep apnea)
- suspected cases of eustachian tube obstruction (eg, child with recurrent otitis after tympanic tubes placed)
- evaluation of "pseudoasthma," where stridor and wheezing are due to vocal cord apposition and not bronchospasm (possibly psychiatric in origin)
- suspected nasopharyngeal carcinoma (persistent pain, history of cigarette use, Oriental ancestry, etc)
- suspected nasopharyngeal candidiasis in an immunocompromised patient even if conventional examination reveals a normal oropharynx
- postoperative evaluation of upper airway surgical sites
- evaluation of patients with known or suspected granulomatous disease (sarcoidosis, Wegener disease), to rule out upper airway granulomas or ulcerations in selected cases

Emergency indications include:

- suspected epiglottitis
- laryngeal trauma
- difficult endotracheal intubations, to provide direct visualization for tube placement
- stridor, to rule out foreign body (diagnosis only)

Nasal endoscopy is less useful in:

- uncomplicated allergic rhinitis; procedure is generally not required to establish this diagnosis
- random screening for nasal polyps in asymptomatic patients or patients with simple allergic rhinitis

Contraindications The procedure is contraindicated when a severe, uncontrolled coagulopathy is present. Mucosal trauma is always a possibility (although unusual) and local tamponade of bleeding sites is difficult. In addition, the sphenopalatine artery lies in the posterior nares, and trauma to this vessel may cause serious arterial hemorrhage. Since nasal endoscopy may theoretically induce cardiac arrhythmias or vasovagal syncope, it is contraindicated in the patient with a tenuous cardiopulmonary status. However, serious morbidity or mortality of this nature has yet to be reported.

Patient Preparation Technique and risks of the procedure are discussed with the patient and verbal consent is obtained. (Some experts consider this procedure an extension of the clinical examination and do not obtain formal written

(Continued)

Nasal Endoscopy *(Continued)*

consent.) Nasal endoscopy is generally performed as an elective, outpatient procedure with scheduling issues handled by the allergist or otolaryngologist. Often, endoscopy is carried out during the initial visit to the allergist's office, at physician's discretion. The patient need not be fasting prior to procedure. Routine medications may be taken the morning of endoscopy. Some endoscopists will require the patient to discontinue aspirin products and nonsteroidal anti-inflammatory agents several days beforehand, especially if significant epistaxis is anticipated. Premedication with sedatives is not usually required.

Aftercare Food and water should be avoided until gag reflex returns (gag may be depressed by Xylocaine® solution or spray), otherwise, no specific post-procedure restrictions are necessary.

Complications Nasal endoscopy appears to be a very safe procedure. Rohr (1983) reported no complications out of 230 rhinopharyngoscopies. A similar safety profile was documented by Selner (1985) with a single nosebleed (mild) out of 400 examinations. Transient complications include coughing, sneezing, and nasal comfort, resolving soon after termination of the procedure. Potential complications include:

- epistaxis
- nasal discomfort (<5%)
- bronchospasm
- laryngospasm (avoided by keeping the instrument above the vocal cords)
- syncope/arrhythmias

Equipment A number of fiberoptic nasal endoscopes are available, either rigid or flexible. Currently, the flexible endoscope is the preferred instrument due to its superior safety profile, patient acceptance, and technical convenience. The flexible endoscope is usually 300 mm in length, with a diameter of 3.7-4 mm; deflection angle of the tip is 90° down and 130° up. The rhinolaryngoscope is connected with a cold light source. In some centers, the instrument is part of a camera-mount-cine system, with video camera, monitor, and recorder suspended from the ceiling. The physician views the images on a standard video monitor, which also provides a permanent audiovisual record of the examination.

Technique At the beginning of the procedure, the patient is comfortably seated in a standard examination chair equipped with head supports. A standard nasal speculum exam is performed. Following this, a 4:1 mixture of 4% lidocaine and 1:1000 epinephrine is aerosolized into the nasopharynx. Alternatively, a 4% cocaine aerosol may be used as a topical anesthetic agent and vasoconstrictor. If a detailed examination of the hypopharynx is planned, some physicians will have the patient gargle with a Xylocaine® solution. Others, however, feel this is unnecessary and avoid this step due to frequent patient discomfort. Additional anesthetic effect may be obtained using 2% viscous lidocaine applied directly to the turbinates with a cotton swab. After 3-5 minutes, the examiner guides the endoscope into the nostril, where the septum and turbinates may be clearly seen. The sinus orifices may also be examined for signs of inflammation or discharge. After the nasal fossa examination is completed, the tip of the endoscope is advanced through the choana and into the nasopharyngeal cavity. A number of important structures are visualized, such as the eustachian tube orifice, Rosenmueller's fossa, and adenoids. The patient may be asked to swallow several times to confirm the location of the eustachian tube orifice. Following inspection of the inferior portion of the oropharynx, the instrument is advanced into the hypopharynx. Here, structures such as the lingular tonsil, posterior tongue, piriform sinuses, and epiglottis are visualized. The vocal cords are easily seen and vocal cord function is assessed with the patient phonating. In general, the endoscope is not passed through the vocal cords, thus avoiding bronchospasm. Anatomy can be reviewed as the instrument is withdrawn. The procedure is then repeated through the other nostril. See table and graphic.

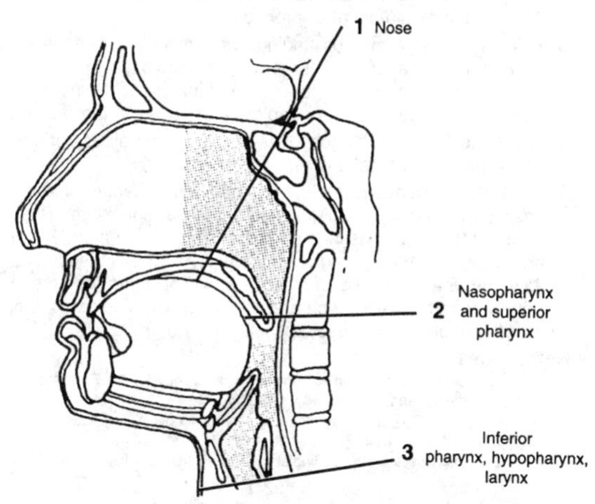

Reproduced with permission, from Selner JC and Koepke JW, "Rhinolaryngoscopy in the Allergy Office", *Ann Allergy*, 1985, 54:480.

Clinical Findings on 400 Consecutive Nasal Endoscopies

		1. Nose
Concha (turbinates)	28	Clefting conchal sinus, polypoidal changes, bullosa, papillary hyperplasia, fibromatous hypertrophy, telangiectasia, atrophy
Septum	42	Deviation, perforation, spurs
Polyps	51	
Inflammatory mucosa	23	Mucous pus, hypertrophy, cystic changes, mucocele, vessel injection, inflammation of ostea of sphenoethmoidal recess, edema
		2. Nasopharynx and Superior Pharynx
Adenoids	63	
Eustachian orifice	5	Torus cyst, lymphoid inclusion, adenoid encroachment
Inflammation — edema	7	Vessel injection, ulceration
Pharyngeal wall	17	Osteophyte, aneurysm, lymphoid hypertrophy
Other	4	Rathke pouch cyst, cystic lymphoid involution
		3. Inferior Pharynx-Hypopharynx-Larynx
Lingular tonsils	28	Significant enlargement
Post tongue	2	Circumvallate papillary cyst
Vallecula	6	Cystic changes, papillomata
Epiglottis	15	Mucocele, inflammation, displacement, petiole prominence
Glottis	24	Erythema, displacement
Vocal cord	23	Polyp papillomata, contact ulceration, paralysis, granuloma, web
Arytenoids	6	Contact ulcer, asymmetry, edema
Other	10	Laryngocele (2), cord trauma (3), inflammatory granuloma (2), paralysis (3)

Reproduced with permission from Selner JC and Koepke JW, "Rhinolaryngoscopy in the Allergy Office," *Ann Allergy*, 1985, 54:480.

(Continued)

Nasal Endoscopy *(Continued)*

Normal Findings No abnormalities seen. A preliminary written report is completed immediately after procedure.

Critical Values Numerous findings of clinical significance may be encountered, including anatomic abnormalities (polyps, hyperplasia, ulcers, carcinoma, cysts), inflammation, edema, and infections. Selner (1985) outlined his findings in 400 consecutive rhinolaryngoscopies in the previous table.

Limitations Rhinopharyngoscopes do not permit biopsy of suspicious lesions or therapeutic interventions (eg, electrocautery)

Additional Information Conventional examination of the upper airways consists of otoscopic evaluation with a nasal speculum. This visualizes only 2.5 cm of the nasal passage due to a short focal length, which leaves significant areas (>11 cm) of the nasopharynx unexamined. Nasal endoscopy allows rapid examination of these areas. The figure depicts the areas of the upper respiratory tract which are difficult to examine using conventional techniques (eg, otoscope, nasal speculum).

References

Rohr A, Hassner A, and Saxon A, "Rhinopharyngoscopy for the Evaluation of Allergic-Immunologic Disorders," *Ann Allergy*, 1983, 50(6):380-4.

Schumacher MJ, "Fiberoptic Nasopharyngolaryngoscopy: A Procedure for Allergists?" *J Allergy Clin Immunol*, 1988, 81(5 Pt 2):960-2.

Selner JC and Koepke JW, "Rhinolaryngoscopy in the Allergy Office," *Ann Allergy*, 1985, 54(6):479-82.

♦ **Oral Provocation Test** *see* Ingestion Challenge Test *on page 125*

Patch Test

Synonyms Contact Dermatitis Skin Test; Epicutaneous Patch Test

Procedure Commonly Includes Application of multiple test materials to the skin surface in order to demonstrate allergic contact dermatitis (ACD). Suspected allergens are taped in rows onto the patient's back and the underlying skin is examined 48 hours later for erythema, signifying delayed-type hypersensitivity.

Indications In general, this procedure is used diagnostically to identify causes of ACD.

The patch test is most useful in the following situations:

- confirm the diagnosis of ACD already suspected from history and physical exam
- determine the individual allergen causing ACD when many are suspected
- explore causes of chronic dermatitis unresponsive to usual therapies
- exclude the presence of ACD in complicated dermatological cases (by means of negative patch testing)

Contraindications Patch testing with a substance previously implicated in an anaphylactic reaction in a particular patient represents a relative contraindication; physician supervision is necessary.

Patient Preparation No special skin preparation is required. Whenever possible, patient should bring additional suspected allergens (eg, personal cosmetics) to the testing area for physician review.

Aftercare The following instructions should be given to the patient. Patch test sites must be kept dry initially. Heavy exercise is not permitted in order to avoid excess perspiration. Any test material causing severe pruritus or pain must be removed promptly and the physician notified. On the evening prior to follow-up appointment, patch tests should be entirely removed by the patient and discarded. Following this, bathing is permissible but vigorous rubbing of test sites should be avoided.

Special Instructions Patch testing requires large areas of normal appearing skin. Thus, patients with known pre-existing dermatitis must undergo careful skin examination prior to patch testing.

Complications Adverse reactions may be broadly divided into two categories, nonimmunologic and immunologic (allergic) reactions. The "irritant skin reaction" is considered nonimmunologic; certain materials may be intrinsically damaging to the skin, causing an early onset, painful, macular dermatitis. Another nonimmunologic complication is bacterial or viral infection involving strongly reacting test sites. Adverse reactions which are immunologic are mediated by either immediate or delayed hypersensitivity mechanisms. Contact urticaria is possible within minutes of applying the standard test battery, but is unusual. Rarely, immediate life-threatening anaphylaxis has been reported but this appears most often associated with patch testing drugs and not with commercial test materials. Examples of delayed hypersensitivity complications include the following:

- severe skin reactions (pustules, necrosis) when an allergen causes a flare of underlying contact dermatitis
- persistent positive reactions
- active sensitization to a test material (ie, ACD may actually be induced by a test substance - incidence unclear)

Overall, however, the incidence of all complications is low and serious complications are reportable.

Equipment Patch test materials are standardized and available commercially. Test allergens are available as a standardized battery consisting of approximately 30 items (benzocaine, neomycin, fragrance mix, wood alcohols, etc). Additional allergen batteries are available for specific occupations such as printers, hairdressers, or medical practitioners. Delivery systems are also standardized and several are available. Commonly, an aluminum cup or round cellulose disk is used to affix each test allergen to the surface of the skin. An ultraviolet marking pen or gentian violet is required to label test sites.

Technique Testing is performed on normal appearing skin. The patient's back is premarked in vertical rows using a fluorescent pen. A small amount of test allergen is applied to the disk (or aluminum cup) and affixed to the skin with nonallergenic tape. Patches remain in place 48 hours and are then removed by the patient. Tape irritation is allowed to resolve for 12-24 hours. Skin response is recorded by the physician by means of a graded scoring system at 24 and 48 hours after patch removal. Certain substances require additional readings at 72 hours (eg, neomycin). The previous steps are only guidelines and subject to physician modification.

Normal Findings The skin underlying each test substance is examined and graded. Normal skin is graded "-".

Critical Values Several grading schemes for evaluating positive skin reactions have been proposed. One popular scheme is as follows:[1]

+: weak positive (faint erythema, no vesicles)
++: strong positive (vesicles, edema, papules)
+++: extreme positive (spreading, bullous)
?: doubtful reaction
IR: irritant reaction

The physician must distinguish primary irritant skin reactions (ie, chemical burns) from true allergic reactions. The former tend to occur early and diminish over days and are more painful, demarcated, and erosive.

Limitations Spurious results from patch testing are well acknowledged in the literature and represent a major clinical challenge. False-positive rates are significant, the most common cause being the use of excessively high concentrations of test material. Other false-positives include misinterpretation of irritant reactions, misinterpretation of contact urticaria, and the so-called "angry back" syndrome (generalized erythema of the entire back). False-negative results are often related to technical errors in allergen placement, concentration, or timing of readings. In some instances, false-negative results stem from the failure to mimic real-life conditions at the workplace; factors such as perspiration and friction are not considered routinely.

Additional Information The economic and social consequences of contact dermatitis are significant. Forty percent to 60% of occupational absenteeism is attributed to some form of contact dermatitis.[2] Patch testing evaluates delayed-type hypersensitivity to various allergens by means of classic type IV

(Continued)

Patch Test *(Continued)*

immunologic reaction (helper T-lymphocyte mediated). Given this, patch testing does not evaluate either immediate hypersensitivity reactions (contact urticaria) or irritant dermatitis. At present, patch testing is the only objective means of establishing ACD. In practicality, frequency of patch testing varies considerably among physicians; some rarely patch test while others routinely test any patient with eczema. It should be noted that the physician's history and physical exam alone is often inadequate in pinpointing even the more common etiologies of ACD.[3] Thus, despite its limitations, patch testing remains an indispensable tool.

Footnotes

1. Fregert S, *Manual of Contact Dermatitis*, 2nd ed, Copenhagen: Munksgaard, 1981.
2. Johnson MLT, Burdick AE, Johnson KG, et al, "Prevalence, Morbidity, and Cost of Dermatological Diseases," *J Invest Dermatol*, 1979, 73:395-401.
3. Kieffer M, "Nickel Sensitivity: Relationship Between History and Patch Test Reaction," *Contact Dermatitis*, 1979, 5(6):398.

References

Adams RM, "Patch Testing - A Recapitulation," *J Am Acad Dermatol*, 1981, 5(6):629-46.

Fischer T and Maibach HI, "Patch Testing in Allergic Contact Dermatitis: An Update," *Semin Dermatol*, 1986, 5:214-24.

Fransway AF, "Epicutaneous Patch Testing: Current Trends and Controversial Topics," *Mayo Clin Proc*, 1989, 64(4):415-23.

Young E and Houwing RH, "Patch Test Results With Standard Allergens Over a Decade," *Contact Dermatitis*, 1987, 17(2):104-7.

Penicillin Allergy Skin Testing

Related Information

Allergy Testing, Intracutaneous (Intradermal) *on page 103*

Allergy Testing, Percutaneous *on page 106*

Synonyms Penicillin Skin Tests; Skin Tests for Penicillin Allergy

Procedure Commonly Includes Skin testing patients with suspected IgE-mediated penicillin allergy. The reagents used in this procedure are derivatives of the basic benzylpenicillin molecule. They are introduced into the epidermis by a skin prick or into the dermis by an intracutaneous (intradermal) injection. An immediate wheal-and-flare reaction confirms immediate hypersensitivity (Gell and Coombs' type I reaction). This is an important procedure in clinical practice and accurately identifies those individuals at high risk for a severe allergic reaction to penicillin.

Indications Theoretically, all patients about to receive a beta-lactam antibiotic should be skin tested. However, it has been demonstrated that such a comprehensive testing policy has a low yield and is not cost-effective. Most authorities recommend skin testing in the following situations:

- patients with a history of penicillin allergy who require penicillin as the drug of choice (eg, treatment of central nervous system syphilis)
- patients with a history of penicillin allergy who require a beta-lactam antibiotic (eg, semisynthetic penicillin, cephalosporin)
- patients with a history of multiple "antibiotic allergies;" skin testing can determine if a beta-lactam drug is a safe treatment option.

Contraindications

- documented history of penicillin-induced anaphylaxis, Stevens-Johnson syndrome, exfoliative dermatitis, or status asthmaticus. These conditions are life-threatening and contraindicate the use of penicillins in general; thus, there is little need to skin test.
- recent use of medications known to inhibit the IgE-mediated skin response (wheal and flare); this includes antihistamines, hydroxyzine, tricyclic antidepressants, and phenothiazines

Patient Preparation In some medical centers, penicillin skin testing is permitted only after formal consultation with the allergist performing the procedure. If the procedure appears necessary, the technique, risks, and benefits should be explained to the patient. As a preliminary screening measure, the physician should perform a brief dermatologic exam to ensure adequate areas of normal-appearing skin and to identify the rare patient with dermographism. The patient should be instructed to discontinue the following medications several days prior to testing: antihistamines, tricyclic antidepressants, hydroxyzine, phenothiazines. Newer antihistamines with extended half-lives may interfere with testing for over 1 week. All medication changes should be approved by the primary physician.

Aftercare If no complications have occurred, the patient may be discharged from the testing center following completion of the test. Skin sites should be kept clean but remain uncovered. Physician should be contacted immediately if symptoms of wheezing, lightheadedness, or shortness of breath develop several hours later (the unusual case of the "late phase response").

Special Instructions If skin testing is performed by a nurse or physician-assistant, a physician should be immediately available for the rare case of anaphylactic shock. Emergency equipment must be in the testing area, including defibrillation equipment, intubation blades, lidocaine (and other cardiac medications), aqueous epinephrine for injection needles, syringes, and tourniquets.

Complications When properly performed, serious adverse reactions are unusual. The incidence of systemic reactions has been estimated at <1%, with the majority of these being mild or self-limited. Local complications are more common, but generally resolve within hours. These include subcutaneous hemorrhage, localized pruritus, and nonspecific irritant reactions. The risk of hepatitis B, local infection, or human immunodeficiency virus (HIV) transmission is diminishingly small since needles are not reused between patients. The "late response" is a rare but reported complication of allergy skin testing (see Allergy Testing, Intracutaneous (Intradermal) *on page 103*).

Equipment The reagents used for skin testing include:

- The "major determinant," a derivative of the benzylpenicillin molecule called benzylpenicillin-polylysine. It is standardized, commercially available, and routinely used.
- The "minor determinant mixture (MDM)," either benzylpenicillin itself or another derivative (such as penicillonate or penicilloyl-amine). The MDM has not yet been standardized and is not commercially available. Nonetheless, the MDM is widely employed by many allergists and is clinically relevant.

Both the major and minor determinants are administered, in most cases. If the major determinant is used alone, 10% to 25% of allergic individuals could be missed. If the minor determinant is used alone, perhaps 5% to 10% of cases could remain undetected, including potential cases of anaphylaxis. In addition to these two reagents, positive (histamine) and negative (diluent) controls are often given. Standard tuberculin syringes, 27-gauge needles, and prick test equipment are also needed.

Technique Ideally, skin test reagents are applied first by the prick test, followed by an intradermal test if the prick test is negative. The prick test is carried out by placing a drop of the reagent in a predetermined location on the skin, usually the forearm. A small needle is passed through the drop and into the epidermis, then removed. (For details, see Allergy Testing, Percutaneous *on page 106*.) For intracutaneous testing, each reagent is individually drawn up into a tuberculin syringe. Again, the volar aspect of the forearm is the preferred site for testing. The reagent (or control) is injected into the dermis, using a 27-gauge needle. A small bleb is raised, usually 0.01-0.02 mL. (For details, see Allergy Testing, Intracutaneous (Intradermal) *on page 103*.)

Data Acquired Test sites are examined at 15-20 minutes for a local wheal-and-flare reaction. The largest diameter of the wheal and/or erythema is measured and recorded in millimeters.

Normal Findings No wheal or erythema after the major determinant, minor determinant, and diluent control. Administration of histamine control should result in a positive skin reaction, with induration >5 mm diameter.

Critical Values For both the prick test and the intracutaneous test, a wheal >5 mm in diameter (with erythema) is considered a positive test. For proper interpretation, the patient should be questioned regarding a history of penicillin allergy. If a reasonable history of penicillin allergy is obtained, a negative skin test essentially rules out a life-threatening allergic response to therapeutic doses of penicillin. No cases of anaphylaxis have been reported in patients who are skin test negative. However, ≤3% of patients who are skin test negative may develop minor reactions while on therapy, such as rash and pruritus. In the patient who has a positive skin test and a positive history of

(Continued)

Penicillin Allergy Skin Testing *(Continued)*

penicillin allergy, the odds of a serious allergic reaction to penicillin therapy are quite high, perhaps 50% to 70%. If skin tests are administered to patients who provide no history of penicillin allergy, the chances of a positive test are low (about 2%). Unfortunately, anaphylaxis during penicillin therapy has been reported in this patient population, although rare. Skin testing all patients prior to beta-lactam therapy, with or without a history of penicillin allergy, is not practical or cost-effective.

Limitations

- This procedure detects only IgE-mediated allergic reactions. Thus, a variety of adverse drug reactions may still occur in skin test negative patients, including serum sickness, drug fever, antibiotic associated colitis, interstitial nephritis, contact dermatitis, bone marrow suppression, and others.
- A number of factors can cause false-positive and false-negative results, as seen in other forms of skin testing (see Allergy Testing, Intracutaneous (Intradermal) *on page 103*).
- Test results apply to penicillin-type antibiotics (natural penicillins, semisynthetic penicillins), but not to cephalosporins, aztreonam, or imipenem.

References

Sarti W, "Routine Use of Skin Testing for Immediate Penicillin Allergy to 6764 Patients in an Outpatient Clinic," *Ann Allergy*, 1985, 55(2):157-61.

VanArsdel PP Jr, Martonick GJ, Johnson LE, et al, "The Value of Skin Testing for Penicillin Allergy Diagnosis," *West J Med*, 1986, 144(3):311-4.

Weiss ME and Adkinson NF, "Beta-Lactam Allergy," *Principles and Practice of Infectious Diseases*, 4th ed, Chapter 17, Mandell GL, Bennett JE, and Dolin R, eds, New York, NY: Church Livingstone, 1996, 264-9.

Weiss ME and Adkinson NF, "Immediate Hypersensitivity Reactions to Penicillin and Related Antibiotics," *Clin Allergy*, 1988, 18(6):515-40.

♦ **Penicillin Skin Tests** *see* Penicillin Allergy Skin Testing *on page 140*

♦ **Percutaneous Allergy Testing** *see* Allergy Testing, Percutaneous *on page 106*

♦ **PPD Test** *see* Tuberculin Skin Testing, Intracutaneous *on page 144*

♦ **Prick Test** *see* Allergy Testing, Percutaneous *on page 106*

♦ **Prong Test** *see* Tuberculin Skin Testing, Multiple Puncture *on page 147*

♦ **Puncture Test** *see* Allergy Testing, Percutaneous *on page 106*

♦ **Purified Protein Derivative (PPD) Test** *see* Tuberculin Skin Testing, Intracutaneous *on page 144*

♦ **Renal Biopsy** *see* Kidney Biopsy *on page 126*

♦ **Rhinolaryngoscopy** *see* Nasal Endoscopy *on page 134*

♦ **Rhinopharyngoscopy** *see* Nasal Endoscopy *on page 134*

♦ **Schirmer 1 Test** *see* Schirmer Test *on page 142*

♦ **Schirmer 2 Test** *see* Schirmer Test *on page 142*

Schirmer Test

Synonyms Schirmer 1 Test; Schirmer 2 Test

Procedure Commonly Includes *In vivo* measurement of total tear production, both basal and reflex tear output. A strip of filter paper is placed in the lower conjunctival sac. After 5 minutes, the amount of moisture on the paper is determined and compared against normal values. Although the technique is somewhat crude, this is a simple and well-established means of assessing the patient with "dry eyes".

Indications

- evaluate patients with suspected Sjögren syndrome in order to confirm decreased tear secretion objectively
- evaluate the "dry eye" syndrome, which encompasses a wide variety of conditions (medications, autoimmune diseases, chronic blepharoconjunctivitis, allergies, etc)

Contraindications None reported

Patient Preparation The patient may take routine oral medications on the day of examination but the specific drugs should be recorded in the chart. "Artificial tears" eye drops (or similar ophthalmics) should be discontinued prior to procedure.

Aftercare The patient may resume previous activity level.

Equipment Standardized, calibrated filter paper strips measuring about 25 mm in length are available for Schirmer testing.

Technique It is usually performed by an ophthalmologist. As noted by Mackie and Seal (1980), the Schirmer test has been performed in a variety of ways. In the Schirmer 1 test, the patient is seated in a well-lit room. The 5 mm top end of a filter paper strip is folded back and placed in the lower palpebral conjunctival sac of each eye. Most prefer an open-end technique. After 5 minutes, the filter paper is removed and the length of the filter paper which has been moistened by tears is recorded in millimeters. Several variations of this basic procedure have been described. In the basal secretion test, topical anesthetic eye drops are placed in the conjunctival sac. After the anesthetic has taken effect, the Schirmer 1 test is repeated with the room somewhat darkened. (Note that some authors refer to this as the "Schirmer 2" test, a potential source of confusion). In the Schirmer 2 test, anesthetic eye drops are again instilled in the conjunctival sac and filter paper strips are positioned as before; a cotton tipped swab is inserted high into the nasal passage. By irritating the nasal mucosa, reflex tear secretion is stimulated.

Normal Findings

- Schirmer 1 test (basic test): 10-30 mm of filter paper moistened at 5 minutes
- Basal secretion test (with anesthetic eye drop): ≥8 mm of moisture at 5 minutes
- Schirmer 2 test: ≥15 mm of moisture at 5 minutes

Critical Values

- Schirmer 1 test: <10 mm of filter paper moistened is considered abnormal; <5 mm is consistent with Sjögren syndrome; this test measures abnormalities in both reflex and/or basal secretions
- Basal secretion test: <8 mm; suggests impaired basic tear secretion
- Schirmer 2 test: <15 mm; suggests impaired reflex tear secretion

Limitations Although test results are quantitative, technique is relatively imprecise. The Schirmer test offers only an approximation of total tear production and other procedures are available, such as fluorescein dye staining and rose bengal staining. The Schirmer test is less reliable in evaluating the moderately dry eye. The ability of this procedure to separate basal from reflex tear secretion has been disputed by some.

Additional Information The patient who presents with dry eyes is a common problem for the general practitioner. The differential diagnosis of xerophthalmia is broad, and includes:

- Sjögren syndrome (keratoconjunctivitis sicca)
- medications
- aging (this has been disputed by some)
- sarcoidosis
- others

Recognition of Sjögren syndrome as a cause of the dry eye is particularly important for future clinical management and the potential association between Sjögren syndrome and other connective tissue diseases. However, even patients with Sjögren syndrome may present with a normal ocular examination and absent (or confusing) ocular symptoms. In these situations, the Schirmer test is most useful as a rapid and inexpensive screen for Sjögren syndrome, particularly when markedly decreased tear production is found (≤5 mm of wetting).

A number of diagnostic criteria for Sjögren syndrome have been proposed by various study groups over recent years.[1] The Schirmer test is one of the key criteria for assessing ocular involvement by Sjögren syndrome, and has been included in the diagnostic criteria put forth by groups from California ("San Diego criteria"), Copenhagen, Greece, Japan, and Europe (revised European criteria).

Footnotes

1. Bell M, Askari A, Bookman A, et al, "Sjögren Syndrome: A Critical Review of Clinical Management," *J Rheumatol*, 1999, 26(9):2051-61.

(Continued)

Schirmer Test *(Continued)*

References

Fox RI, Tornwall J, and Michelson P, "Current Issues in the Diagnosis and Treatment of Sjögren Syndrome," *Curr Opin Rheumatol*, 1999, 11(5):364-71.

Friedlaender MH, "Ocular Manifestations of Sjögren Syndrome: Keratoconjunctivitis Sicca," *Rheum Dis Clin North Am*, 1992, 18(3):591-608.

Mackie IA and Seal DV, "Confirmatory Tests for the Dry Eye of Sjögren Syndrome," *Scand J Rheumatol Suppl*, 1986, 61:220-3.

♦ **Scratch Test** *see* Allergy Testing, Percutaneous *on page 106*

♦ **Skin Prick Test** *see* Allergy Testing, Percutaneous *on page 106*

♦ **Skin Test Battery** *see* Anergy Skin Test Battery *on page 110*

♦ **Skin Tests for Histoplasmosis, Blastomycosis, Coccidioidomycosis** *see* Fungal Skin Testing *on page 122*

♦ **Skin Tests for Penicillin Allergy** *see* Penicillin Allergy Skin Testing *on page 140*

♦ **Tine Test** *see* Tuberculin Skin Testing, Multiple Puncture *on page 147*

♦ **Tuberculin Skin Testing** *see* Tuberculin Skin Testing, Intracutaneous *on page 144*

Tuberculin Skin Testing, Intracutaneous

Related Information

Anergy Skin Test Battery *on page 110*
Fungal Skin Testing *on page 122*
Tuberculin Skin Testing, Multiple Puncture *on page 147*

Synonyms Mantoux Test; PPD Test; Purified Protein Derivative (PPD) Test; Tuberculin Skin Testing

Procedure Commonly Includes Intradermal injection of culture extracts of *Mycobacterium tuberculosis* (MTB). This is an *in vivo* means of evaluating delayed hypersensitivity to MTB. Skin test sites are examined at 24, 48, and 72 hours for signs of induration and erythema. A positive skin test indicates prior exposure to MTB (either recent or remote), with an adequate cell-mediated immune response.

Indications The tuberculin skin test can be used in two ways: 1) as an aid in the diagnosis of individuals with clinically suspected active MTB infection (ie, fever, cough, hemoptysis, weight loss, pulmonary infiltrates) who require multidrug treatment, or 2) as a means of screening for latent MTB infection in asymptomatic persons who belong to certain groups at high risk for MTB, in order to identify persons who may benefit from preventative treatment with isoniazid. PPD testing is indicated in the following high-risk groups as part of routine evaluation, even if asymptomatic:

- HIV-infection, or persons with risk factors for HIV but in whom the HIV status is unknown
- persons who have been recently exposed to a proven (index) case of active tuberculosis; this includes close household contacts and healthcare workers with significant exposure
- injection drug users, even if HIV-seronegative
- foreign-born persons from areas where TB is endemic (eg, Asia, Africa, and Latin America)
- medically underserved, low-income populations, including high-risk racial and ethnic groups (eg, Asians and Pacific Islanders, African-Americans, Hispanics, and Native Americans)
- persons with ongoing exposure to TB, such as residents of correctional facilities and nursing homes
- other groups with an increased prevalence of TB (eg, migrant farm workers or homeless persons)

Certain medical conditions are associated with significantly higher risk for TB than the general population and should undergo PPD testing as a part of routine care. These include:

- diabetes mellitus
- silicosis
- prolonged corticosteroid therapy

- other immunosuppressive therapy including chemotherapy, cytotoxic agents, and medications used to prevent transplant rejection in organ recipients
- head and neck malignancies
- hematologic and reticuloendothelial cancers (eg, leukemia and Hodgkin disease)
- end-stage renal disease
- intestinal bypass or gastrectomy
- chronic malabsorption syndromes
- chest radiograph findings suggestive of previous TB (in a person who received inadequate or no treatment)
- low body weight (10% or more below the ideal)

PPD skin testing should be part of an organized TB screening program for health care workers, who should be skin tested on employment and afterwards at regular intervals. The CDC also recommends PPD testing for staff of long-term care facilities who may be exposed to TB patients on the job, such as guards at prisons, and for staff who would pose a risk to large numbers of susceptible persons if they developed infectious TB, such as staff at AIDS hospice houses, or staff at daycare facilities. Such persons should also be skin tested upon employment and at regular intervals afterwards.

Contraindications PPD skin testing should not be performed on persons who have documented history of a positive PPD skin test in the past, due to the severity of the skin reaction that may be seen in highly sensitive persons. Such hyperimmune responses include vesiculation and local skin necrosis. Note that the development of local skin erythema (without induration) from a tuberculin skin test done in the past does not usually constitute a true hypersensitivity reaction. Some clinicians will use a 1 tuberculin unit (1 TU) PPD skin test in a person with a questionable history of a positive PPD.

The tuberculin skin test is available in three concentrations: 1 tuberculin unit (TU), 5 TU, and 250 TU. The 5 TU PPD is the most commonly administered. **The 250 TU dose should never be used for the initial injection.**

PPD skin test reactivity may be depressed up to 6 weeks in persons who have received certain vaccinations, such as measles and influenza, and in those who have had recent viral infections (influenza, mumps, and others). The PPD skin test is not contraindicated under these circumstances but should be administered after 6 weeks if being performed on a routine basis.

Patient Preparation The procedure is explained to the patient. Inquiries should be made regarding past PPD reactions. No specific skin preparation is necessary; however, patients with severe skin disease, such as psoriasis, should be examined beforehand to ensure that there are suitable areas of normal appearing skin. Although testing need not be performed by a physician, one should be immediately available for systemic reactions.

Aftercare If no adverse reaction has occurred within several minutes, the patient may be discharged from the testing center. In some centers, patients are given written instructions on measurement and recording of a positive skin reaction at home. Other centers prefer patients to return to the test center at 48 and 72 hours for formal skin test reading by a nurse or physician. Test sites should be kept clean for 72 hours. No bathing restrictions are necessary. The patient should contact a physician if a severe local reaction develops or if fever and dyspnea occurs.

Special Instructions If skin testing is performed in a separate department, requisition should state:

- the strength of tuberculin test (1 TU, 5 TU, 250 TU)
- whether an anergy skin battery is also desired

Complications In general, adverse reactions are uncommon. Rare complications include fever, lymphangitis, adenopathy, and local ulcers or vesicles. If local lesions develop, these should be treated with dry sterile dressings. The use of topical ointments is optional.

Equipment Culture extracts of MTB (tuberculins) are available for injection in preparations termed "purified protein derivatives" or PPD. Commercial preparations of PPD are available in different doses, standard test dose being 5
(Continued)

Tuberculin Skin Testing, Intracutaneous *(Continued)*

tuberculin unit dose (5 TU). Also required are a disposable glass or plastic tuberculin syringe, a short 1/4" to 1/2" 26- or 27-gauge needle.

Technique The standard 5 TU tuberculin test is performed as follows. A skin site on the volar surface of the forearm is cleaned. 0.1 mL 5 TU PPD is drawn up into a tuberculin syringe and the needle is inserted bevel upwards intradermally and a discrete wheel (5-10 mL) is produced. If the test is improperly performed, a second dose can be given at an alternate location. Test sites are examined at 24, 48, and 72 hours for the presence of induration, by palpation and inspection. The largest transverse diameter of induration is measured along the long axis of the forearm. Areas of erythema are disregarded. The following should be **carefully** recorded in the chart: Strength of PPD used, date of testing, date of reading, and size of induration. The applied method described also applies to testing with nonstandard tuberculin doses (1 TU or 250 TU).

Normal Findings In general, the <5 TU PPD test is considered "insignificant" when induration is <10 mm, however, this breakpoint is controversial.

Critical Values The CDC has recommended the following interpretation of the 5 TU skin test (does not apply to the 1 TU or 250 TU skin tests):

Induration ≥5 is considered a positive tuberculin skin test in the following groups:

- HIV infection, or persons suspected of having HIV infection
- close contacts of a person with infectious TB (eg, household contacts)
- persons with chest x-ray findings suggestive of previous TB and who have received inadequate or no treatment
- injection drug users whose HIV status is unknown

Induration ≥10 is considered positive in persons who do not meet the above criteria but who have other risk factors which include:

- persons with certain medical conditions such as diabetes mellitus, silicosis, prolonged corticosteroid therapy, other immunosuppressive therapy, head and neck malignancies, hematologic and reticuloendothelial diseases, end-stage renal disease, intestinal bypass or gastrectomy, chronic malabsorption syndromes, and low body weight (10% or more below the ideal)
- injection drug users, HIV seronegative
- foreign-born persons from areas where TB is endemic (eg, Asia, Africa, and Latin America)
- medically underserved, low-income populations, including high-risk racial and ethnic groups (eg, Asians and Pacific Islanders, African-Americans, Hispanics, and Native Americans)
- persons with ongoing exposure to TB such as residents of correctional facilities and nursing homes
- other groups with an increased prevalence of TB (eg, migrant farm workers or homeless persons)
- children younger than 4 years of age

Induration ≥15 is considered a positive skin test in all persons, including those with no known risk factors for TB.

The foregoing discussion applies only to the 5 TU PPD test. No standardization has yet been devised for the 1 TU or 250 TU PPD test. However, the 1 TU test is commonly used in patients with a history of a significant local reaction to a 5 TU PPD test. The 250 TU test is used to rule out exposure to any mycobacterial organisms (tuberculosis or nontuberculosis). Some experts feel that a negative 250 TU PPD essentially excludes tuberculosis exposure, providing the patient has a fully reactive anergy panel.

Limitations For best results, trained personnel are necessary for administering and reading the test.

Additional Information The tuberculin test is a measure of delayed (cellular) immunity to MTB. As such, a positive test indicates only exposure to MTB and does not distinguish current from past infections. False-positive tests may be seen with exposure to nontuberculous (atypical) *Mycobacterium* or previous inoculation with BCG vaccine. False-negative tests are common and can be difficult to interrupt. Causes for false-negative tests relate not only to the technique of administration, but also the age and immune status of the person being tested. Insignificant reactions are commonly seen secondary to anergy from immunosuppressive therapy, neoplastic disease, various bacterial or viral infections, and vaccinations. Thus, the tuberculin test is often performed along with skin tests for common antigens, such as *Candida* and mumps, to assess possible anergic states. In addition, hypersensitivity to tuberculin may diminish gradually with age. A "booster phenomenon" has been described in the elderly whereby waning tuberculin sensitivity is augmented by repeating 5 TU skin testing at 1 week intervals. Although controversy exists concerning the interpretation of both the booster phenomenon and of the standard tuberculin test itself, this test remains an invaluable aid in diagnosing tuberculous infection.

References

Centers for Disease Control and Prevention, "Core Curriculum on Tuberculosis: What the Clinician Should Know," U.S. Department of Health and Human Services, Public Health Service, National Center for Prevention Services, Division of Tuberculosis Elimination, Atlanta, Georgia, 3rd edition, 1994.

Centers for Disease Control and Prevention. "Prevention and Treatment of Tuberculosis Among Patients With Human Immunodeficiency Virus: Principles of Therapy and Revised Recommendations," *MMWR Morb Mortal Wkly Rep* , 1998, 47(RR-20):1-78.

Graham NM, Nelson KE, Solomon L, et al, "Prevalence of Tuberculin Positivity and Skin Test Anergy in HIV-1-Seropositive and -Seronegative Intravenous Drug Users," *JAMA*, 1992, 267(3):369-73.

Huebner RE, Schein MF, Bass JB Jr, "The Tuberculin Skin Test," *Clin Infect Dis*, 1993, 17(6):968-75.

Huebner RE, Villarino ME, and Snider DE Jr, "Tuberculin Skin Testing and the HIV Epidemic," *JAMA*, 1992, 267(3):409-10.

Rosenberg T, Manfreda J, and Hershfield ES, "Two-Step Tuberculin Testing in Staff and Residents of a Nursing Home," *Am Rev Respir Dis*, 1993, 148(6 Pt 1):1537-40.

Tuberculin Skin Testing, Multiple Puncture

Related Information

Tuberculin Skin Testing, Intracutaneous *on page 144*

Synonyms Prong Test; Tine Test

Procedure Commonly Includes Extracts of *Mycobacterium tuberculosis* (MTB) are introduced into the skin by means of a disposable, multiple-point applicator. The applicator has several triangular shaped prongs (tines) which are coated with tuberculin (either purified protein derivative (PPD) or old tuberculin (OT)). The multiple puncture device is standardized to deliver an amount of tuberculin ≥5 tuberculin units (TU) of PPD by the Mantoux method (see Tuberculin Skin Testing, Intracutaneous *on page 144*). The skin test site is examined at 48 and 72 hours for induration or vesiculation. The tine test is most useful as a screening tool for MTB but lacks the precision of the Mantoux test.

Indications The tine test is a screening test used to identify persons who have been previously exposed to MTB. It is a relatively inexpensive way of evaluating large numbers of asymptomatic individuals for tuberculin sensitivity. The tine test may be useful in some public health programs to identify individuals who would require further evaluation for MTB infection (eg, sputum culture, chest x-ray, etc) and is useful in epidemiologic studies to determine the prevalence of MTB infection in specific populations. The tine test is not useful in making decisions regarding antituberculous prophylaxis or treatment for a given patient.

Contraindications Previously known sensitivity to tuberculin from a prior Mantoux test or tine test. Commercial preparations of PPD for tine testing also contain some acacia as a stabilizer and should not be used in the rare individual allergic to acacia.

Aftercare The patient should be instructed to keep the test site clean.

Special Instructions Requisition must state medications patient is currently receiving, especially any steroid preparations or other immunosuppressives.

Complications Adverse reactions are uncommon. Rarely, fever, adenopathy, and local ulceration may be seen. Data derived from more than 3000 persons receiving the tine test have shown a rate of slight to mild vesiculation at the

(Continued)

Tuberculin Skin Testing, Multiple Puncture *(Continued)*

test site of <2%. One individual reported a slight ulceration. These rates are similar to those of the Mantoux test. Local vesiculation is usually treated only with dry sterile dressings. The use of topical steroids is optional.

Equipment Several types of applicators are available commercially. Concentrated tuberculin is used in all applicators in either one of two forms: old tuberculin (OT) or purified protein derivative (PPD). The device consists of an applicator with points coated with dried tuberculin.

Technique Tuberculin is introduced into the skin by pressing an applicator firmly onto a clean skin surface, preferably the volar aspect of the forearm. Test site is examined at 48 and 72 hours for evidence of papules or vesicles. In the first case, if a papular reaction occurs, the largest single papule is examined and the diameter of induration recorded. If several papules are found coalesced, the largest diameter of induration is recorded. In the second case, if a vesicular reaction occurs, it is not necessary to record the diameter of induration; documentation of a significant vesicular reaction is sufficient.

Normal Findings When interpreting the skin test, areas of erythema should be ignored. No papular or vesicular skin reaction is considered a normal finding. An area of induration ≤2 mm is also considered a negative skin test.

Critical Values

- Papular reaction, or area of induration present. If either is ≥2 mm, the test is considered positive. In general, this requires further confirmation with a 5 TU PPD test using the Mantoux method.
- Vesicular reaction. This is considered a significantly positive test and no further confirmatory testing by the Mantoux method is necessary.

Limitations The tine test shares many of the same limitations as the intracutaneous tuberculin test, including false-negative reactions in patients with impaired immune systems. In addition, the tine test delivers a variable dose of highly concentrated tuberculin and thus, false-positive reactions are relatively common. It is not intended for strict diagnostic use and thus, few management decisions can be made using isolated tine test results.

Additional Information Tuberculin skin testing remains an invaluable tool in the diagnosis of tuberculosis. Infection with MTB results in skin sensitivity to culture extracts of MTB (tuberculins), an example of delayed or cellular hypersensitivity. The tine test has several advantages over the intracutaneous test. These include:

- little equipment necessary
- less expensive
- no training required for administration

The tine test is most useful when screening large numbers of asymptomatic individuals in whom the suspicion for tuberculous infection is low. In general, completely negative tine tests are felt to correlate highly with negative Mantoux tests; tine tests with vesicular reactions are felt to correlate strongly with significant (>15 mm) Mantoux tests. Interpretation of a papular reaction with a tine test is more problematic. Since doses of delivered tuberculin are uncontrolled with a multiple point applicator, false-positive cross reactions with nontuberculous *Mycobacterium* are common. Further testing using the Mantoux test with its attendant cost and time is necessary to interpret the papular reaction. Clinical studies which have compared the PPD tine test against the 5 TU PPD Mantoux test as the gold standard have shown a false-positive rate of the tine test of 10% and a false-negative rate of 6%. Similar rates have been reported with the tine test using old tuberculin (OT).

References

Anand JK and Roberts JT, "Disposable Tuberculin Tests: Available and Needed. A Review," *Public Health*, 1991, 105(3):257-9.

Higgis SP, Bradbeer CS, and Bateman NT, "Tine Testing in HIV Positive Patients," *Thorax*, 1993, 48(8):831-4.

The American Thoracic Society, "The Tuberculin Skin Test," *Am Rev Respir Dis*, 1981, 124:356-63.

Widefield Capillary Microscopy

Synonyms Nailfold Capillaroscopy; Nailfold Capillary Microscopy

Procedure Commonly Includes Examination of finger nailfold capillaries with a wide-angle microscope or ophthalmoscope. Abnormalities in the magnified appearance of nailfold capillaries have been described in several connective tissue diseases, especially systemic sclerosis (scleroderma) and related diseases, such as dermatomyositis and mixed connective tissue disease (MCTD). A distinctive capillary pattern of capillary enlargement accompanied by avascular areas has been reported in >80% of patients with systemic sclerosis.

Indications Clinical applications for this procedure are still evolving. Common indications include:

- early recognition of scleroderma
- evaluation of the patient with isolated Raynaud phenomenon (ie, not associated with signs or symptoms of other connective tissue diseases). Isolated Raynaud phenomenon can precede the development of connective tissue disease by years. A negative capillaroscopy examination in such an individual suggests a benign course. Abnormal capillaroscopy in patients with isolated Raynaud phenomenon are at high risk for the development of a scleroderma-spectrum disorder months or years later. Some centers perform capillaroscopy routinely on all Raynaud patients.
- evaluation of the patient with mixed connective tissue disease (MCTD), where there are combined features of scleroderma, systemic lupus erythematosus (SLE), and polymyositis. Nailfold capillaroscopy may predict the subset of patients with MCTD who will go on to manifest diffuse systemic sclerosis.
- evaluation of the patient with known scleroderma, in order to estimate the severity of visceral involvement. Severity of capillary lesions correlates reasonably well with the degree of multisystem organ disease and survival.

Nailfold capillaroscopy has also been reported to be useful in other diseases including Sjögren syndrome[1], hypothyroidism[2], hypertension[3] (to assess the effects of antihypertensive agents on the microcirculation), and others.

Contraindications None reported; however, extensive nail disease (eg, onychomycosis) may preclude a thorough examination and represents a relative contraindication.

Patient Preparation Technique is explained to the patient and verbal consent is obtained. Female patients should remove fingernail polish beforehand.

Complications None reported; this procedure is risk-free.

Equipment A variety of instruments have been advocated for microscopy, including a handheld magnifying glass, ophthalmoscope, an inverted 10x microscope eyepiece, and a stereomicroscope. Some authorities advocate the conventional ophthalmoscope due to its effectiveness and easy availability but the viewing field is quite narrow. Maricq (1981) argues for the stereomicroscope with magnification of 12-16x which allows depth perception and wide-angle viewing. Recently, semiautomated image analyzing systems[4] and videomicroscopy have also been reported.

Technique In some centers, all 10 nailfolds are routinely examined; others advocate testing of the fourth nailfolds only. A drop of oil is placed on the nailfold, usually grade B immersion oil (fairly viscous). Nailfold capillaries are examined with the magnifying instrument of choice; incident lighting usually is provided by a fiberoptic cool light source. Photographs of abnormal capillary anatomy may be obtained using specialized techniques.

Normal Findings Nailfold capillaries have a tight, hairpin appearance and are found in parallel arrays. There are usually three components to the capillary: an afferent limb of about 10 uM width, an efferent limb of 20 uM width, and an apical portion. The mean length of the capillary is 215-235 uM in various studies. Normal nailfold capillaroscopy findings have recently been described for children and adolescents[5].

Critical Values The pattern of capillary abnormalities seen in scleroderma is characterized by:

(Continued)

Widefield Capillary Microscopy *(Continued)*

- "megacapillaries," which are enlarged capillary loops >10x normal size. All three components of the capillary loop may be enlarged or only the apical portion.
- loss of capillaries (reduction in number)
- regions of avascularity; this is usually seen in advanced scleroderma
- increased tortuosity and disorganization of the remaining capillaries
- capillary hemorrhages

Some of these features may be absent in a given patient and nail-to-nail variability is not uncommon. Rating scales have been developed (semiquantitative) to classify the degree of capillary involvement. The complete "scleroderma pattern" described above is found in 80% to 90% of persons with scleroderma, but is seldom seen in other connective tissue diseases. Megacapillaries are seen in the CREST syndrome variant of scleroderma, as well as dermatomyositis and MCTD. However, diseases such as SLE do not have a typical nailfold capillaroscopic pattern, although tortuous capillaries, increased length of the capillaries, and prominent subpapillary plexus have all been described in SLE. Megacapillaries are typically absent in both SLE and rheumatoid arthritis.

Additional Information Although the technique of capillary microscopy has gained clinical acceptance in the past decade, it was first described as far back as 1912. The pathologic basis of this procedure - anatomic derangements of cutaneous microvessels in systemic sclerosis - was originally documented in the 1920s; this included the existence of "giant" nailfold capillaries. The introduction of Widefield technique helped popularize this noninvasive procedure in recent years. A high degree of correlation has been demonstrated between findings on capillary microscopy and histologic features on nailfold biopsy.

Footnotes

1. Tektonidou M, Kaskani E, Skopouli FN, et al, "Microvascular Abnormalities in Sjögren Syndrome: Nailfold Capillarscopy," *Rheumatology* (Oxford), 1999, 38(9):826-30.
2. Pazos-Moura CC, Moura EG, Breitenback MM, et al, "Nailfold Capillaroscopy in Hypothyroidism and Hyperthyroidism: Blood Flow Velocity During Rest and Postocclusive Reactive Hyperemia," *Angiology*, 1998, 49(6):471-6.
3. Martina B, Surber C, Jakobi C, et al, "Effect of Moxonidine and Cilazapril on Microcirculation as Assessed by Finger Nailfold Capillaroscopy in Mild-to-Moderate Hypertension," *Angiology*, 1998, 49(11):897-901.
4. Hu Q and Mahler F, "New System for Image Analysis in Nailfold Capillaroscopy," *Microcirculation*, 1999, 6(3):227-35.
5. Terreri MR, Andrade LE, Puccinelli ML, et al, "Nail Fold Capillaroscopy: Normal Findings in Children and Adolescents," *Semin Arthritis Rheum*, 1999, 29(1):36-42.

References

Blockmans D, Beyens G, and Verhaeghe R, "Predictive Value of Nailfold Capillaroscopy in the Diagnosis of Connective Tissue Diseases," *Clin Rheumatol*, 1996, 15(2):148-53.

Kabasakal Y, Elvins DM, Ring EF, et al, "Quantitative Nailfold Capillaroscopy Findings in a Population With Connective Tissue Disease and in Normal Healthy Controls," *Ann Rheum Dis*, 1996, 55(8):507-12.

Lee P, Leung FY, Alderdice C, et al, "Nailfold Capillary Microscopy in the Connective Tissue Diseases: A Semiquantitative Assessment," *J Rheumatol*, 1983, 10(6):930-8.

Lee P, Sarkozi J, Bookman AA, et al, "Digital Blood Flow and Nailfold Capillary Microscopy in Raynaud Phenomenon," *J Rheumatol*, 1986, 139(3):564-9.

Lovy M, MacCarter D, and Steigerwald JC, "Relationship Between Nailfold Capillary Abnormalities and Organ Involvement in Systemic Sclerosis," *Arthritis Rheum*, 1985, 28(5):496-501.

Maricq HR, "Widefield Capillary Microscopy," *Arthritis Rheum*, 1981, 24(9):1159-65.

McGill NW and Gow PJ, "Nailfold Capillaroscopy: A Blinded Study of its Discriminatory Value in Scleroderma, Systemic Lupus Erythematosus, and Rheumatoid Arthritis," *Aust N Z J Med*, 1986, 16(4):457-60.

NEUROLOGY

Brainstem Auditory Evoked Responses

Related Information

Electroencephalography *on page 154*

Synonyms BAEP; BAER; Brainstem Auditory Evoked Potentials

Procedure Commonly Includes Brainstem auditory evoked responses (BAER) evaluate the functional integrity of the auditory pathway from the eighth cranial nerve through the medulla, pons, and midbrain. The auditory nerve is stimulated by a series of clicks 50-100 milliseconds in duration through headphones that allow the stimulus to be presented to one ear at a time. Electrical potentials are produced by auditory neurons in response to these stimuli. They are called auditory evoked responses or potentials. The electrical activity is detected and recorded by electrodes placed on the scalp over the mastoid bone and the vertex of the skull. Immediately after each click stimulus is presented, seven consecutive potentials are normally recorded, waves I through VII. Each waveform corresponds to a specific brainstem relay station. For example, wave I corresponds to the acoustic nerve, wave II to the cochlear nucleus, wave III to the superior olivary nucleus, and so on. This relationship between electrical potential and anatomic structure allows localization of auditory lesions to within several millimeters. BAER testing is a safe, objective means of diagnosing and localizing early, subclinical lesions of the auditory system.

Indications BAER is helpful indicated in the following clinical situations:

- diagnose acoustic neuromas
- diagnose intrinsic brainstem lesions (including MS, though less sensitive than visual evoked potentials)
- evaluate compressive or infiltrative lesions of the posterior fossa
- evaluate hearing in infants and uncooperative patients
- evaluate various degenerative disorders of the CNS (olivopontocerebellar degeneration, Charçot-Marie-Tooth disease, Wilson disease)
- evaluate dysfunction resulting from brainstem ischemia
- an ancillary study in the evaluation of coma
- diagnose brain death when EEG is inconclusive

Note: BAER is generally **normal** (or minimally abnormal) in the following: trigeminal neuralgia, brainstem transient ischemic attacks (TIAs), "locked-in" syndrome, lateral medullary infarcts, and factitious hearing loss.

Contraindications Absolute contraindications to BAER testing have not been reported. BAER may be performed in patients with mild to moderate degrees of peripheral hearing loss (eg, otosclerosis). Patients with severe peripheral hearing loss may still undergo BAER testing but there is a possibility that the acoustic nerve may not be sufficiently activated by click stimuli. Impacted cerumen represents a relative contraindication and should be removed prior to

(Continued)

Brainstem Auditory Evoked Responses *(Continued)*

the study. Similarly, BAER testing should be postponed in the patient with acute serous otitis media. Patient cooperation, while helpful, is not absolutely necessary. This procedure may be performed on the deeply comatose patient. Severe spasms of the head and neck musculature may interfere with EEG tracings.

Patient Preparation Procedural details should be explained and informed consent obtained. Routine medications, including ear drops, may be taken the morning of the procedure. Patients should be instructed to wash their hair the night before the procedure. There are no dietary restrictions; fasting is not required.

Aftercare There are no restrictions to physical activity following this test. No sedation is used and, therefore, patients may drive themselves home.

Special Instructions It is helpful for the examiner to have a brief clinical history, pertinent neurologic findings, and diagnostic impression at the time of testing. The laboratory should be informed in advance of tests to be performed on infants and neonates.

Equipment

- scalp electrodes (same as those used for EEG)
- earphones
- tone stimulator capable of producing "clicks" at different decibel levels and polarities
- signal amplifier and filter
- computer system for signal averaging

Technique BAER is performed with the patient seated in a sound-dampened room. Surface electrodes are placed on the scalp at the vertex and mastoid or earlobe of the ear being tested. Each ear is tested separately and a masking noise (white noise) is presented to the contralateral ear to avoid cross-over stimulation of both ears. The hearing threshold is determined and a series of clicks 60-70 dB over that threshold are presented. These consist of brief 50-100 msec square waves that are repeated at a frequency of 10 Hz. Electrical activity in the auditory pathways is detected by the scalp electrodes and recorded for a 10 msec interval following each click. Typically, the amplitude of evoked responses is low and therefore requires amplification. Computer signal averaging is used to diminish random, background electrical noise from surrounding neurons. In total, more than 500 clicks are presented to each ear amounting to more than 000 consecutive trials. The evoked potentials for each trial are transmitted to a computer and the signals are averaged. The composite waveform generated appears as seven discernible waves, (I-VII). The procedure requires 60-90 minutes.

Data Acquired Auditory evoked responses for each ear, signal averaged by the computer. These responses appear graphically as a plot of electrical potential on the Y-axis versus time on the X-axis.

Normal Findings The normal auditory evoked response produces a series of impulses that are graphed as a tracing with seven distinct waves. An experienced neurologist then interprets the results. A tracing from a normal BAER is shown in the following figure with electrical potential on the vertical axis and time on the horizontal axis. From this computer-generated wave several important parameters are evaluated:

- absolute latency - the time interval from stimulus presentation to the wave peak
- interpeak latency - the time interval between the peaks of any two waves
- wave amplitude
- wave duration

Normal values have been published based on studies of healthy individuals. However, precise cutoffs are determined by each laboratory depending on equipment, technique, etc. The seven waves of a normal BAER tracing correspond to discrete anatomical structures as follows:

- wave I - acoustic nerve (pons)
- wave II - cochlear nucleus (pons)
- wave III - superior olivary nucleus (pons)
- wave IV - lateral lemniscus (pons)

- wave V - inferior colliculus (midbrain)
- wave VI - medial geniculate (thalamus)
- wave VII - auditory radiations (thalamocortical)

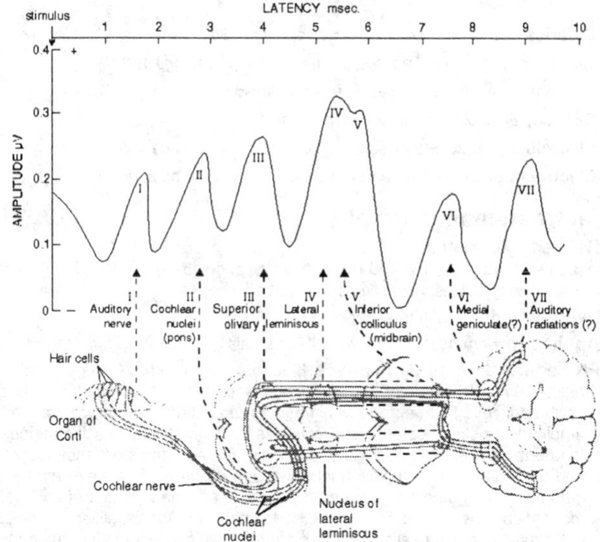

Far-field brainstem auditory evoked responses (BAER). Diagram of the proposed electrophysiologic-anatomic correlations in humans. Reproduced with permission from Adams RD and Victor M, *Principles of Neurology*, 3rd ed, "Part 1/Approach to the Patient With Neurologic Disease," New York, NY: McGraw-Hill Book Co, 1985, 28.

Critical Values In general, an abnormality in a specific wave suggests a lesion in the corresponding nuclear "relay station." Abnormalities in interpeak latency are the most helpful in interpretation of the data (although in some cases, a wave may be absent). Prolongation of the interpeak latencies involving waves I-III, for example, is suggestive of an acoustic neuroma. In contrast, prolongation of the absolute latency is less useful diagnostically and usually represents a disorder of the peripheral auditory apparatus. Idealized evoked responses in various conditions are listed in the following table.

Brainstem Auditory Evoked Responses

Lesion	BAER Abnormality
Acoustic neuroma	↑ interpeak latency, especially waves I-III, ipsilateral
Multiple sclerosis	↓ amplitude wave V and/or ↑ interpeak latency
Elevated intracranial pressure	Absent wave V
Brain death	Waves II-VII absent or waves I-VII absent, bilaterally (difficult to interpret when wave I is absent)
Traumatic damage to the cochlea	Waves I-VII absent, ipsilateral

References

Adams RD and Victor M, *Principles of Neurology: Companion Handbook*, 6th ed, New York, NY: McGraw-Hill Book Co, 1997.

Aminoff MJ, *Electrodiagnosis in Clinical Neurology, 4th ed*, New York, NY: Churchill-Livingstone, 1999.

(Continued)

Brainstem Auditory Evoked Responses *(Continued)*

Chiappa KH, *Evoked Potentials in Clinical Medicine*, 3rd ed, Philadelphia, PA: Lippincott Williams & Wilkins, 1997.

Kveton JF, "The Efficacy of Brainstem Auditory Evoked Potentials in Acoustic Tumor Surgery," *Laryngoscope*, 1990, 100(11):1171-3.

♦ **Calorics** *see* Electronystagmography *on page 160*

♦ **Cerebrospinal Fluid Tap** *see* Lumbar Puncture *on page 160*

♦ **Diagnostic Audiometry** *see* Pure Tone Audiometry *on page 170*

♦ **EEG** *see* Electroencephalography *on page 154*

♦ **Electrodiagnostic Study** *see* Electromyography *on page 156*

♦ **Electroencephalogram** *see* Electroencephalography *on page 154*

Electroencephalography

Related Information

Brainstem Auditory Evoked Responses *on page 151*
Visual Evoked Responses *on page 182*

Synonyms EEG; Electroencephalogram

Applies to Somatosensory Evoked Potentials

Procedure Commonly Includes Electroencephalogram (EEG) records the electrical activity of the brain using scalp electrodes. The procedure is based on the principle that neurons within the cerebral cortex normally generate low amplitude electrical potentials. Electrodes positioned over specific regions of the cortex are able to detect these signals. Brain rhythms are then amplified and transmitted to a multichannel polygraph which records wave forms with automatic pens on moving paper. It provides a continuous plot of voltage on the vertical axis versus time on the horizontal axis. Abnormalities in the EEG pattern may be diagnostic of specific neurologic diseases. It offers a means of evaluating gray matter disease and is the only electrophysiologic measure of ongoing cortical function.

Indications Common indications for EEG in general practice include:

- evaluate of the patient with a suspected seizure disorder; EEG is able to objectively document the presence of seizure activity. It is also important in its ability to localize the site of a seizure focus and classify the nature of the epileptiform discharges. EEG is nearly always abnormal during an acute generalized seizure and frequently abnormal during an acute focal seizure. The EEG may also have diagnostic utility during the interictal period with abnormal discharges seen in 80% of patients with petit mal and 60% of patients with grand mal seizures. It is important to note that seizure disorder is a clinical diagnosis and not and EEG diagnosis. EEG is specific in only a few forms of epilepsy and a normal EEG does not rule out seizure disorder.
- assess coma and other impairments in mental status; the EEG is abnormal in nearly every case of metabolic encephalopathy or ischemic encephalopathy but is normal in most psychiatric conditions. In general, metabolic encephalopathies produce a diffuse slowing or triphasic pattern. EEG may also be helpful in identifying subclinical status epilepticus.
- diagnosis of certain infections of the central nervous system; diffuse slow patterns are seen in diffuse cerebral disease such as Alzheimer disease. Creutzfeldt-Jakob disease and subacute sclerosing panencephalitis often manifest an unusual high amplitude slow and spike pattern. Infectious encephalitis caused by herpes simplex tends to produce periodic lateralizing epileptiform discharges emanating from the temporal lobes.
- evaluate sleep disorders; overnight EEG is an integral part of the polysomnogram.
- evaluate pseudoseizures; EEG is normal in spite of tonic clonic movements.
- intraoperative monitoring of cerebral activity; EEG may be used during certain neurosurgical procedures, carotid endarterectomies, and some non-neurologic surgeries.

Additional roles for EEG include:

- diagnose intracranial mass lesions; EEG may assist in diagnosing and localizing lesions such as brain tumors and abscesses but it cannot reliably distinguish between these entities. CT scan and MRI have supplanted EEG in the evaluation of space occupying lesions.
- evaluation of cerebrovascular disease; EEG can demonstrate regional electrical abnormalities in the distribution of a thrombosed vessel in patients who have suffered recent cortical strokes. In the setting of a subcortical stroke ("lacunar stroke"), the EEG is generally normal even though the patient may be hemiplegic. In this way, EEG may play a role in distinguishing cortical from subcortical stroke syndromes. It has also had a role in the localization of subarachnoid hemorrhages. However, CT scan, MRI, and diffusion weighted MR (MRD) have become the diagnostic tests of choice for stroke and subarachnoid hemorrhage.
- assess head injury; following cerebral concussion, EEG is generally normal but after a cerebral contusion EEG is usually abnormal although nonspecific. EEG has also been used in the past to predict the subset of patients with head trauma who will go on to develop a seizure disorder.

Contraindications There are no absolute contraindications for EEG.

Patient Preparation Details of the procedure are discussed with the patient and informed consent is obtained. Patients should be instructed to wash their hair the night before testing and to avoid the use of hair oils, sprays, or creams. Fasting is not necessary prior to EEG and, in fact, relative hypoglycemia has been reported to alter the EEG. The patient should also be reasonably well rested since sleep deprivation has been known to cause alpha-rhythm abnormalities. When possible, sedative medications should be discontinued well in advance of testing. Such medications include benzodiazepines, barbiturates, ethanol, etc. If the patient is already receiving anticonvulsants such as carbamazepine and phenytoin, decisions regarding discontinuation of the medications is left to the clinician.

Aftercare If an overnight sleep study has been performed, the patient is not permitted to drive home afterwards. In the case of a routine (wake) EEG, no specific postprocedure restrictions are necessary. If anticonvulsant medications were discontinued for the study, the patient should be instructed to restart medications unless specifically instructed to the contrary by a physician.

Special Instructions Requests for EEG from the ordering physician should state the patients age, brief clinical history, overall impression, and reason for the study. Special requests can be made for overnight study, sleep study, nasopharyngeal leads, activation procedures, and evoked response testing.

Complications EEG is considered a safe procedure and is well tolerated.

Technique After the scalp is cleaned, surface electrodes are placed and secured with an adhesive. From 8-20 electrodes are placed in a pattern designated by convention. Each electrode is approximately 0.5 cm in diameter. The underlying electrical activity of the brain is then recorded. The signals are amplified, filtered, and transmitted to a polygraph. Activity within anatomically different areas of the brain are recorded on separate "channels" producing a continuous graph on a moving paper with voltage on the vertical axis and time on the horizontal axis. Testing generally requires approximately 1 hour during which several "activation" measures may be attempted in order to induce seizure activity under controlled laboratory conditions. These include:

- Hyperventilation - produces respiratory alkalosis and cerebral vasoconstriction often resulting in generalized epileptiform activity that precipitates absence seizures.
- Photic stimulation - a strobe light flashing at 1-50 Hz is placed 30 cm from the patient's eyes to elicit epileptiform activity.
- Sleep EEG - for suspected temporal lobe epilepsy

Ambulatory EEG monitoring is now available and is useful in detecting frequent but atypical episodes.

References

Adams RD and Victor M, *Principles of Neurology: Companion Handbook*, 6th ed, New York, NY: McGraw-Hill Book Co, 1997.

(Continued)

Electroencephalography *(Continued)*

Aminoff MJ, *Electrodiagnosis in Clinical Neurology*, 4th ed, New York, NY: Churchill-Livingstone, 1999.

Aminoff MJ "Electrophysiologic Studies of the Central and Peripheral Nervous Systems," *Harrison's Principles of Internal Medicine*, 14th ed, Fauci AS, Braunwald E, Isselbacher KJ, et al, eds, New York, NY: McGraw-Hill Book Co, 1998, 2282-97.

Davis TL and Freemon FR, "Electroencephalography Should not Be Routine in the Evaluation of Syncope in Adults," *Arch Intern Med*, 1990, 150(10):2027-9.

Niedermeyer E and DaSilva FL, *Electroencephalography*, 4th ed, Baltimore, MD: Williams & Wilkins, 1999.

Spehlmann R, *EEG Primer*, Elsevier, North Holland: Biomedical Press, 1981.

Wee AS, "Is Electroencephalography Necessary in the Evaluation of Syncope?" *Arch Intern Med*, 1990, 150(10):2007-8.

Electromyography

Related Information

Nerve Conduction Studies *on page 164*
Neuromuscular Junction Testing *on page 168*
Single Fiber Electromyography *on page 174*

Synonyms Electrodiagnostic Study; EMG

Procedure Commonly Includes Insertion of a needle electrode into skeletal muscle to measure electrical activity and assess physiologic function. Percutaneous, extracellular needle electrodes are placed into a selected muscle group. Muscle action potentials (AP) are detected by the electrodes then amplified and displayed on a cathode ray oscilloscope. Fluctuations in voltage are heard as "crackles" over a speaker permitting both auditory and visual analysis of the muscle APs. Testing is performed with the muscle at rest, with a mild voluntary contraction, and with maximal muscle contraction (where recruitment pattern and interference are noted). Unlike nerve conduction studies, EMG does not involve external electrical stimulation. Muscle APs, normal and abnormal, are physiologically generated. In various diseases of the motor system typical electrical abnormalities may be present:

- increased insertional activity
- abnormal motor unit potentials
- fibrillations
- fasciculations
- positive sharp waves
- decreased recruitment pattern

EMG assesses the integrity of upper motor neurons, lower motor neurons, the neuromuscular junction, and the muscle itself. It is seldom diagnostic of a particular disease entity. Its major use lies in differentiating between the following disease classes:

- primary myopathy
- peripheral motor neuron disease
- disease of the neuromuscular junction

As with nerve conduction velocity studies (with which EMG is usually paired), EMG should be considered an extension of the history and physical examination.

Indications In the neurologic literature, EMG has been performed in a wide variety of clinical situations. Common indications for EMG in general practice include the following.

Evaluate the patient with clinical features of primary muscle disease - symmetric and proximal weakness, muscle atrophy, intact sensory system. Examples include:

- muscular dystrophy
- glycogen storage disease
- myotonia
- inflammatory myopathies (systemic lupus, sarcoidosis, infectious myopathies)
- polydermatomyositis
- alcoholic myopathy
- endocrine myopathies, and others

Evaluate the patient with lower motor neuron disease including:

- suspected peripheral nerve lesions, such as diffuse peripheral neuropathies, spinal root lesions, and trauma
- suspected disease of the anterior horn cells characterized by asymmetric weakness, muscle atrophy, and fasciculations as seen in amyotrophic lateral sclerosis and poliomyelitis

Assess the patient with suspected upper motor neuron disease, when prior imaging studies are inconclusive:

- occult lesions of the corticospinal tract (syringomyelia, tumor) and, less commonly, lesions of the cerebral tract (tumor, CVA).

Evaluate the patient with suspected neuromuscular junction (NMJ) disease:

- myasthenia gravis (conventional EMG is not the diagnostic test of choice for myasthenia gravis; however, other forms of EMG such as single fiber EMG and repetitive stimulation tests are highly specific for NMJ disease.)
- paraneoplastic syndromes including Eaton-Lambert
- assessment of the patient with severe and persistent muscle cramps
- serial documentation of response to therapy for known cases of myopathy or neuropathy
- identification of significantly diseased muscle groups to help guide muscle biopsy (if clinical examination is inconclusive)

EMG is less useful in:

- restless leg syndrome
- transient, self-resolving muscle cramps
- uncomplicated cases of polymyalgia rheumatica unless the diagnosis is in doubt or underlying myositis is suspected
- routine cases of fibrositis/fibromyalgia

Contraindications The following situations represent relative contraindications:

- severe coagulopathy, including hemophilia and marked thrombocytopenia. (EMG has been performed safely with platelet counts as low as 20,000/mm^3, but this is not recommended).
- systemic anticoagulation including intravenous heparin, low molecular weight heparin formulations, and warfarin
- patients with an unusual susceptibility to systemic infections since EMG has been known to cause transient bacteremia
- patients undergoing a muscle biopsy after EMG require special consideration. Needle insertion and manipulation during EMG may cause local microscopic tissue damage secondary to trauma. Histologically, this damage may be confused with a focal myopathy. Therefore, some experts avoid detailed needle examinations of the specific muscle groups that are to be biopsied although EMG testing of surrounding muscle groups is frequently performed.

Patient Preparation Details of the procedure are reviewed with the patient. Considerable patient apprehension often accompanies "needle tests" and calm reassurance from the medical team can help allay such anxieties. Aspirin products and nonsteroidal anti-inflammatories (NSAIDs) should be discontinued 7 days prior to the procedure. Routine medications may be taken on the morning of the examination. If a coagulopathy is suspected, appropriate hematologic testing should be ordered (eg, PT, PTT, CBC, bleeding time, etc). If a primary muscle disease is suspected, a creatine phosphokinase (CPK) level should be drawn prior to needle examination. Routine EMG testing may cause minor elevations in CPK of up to one to one and one-half times baseline. However, striking elevations in CPK, as seen with polymyositis or muscular dystrophy, are not associated with EMG testing.

Aftercare No specific activity restrictions are necessary. The patient may resume previous activity level.

Special Instructions The requisition from the ordering physician should include a brief clinical history, tentative neurologic diagnosis, and the specific limb(s) or muscle group(s) in question. The physician should also state whether nerve conduction studies are desired, although in some centers these may be added at the neurologist's discretion.

(Continued)

Electromyography *(Continued)*

Complications Local discomfort at the site of needle insertion is the most common complication. Generally, severity of discomfort is mild and there are no significant sequelae. Pneumothorax has been rarely documented in the literature in association with needle examination of the paraspinal muscles. Transient bacteremia has been reported but routine antibiotic prophylaxis for patients with high-risk cardiac lesions is not generally recommended.

Equipment EMG is generally performed in a specially equipped procedure room reserved for electrodiagnostic studies. Basic instruments include:

- needle electrodes - these may be monopolar (sharpened, coated steel wires), coaxial, or bipolar (two wires within a needle). The needles record electrical activity from muscle fibers directly contacting the tip as well as fibers within a several millimeter radius.
- amplifier with filters
- cathode ray oscilloscope with the vertical axis measuring voltage and the horizontal axis measuring time. This device usually has an audio amplifier and loudspeaker, which converts action potentials to sound energy.
- data storage apparatus

Technique A brief neurologic examination is performed prior to the start of the procedure. For EMG of the extremities, the patient lies recumbent on the examination table. When paraspinal muscles are tested, the patient is placed in a prone position. No intravenous sedation, analgesia, or local anesthesia is used. The skin is cleansed thoroughly with alcohol pads and the patient is instructed to relax as much as possible. The process is as follows.

Recording needle electrode is inserted percutaneously into the muscle being tested. The initial electrical activity of the muscle, as seen on the oscilloscope and heard over the loudspeaker, is called the **insertional activity**.

The needle is then held stationary and the muscle action potentials during voluntary relaxation are recorded.

The patient is then asked to perform a mild, submaximal contraction of the test muscle. The summed muscle action potentials - the motor unit potential - are observed on the oscilloscope.

Finally, a maximal muscle contraction is performed. The compound action potentials generated during this maneuver are studied for **interference** and **recruitment pattern**.

Needle examination is, by nature, a slow and labor-intensive process. Numerous muscles must be tested individually including both symptomatic and clinically asymptomatic muscles. Within a specific muscle, several independent sites may need to be examined, particularly when the muscle has a large surface area. A number of myopathic processes are focal and sampling errors even within an individual muscle are possible (ie, disease process may effect proximal portions of a muscle, sparing distal fibers).

Normal Findings Results are interpreted by a neurologist or physiatrist with preliminary impression written in the chart on completion of the examination. A formal, typed report is completed several days later. The fundamental principles underlying test interpretation are as follows.

- Insertional activity: Immediately upon needle insertion, there is a brief burst of electrical activity lasting <300 milliseconds. This "insertional activity" is heard over the loudspeaker and may be increased or decreased in various disease states.
- Electrical activity at rest: Muscle tissue is normally silent at rest. No action potentials are seen on the oscilloscope.
- Minimal muscle contraction: When a minimal contraction is performed, several motor units are activated. Several individual action potentials are normally visible on the oscilloscope at a rate of 4-5/second. The idealized configuration of a single motor unit potential is shown in the following figure.
- Full voluntary contraction: As the strength of the muscle contraction increases, further muscle units are recruited. On the oscilloscope the action potentials appear more disorganized and individual action potentials are no longer recognized. This represents a compilation of motor unit

potentials firing asynchronously. The normal interference pattern is considered "full," that is, the amplitude of the action potentials is high (≤5 millivolts and the first rate is fast (40/second)).

EMG FINDINGS

	EMG Steps / LESION	NORMAL	NEUTOGENIC LESION		MYOGENIC LESION		
			Lower Motor	Upper Motor	Myopathy	Myotonia	Polymyositis
1	Insertional Activity	Normal	Increased	Normal	Normal	Myotonic Discharge	Increased
2	Spontaneous Activity	—	Fibrillation Positive Wave	—	—	—	Fibrillation Positive Wave
3	Motor Unit Potential	0.5-1.0 mV 5-10 ms	Large Unit Limited Recruitment	Normal	Small Unit Early Recruitment	Myotonic Discharge	Small Unit Early Recruitment
4	Interference Pattern	Full	Reduced Fast Firing Rate	Reduced Slow Firing Rate	Full Low Amplitude	Full Low Amplitude	Full Low Amplitude

Idealized EMG findings, normal, neurogenic lesions, and myogenic lesions. Reproduced with permission from Kimura J, Chapter 13, "Types of Abnormality," *Electrodiagnosis in Diseases of Nerve and Muscle: Principles and Practice*, 2nd ed, Philadelphia, PA: FA Davis, 1989, 263.

Critical Values Abnormalities may be found in one or more of the previously outlined areas.

Insertional activity: Electrical activity is increased in both neurogenic disorders (eg, lower motor nerve disease) and myogenic disorders (eg, Polymyositis), and thus is considered a nonspecific finding. Decreased insertional activity is less common but may be associated with far-advanced denervation or myopathy, especially when fat or collagen replaces muscle. A distinctive insertional pattern is seen with myotonia, an unusual neurologic disorder, and is termed "myotonic discharge."

Abnormal activity at rest: Instead of the electrical silence which characterizes the muscle at rest, spontaneous action potentials in single muscle fibers (fibrillation potentials) may be observed in several disease states.

Fibrillations are seen 1-3 weeks after destruction of a lower motor neuron. Denervated muscle fibers develop heightened chemosensitivity and individual muscle fibers contract spontaneously. The phenomenon of "positive sharp waves" may also be seen. Fibrillations may also occur with severe polymyositis when extensive areas of necrosis interrupt nerve innervation. The eye is unable to perceive these fibrillations.

Fasciculations represent random contractions of a full motor unit, often visible through the skin. (A motor unit consists of an anterior horn cell, axon, neuromuscular junction, and the numerous muscle fibers supplied by the axon.) Fasciculations may be benign and not associated with any other EMG abnormalities. They may also be associated with amyotrophic lateral sclerosis, other anterior horn cell diseases, nerve root compression, herniated nucleus pulposus syndrome, acute polyneuropathy, and others.

Abnormalities during submaximal contraction: Individual motor unit potentials are distinguishable during this phase of testing and include abnormalities in amplitude, shape (number of phases, serrations, configuration), and/or duration. Increased motor unit potential amplitude is seen in lower motor neuron disease but is normal in upper motor neuron disease. Decreased motor unit potential amplitude is characteristic of polymyositis and other myopathies and is also associated with decreased duration of MUP.

Abnormalities during maximal muscle contraction: At full recruitment, abnormalities in interference patterns may be observed. In myogenic lesions, such as polymyositis and myotonia, the amplitude of the MUPs is significantly

(Continued)

Electromyography *(Continued)*

decreased but the recruitment pattern is normal (ie, the number of activated motor units is normal but the number of muscle fibers per motor unit is diminished). In lower motor neuron lesions, the number of motor units recruited is decreased. In severe cases of neuropathy, the maximum interference pattern resembles that of a single MUP, with individual potentials visible. Amplitude of MUPs may be normal.

References

Adams RD and Victor M, *Principles of Neurology: Companion Handbook*, 6th ed, New York, NY: McGraw-Hill Book Co, 1997.

Aminoff MJ, *Electromyography in Clinical Practice*, 4th ed, New York, NY: Churchill-Livingston, 1999.

Goodgold J and Eberstein A, *Electrodiagnosis of Neuromuscular Diseases*, 3rd ed, Baltimore, MD: Williams & Wilkins, 1983.

Kimura J, *Electrodiagnosis in Diseases of Nerve and Muscle: Principles and Practice*, 2nd ed, Philadelphia, PA: FA Davis Co, 1989.

Martin JB and Hauser SL, "Approach to the Patient With Neuromuscular Disease," *Harrison's Principles of Internal Medicine*, 14th ed, Fauci AS, Braunwald E, Isselbacher KJ, et al, eds, New York, NY: McGraw-Hill Book Co, 1998, 2277-93.

Electronystagmography

Synonyms Calorics; ENG; Vestibular Test

Procedure Commonly Includes Vertical and horizontal occular recording of saccades, gaze, optokinetics, pendulum pursuit, head positions, Hallpike maneuvers, spontaneous nystagmus, calorics, and fixation suppression.

Indications Provide information to aid in the diagnosis of disorders of the auditory and vestibular systems

Patient Preparation The patient's ear canals must be free of excessive cerumen, irritation, and tympanic membrane perforation. Sedatives and tranquilizers are to be withheld for 48-72 hours prior to testing if approved by attending physician. The patient must be alert and cooperative to instructions and should bring eyeglasses and hearing aids. The patient may have breakfast or lunch prior to testing.

Turnaround Time Final report is given within 24 hours.

Causes for Rejection Uncooperativeness or refusal by patient, excessive cerumen, tympanic membrane perforation or irritated auditory canal, blindness or severely impaired visual acuity, uncontrollable muscle artifact, nausea and emesis

Limitations Patient's failure to understand test instructions, nausea and vomiting following caloric stimulation

♦ **EMG** *see* Electromyography *on page 156*

♦ **ENG** *see* Electronystagmography *on page 160*

♦ **Hearing Test** *see* Pure Tone Audiometry *on page 170*

♦ **Latency Studies** *see* Nerve Conduction Studies *on page 164*

♦ **LP** *see* Lumbar Puncture *on page 160*

Lumbar Puncture

Related Information

Myelogram *on page 381*

Synonyms Cerebrospinal Fluid Tap; LP; Spinal Tap

Procedure Commonly Includes Cerebrospinal fluid (CSF) is collected for chemical, microbiologic, and cellular analysis. CSF flows through the subarachnoid space and surrounds the structures of the central nervous system. It is formed in the choroid plexus in the lateral, third, and fourth ventricles of the brain at a rate of about 500 cm^3/day. The adult CNS contains approximately 120 cm^3 of CSF and can be completely replaced in approximately 5 hours. The procedure can be performed with local anesthesia either at the bedside or in the Radiology Department with CT or fluoroscopic guidance. A spinal needle is passed into the intervertebral space, generally between the 4th and 5th lumbar vertebrae, and the CSF drains passively into sterile collection tubes.

Indications CSF examination is often diagnostic in patients with encephalitis, meningitis, metastatic leptomeningitis, subarachnoid hemorrhage, and some inflammatory processes. The threshold for performing CSF sampling is variable among clinicians. However, there are clear indications for the procedure in the following settings:

- clinically suspected meningitis, (acute, subacute, or chronic), encephalitis, or meningoencephalitis
- suspected syphilis involving the central nervous system (tertiary syphilis)
- evaluation of possible CNS malignancies including lymphoma, leukemia, and meningeal carcinomatosis
- lymphoma staging
- possible demyelinating diseases such as multiple sclerosis and Guillain-Barré syndrome
- suspected subarachnoid hemorrhage

For the above indications, CSF findings are fairly distinctive which clearly aids in diagnosis. For other diseases, although the CSF findings may be abnormal, they are nonspecific, resulting in a low sensitivity and specificity. This latter group includes primary brain tumor, tumors metastatic to the CNS, brain abscess, subdural empyema, connective tissue disease (eg, lupus or Sjögren syndrome), and subdural or epidural hematoma. For these conditions, lumbar puncture should be deferred in favor of more sensitive and specific, less invasive testing. Although more controversial, lumbar puncture has also be used in the setting of acute stroke to determine whether hemorrhage is present, in the evaluation of dementia to exclude chronic meningitis and syphilis, in the evaluation of asymptomatic patients with positive serology for syphilis, and in cases of suspected epidural abscess.

Contraindications The only absolute contraindication to LP is a lumbar infection, such as epidural abscess, that prevents access to the subarachnoid space without tracking the needle through infected tissue. Increased intracranial pressure or a space-occupying lesion should be considered major relative contraindications. The most dangerous situations are those in which there is massive swelling that is rapid in onset. Relative contraindications include the following.

- Coagulopathies predispose to local hemorrhagic complications. Impaired coagulation may be either endogenous or iatrogenic. Optimally, at least 6 hours should elapse between discontinuation of heparin and LP. Heparin can be restarted 3-4 hours after LP. Coumadin® can be reversed with vitamin K or, if LP must be done urgently, with fresh frozen plasma.
- Thrombocytopenia also predisposes to hemorrhage. Platelets should be ≥40,000 if their function is impaired by systemic disease, eg uremia. Thrombocytopenia can be corrected by transfusion of platelets. In the absence of splenic sequestration or platelet antibodies, each unit should increase the platelet count by $6000/mm^3$.
- Severe scoliosis

Septicemia is not a contraindication to lumbar puncture. Retrospective studies have not demonstrated an increased incidence of meningitis in septic patients undergoing LP when compared with septic patients who did not undergo the procedure.

Patient Preparation The risks, benefits, and alternatives to the procedure are explained to the patient and informed consent is obtained. The procedure can be performed with the patient in a seated position leaning over a table or other object or in the lateral decubitus position. Intravenous sedation, anxiolytics, and narcotics are not generally necessary and may interfere with assessment of mental status following the procedure.

Aftercare Patients should be kept at bedrest for 3-4 hours following the procedure. Opinions vary regarding the optimal positioning. Some favor the prone position based on a study that demonstrated significantly fewer occurrences of spinal headache. However, the prone position may not be as well tolerated by the patient and can make assessment more difficult. The frequency of vital signs and neurologic checks should be based on the patient's overall status.

Complications LP is a relatively safe procedure and serious complications are uncommon. Complications include the following.

- Headache is the most common complication occurring in approximately 1 out of 10 patients - more commonly in younger and female patients. It is also more likely to occur with use of larger needles. The headache is

(Continued)

Lumbar Puncture *(Continued)*

typically frontal and is relieved by lying supine. They may be associated with nausea, vomiting, tinnitus, and cold sweats. Onset is anywhere from 15 minutes to 4 days postprocedure but most commonly occurs 12-24 hours after LP. The headache generally resolves within a few days but may last as long as 4 weeks or more. It is believed that the headache results from traction on the meninges and pain sensitive blood vessels with leak of CSF from the torn dura. It is not related to the amount of spinal fluid removed at the time of LP but may be related to the size of the dural tear. Treatment of headaches generally includes bedrest and analgesia. Persistent headaches may be relieved with blood patches placed by an anesthesiologist.

- Low backache may arise from root irritation and/or trauma to the periosteum, local extravasation of CSF or blood, minor injury to the annulus fibrosus, or disc herniation. Repeated puncture may increase the frequency of back pain.
- Infection is associated with inadequate attention to sterile technique and to tracking of the needle through infected tissue. Signs and symptoms of meningitis generally occur within the first 12-24 hours after contaminated LP.
- Hemorrhage / excessive bleeding most often occurs in the presence of coagulopathy. It can result in spinal subdural hematoma causing cord compression. Blood in the subarachnoid space and result in arachnoiditis. Most local bleeding is of little clinical significance though it may complicate the interpretation of cell counts.
- Brainstem herniation (uncus or cerebellar tonsils) is a rare life-threatening complication of LP. It occurs when free communication of CSF and rapid equilibration of pressure throughout the subarachnoid space is impaired. The risk is greatest with posterior fossa masses.
- Diplopia resulting from abducens nerve palsy is a rare complication. It is thought to be caused by stretching of the nerve across the petrous portion of the temporal bone.

Equipment Commercial LP trays are available. The required items include iodine swabs, alcohol pads, sterile gloves and drapes, local anesthesia (usually lidocaine 1% or 2%) with syringes and needles, spinal needle with stylette (20- or 22- gauge), four sterile collecting tubes, manometer, connecting tube, and three-way stopcock.

Technique Fundoscopic and neurological examinations should be performed to rule out papilledema and focal neurological defects. If either is present, CT scan should be performed to evaluate for mass lesions. Blood samples should be obtained to measure serum glucose and protein for comparison with spinal fluid concentrations. Proper positioning of the patient is essential for a successful LP. The most common positioning is with the patient in the lateral decubitus position with knees and hips flexed, chin touching the chest. The L4-L5 interspace is located by drawing an imaginary line between the iliac crests. The area is prepared and draped in sterile fashion and infiltrated with local anesthetic. The spinal needle is inserted in the midline of the interspace along an imaginary line between the interspace and the umbilicus (slight cephalad). (The L3-L4 interspace can also be used safely as the spinal cord extends no further than the L2 vertebral body.) The needle should be advanced slowly and the stylette withdrawn frequently to check for spinal fluid. Firm resistance is usually felt as the needle contacts the ligamentum flavum, followed by a sudden release of resistance as the dura and arachnoid are penetrated. When the first spinal fluid is obtained, the manometer is attached and opening pressure measured. If opening pressure is initially elevated, make sure that the patient is relaxed. Increased abdominal and central venous pressure can elevate CSF pressure. If pressure is markedly elevated, collect only the fluid already in the manometer, disconnect it, replace the stylette, and consider neurosurgical consultation. If pressure is normal, collect the CSF sequentially in four tubes. Following collection, the manometer is reattached to measure closing pressure. The stylette is reinserted and both needle and stylette are removed together. Pressure is held over the LP site until bleeding has stopped. Alternatively, the LP can be performed with the patient in a seated position leaning over a bedside table. The neck and spine are maximally flexed with arms folded across the chest.

Data Acquired In addition to estimation of spinal fluid pressure as noted above, appearance of the fluid is also important and should be described in the procedure note. In pathologic states, fluid may be yellow, bloody, xanthochromic, or purulent. The choice of tests to be performed on spinal fluid depends upon the clinical setting. Routine tests include cells counts, protein, and glucose. Additional tests depend upon the clinical setting. In suspected infectious processes, additional tests may include VDRL, various bacterial and fungal antigens, cultures (bacterial, fungal, viral, and tuberculous), India ink preparation (*Cryptococcus*), antibody titers, Gram stain, and acid-fast bacilli (AFB) smear. When malignancy is suspected, cytology may be helpful. In addition, antibodies against Purkinje cell cytoplasm (Yo antibodies) and CNS neurons (Hu antibodies) are associated with paraneoplastic cerebellar syndromes. CSF IgG/albumin ratio, IgG index, oligoclonal bands, and myelin basic protein may be useful in the diagnosis of multiple sclerosis.

Specimen 12-14 cm^3 of spinal fluid can be removed from an adult and is sufficient for most tests. Smaller volumes are generally adequate for basic testing.

Container Four sterile tubes labeled 1-4.

Collection Tube 1 (2 cm^3) for cell count and for comparison with tube 4 if the tap is traumatic Tube 2 (5-7 cm^3) for protein, glucose, oligoclonal bands, serology, and other biochemical tests Tube 3 (3-5 cm^3) for microbiologic stains and cultures and Tube 4 (3-5 cm^3) for cell count and optional studies

Storage Instructions Specimen should be hand-carried to the laboratory immediately after collection.

Normal Findings Normal opening pressure in the recumbent position is 8-20 cm of H_2O and 10-25 cm of H_2O in the sitting position. Pressures vary with respiration 4-10 mm H_2O. CSF is normally clear and contains 60%-70% of serum glucose (unless serum glucose is 300 mg/dL). Protein content is 15-55 mg/dL. Normally, the CSF can contain 0-5 mononuclear white blood cells/mm^3 (lymphocytes and monocytes). The presence of even 1 or 2 polymorphonuclear leukocytes (PMNs) is considered abnormal. There should be no red blood cells (RBCs) and Gram stain and culture should be negative.

Critical Values The interpretation of CSF findings should always be made in conjunction with the clinical presentation. Considerable overlap exists between the different disease entities. LP is of greatest value in the diagnosis of **bacterial meningitis**. The classic findings include increased WBCs (often >500/mm^3), predominance of PMNs on differential (>5/mm^3 is highly sensitive but not specific), decreased glucose (<40 mg/dL, 58% sensitivity), low CSF glucose to blood ratio (<.3, sensitivity 70%). Gram stain is positive in 60% to 90% of cases as is the culture (80%). **Viral meningitis** rarely presents with CSF WBC counts >1000/mm^3, CSF protein levels >100 mg/dL, or glucose 40 mg/dL. These patients should be treated as bacterial meningitis until proven otherwise. **Fungal meningitis** rarely presents with a normal CSF picture but the abnormalities are nonspecific (elevated glucose, decreased protein, and lymphocytic pleocytosis). In cases of cryptococcal meningitis, antigen detection tests are accurate early in the course of the illness. **Tuberculous meningitis** similarly presents with an abnormal but nonspecific CSF profile and may sometimes mimic bacterial meningitis. AFB smears have a low sensitivity (<25%) but AFB culture has a 90% sensitivity. **Malignancy** involving the meninges (primary or metastatic) often results in a CSF profile that resembles infectious meningitis. Typically, there is leukocytosis, elevated protein, and glucose may range from normal to markedly decreased. A normal CSF profile makes malignancy highly unlikely. Sensitivity of CSF cytology varies significantly among studies with ranges from 60%-90% independent of variables such as cell type and primary versus metastatic process. LP may be helpful in the diagnosis of **subarachnoid hemorrhage** (SAH), particularly where CT scan is equivocal. However, difficulty in interpretation in the face of possible traumatic taps limits its usefulness. The presence of xanthochromia suggests SAH but it is also present in 33% of traumatic taps. Decease in RBCs between tubes 1 and 4 suggest traumatic tap but studies have shown this observation to have a specificity of only 56%. As a result of these limitations and the

(Continued)

Lumbar Puncture *(Continued)*

potential complications of LP, CT scan has supplanted LP in the diagnosis of SAH. The diagnosis of **multiple sclerosis** may be supported by the presence of oligoclonal bands and myelin basic protein in the CSF. Sensitivity and specificity of these findings is variable. **Guillain-Barré** syndrome is characterized by an isolated CSF protein >200 mg/dL with the remainder of the parameters within the normal range. The absence of an elevated protein level all but excludes **Guillain-Barré**. In general, LP is more helpful for this entity than for multiple sclerosis.

Limitations In the presence of a traumatic tap, WBCs may be passively transferred to the CSF sample. When evaluating CSF cell counts in the presence of a traumatic tap, for every 700 RBCs, 1 WBC is expected. If the ratio of WBCs to RBCs exceeds 1 in 700, pathology should be suspected.

Additional Information Because of the risk of tonsillar herniation following LP, controversy exists concerning the routine use of head CT prior to LP. Data remain incomplete and several clinical approaches are available. The conservative approach is to always perform a head CT prior to LP regardless of the neurologic findings. Other clinicians follow a more flexible approach and argue that herniation only occurs when papilledema or focal neurologic deficits are present. In the absence of these findings LP can be safely performed without CT scan. A middle ground approach has been advocated whereby CT scan is performed prior to LP in the presence of papilledema, focal neurologic deficits, recent history of sinusitis or otitis media, severe and progressive headache, and deterioration of mental status. In our institution we generally adopt the conservative approach and treat acute meningitis empirically prior to CT and LP.

References

"Clinical Policy for the Initial Approach to Patients Presenting With Altered Mental Status," *Ann Emerg Med*, 1999, 33(2):251.

Fishman RA, *Cerebrospinal Fluid in Diseases of the Nervous System*, Philadelphia, PA: WB Saunders Co, 1980.

Hall JB, Schmidt GA, and Wood LD, eds, *Principles of Critical Care*, 2nd ed, New York, NY: McGraw-Hill Book Co, 1998.

Martin JB and Hauser SL, "Approach to the Patient With Neurologic Disease," *Harrison's Principles of Internal Medicine*, 14th ed, Fauci AS, Braunwald E, Isselbacher KJ, et al, eds, New York, NY: McGraw-Hill Book Co, 1998, 2277-93.

♦ **NCV** *see* Nerve Conduction Studies *on page 164*

Nerve Conduction Studies

Related Information

Electromyography *on page 156*

Synonyms Latency Studies; NCV; Nerve Conduction Velocity

Procedure Commonly Includes Electrical stimulation of a peripheral nerve and recording of the evoked action potentials. Nerve conduction studies may be performed on either sensory nerves or mixed (sensorimotor) nerves. Following percutaneous electrical stimulation of an axon, a physiologic action potential (AP) is generated. This signal propagates down the axon where it is detected at a distant site by surface electrodes. If a motor nerve is tested, the AP of the corresponding muscle is recorded. If a sensory nerve is examined, the AP of the identical nerve is recorded. In either case, the evoked AP is displayed on an oscilloscope where amplitude (in millivolts) and duration (in milliseconds) are read directly. From this, several important parameters are calculated including the **latency period** (the time interval between stimulus presentation and initiation of AP) and maximum **nerve conduction velocity** (speed of impulse propagation). This technique provides objective information regarding nerve function not readily obtained from conventional electromyography. NCV testing is considered the procedure of choice in evaluating the patient with peripheral nerve dysfunction and should be considered an extension of the history and physical examination.

Indications Nerve conduction velocity (NCV) testing is useful in the following situations:

- confirm the presence of a sensory deficit in an objective manner, especially when the physical examination is inconclusive or malignancy is suspected

- evaluate the patient with diffuse polyneuropathy to determine severity and extent of disease and distinguishing demyelinating from axonal processes
- assess the patient with muscle weakness in order to distinguish a neuropathic process from primary muscle disease
- evaluate the patient with acute ascending paralysis to confirm the diagnosis of Guillain-Barré syndrome rapidly prior to plasmapheresis
- confirm the diagnosis of mononeuritis multiplex
- assess nerve entrapment syndromes (mononeuropathies) such as carpal tunnel syndrome; determine the lesion site, differentiating entrapment from diffuse neuropathy; assess severity, and evaluate response to surgical interventions

Conventional NCV testing may often be **normal** in:

- primary muscle disease
- radiculopathies
- disease involving very proximal segments of a peripheral nerve (if suspected clinically, "H reflex" testing is indicated)
- most axonal-type neuropathies, unless the "fast-fibers" are severely damaged
- anterior horn cell disease, such as any atrophic lateral sclerosis; NCVs are typically normal, or only marginally abnormal
- peripheral nerve lesions of any type if examined early in the disease course. For example, in the first 1-2 weeks of acute Guillain-Barré syndrome, NCVs are usually normal. Even with complete transection of a peripheral nerve, as seen with trauma, NCVs distal to the lesion remain normal for several days.

Contraindications Relative contraindications include:

- agitated, uncooperative patient
- presence of a cardiac pacemaker or implanted cardiac defibrillation device
- presence of an indwelling cardiac catheter, such as Swan-Ganz or central venous line

Patient Preparation Risks and benefits of the procedure are discussed with the patient and informed consent is obtained. The patient should be seen and examined by a physician prior to the procedure since the accuracy of the test depends, in part, on the accuracy of the clinician's impression. The patient may take his/her usual medications on the morning of examination, including analgesics as needed.

Aftercare No specific activity restrictions are required after the procedure. Patients may resume their prior level of activity.

Special Instructions Requisitions from ordering physicians should include a brief clinical history, pertinent neurologic findings, specific disease conditions sought, and specific limbs to be tested. The ordering physician should also state if electromyography or other electrophysiologic testing is desired

Complications NCV testing is safe and well tolerated. Since surface electrodes are preferred over needle electrodes in most instances, the procedure is better tolerated by patients. There have been concerns raised regarding the safety of NCV testing in patients with cardiac pacemakers. Theoretically, an electrical stimulus delivered to the skin in close proximity to the pacemaker site may interfere with its function and increasing the risks of dysrhythmias.

Equipment NCV testing is performed with commercial EMG equipment adaptable to a nerve stimulator. Surface electrodes are found silver plates (0.5-1 cm diameter) placed directly on the skin for nerve stimulation. When two electrodes are contacted by the nerve stimulator, one will act as the cathode and the other as the anode. Current will then flow between the negative and positive poles depolarizing the underlying nerve. The nerve stimulator itself is available in a variety of designs. Commonly, it is bipolar with two metal prongs, 2-3 cm apart, attached to an insulated handle. The electrical impulse produced is a square wave of short duration (0.5-1.0 msec) and of variable intensity (0-600 volts). All stimulators are capable of generating either a threshold stimulus (evoked action potential in a few axons) or a supramaximal stimulus (all axons in a nerve stimulated). Stimuli may be delivered in pairs or as a constant train. The stimulation and cathode ray oscilloscope are coordinated so that the sweep on the oscilloscope precedes the stimulus by a variable delay. In this way, a marker indicating the precise moment of stimulus

(Continued)

Nerve Conduction Studies *(Continued)*

delivery is always visible. The evoked action potentials, whether muscle or nerve, are recorded on surface electrodes. (Occasionally, needle electrodes may be needed, particularly when evaluating small, atrophic muscle fibers.) The compound action potentials detected by the recording electrodes are amplified 1000 times for muscle action potentials and approximately 100,000 times for sensory action potentials. Due to the magnitude of amplification, surrounding "noise" must be reduced, primarily through the use of high frequency, low-pass filters and amplifiers with a high signal-to-noise ratio (100,000:1) and a high impedance (megaohm range). The amplified action potential is displayed on a cathode ray oscilloscope (frequency range 10 Hz to 10 kHz). Action potentials may be photographed using a synchronized shutter mechanism and/or stored on magnetic tape. The oscilloscope is also capable of displaying multiple, serial action potentials on the screen for simultaneous comparison (each succeeding AP is placed on a higher baseline). The oscilloscope screen is calibrated for electrical potential on the vertical axis (eg, 1 cm = 1 volt) and time on the horizontal axis (in msec). Some devices calculate the values for latency automatically and provide an automatic digital readout.

Technique Techniques differ somewhat between laboratories. The following summary outlines common principles. Initially, a brief neurologic examination is conducted. The patient is asked to rest comfortably with muscles relaxed. For evaluation of a motor nerve, the axon must be stimulated at two or more sites. For example, when testing the median nerve, the electrical stimulus is delivered to the wrist (distal site) and the antecubital fossa (proximal site); each site is tested separately. The positive lead of the bipolar stimulator depolarizes the nerve and the resultant action potential propagates down the axon in one direction (the anode hyperpolarizes the nerve and blocks conduction in the opposite direction). Recording electrodes located over the innervated muscle sense the compound muscle action potential that eventually results. This entire sequence is displayed on the oscilloscope, starting from the original stimulus presentation (indicated by a "stimulus artifact" marker), followed by a delay prior to the start of the muscle action potential. Paired stimuli or a train of stimuli are presented. These steps are repeated at separate sites along the same axon. The **latency** (in msec) is defined as the time delay between the stimulus artifact and the first (negative) deflection of the muscle action potential. Both the proximal and distal stimulation sites with the recording electrode sites kept constant determine values for latency. Latency in motor nerve testing reflects the sum of pure nerve conduction time and the delay at the neuromuscular junction. Since conduction velocity for the nerve alone is desired, the delay at the neuromuscular junction must be factored out. This is the basis for testing at both proximal and distal stimulating sites. Maximum NCV is calculated by the following:

NCV (motor) = distance (mm) between proximal and distal sites / proximal latency (msec) - distal latency (msec)

NCV is an estimation of action potential propagation between the two sites of electrical stimulation. It does not measure nerve function past the distal site or closer than the proximal site. The nerve conduction time from stimulus presentation at the distal electrode to the start of the muscle action potential, the **distal** or **terminal latency**, is often recorded separately from the maximum NCV. Distal latency reflects both nerve conduction and NMJ transmission. Sensory nerves may be tested in an analogous fashion. NCVs may be obtained in two ways: 1) orthodromic testing - stimulating electrodes are placed distally and sensing electrodes are placed proximally or 2) antidromic testing - stimulating electrodes are placed proximally and sensing electrodes distally; this mimics physiologic impulse propagation. **Latency** is the time delay between electrical stimulation and the appearance of a nerve action potential at the sensing electrode. Testing of sensory nerves does not involve muscle action potentials or neuromuscular junction delays. Calculation of sensory nerve latencies is simpler than motor latencies since stimulation is required at only one site along the axon:

NCV (sensory) - distance (mm) between stimulation point and recording electrode / sensory latency (msec)

Other important variables are the **amplitude** of the action potentials (in mV), **dispersion** of the action potentials, and the presence of **conduction blocks**. NCV may be determined for any peripheral nerve accessible to surface electrical stimulation. Only a limited number of nerves can be tested, in practicality, and the examination must be tailored to the clinical impression. In most centers, nonaffected limbs are also screened for generalized neuropathy (or to serve as internal controls). Commonly evaluated nerves include:

- upper extremity - median, ulnar, radial nerves (both sensory and motor)
- lower extremity - peroneal, tibial, superficial peroneal, sural nerves

Less accessible nerves in the upper extremity include the brachial plexus and shoulder girdle nerves. In the lower extremity, the lumbosacral plexus, saphenous nerve, and lateral femoral cutaneous nerve are relatively difficult to test and are not generally used for asymptomatic screening.

Normal Findings A preliminary written impression is generally provided by the examining physician the same day. Normal values for distal latency, conduction velocity, and amplitudes of evoked action potential have been established. These values are dependent on age and gender. Since equipment and technique vary from one laboratory to another, each laboratory develops its own set of normal values. Published normal values for median nerve motor conduction are:

- distal latency 3.7 msec
- conduction velocity, elbow to wrist, 58 msec
- amplitude (wrist stimulation), 13.2 mV

Normal values vary for each peripheral nerve.

Critical Values In addition to objectively confirming the existence of a peripheral neuropathy, NCV testing can usually distinguish between the two major pathologic forms of neuropathy - axonal and demyelinating neuropathy. It is difficult to distinguish these disorders on the basis of history and physical examination alone. In addition, management strategies for these disorders are quite divergent. NCV testing allows initial categorization of a neuropathic process as a mononeuropathy, mononeuritis multiplex, or polyneuropathy. Within these broad categories, the pathologic process may be further divided into axonal or demyelinating lesions. In general, demyelinating diseases are characterized by decreased conduction velocities, markedly prolonged distal latencies, and normal (or slightly decreased) action potential amplitude. In addition, two may be variably present: 1) action potential dispersion (temporal variability of action potentials), and 2) conduction block (markedly decreased or absent action potential amplitude with proximal nerve stimulation but not with distal site stimulation). NCV testing is often effective in diagnosing demyelinating disorders. Polyneuropathies due to demyelinating diseases include Guillain-Barré syndrome, diphtheric polyneuritis, demyelinating neuropathy associated with carcinoma, and several rare genetic neuropathies, Dejerine-Sottas disease, metachromatic leukodystrophy, and others. Axonal neuropathies are characterized by normal conduction velocity but decreased action potential amplitude. Usually only a fraction of the axons in a nerve undergo degeneration. The fastest conducting axons in a nerve may be relatively spaced (unless disease is severe). Since nerve conduction velocities reflect only the fast fibers and not the slow or medium, conduction velocities are typically normal in spite of extensive axonal degeneration. Polyneuropathies are due to axonal degeneration are common and include neuropathies due to the following:

- systemic disease - uremia, porphyria, vitamin B_{12} deficiency, systemic amyloidosis, severe hypothyroidism, and chronic liver disease
- medications - cis-platinum, vincristine, and metronidazole
- toxins - alcohol, arsenic, lead, etc.
- hereditary neuropathies - ataxia-telangiectasia syndrome, Friedreich's ataxia

Many neuropathies are due to mixed axon-demyelinating processes. Examples include diabetic neuropathy, neuropathy associated with multiple myeloma or lymphoma, and several drugs. Characteristic features of the neuropathies are shown in the following table.

(Continued)

Nerve Conduction Studies *(Continued)*

Nerve Conduction Studies

	Axonal Neuropathy	Severe Axonal Neuropathy	Demyelinating Neuropathy
Conduction velocity	N	N or ↓	↓↓
Distal latency	N or ↑	↑	↑↑
Action potential amplitude	↓	↓↓	N
Dispersion of APs	—	—	Possible
Conduction blocks	—	—	Possible
Examples	Uremic, alcoholic		Guillain-Barré syndrome

NCV testing is also useful in the diagnosis of mononeuropathy multiplex, a condition in which neuropathy develops in multiple, but noncontinuous nerves, either simultaneously over a prolonged period of time. Individual nerve trunks appear to be afflicted in a random fashion. NCV testing can determine if mononeuritis multiplex is being caused by an axonal or demyelinating neuropathy. Axonal processes potentially leading to mononeuritis multiplex are polyarteritis nodosum and vasculitic syndromes associated with connective tissue diseases such as systemic lupus erythematosus, rheumatoid arthritis, and others. Demyelinating mononeuritis multiplex is most often due to chronic inflammatory demyelinating polyradiculoneuropathy. The distinction between axonal and demyelinating processes is significant for clinical decision making. Focal involvement of a single nerve or mononeuropathy is frequently encountered in general practice. This implies local nerve compression usually secondary to trauma or entrapment. NCV testing reveals localized slowing of nerve conduction at the point of compression due to localized demyelination that precedes distal axon degeneration. Carpal tunnel syndrome is a common entrapment syndrome involving the median nerve. Testing can localize the lesion, exclude polyneuropathy, and assess severity. The presence of axonal degeneration distal to the compression site may warrant surgical intervention.

References

Adams RD and Victor M, *Principles of Neurology: Companion Handbook*, 6th ed, New York, NY: McGraw-Hill Book Co, 1997.

Aminoff MF, *Electrodiagnosis in Clinical Neurology*, 4th ed, New York, NY: Churchill-Livingstone, 1999.

Asbury AK, "Disease of the Peripheral Nervous System," *Harrison's Principles of Internal Medicine*, 14th ed, AS Fauci, E Braunwald, KJ Isselbacher, et al, New York, NY: McGraw-Hill, 1998, 2457-69.

Kimura J, *Electrodiagnosis in Diseases of Nerve and Muscle: Principles and Practice*, 2nd ed, Philadelphia, PA: FA Davis Co, 1989.

♦ **Nerve Conduction Velocity** *see* Nerve Conduction Studies *on page 164*

Neuromuscular Junction Testing

Related Information

Electromyography *on page 156*

Single Fiber Electromyography *on page 174*

Synonyms Neuromuscular Transmission Study; Repetitive Stimulation Testing

Procedure Commonly Includes Stimulation of an individual motor nerve by means of repetitive electrical impulses with measurement of muscle electrical activity. Supramaximal electrical stimuli are delivered to the skin overlying a motor nerve. A percutaneous electrode, placed over the corresponding muscle, records the evoked muscle action potentials using standard EMG technique. This procedure is unique in that electrical stimuli are delivered in a repetitive train (1-4 Hz). In diseases of the neuromuscular junction, characteristic changes in the compound action potential may be seen on repetitive stimulation.

Indications Evaluation of the patient with a disorder of the neuromuscular junction suspected on clinical grounds. This includes both postsynaptic disorders such as myasthenia gravis and presynaptic disorders such as the Eaton-Lambert myasthenic syndrome (associated with oat cell carcinoma) and botulism.

Contraindications There are no absolute contraindications for this procedure.

Patient Preparation The risks and benefits of the procedure should be discussed with the patient and informed consent should be obtained. Patients generally express considerable anxiety about tests involving multiple needlesticks. A thorough explanation of the procedure is important to help allay these fears. Patients may take all of their routine medications, including anticholinesterases, on the morning of the procedure.

Aftercare There are no specific activity restrictions following the procedure.

Special Instructions The ordering physician should state the clinical history, pertinent findings, overall neurologic impression, and all electrophysiologic tests desired.

Complications Neuromuscular junction testing is a safe procedure without serious complications. With myasthenia gravis, the patient may experience transient weakness in the tested muscles but the procedure does not induce myasthenic crisis. Minor discomfort may be associated with needle puncture and electrical stimulation but is generally well tolerated.

Equipment Standard EMG equipment is employed including surface recording electrodes, preamplifier, electrical stimulus generator, cathode ray oscilloscope, and loudspeaker. The procedure is carried out in a fully equipped electrodiagnostic testing room.

Technique The patient is placed in a comfortable sitting or recumbent position. The examiner selects the skeletal muscles to be tested based on information provided in the history. Muscles of the hand are often tested first. The motor nerve innervating the selected muscle is stimulated with brief, supramaximal electrical pulses delivered through the skin. Initially, stimuli are presented slowly, from 1-10/second (optimally 2-4/second) and the evoked muscle action potentials are observed on the oscilloscope. If the muscle activity is felt to be normal, the rate may be increased (<50/second). If testing remains normal, the procedure should be repeated on several other muscles including large proximal muscles such as the deltoid. Provocative measures have been employed in some centers to increase test sensitivity. These are optional and involve priming the myoneural junction (exercise, curare).

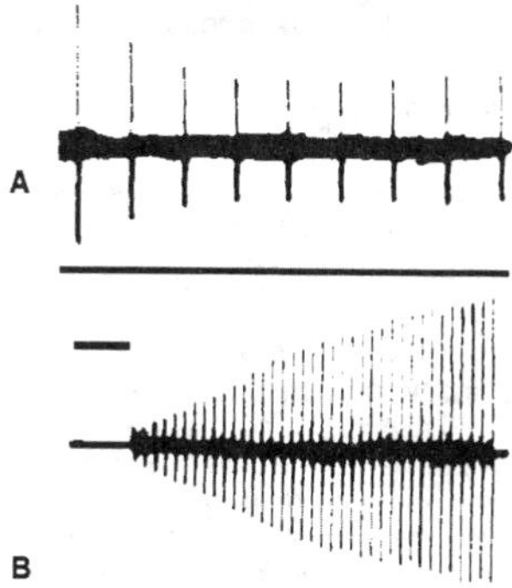

Action potentials obtained by neuromuscular function testing in (A) myasthenia gravis and (B) Eaton-Lambert syndrome. Reproduced with permission from Adams RD and Victor M, "Part V/Diseases of Peripheral Nerve and Muscle," *Principles of Neurology*, 4th ed, New York, NY: McGraw-Hill, 1989, 956.

(Continued)

Neuromuscular Junction Testing *(Continued)*

Normal Findings When repetitive stimuli are delivered at 1-10 impulses/second, muscle action potentials appear uniform and amplitudes high. Even when stimuli are maintained for 60 seconds, amplitudes do not diminish significantly. The same holds true for rapid rates of stimulation. Normal muscle can tolerate 25 stimuli/second without fatiguing. The neurologist's impressions are recorded in the chart immediately after the procedure.

Critical Values In myasthenia gravis, slow rates of nerve stimulation (2-3/second) produce a characteristic funnel-shaped decrement in muscle action potentials over time. As depicted in the diagram, the action potential amplitudes decrease over the first five stimuli, but do not reach zero. This is called the "M response". The effect plateaus almost immediately and subsequent amplitudes may increase slightly. This pattern of early electrical decrement with subsequent stabilization is highly specific for myasthenia gravis. In presynaptic disorders such as Eaton-Lambert syndrome and botulism, a nearly opposite pattern is produced. When stimuli are presented at a rapid rate (20/second), action potentials initially have low amplitudes. With subsequent stimuli, the voltage increases in a continuous fashion as shown in the tracing on the previous page. This finding is felt to be fairly specific for presynaptic disorders.

Limitations

- Decremental response of the action potential is nonspecific. It has been described with myotonia, amyotrophic lateral sclerosis, and other diseases. However, the decrement-plateau pattern is believed to be unique to myasthenia gravis
- Results may be falsely negative if minimally involved muscle groups are examined.
- The "M response" may not be seen early in the course of myasthenia gravis.

References

Adams RD and Victor M, "Laboratory Aids in the Diagnosis of Neuromuscular Disease," *Principles of Neurology: Companion Handbook*, 6th ed, New York, NY: McGraw-Hill Book Co, 1997.

Johnson EW and Wiechers D, "Electrodiagnosis," *Krusen's Handbook of Physical Medicine and Rehabilitation*, 4th ed, Kottke FJ and Lehmann JF, eds, Philadelphia, PA: WB Saunders Co, 1990, 72-107.

Rowland LP, ed, *Merritt's Textbook of Neurology*, 9th ed, Baltimore, MD: Williams & Wilkins, 1995.

Shahani BT and Young RR, "Clinical Electromyography", *Clinical Neurology*, Baker AB, ed, Philadelphia, PA: Harper and Row, 1985, 1-52.

♦ **Neuromuscular Transmission Study** *see* Neuromuscular Junction Testing *on page 168*

♦ **Pattern-Shift Visual Evoked Responses** *see* Visual Evoked Responses *on page 182*

Pure Tone Audiometry

Related Information

Speech Audiometry, Threshold Only *on page 176*
Speech Discrimination Audiometry *on page 179*

Synonyms Audiogram; Audiologic Assessment; Diagnostic Audiometry; Hearing Test

Applies to Basic Comprehensive Audiometry; Tympanometry

Procedure Commonly Includes Audiometry involves assessment of overall hearing sensitivity by means of a standardized set of pure tones, electronically generated by an audiometer. The patient with clinically suspected hearing loss is presented with a series of pure tones over a range of frequencies. The "auditory threshold," the minimal intensity of sound required for audibility, is determined for each frequency. Both air conduction (using earphones) and bone conduction (using a bone vibrator) may be tested.

Using the data acquired during testing, the threshold hearing level (in decibels) is plotted against the frequency (in Hertz) for each pure tone. Four separate curves are generated - right ear air conduction (AC), right ear bone conduction (BC), left ear AC, and left ear BC. These four curves comprise the pure tone audiogram. In addition to quantifying the degree of hearing loss, the pattern of the audiogram may point to the etiology of the loss - conductive hearing loss, sensorineural loss, or mixed deficits. Pure tone audiometry is regarded by some as the initial screening test of choice for audiologic dysfunction.

Indications

- evaluate hearing loss, suspected from either the patient's reported symptoms or abnormalities identified on examination
- periodic screening for hearing loss during prolonged ototoxic drug therapy
- periodic industrial screening for individuals at risk for noise-induced hearing loss
- selected cases of tinnitus, particularly when the neurologic examination is normal and entities such as acoustic neuroma, vascular compression, Ménière syndrome, etc suspected

Contraindications Audiometry is essentially without risk and, therefore, there are no contraindications. However, the accuracy of the test depends upon truthful, voluntary responses from the patient. Diagnostic yield may be limited in elderly patients with dementia and in very young children. Since both groups frequently require testing, audiometry results should be carefully interpreted and more sophisticated testing may be required.

Patient Preparation Patients should undergo clinical examination by a physician prior to audiometry. Reversible or self-limited causes for hearing loss, such as cerumen impaction, acute otitis media, and labyrinthitis, are ruled out prior to initiation of testing. The procedure is explained to the patient and informed consent is obtained. No dietary or activity restrictions are necessary and the patient may take usual medications on the day of the examination. Hearing aid, if worn, should be brought to the testing site.

Equipment The audiometer is an electronic device capable of generating pure tones at a specific frequency, specific intensity, and duration, either singly or in series. As such, pure tones are nonenvironmental (are not heard outside the laboratory environment). For air conduction testing, tones are presented to each ear independently with specialized earphones. For bone conduction testing, a bone vibrator is placed onto the mastoid process of either right or left temporal bone; external auditory canals are not generally occluded. All equipment must be continually calibrated to conform to international standards. This ensures that a gradual loss of hearing noted on serial testing is truly valid and not due to testing error. Parameters regarding pure tone stimulus are as follows.

- Pulsed or intermittent pure tones are preferred to continuous tones. This avoids the phenomenon of "threshold adaptation."
- Optimal duration of each tone is from 200-500 msec based on signal theory.
- When tones are presented in rapid series, "off-time" intervals of 200 msec are generally maintained between stimuli.
- Characteristics of tones may be manually adjusted by the audiologist.

Audiometry is performed in an isolated sound-dampened environment. As with other psychoacoustic testing, all audiometric equipment is discretely arranged so that visual cues are minimized.

Technique The patient is instructed to signal the audiologist each time a tone is perceived. A variety of response signals may be employed - responding "yes" with each tone, tapping the rhythm of tones, or pointing to the ear where the tone is heard. For air conduction thresholds, earphones are comfortably positioned and the better ear, if known, is tested first. Some audiologists quickly screen each ear using the same initial frequency in order to tentatively determine the better ear. Tones are often presented in an ascending series from low to high frequency. Although the range of human hearing may span from 20-20,000 Hz, the frequencies of 200-6000 Hz are most relevant for the comprehension of speech. Standardized frequencies tested include 125, 250, 500, 1000, 1500, 2000, 3000, 4000, 6000, and 8000 Hz. This represents octave intervals by convention but intervening frequencies may be tested. At a given frequency, tones are initially presented at a low intensity and incrementally increased by approximately 5 dB steps. More than 50% of tones heard are conventionally accepted as the threshold for that particular frequency. For example, a series of pure tones at 1000 Hz is presented to the left ear at an initial intensity of 0 dB, then 10 dB, etc. At 25 dB the patient responds to 50% of the tones and this is tentatively considered the auditory

(Continued)

Pure Tone Audiometry *(Continued)*

threshold. Often, tone intensities slightly above and below this auditory threshold are tested to verify and accurately identify the precise threshold value. If responses are consistent, the auditory threshold for left ear air conduction is taken as 25 dB at a frequency of 1000 Hz. Specific situations are as follows.

- If profound hearing loss is expected, frequencies from 125-500 Hz are tested first.
- If a tone is not audible even at maximum audiometer output, "no response" is recorded.
- If 100% correct response occurs at a minimal intensity, testing below 0 dB is possible. The "0 dB" hearing level in audiometry is a modal value derived from a large population of normals. Thus, certain individuals may demonstrate greater hearing sensitivity and thresholds down to -20 dB are measurable.

In order to minimize the problem of tone perception in the nontest ear, "masking" techniques have been developed. Continuous white noise of a narrow bandwidth is channeled into the nontest earphone. Masking noise is designed to avoid distortion of pure tones in the test ear ("overmasking"), while decreasing the signal-to-noise ratio in the nontest ear. For bone conduction thresholds, the technique is similar. A bone vibrator is placed over the mastoid process of the appropriate ear and pure tones are transmitted. Factors such as vibrator placement and pressure may influence results. Fewer frequencies are tested: 250, 500, 1000, 2000, 3000, and 4000 Hz. In addition, audiometer output is limited to approximately 80 dB due to distortion and other technical factors. Interrupted signals in an ascending series are preferred. Masking of the nontest ear is even more significant with bone conduction testing. Each ear is tested separately for air and bone conduction yielding four independent sets of data.

Normal Findings Normal values for auditory thresholds were defined by the International Standards Organization (ISO) in 1984. These values are derived from large population studies of normal adults 18-30 years of age. In most instances, a licensed audiologist or otologist completes a written interpretation on the day of testing. For both AC and BC, normal threshold levels at each pure tone frequency have been designated as "0 dB hearing level". Audiometers have been calibrated to this scale. The audiogram is a plot of tone intensity (dB) on the vertical axis against frequency (Hz) on the horizontal axis. A normal audiogram is illustrated in the figure "a" below where most thresholds are approximately 0 dB. In normal individuals, a small discrepancy is often seen between air and bone conduction thresholds, the "AC-BC gap". At any given frequency the threshold for AC is somewhat lower than BC (ie, a stronger signal is required for BC).

Critical Values Abnormalities in the audiogram are characterized in terms of severity of hearing loss, specific frequencies most effected, unilateral or bilateral loss, and relative air versus bone conduction loss. From this analysis the audiologist may be able to quantify the general degree of loss and classify hearing loss in clinical terms - conductive hearing loss versus sensorineural loss versus nonorganic loss. This is termed "site of lesion" testing. Several principles of interpretation deserve mention.

- For site of lesion testing, "conductive" loss implies a lesion in the external auditory meatus, tympanic membrane, and/or middle ear. "Sensorineural" loss usually implies a lesion in the cochlea or acoustic nerve (cranial nerve VII), but not the cortex. "Central" hearing loss refers to a lesion in the brainstem or auditory cortex. This cannot be adequately evaluated by pure tone audiometry. "Nonorganic" hearing loss implies an intact auditory circuit with deafness due to other factors (eg, malingering, psychosis).
- Mixed lesions are not uncommon.
- Normal AC thresholds imply normal auditory structures from external ear to acoustic nerve and BC thresholds are presumed normal as well.
- Loss of AC sensitivity is nonspecific and BC thresholds are necessary to differentiate conductive from sensorineural loss.

gle Fiber Electromyography *(Continued)*

itical Values In disorders of the neuromuscular junction, such as myas-henia gravis, jitter is markedly increased. The phenomenon of "blocking" may be seen as well. When two single fibers are being tested for jitter, the second iber may intermittently fail to fire. These blocked action potentials represent ailure of impulse conduction. In normal individuals, the value for jitter stays constant even through repeated muscle contractions. With myasthenia gravis, jitter continually increases with repetitive muscle contractions. With Eaton-Lambert syndrome, jitter is also increased when tested initially, but with repetitive muscle contraction jitter decreases over time. Fiber density is increased early in neuropathic processes that are characterized by reinnervation. However, some authors have argued that fiber density is also increased in a variety of myopathic conditions, particularly when segmental muscle necrosis has occurred with subsequent regeneration. Thus, some experts feel that fiber density lacks that diagnostic specificity to distinguish neuropathy from myopathy. Others point out that both fiber density and jitter are usually normal or only slightly increased in myopathic conditions.

Limitations

- Procedure requires some degree of patient training. The patient must perform a minimal muscular contraction.
- When a significant baseline tremor or movement disorder exists, test results may be difficult to interpret.
- Increased jitter or fiber density cannot be used to reliably differentiate neuropathy from myopathy.
- SF-EMG should not be used as the sole diagnostic test in evaluating neurologic disorders.

Additional Information SF-EMG is a rapid and well-tolerated means of assessing neuromuscular junction disease. Although SF-EMG has limited diagnostic specificity, the sensitivity is outstanding for diseases such as myasthenia gravis. SF-EMG may be the first objective marker of neurologic disease when both physical examination and conventional EMG are normal.

References

Adams RD and Victor M, *Principles of Neurology: Companion Handbook*, 6th ed, New York, NY: McGraw-Hill Book Co, 1997.

Johnson EW and Wiechers D, "Electrodiagnosis," *Krusen's Handbook of Physical Medicine and Rehabilitation*, 4th ed, Kottke FJ and and Lehmann JF, eds, Philadelphia, PA: WB Saunders Co, 1990, 72-107.

Martin JB and Hauser SL, "Approach to the Patient With Neuromuscular Disease," *Harrison's Principles of Internal Medicine*, 14th ed, Fauci AS, Braunwald E, Isselbacher KJ, et al, eds, New York, NY: McGraw-Hill Book Co, 1998, 2277-93.

Rowland LP, ed, *Merritt's Textbook of Neurology*, 9th ed, Baltimore, MD: Williams & Wilkins, 1995.

Shahani BT and Young RR, "Clinical Electromyography," *Clinical Neurology*, Baker AB, ed, Philadelphia, PA: Harper and Row, 1985, 1-52.

♦ **Single Fiber EMG** *see* Single Fiber Electromyography *on page 174*

♦ **Somatosensory Evoked Potentials** *see* Electroencephalography *on page 154*

♦ **Speech Audiometry, Threshold and Discrimination** *see* Speech Discrimination Audiometry *on page 179*

Speech Audiometry, Threshold Only

Related Information

Pure Tone Audiometry *on page 170*

Speech Discrimination Audiometry *on page 179*

Synonyms Speech Reception Threshold (SRT); Speech Threshold; Spondee Threshold

Procedure Commonly Includes Determining the lowest hearing level necessary for the detection and comprehension of human speech. The listener is presented with a series of selected test words, either disyllabic words (spondees) or running speech, using earphones in a sound-attenuated room. The speech reception threshold (SRT) is defined as the lowest hearing intensity (in audiometric decibels) at which the listener correctly repeats 50% of the words. The SRT for an individual is compared against population norms in order to grade the degree of relative hearing loss. This test is also useful in

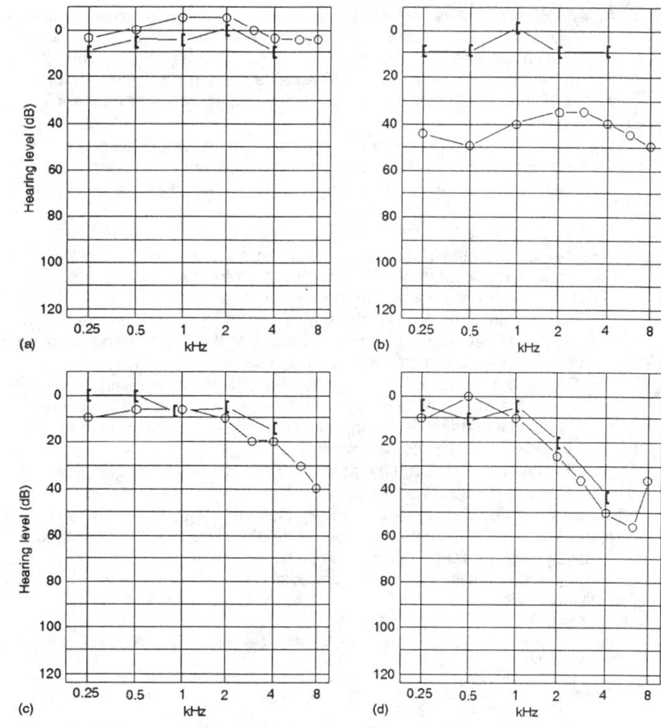

Idealized pure tone audiograms, right ear only. Symbols: o = air conduction, [= bone conduction. Figure (a) represents a normal audiogram. Figure (b) represents pure conductive hearing loss. Figure (c) depicts hearing loss associated with aging. Figure (d) depicts typical noise-induced hearing loss. Reproduced with permission from Lutman ME, "Diagnostic Audiometry," *Scott-Brown's Otolaryngology*, 5th ed, Chapter 7, Stephens D, ed, London, England: Butterworth's, 1987.

- In theory, BC thresholds reflect events in the cochlea or acoustic nerve alone, bypassing pathology in the external and middle ear. Please note that numerous exceptions exist.
- The difference between AC and BC thresholds at a given frequency reflects conductive hearing loss.
- The difference between BC thresholds and 0 dB reflects sensorineural loss.

Examples of idealized audiograms are shown in figures b, c, and d. Figure "b" show a marked decrease in sensitivity for AC thresholds with BC relatively spared. Both low and high frequencies are equally impaired. This pattern is classically seen with pure conductive hearing loss. If a large mass component is playing a role (serous otitis media), thresholds may be more impaired at higher frequencies. Other examples of conductive loss include eustachian tube dysfunction, otitis media, and impacted cerumen. With most cases of sensorineural loss, both AC and BC are significantly impaired and hearing loss is more pronounced as the frequency increases. Figure c depicts a constant loss of sensitivity for AC and BC that steadily worsens from low to high frequency. This pattern is often seen with the normal aging process. Figure d demonstrates the pattern seen with noise-induced hearing loss. Both

(Continued)

Pure Tone Audiometry *(Continued)*

AC and BC are impaired equally but sensitivity appears to be most effective at 4000 Hz. Hearing loss declines steadily from 250-4000 Hz (typical of sensorineural loss) but then improves from 4000-8000 Hz (atypical). Another exception to the classic pattern of sensorineural is seen in early Ménière disease where AC and BC thresholds are most elevated in the lower frequencies.

Limitations

- Test is highly dependent on patient cooperation and reliability.
- Only nonenvironmental sounds are tested, not human speech.
- Only threshold levels of hearing are evaluated; there is no testing of suprathreshold sounds.
- Issues such as perceived clarity of sounds are not addressed.
- The effect of the stimulus on the listener's brain and auditory system cannot be measured directly and must be inferred
- Nonorganic hearing loss may be difficult to rule out.
- The assumption that BC thresholds are independent of external and middle ear pathology is incorrect. Disease in the external and middle ear may elevate BC thresholds, often unpredictably.
- The problem of cross-hearing may be significant, particularly with BC thresholds where the skull readily transmits vibrations to both cochlea.
- If sensorineural loss is found, cochlear and retrocochlear lesions cannot be reliably differentiated.
- Only the site of lesion may be inferred, not any specific etiologies
- Technical limitations

Additional Information Pure tone audiometry, despite its limitations, is extremely useful in screening for loss of hearing sensitivity. The procedure is relatively simple, fast (20-30 minutes), and has high reliability and reproducibility. In most cases. Pure tones are easily generated and audiologist may individualize each case easily.

References

Bess FH and Humes LE, *Audiology: The Fundamentals*, 2nd ed, Baltimore, MD: Williams & Wilkins, 1995.

Conijn EA, Van der Drift JF, Brocaar MP, et al, "Conductive Hearing Loss Assessment in Children With Otitis Media With Effusion. A Comparison of Pure Tone and BERA Results," *Clin Otolaryngol*, 1989, 14(2):115-20.

Durrant JD and Lovrinic JH, *Bases of Hearing Science*, 3rd ed, Baltimore, MD: Williams & Wilkins, 1995.

Katz J, ed., *Handbook of Clinical Audiology*, 4th ed, Baltimore, MD: Williams & Wilkins, 1994.

Lovrinic JH, "Pure Tone and Speech Audiometry," *Audiology for the Physician*, Chapter 2, Keith RW, ed, Baltimore, MD: Williams & Wilkins, 1980, 13-31.

Lutman ME, "Diagnostic Audiometry," *Scott-Brown's Otolaryngology*, 5th ed, Chapter 7, Kerr AG, ed, London, England: Butterworth's Publishers, 1987, 244-71.

♦ **Repetitive Stimulation Testing** *see* Neuromuscular Junction Testing *on page 168*

♦ **Repetitive Stimulation Tests** *see* Single Fiber Electromyography *on page 174*

♦ **SF-EMG** *see* Single Fiber Electromyography *on page 174*

Single Fiber Electromyography

Related Information

Electromyography *on page 156*
Neuromuscular Junction Testing *on page 168*

Synonyms SF-EMG; Single Fiber EMG

Applies to Repetitive Stimulation Tests

Procedure Commonly Includes Recording the electrical activity of a single motor fiber using conventional electromyographic techniques. A specialized electrode is inserted percutaneously into a selected muscle and the electrical activity of the muscle fiber is displayed as an action potential wave on a cathode ray oscilloscope. Unlike conventional EMG, the electrode is small enough to pick up activity in only one or two muscle fibers, an almost "pure" action potential. SF-EMG is used to diagnose diseases of the neuromuscular junction such as myasthenia gravis. This technique estimates **muscle jitter** (the electrical variability between two muscle fibers in the same motor unit) and **fiber density** (the number of individual muscle fibers in a single motor

unit). SF-EMG is a sensitive means of confirming the dia gravis; muscle jitter and fiber density may be abnormal e\ is subclinical.

Indications Diagnosis of diseases of the neuromuscula myasthenia gravis, Eaton-Lambert syndrome (myasthe syndrome associated with small cell carcinoma of the l Some authorities advocate SF-EMG as a means of disting from myopathy but this is controversial.

Contraindications Although there are no absolute contra EMG, test results may be compromised in the patient with gross tremor, or uncontrolled movement disorder. Repetitive may be more appropriate in these situations.

Patient Preparation SF-EMG is often performed along w EMG and the same considerations apply.

Aftercare No specific activity restrictions are necessary follo dure.

Special Instructions The requisition from the ordering ph include a brief clinical history, pertinent neurologic findings, and impression. In many cases, SF-EMG is performed at the neuro tion in conjunction with conventional EMG without an explicit o

Complications SF-EMG is essentially risk-free and no signific tions have been reported. Patients tolerate the procedure well, result of the low number of needle punctures required.

Equipment A small, highly selective electrode is used for SF-EM usually a 25 micron diameter wire within a hollow cutting nee equivalent to approximately 50% of the width of a single muscle fiber action potentials are recorded with minimal distortion and tran standard oscilloscope and a loudspeaker. A 500 Hz filter is oft eliminate background noise from distant muscle fibers.

Technique Any muscle fiber accessible to conventional EMG may using SF-EMG. Several authors advocate routine testing of the digitorum communis due to its accessibility and the ease of volunta control. Initially, the patient is trained to perform a minimal muscle co (eg, raising the third finger). Following this the needle electrode is percutaneously and electrical activity is measured at rest and during a contraction. A crisp "pop" on the loudspeaker and a uniform repro waveform on the oscilloscope signifies a single fiber action potential. T major parameters obtained during SF-EMG are fiber density and muscl The former is based on the observation that a randomly inserted electro record the action potential from a single fiber approximately 70% of the In the remaining 30%, the electrode will pick up electrical activity of tw more fibers. The fiber density is determined by inserting the elect randomly into the same muscle 20 separate times. The number of indivi fibers sensed during each insertion is noted. In other words, the numbe synchronous action potentials is counted at each of 20 different electro positions; the average value of the 20 measurements is the fiber density. Th parameter estimates the number of single muscle fibers in one motor unit Muscle jitter represents the electrical variability between two single muscle fibers in the same motor unit. Although innervated by the same nerve, these two fibers may differ slightly with respect to impulse propagation and electrical potential. If the first fiber is held "still" in time on the oscilloscope, the action potential of the second fiber appears to vary in time with respect to the first fiber. The time difference between the appearance of the two action potentials (in msec) is recorded for 200 consecutive depolarizations. The mean value for these 200 time intervals is termed the mean consecutive difference and is the numerical value that estimates jitter.

Normal Findings Single fiber action potentials resemble fibrillation potentials in terms of configuration and duration. Normal values for fiber density have been established from asymptomatic volunteers and vary for individual muscles. For the extensor digitorum communis, the fiber density is normally 1.3-1.8 microns. Normal value to jitter for the same muscle is approximately 55 msec (expressed as the mean consecutive difference). A neurologist specially trained in this technique does interpretation.

(Continued)

confirming hearing thresholds obtained using pure tone audiometry. SRT is considered a routine component of basic audiologic evaluation.

Indications

- screen for hearing impairment suspected on clinical grounds; some experts consider SRT the initial screening procedure of choice
- confirm hearing thresholds obtained by pure tone audiometry, primarily as a cross-check for test reliability
- follow-up on abnormal pure tone audiometry, usually as a prelude to speech discrimination testing

Contraindications SRT is essentially risk-free and no absolute contraindications have been reported.

Patient Preparation Patients should be examined by a physician prior to speech audiometry. Reversible or self-limited causes of hearing loss should be ruled out prior to testing (eg, cerumen impaction, labyrinthitis, acute otitis media, etc). The procedure is explained to the patient and informed consent is obtained. No dietary or activity restrictions are necessary and the patient may take usual medication, including nasal sprays and decongestants. Hearing aids, if worn, should be brought to the testing center.

Aftercare There are no specific post-test restrictions. Follow-up is arranged by primary physician or audiologist as necessary.

Special Instructions The validity of the procedure depends on patient accuracy and reliability. Diagnostic yield may be limited in the patient with dementia or in very young children.

Complications None reported

Equipment As with pure tone audiometry, an electronic audiometer is used. This is a device capable of transmitting recorded speech via earphones. Alternatively, monitored live voice (MLV) may be used with the audiometer in the "off" position. The audiometer is equipped with a separate voltage unit meter to monitor sound intensity. Several protocols have been published regarding the speech stimuli. The majority of these auditory word lists are composed of disyllabic words called "spondees" (each syllable spoken with equal intensity). Word lists adhere to the following criteria.

- Words must be familiar to the listener.
- Words display phonetic variation.
- A normal sample of speech sounds is used.
- There is homogeneity of audibility.

Prerecorded lists of spondees are commercially available, such as the Psychoacoustic Laboratory (PAL) which consists of two lists of 42 words each and the Central Institute for the Deaf (CID) Tests W-1 and W-2 consisting of 36 spondaic words. In comparison with live speech, the recorded versions may contain psychoacoustic modifications including the following.

- Difficult spondees are presented at a higher intensity (2 dB louder).
- Spondees judged "simple" are 2 dB softer.
- The carrier phrase "say the word" is included before each spondee at a level 10 dB greater than the test spondee.
- Word lists may be scrambled to provide multiple equivalent forms of the test (PAL No 9).
- Automatic attenuation is incorporated. For example, in the W-2 test the sound intensity is automatically decreased by 3 dB every third word.

Monitored live voice (MLV) technique may be employed instead of recorded speech. Either standard spondee lists may be read, or less commonly, "running" speech presented. MLV allows modifications for children and other specialized groups. A widely-accepted children's spondee list has been published for MLV.

Technique The patient is seated in sound-dampened room with earphones comfortably placed. Some audiologists provide the listener with an alphabetized list of spondees to be tested in order to ensure word familiarity. The listener is instructed to simply repeat the word heard through the earphones without a penalty for an incorrect response. Speech signals may be presented in either a descending or ascending fashion. A common descending clinical protocol follows.

(Continued)

Speech Audiometry, Threshold Only *(Continued)*

1. A spondaic word is presented approximately 40 dB above the estimated speech threshold.
2. If the listener responds correctly, decrease by 10 dB and present a different spondaic word.
3. Repeat step 2 until a word is repeated incorrectly, at which point a second spondaic word is presented at the same intensity. If this second word is correctly repeated, continue to decrease intensity by 10 dB until two consecutive spondaic words are correctly identified. If, however, an error is made on the second word, increase intensity by 10 dB and proceed to the next step.
4. Once the intensity is increased, threshold exploration is begun. This involves a somewhat complex series of steps using longer spondee lists and smaller increments or decrements in intensity (2-5 dB steps). The SRT in this method must be calculated by the audiologist and approximately with the same criteria traditionally used to define SRT (50% correct responses). Speech signals may also be presented in an ascending protocol. This technique begins with a spondee at the lowest possible intensity with a stepwise increase in intensity.

SRTs are obtained for each ear independently. As with pure tone audiometry, masking techniques are necessary. White noise is presented to the nontest ear. Contralateralization of speech stimuli may occur via bone conduction, especially when SRT of the test ear is greater than the bone conduction threshold of the nontest ear by 40 dB or more, or when SRT differs by >40 dB between ears.

Normal Findings Interpretation is done by an audiologist or otologist on the day of testing. Normal values for auditory thresholds have been derived from population studies of healthy adults. The average threshold level (for both pure tone and speech audiometry) within this population has been calculated and defines audiometric "0 dB." Thus, an average SRT would be 0 dB for both right and left ears in a young, healthy adult. "Normal" hearing thresholds vary somewhat depending upon the author. Hearing level loss from 0-25 dB is considered normal in most classification systems. Such individuals display no difficulties in speech comprehension and hearing aid evaluation is not necessary. Negative SRT values (eg, -5 dB) are possible in some normal individuals since 0 dB represents only a population mean. Clinical trials have demonstrated that SRT correlates closely with threshold for pure tones. The threshold for pure tones should agree with the threshold for speech to within 5-6 dB, provided the pure tone curve is flat. (If the curve is sloping, the pure tone thresholds at 500 and 1000 Hz may be averaged and compared with SRT.)

Critical Values The speech reception threshold in each ear may be compared with established population norms. A variety of hearing impairment scales have been devised to classify the degree of loss: mild, moderate, severe, and profound. These scales are listed in the figure and apply to both speech reception thresholds and pure tone thresholds. SRT levels are elevated in both conductive and sensorineural types of hearing loss and do not discriminate. A discrepancy between SRT and pure tone threshold of 12 dB or more is considered significant and deserves further evaluation. A discrepancy of this magnitude suggests a severe defect in speech discrimination as seen in:

- certain central nervous system lesions
- presbycusis
- inappropriate spondee selection (eg, unfamiliar words)

In addition, discrepancy may also be due to tinnitus (pure tone threshold more affected than speech), problems with equipment calibration, and patient artifacts including malingering.

Limitations

- Speech signals are technically more difficult to calibrate than pure tones.
- Listener response is relatively complicated.
- Results may be influenced by familiarity of the patient with the specific word lists used.
- Speech comprehension at suprathreshold levels is not assessed.

Hearing level (loss) in dB re:ANSI-1969

0 10 20 30 40 50 60 70 80 90 100 110 120

	Profoundly deaf					Clarke (1957)
	Slight deafness	Partial deafness	Severe deafness	Profound deafness		Dale (1962)
Class A: Not significant	Class B: Slight	Class C: Mild	Class D: Marked	Class E: Severe	Class F: Extreme	Davis & Silverman (1970)
Normal	Mild	Moderate	Severe	Profound		Pauls & Hardy (1953)
Normal	Mild	Moderate	Moderately severe	Severe	Profound	Goodman (1965)
Normal	Class 1: Mild losses	Class 2: Marginal losses	Class 3: Moderate losses	Class 4: Severe losses	Class 5: Profound losses	Streng et al (1955)
Normal	Hard of hearing	Educationally or partially deaf	Deaf			Streng at al (1955)

Hearing impairment scales, classifying degree of severity. Applies to both speech reception thresholds and pure tone thresholds. Reproduced with permission from Lloyd LL and Kaplan H, Audiometric Interpretation: *A Manual of Basic Audiometry*, Baltimore, MD: University Park Press, 1978, 16.

Additional Information Some authorities recommend SRT as the first test to be administered to patients with clinical hearing loss. Arguments include the following.

- The stimuli used with SRT (spondaic words) are more concrete and familiar for many patients than pure tones.
- Spondees are more clinically relevant than nonenvironmental tones since a day-to-day function (speech reception) is being evaluated.
- It is more difficult for the patient with factitious hearing loss to consistently produce falsely elevated speech reception thresholds.
- Even less time is needed than pure tone audiometry.

References

Bess FH and Humes LE, *Audiology: The Fundamentals*, 2nd ed, Baltimore, MD: Williams & Wilkins, 1995.

Durrant JD and Lovrinic JH, *Bases of Hearing Science*, 3rd ed, Baltimore, MD: Williams & Wilkins, 1995.

Katz J, ed, *Handbook of Clinical Audiology*, 4th ed, Baltimore, MD: Williams & Wilkins, 1994.

Lovrinic JH, "Pure Tone and Speech Audiometry," *Audiology for the Physician*, Chapter 2, Keith RW, ed, Baltimore, MD: Williams & Wilkins, 1980, 13-31.

Lutman ME, "Diagnostic Audiometry," *Scott-Brown's Otolaryngology*, 5th ed, Chapter 7, Kerr AG, ed, London, England: Butterworth's Publishers, 1987, 244-71.

Schill HA, "Thresholds for Speech," *Handbook of Clinical Audiology*, 3rd ed, Katz J, ed, Baltimore, MD: Williams & Wilkins, 1985, 224-34.

Speech Discrimination Audiometry

Related Information

Pure Tone Audiometry *on page 170*

Speech Audiometry, Threshold Only *on page 176*

Synonyms Speech Audiometry, Threshold and Discrimination

Procedure Commonly Includes Testing speech comprehension at suprathreshold, conversational levels. A series of phonetically balanced words is presented to the listener at a specific sound intensity level. The listener repeats this list of words back to the examiner and the percentage of correct responses is determined at that intensity level. The procedure is repeated at different intensity levels with new word lists. Each time, the percentage of correct responses is recorded as the "discrimination score." Data accumulated in this manner is plotted as a performance-intensity function, the "articulation curve," with discrimination score on the vertical axis and sound pressure level (in dynes/cm^2) on the horizontal axis. From this curve several useful points may be read directly including:

- optimal discrimination score, "PB_{max}," the highest point on the articulation curve

(Continued)

Speech Discrimination Audiometry *(Continued)*

- speech reception threshold, the speech intensity corresponding to a 50% correct response rate
- the discrimination loss, the difference of PB_{max} from 100%

These parameters, along with the shape of the articulation curve, are compared with established norms. Both the degree and nature of hearing loss may be characterized. Speech discrimination testing is an integral part of the standard audiologic battery and plays an important role in evaluating conversation-level hearing.

Indications Speech discrimination tests have been applied to a number of clinical situations, with variable degrees of success. Among these are:

- evaluation of hearing skills necessary for day-to-day conversation and social adequacy
- determination of the site of an audiologic lesion (of somewhat limited values and must be combined with other forms of testing)
- selection of patients who might benefit from otologic surgery
- assessment of aural rehabilitation
- screening for central auditory disorders (procedure well-suited due to complexity of stimuli)
- selection of candidates eligible for hearing aids

Contraindications There are no absolute contraindications for this procedure.

Patient Preparation Patients should be examined by a physician prior to speech audiometry. Reversible or self-limited causes of hearing loss such as impacted cerumen, labyrinthitis, and acute otitis media should be ruled out. The procedure is then explained to the patient. There are no dietary or activity restrictions and the patient may take usual medications, including nasal sprays and decongestants, prior to the test. Hearing aids, if worn, should be brought to the test center.

Equipment Speech discrimination testing is performed using a standard audiometer, an electronic device capable of transmitting recorded speech to each ear independently via earphones. Instead of recorded speech, monitored live voice (MLV) may be alternatively employed for speech stimulus presentation. Speech discrimination tests are of four basic types:

- monosyllabic words with open response (repeat the words)
- monosyllabic words with closed response (multiple choice answers)
- sentences with open response
- sentences with closed response

Technique The patient is seated in a sound dampened room and earphones are placed. The listener is instructed to repeat the words heard through the earphones and instructed that there is no "penalty" for an incorrect response. Each ear is tested separately (monaurally) as well as together (binaurally). The audiologist selects a word list appropriate for the listener and presents the list using either a recording or MLV technique. Stimuli are presented at a sound level approximating normal conversational speech. On average, this is 70 dB sound pressure level (dynes/cm^2 x 0.0002). For soft speech at 1 meter, intensity would be 60 dB SPL. Generally, the intensity levels chosen reflect this 60-80 dB range. The percentage of correct responses is determined at a specific frequency. A new list of words is then presented at a different frequency and the discrimination score is again noted. This procedure is continued at the discretion of the audiologist. If a wide range of sound intensity levels is assessed, then an articulation curve may be plotted. This curve plots the discrimination score on the vertical axis and the sound pressure level (SPL) on the horizontal axis. The maximum discrimination score, PB_{max}, may be read directly from the curve (the highest point) as can the speech reception threshold (intensity at which discrimination score is 50%). During monaural testing, speech stimuli presented to the test ear may also be perceived in the nontest ear primarily via bone conduction. Therefore, as with other forms of audiometric testing, masking techniques are necessary to offset this problem. Filtered white noise is transmitted to the contralateral ear while the word list is being transmitted to the test ear. Speech discrimination testing may also be performed with competing noise in the test ear, "discrimination in noise." This technique is felt to better simulate day-to-day social communication. Various types of competing noise may be used: cafeteria noise, filtered white noise, competing voice, or voice babble. Both the speech stimulus (word list) and the completing noise are presented to the same ear simultaneously. This technique is particularly useful in hearing aid evaluation.

Data Acquired

- performance - intensity function for both right and left ears; if testing is extensive a complete articulation curve may be plotted
- PB_{max}
- speech reception threshold
- discrimination in noise (optional)

Normal Findings Interpretation is done by an audiologist or otologist, generally on the day of testing. Normal values for the articulation curve have been derived from testing normal hearing young adults. However, depending on the particular speech discrimination test selected, normal curves may differ substantially. Therefore, scores from different tests should not be compared directly. In the following figures, a normal performance-intensity function is shown. The normal value for PB_{max} is 100% for most tests, and this is generally achieved at 40-50 dB SPL. Once this maximum discrimination score is obtained, the normal listener will maintain the 100% score as sound intensity is increased. The normal value for the speech reception threshold (discrimination score of 50%) is approximately 30 dB SPL but varies considerably depending on the specific word list chosen. Speech reception threshold obtained directly from a formal articulation curve is the gold standard. The techniques described in Speech Audiometry, Threshold Only *on page 176* are approximations of this value. It should be noted that the decibel scale on the performance-intensity graph represents actual SOL in units of dynes/cm^2. In contrast, the decibel scale used for pure tone audiometry and speech threshold audiometry is a relative value scale without physical units. This latter scale defines 0 dB hearing level (HL) as the average hearing acuity for a normal population, the "audiometric zero." The value of 0 dB HL (audiometric zero) corresponds to 24.5 dB SPL at 250 Hz. Another parameter is "discrimination loss," the difference between PB_{max} and 100%. The normal value is zero.

Critical Values The figure on the following page depicts idealized curves seen with conduction loss, cochlear loss, or retrocochlear loss.

General principles for interpretation are as follows.

- For pure conductive hearing loss, PB_{max} will eventually reach 100% but only at high intensity levels. Speech reception threshold is elevated. Clinically, an afflicted individual will display adequate speech discrimination if the stimulus is sufficiently loud.
- For sensorineural loss in the cochlea, PB_{max} is reduced (best discrimination score is <100%) and this value is achieved only at high sound intensity levels. When sound intensity is increased even further, speech discrimination does not worsen (the articulation curve reaches a plateau).
- For retrocochlear, cranial nerve VIII loss, a characteristic "rollover phenomenon" is observed. After PB_{max} is reached, further increases in sound intensity actually cause a worsening of speech discrimination. "Rollover" refers to the shape of the curve. In the example shown, PB_{max} is 55% at 75 dB SPL. When word lists are presented at a higher sound intensity - 80 dB and above - more errors are made. Discrimination scores worsen to 20% correct at 90 dB.
- For auditory dysfunction (lesion in the brainstem or brain), the curve may resemble that of retrocochlear loss with rollover, but often the curve is not predictable.

These guidelines apply to the majority of cases but many exceptions have been noted. Considerable overlap may exist between diagnostic groups and this limits diagnostic utility. Speech discrimination alone should not be relied upon for site of lesion determination. Other supporting tests are needed. Several classification schemes have been published to grade the loss in speech discrimination at any given intensity. These are based on the discrimination score. Categories include normal slight discrimination difficulty, moderate difficulty, poor discrimination (50% to 60% correct responses) and very poor discrimination (<50% correct).

(Continued)

Speech Discrimination Audiometry *(Continued)*

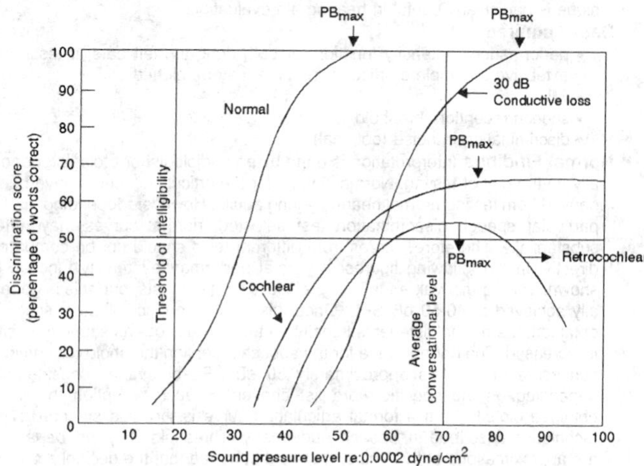

Idealized articulation curves for normal hearing, cochlear hearing loss conductive loss, and retrocochlear loss. Reproduced with permission from Lloyd LL and Kaplan H, Audiometric Interpretation: *A Manual of Basic Audiometry*, Baltimore, MD: University Park Press, 1978, 93.

References

Bess FH and Humes LE, *Audiology: The Fundamentals*, 2nd ed, Baltimore, MD: Williams & Wilkins, 1995.

Durrant JD and Lovrinic JH, *Bases of Hearing Science*, 3rd ed, Baltimore, MD: Williams & Wilkins, 1995.

Katz J, ed, *Handbook of Clinical Audiology*, 4th ed, Baltimore, MD: Williams & Wilkins, 1994.

Lovrinic JH, "Pure Tone and Speech Audiometry," *Audiology for the Physician*, Chapter 2, Keith RW, ed, Baltimore, MD: Williams & Wilkins, 1980.

Lutman ME, "Diagnostic Audiometry," *Scott-Brown's Otolaryngology*, 5th ed, Chapter 7, Kerr AG, ed, London, England: Butterworth's Publishers, 1987, 244-71.

Penrod JP, "Speech Discrimination Testing," *Handbook of Clinical Ideology*, 3rd Ed, Katz J, ed, Baltimore, MD: Williams & Wilkins, 1985.

♦ **Speech Reception Threshold (SRT)** *see* Speech Audiometry, Threshold Only *on page 176*

♦ **Speech Threshold** *see* Speech Audiometry, Threshold Only *on page 176*

♦ **Spinal Tap** *see* Lumbar Puncture *on page 160*

♦ **Spondee Threshold** *see* Speech Audiometry, Threshold Only *on page 176*

♦ **Tympanometry** *see* Pure Tone Audiometry *on page 170*

♦ **VERs** *see* Visual Evoked Responses *on page 182*

♦ **Vestibular Test** *see* Electronystagmography *on page 160*

♦ **Visual Evoked Potentials** *see* Visual Evoked Responses *on page 182*

Visual Evoked Responses

Related Information

Electroencephalography *on page 154*

Synonyms Pattern-Shift Visual Evoked Responses; VERs; Visual Evoked Potentials

Procedure Commonly Includes Stimulation of the retina and optic nerve with a shifting checkerboard pattern. This external visual stimulus causes measurable electrical activity in neurons within the visual pathways. This is called the visual evoked response (VER) and is recorded by EEG electrodes located over the occiput. Using special computer techniques, the evoked responses are measured over multiple trials, amplified, and averaged. As with conventional EEG, a waveform may be plotted (electrical potential versus time). With pattern-shift VER, the waveform normally appears as a straight line with a single positive peak (100 msec after stimulus presentation). Abnormalities in this characteristic waveform may be seen in a variety of pathologic processes involving the optic nerve and its radiations. Pattern-shift VER is a highly sensitive means of documenting lesions in the visual system. It is especially useful when the disease process is subclinical as when the ophthalmologic exam is normal and the patient lacks visual symptoms.

Indications The indications of VER are summarized below.

- suspected optic or retrobulbar neuritis
- confirm the diagnosis of multiple sclerosis suspected on clinical grounds; may be helpful in a young adult with transverse myelitis to establish more extensive demyelinating disease
- evaluate lesions of the optic nerve; VERs are abnormal in a number of diseases including glaucoma, ischemic optic neuropathy, pseudotumor cerebri, toxic amblyopias, nutritional amblyopias and neoplasms compressing the anterior visual pathways. The VER may be abnormal in other conditions involving the central nervous system (primary or secondary) such as sarcoidosis, pernicious anemia, and Friedreich's ataxia. However, abnormalities are nonspecific and are **not** diagnostic of a specific disease entity.
- assess visual function in the infant or child
- evaluate for possible hysterical blindness
- monitor the visual system during optic nerve or related surgery
- assess visual acuity in special circumstances such as amblyopia

The reliability of VER in the diagnosis of retrochiasmic lesions remains questionable. VERs to full field pattern recognition stimuli are usually normal in patients with unilateral hemispheric lesions.

Contraindications VER can be reliably performed in patients with mild to moderate loss of visual acuity. In the severely myopic patient (visual acuity <20/200), the checkerboard pattern cannot be seen adequately and testing should not be performed. The patient must also be reasonably cooperative and attentive enough to watch the visual stimulus for a period of several minutes. Muscle spasms involving the head and neck will compromise test results. If this is a problem, appropriate medications can be administered.

Patient Preparation The procedure is explained and informed consent should be obtained. Routine medications may be taken on the morning of the procedure, including prescription ophthalmologic medications. The patient should be instructed to wash his/her hair the night before testing in order to facilitate electrode placement. There are no dietary restrictions prior to testing and, in fact, it is suggested that the patient eat something shortly before testing to avoid relative hypoglycemia. Corrective lenses, if worn, should be brought to the testing area.

Aftercare There are no activity restrictions following the procedure and the patient may resume previous activity levels. Since sedation is not administered, outpatients may drive themselves home.

Special Instructions In most cases, this procedure is ordered directly by a neurologist. If ordered by another physician, the requisition should include a brief clinical history, pertinent neurologic findings, and overall impression. When testing children and neonates, special techniques are necessary and the laboratory should be notified of this in advance.

Complications VER testing is a safe, pain-free procedure. There is a theoretical risk of inducing seizure activity in susceptible patients as a result of the flashing checkerboard. However, this risk appears clinically negligible. The stimulus used for VER testing is quite different from the flashing strobe light that is used for seizure "activation" in EEG testing. The alternating checkerboard maintains a constant level of luminescence unlike a strobe light.

Equipment

- surface scalp electrodes (the same as those used for conventional EEG)
- pattern-shift stimulator, either a television screen or projected image
- signal amplifier with filters
- computer system for signal averaging

(Continued)

Visual Evoked Responses *(Continued)*

Technique VER is performed in a specially equipped electrodiagnostic procedure room. The patient is seated comfortably approximately one meter away from the pattern shift screen. Surface electrodes are placed on the scalp overlying the occipital and parietal regions with reference electrodes in the front region and ear. The patient is asked to focus his/her gaze onto the center of the screen. Each eye is tested separately (monocular testing). A shifting checkerboard is presented on the screen, with the squares reversing colors every 0.5-1 second. In general, 100 or more pattern shifts are presented. Each pattern alteration is considered a separate stimulus. The scalp electrodes detect electrical activity in the optic nerve and its radiations. Electrical potentials are recorded for a 500 msec interval following a stimulus. Characteristically, VERs are of low amplitude and require considerable amplification. Computer signal averaging must be used to diminish random, background electrical signals and isolate the VER. Conventional EEG does not utilize this technology. It is unable to distinguish VERs (from strobe light stimuli) from background "noise." The results of the numerous consecutive trials are computer average. The composite signal appears as a waveform with potential on the vertical axis and time on the horizontal axis.

Data Acquired A computer averaged visual evoked response at each electrode

Normal Findings Data are interpreted by an experienced neurologist, usually on the day of testing. The normal visual evoked response is a single, triphasic wave. This is shown in the following figure. The peak of the wave occurs approximately 100 msec after stimulus presentation and is referred to as "P-100". Several parameters of the evoked response are measured including:

- absolute P-100 latency - the time interval between the stimulus and the first large positive (downward) peak of P-100. Normal range is 90-110 msec.
- interocular latency - the difference in P-100 latency between the right and left eyes. Normally, the latency difference is <8-10 msec.
- amplitude of the VER
- duration of the triphasic wave

Normal values for these parameters are established for each laboratory and are age and gender dependent.

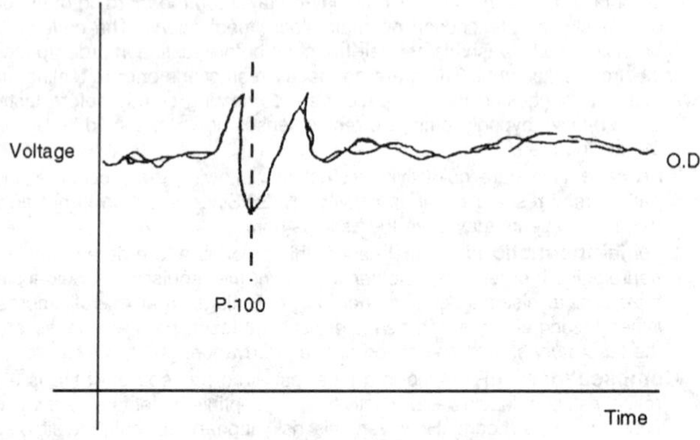

Visualized evoked response for one eye, depicting "P-100," Stimulus is presented at time 0.

Critical Values Any disease that slows conduction of optic nerve fibers will prolong the absolute P-100 latency. For example, in unilateral optic neuritis form multiple sclerosis, the P-100 wave may be detected as late as 200 msec after the stimulus. Both the absolute P-100 latency and the difference in latency between the two eyes would be abnormal. The advantage of VER testing lies in its sensitivity, not its specificity. Only limited information can be obtained regarding the nature of the visual lesion. P-100 latencies may be prolonged in multiple sclerosis, ischemic optic neuropathy, tumors, etc. VER testing may be useful in localizing the site of the lesion as shown in the following table. Abnormalities of P-100 duration or amplitude have more limited diagnostic utility due to the lack of specificity.

Visual Evoked Responses

VER Abnormality	Lesion Site
Prolonged latency, right eye only	Right optic nerve, anterior to the optic chiasm
Prolonged latency, left eye only	Left optic nerve, anterior to the optic chiasm
Prolonged latencies, right and left eye symmetrically	Localization not possible
Normal latency, midline electrodes	Either no lesions, or lesion is posterior to optic chiasm, or false-negative / technical error

Additional Information The pattern ship VER is useful in the confirmatory diagnosis of multiple sclerosis. Studies have shown that PS-VER is abnormal in a significant number of multiple sclerosis patients whose formal ophthalmologic examinations are normal. The rate of false negativity with pattern shift VER is relatively low. Some experts feel that VER may be used to rule out optic neuritis.

References

Aminoff MJ, "Electrophysiologic Studies of the Central and Peripheral Nervous Systems," *Harrison's Principles of Internal Medicine*, 14th ed, Fauci AS, Braunwald E, Isselbacher KJ, et al, eds, New York, NY: McGraw-Hill Book Co, 1998, 2282-97.

Celesia GG, "Visual Evoked Potentials in Clinical Neurology," *Electrodiagnosis in Clinical Neurology*, 4th ed, Aminoff MJ, ed, New York, NY: Churchill Livingston, 1999.

Chiappa KH, *Evoked Potentials in Clinical Medicine*, 3rd ed, Philadelphia, PA: Lippincott Williams & Wilkins, 1997.

Emerson RG, Walczak TS, and Turner CA, "EEG and Evoked Potentials," *Merritt's Textbook of Neurology*, 9th ed, Roland LP, ed, Baltimore, MD: Williams & Wilkins, 1995.

Shahroki F, Chiappa KH, and Young RR, "Pattern Shift Visual Evoked Response: Two Hundred Patient With Optic Neuritis and/or Multiple Sclerosis," *Arch Neurol*, 1978, 35:65-71.

(Continued)

PULMONARY MEDICINE AND CRITICAL CARE

♦ **A-a Gradient** *see* Alveolar to Arterial Oxygen Gradient *on page 188*
♦ **(A-a)O_2** *see* Alveolar to Arterial Oxygen Gradient *on page 188*
♦ **ABG** *see* Arterial Blood Gases *on page 191*

Airway Resistance

Related Information

Thoracic Gas Volume *on page 265*

Applies to Conductance; Specific Airways Resistance; Specific Conductance

Procedure Commonly Includes Airways resistance (R_{aw}) reported in cm H_2O pressure/L/second flow, specific airways resistance (SR_{aw}) reported in cm H_2O pressure/L/second flow/L FRC, airways conductance (G_{aw}) reported in L/second flow/cm H_2O pressure, and specific airways conductance (SG_{aw}) reported in L/second flow/cm H_2O/L FRC.

Indications Airway resistance is a measure of the resistance (measured in cm H_2O) to airflow (measured in L/second) afforded by all anatomical structures between the atmosphere and the lung alveoli, including the mouth, nasopharynx, and the central and peripheral airways. Evaluation of airway responsiveness, provocation testing, characterization of various types of obstructive lung disease, localization of the primary site of flow limitation, and evaluation of localized obstruction.

Contraindications

- patient unable to follow necessary instructions
- uncooperative patient

Patient Preparation The patient should avoid heavy meals 3 hours prior to testing. The patient should be conscious and able to follow simple instructions. The patient's height and weight should be measured without shoes. Loose comfortable clothing that does not restrict chest expansion should be worn. Smoking history, including last cigarette smoked, should be obtained. Current medications should be obtained with particular emphasis on bronchodilators and steroids. Indicate time period prior to testing that medication was last taken.

Aftercare Usually none. Patients complaining of lightheadedness and dizziness should be observed for 5 minutes after recovering and may benefit from rebreathing CO_2 from a paper bag.

Special Instructions Patients almost always have to be instructed to place palms flat against their cheeks during the closed shutter panting to avoid hysteresis of the mouth pressure signal from bulging cheeks when measuring TGV (thoracic gas volume). Thoracic gas volume value used in calculation of specific airways resistance and specific conductance must be measured just prior to measurement of airways resistance to ensure correct normalization of airway resistance and/or conductance to volume. Some body plethysmographs measure airways resistance during normal tidal breathing without requiring the patient to pant.

Equipment Body plethysmograph

Technique After proper instructions are given, the patient is seated in a calibrated body plethysmograph, noseclips and mouthpiece are adjusted, and the door is sealed. Allow box pressure to stabilize (temperature equilibration) then instruct the patient to breathe normally. Measurements are made in triplicate of the change in box pressure (delta P_{box}). versus flow. Mouthpiece shutter is

(Continued)

Airway Resistance *(Continued)*

closed at end tidal expiration, the patient is instructed to pant lightly against the closed shutter at a rate of approximately 1-2 breaths/second, and triplicate measurements are made of delta P_{box} versus P_{mouth}. The mean of three angles of P_{mouth}/P_{box} are used in the calculation of TGV. The airway resistance should not be made from the mean angle of flow/P_{box}, but rather the mean of the values for R_{aw}. Measurements of box pressure are made at point of inspiratory and expiratory flow of 0.5 $liter_{BTPS}$/second. A shutter at the mouthpiece is closed and the subject is asked to pant against the closed shutter. Angle of change in mouth pressure [delta P_{mouth}] (Y axis) during closed shutter panting plotted against changes in box pressure [delta P_{box}] (X axis) is representative of thoracic gas volume at which measurement of airways resistance is made. This allows reporting of specific resistance (normalized to lung volume).

Turnaround Time Preliminary report usually ready in 1 day, interpreted report in 1 day.

Causes for Rejection Glottis closure during airways resistance measurement, cheeks bowing in or out during closed shutter panting, nonreproducible results.

Normal Findings The normal range for airway resistance is 0.6-2.8 cm H_2O/L/second. The normal range for airway conductance is 0.36-1.7 L/second/cm H_2O. The normal range for specific conductance (conductance normalized to the lung volume at which it is measured) is 0.114-0.404 L/second/cm H_2O/L.

Limitations Lack of established criteria for measuring the angle of a resistance loop when there is significant hysteresis, which often occurs in the face of advanced obstructive lung disease. An accepted practice is to measure the slope of a best fit line drawn through the curve at the more linear (low flow) portion of the curve.

Additional Information Volume standardization of the airway resistance may be accomplished by dividing the conductance, SG_{aw} (the reciprocal of the resistance) by the TGV at which the resistance measurement was made. Changes in conductance values of >40% and resistance values >50% are considered significant when evaluating airway responsiveness to medication or challenge tests.

Airway Resistance and Conductance

		Normal Values
Airway resistance	R_{aw}	0.6-2.8 cm H_2O / LPS_{BTPS}
Airway conductance	G_{aw}	0.36-1.7 LPS_{BTPS} / cm H_2O
Specific conductance	SG_{aw}	0.114-0.404 LPS_{BTPS} / cm H_2O / L_{BTPS} TGV

Categorization of Severity (FRC >2 L)

Severity	R_{aw} (cm H_2O / LPS)
Mild	2.8-4.5
Moderate	4.5-8.0
Severe	>8.0

References

Ducharme FM and Davis GM, "Respiratory Resistance in the Emergency Department: A Reproducible and Responsive Measure of Asthma Severity," *Chest*, 1999, 116(1):268.

Exar EN and Collop NA, "The Upper Airway Resistance Syndrome," *Chest*, 1999, 115(4):1127-39.

Haavisto L, Sipila J, and Suonpaa J, "Nonspecific Nasal Mucosal Reactivity, Expressed as Changes in Nasal Airway Resistance After Bilateral Saline Provocation," *Am J Rhinol*, 1998, 12(4):275-8.

Alveolar to Arterial Oxygen Gradient

Related Information

Arterial Blood Gases *on page 191*
Shunt Determination *on page 247*

Synonyms A-a Gradient; (A-a)O_2; P(A-a)O_2

Procedure Commonly Includes Results generally include the measured and calculated parameters of an arterial blood gas test plus the calculated gradient of the partial pressure of alveolar to arterial dissolved oxygen expressed in millimeters of mercury (mm Hg).

Indications The A-a gradient is used to assess oxygenation. It compares the arterial pO_2 (PaO_2) to the theoretical maximum alveolar pO_2 (PAO_2).

Patient Preparation Patient preparation includes assessment of peripheral circulation on both sides, the Allen test. Both the radial and ulnar arteries should be compressed at a level approximately 1 centimeter proximal to the wrist joint while the patient makes a tight fist for approximately 5 seconds. The patient is then instructed to open the fist in a relaxed fashion. The palmar surface of the hand should be blanched. Release compression on the ulnar artery. The palmar surface should flush within 5 seconds. Prolonged delay before flushing indicates decreased ulnar artery flow. Radial arteries lacking collateral ulnar circulation should be avoided as puncture sites if possible. The skin over the puncture site should be swabbed with a Betadine® solution followed by an alcohol swab.

Aftercare The puncture site should be compressed for a minimum of 5 minutes, longer if the patient is taking anticoagulant therapy, aspirin or has a prolonged prothrombin time. After 5 minutes, the puncture site should be inspected for several seconds to ensure that clotting has taken place. During this inspection, palpate the pulse proximal and distal to the puncture site to assess the presence of arterial spasm. A sterile bandage should be placed over the puncture site to keep the puncture site clean while healing. **Warning:** A bandage is **not** a substitute for compression of the puncture site.

Technique The calculated alveolar oxygen tension is generally obtained from the alveolar air equation:

$$PAO_2 = ((Pb - 47) \times FiO_2) - PaCO_2/0.8$$

where:

- PAO_2 = alveolar oxygen tension (mm Hg or torr)
- Pb = barometric pressure (mm Hg or torr)
- FiO_2 = fractional concentration of inspired oxygen
- $PaCO_2$ = partial pressure of dissolved CO_2 in arterial blood (mm Hg or torr)
- 0.8 = average, normal respiratory exchange ratio, the ratio of CO_2 output to O_2 intake.

The following parameters are needed for calculation of the A-a gradient:

- barometric pressure (Pb) in mm Hg
- arterial pCO_2 ($PaCO_2$) in mm Hg
- arterial pO_2 (PaO_2) in mm Hg
- fractional concentration of inspired oxygen (FiO_2)

$$\text{A-a gradient (mm Hg)} = [((Pb - 47) \times FiO_2) - pCO_2/0.8] - PaO_2$$

where:

- 47 = H_2O pressure at 37°C in mm Hg
- 0.8 = assumed normal respiratory exchange ratio.

If the patient is breathing inspired oxygen concentrations >60%, the product ($PaCO_2/0.8$) can be eliminated from the alveolar air equation.

Turnaround Time Analysis of arterial blood gas typically takes less than 5 minutes, calculation of A-a gradient can be accomplished within 1 minute.

Specimen Heparinized arterial blood

Container Glass or plastic syringes (3-10 mL) may be used. Glass is preferred if sample measurement is delayed more than 1 hour. Glass capillary tubes are used for microsamples. It is impossible to maintain anaerobic integrity of a sample if evacuated glass tubes are used and their use is discouraged.

Collection Personnel performing the arterial puncture should wear rubber gloves. Perform necessary tests to assess collateral circulation. After choosing the optimal puncture site, clean site with Betadine® solution followed by alcohol. Allow alcohol to air dry. Slight hyperextension of the brachial and radial puncture sites by placement of a rolled up towel under the elbow or wrist may facilitate palpation of the pulse. Draw up approximately 0.3 mL sodium heparin (1000 units/mL) into syringe. Replace needle with a sterile one.

(Continued)

Alveolar to Arterial Oxygen Gradient *(Continued)*

Needle sizes of 23- to 25-gauge x 5/8" to 1" in length are commonly used. Holding the syringe with the needle pointing upward, pull the syringe plunger back to the end of the syringe to allow the liquid heparin to come in contact with the internal surface of the syringe. Expel excess heparin into the needle cap, making sure that the dead space of the syringe and needle do not contain any air. Palpate the artery with the index finger and puncture the artery, holding the needle at an angle of approximately 25° to the surface of the skin. Allow the pressure of the artery to fill the syringe. Withdraw the needle and immediately apply pressure using a sterile gauze pad. Insert needle into rubber stopper. Hold pressure for a minimum of 5 minutes. Include collection procedures for capillary sampling and arterial mean line and catheter collection.

Storage Instructions Samples not analyzed within 10 minutes should be stored in an ice-slush mixture (approximately 2°C). Syringe barrel plunger assembly should be sufficiently tight to prevent sample dilution with the ice-slush mixture.

Causes for Rejection Large air bubbles will cause all values to be erroneous. The magnitude of the error will be determined by the size of the air bubble, sample and sample air bubble interface, length of time bubble was in contact with sample before analysis and the gradient between sample gas tensions and room air gas tensions. Small bubbles, if immediately expelled will generally not cause any significant error. Samples with large (more than 0.2 mL) bubbles should be discarded and a new, anaerobic sample obtained.

Normal Findings <15 mm Hg in young adults, gradient increases with age. The following equations can be used to predict a resting A-a gradient while breathing room air:

Predicted A-a gradient on room air = (age + 4) / 4

Low arterial PaO_2 in the presence of a normal A-a gradient indicates that the patient is not ventilating adequately but the transfer of oxygen from the alveoli to the alveolar capillaries is normal (alveolar hypoventilation).

An elevated A-a gradient indicates ventilation/perfusion mismatching in the lung, a diffusion defect, or the presence of a right-to-left circulatory shunt.

Limitations While the alveolar to arterial oxygen gradient should always yield a positive number, there are several assumptions made which, if deviated from, may cause the equation to yield a negative number. The major assumptions are listed.

- The FiO_2 is often not measured; the assumed FiO_2 may vary widely from that actually received by the patient.
- The barometric pressure is not measured or is not measured at the time the arterial blood gas is obtained (eg, the Pb is measured once at the beginning of the day and this value is used for the entire day).
- The increase in Pb when a patient is artificially ventilated is seldom taken into account.
- A value of 47 mm Hg is typically used to subtract water vapor pressure (PH_2O) from the barometric pressure (Pb). This assumes a constant body temperature of 37°C. Actual body temperature may vary from this and thus change the actual PH_2O.
- The alveolar air equation which solves for the PAO_2 assumes that arterial pCO_2 ($PaCO_2$) is equal to alveolar pCO_2 ($PACO_2$). Although the two may be nearly identical in normal lungs, in diseased lungs there can be a difference of several mm Hg.
- The alveolar air equation also assumes a normal respiratory exchange ratio (R) of 0.8. This is true only when the metabolic R value equals 0.8 and the patient is in a steady-state. Because of either changes in metabolism (largely diet dependent) or deviations from a steady-state (when the respiratory exchange ratio does **not** equal the metabolic exchange ratio, as in acute hyperventilation), the R used in the alveolar air equation can vary widely from 0.8.

Taken together, the assumptions inherent in the use of the alveolar gas equation can cause the calculated PaO_2 (and thus the (A-a) DO_2) to vary several mm Hg above or below the value that would be obtained if everything was precisely measured.

References

Birdi I, Regragui IA, Izzat MB, et al, "Effects of Cardiopulmonary Bypass Temperature on Pulmonary Gas Exchange After Coronary Artery Operations," *Ann Thorac Surg*, 1996, 61(1):118-23.

Cardus J, Burgos F, Diaz O, et al, "Increase in Pulmonary Ventilation-Perfusion Inequality With age in Healthy Individuals," *Am J Respir Crit Care Med*, 1997, 156(2 Pt 1):648-53.

Hupert N, "Use of Alveolar-Arterial Oxygen Gradient," *Am J Med*, 1998, 105(5):458.

Jones JS, Neff TL, and Carlson SA, "Use of the Alveolar-Arterial Oxygen Gradient in the Assessment of Acute Pulmonary Embolism," *Am J Emerg Med*, 1998, 16(4):333-7.

Arterial Blood Gases

Related Information

Alveolar to Arterial Oxygen Gradient *on page 188*
Arterial Blood Oximetry *on page 195*
Arterial Cannulation *on page 17*
Pulse Oximetry *on page 245*
Shunt Determination *on page 247*

Synonyms ABG; Blood Gases, Arterial

Procedure Commonly Includes Measured parameters include: pH, pCO_2, and pO_2; calculated parameters include: bicarbonate (HCO_3), base excess or deficit (BE), standard bicarbonate, standard base excess, alveolar to arterial oxygen gradient ($p[A\text{-}a]O_2$).

Indications Assessment of oxygenation of arterial blood and the blood's acid-base balance

Contraindications Relative contraindications include peripheral artery spasm.

Patient Preparation Patient preparation includes assessment of peripheral circulation on both sides, the Allen test. Both the radial and ulnar arteries should be compressed at a level approximately 1 centimeter proximal to the wrist joint while the patient makes a tight fist for approximately 5 seconds. The patient is then instructed to open the fist in a relaxed fashion. The palmar surface of the hand should be blanched. Release compression on the ulnar artery. The palmar surface should flush within 5 seconds. Prolonged delay before flushing indicates decreased ulnar artery flow. Radial arteries lacking collateral ulnar circulation should be avoided as puncture sites if possible. If the radial artery is unsuitable as a puncture site, the brachial artery is the second choice, followed by the femoral artery. If the need for repeated measurements over several days exists, placement of an arterial catheter is indicated. The skin over the puncture site should be swabbed with a Betadine® solution followed by an alcohol swab. See the illustration on the following page.

Aftercare The puncture site should be compressed for a minimum of 5 minutes, longer if the patient is taking anticoagulant therapy, aspirin or has a prolonged prothrombin time. After 5 minutes, the puncture site should be inspected for several seconds to ensure that clotting has taken place. During this inspection, palpate the pulse proximal and distal to the puncture site to assess the presence of arterial spasm. A sterile bandage should be placed over the puncture site to keep the puncture site clean while healing. **Warning:** A bandage is **not** a substitute for compression of the puncture site.

Turnaround Time Results are available immediately after analysis. Stat results should be available 10 minutes after receipt of the sample.

Specimen Adequately heparinized (sodium or lithium heparinate) arterial or "arterialized" capillary blood sample. Volume and/or concentration of heparin should be adjusted to yield a final blood concentration of 30-100 units/mL blood in a syringe sample or 50-250 units/mL blood in a capillary sample.

Container Glass or plastic syringes (3-10 mL) may be used. Glass is preferred if sample measurement is delayed more than 1 hour. Glass capillary tubes are used for microsamples. It is impossible to maintain anaerobic integrity of a sample if evacuated glass tubes are used and their use is discouraged.

(Continued)

ALLEN'S TEST FOR COLLATERAL CIRCULATION

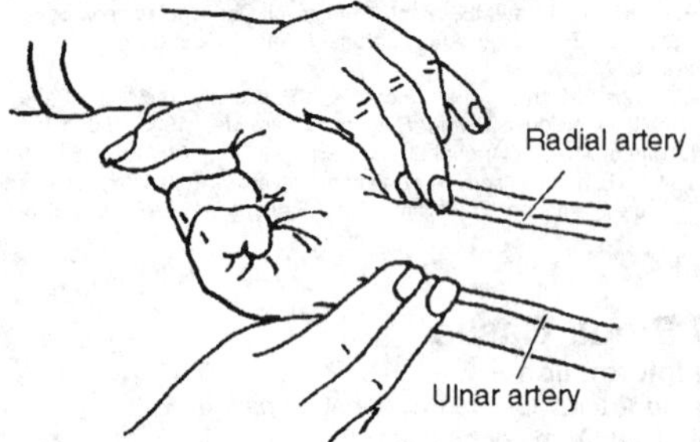

Fist clenched tightly, radial and ulnar arteries compressed

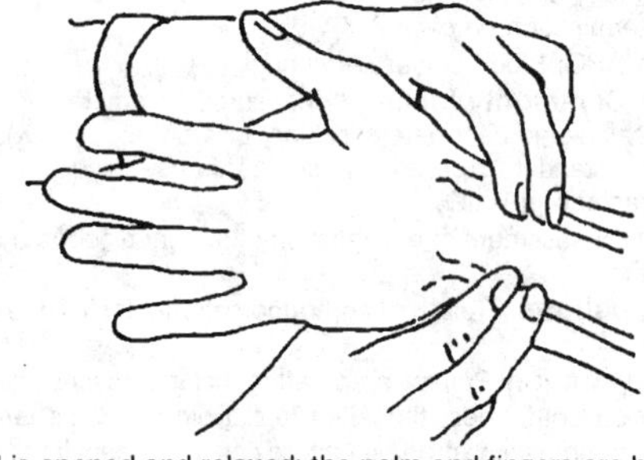

The hand is opened and relaxed; the palm and fingers are blanched

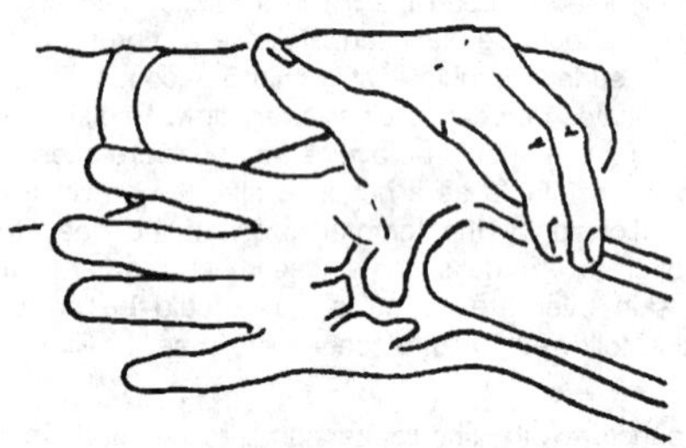

Pressure removed from ulnar artery, entire hand should flush within 15 seconds

Reproduced with permission from Shapiro BA, Harrison RA, and Walton JR, "Guidelines for Sampling and Quality Control," *Clinical Application of Blood Gases*, 2nd ed, Chapter 14, Chicago, IL: Year Book Medical Publishers, Inc, 1977, 148.

Collection Syringe sampling: Assemble the following equipment: syringe; needles (20- to 25-gauge (2)); anticoagulant (eg, sodium heparinate - 1000 units/mL); sterile gauze sponges or cotton; skin antiseptic (eg, 70% alcohol and Betadine® swabs); rubber stopper or needle cap; tourniquet; adhesive bandage. Don disposable rubber gloves as an infection control measure. Preheparinized glass or plastic syringes are available in blood gas kits from several manufacturers. Syringes preheparinized with liquid heparin should be held vertically, needle up, and the liquid heparin should be pushed into the dead space of the syringe and needle, expelling all air out of the dead space.

If preheparinized syringes are not used, the following procedure should be used. Fit a needle onto the syringe and draw 0.5-1 mL anticoagulant into it. Remove the original needle and replace with a sterile needle. Pull and push syringe plunger several times to coat syringe surface. Holding the syringe with the needle up, expel all liquid heparin into needle cap, taking care not to leave any air bubbles in the dead space of the needle. Perform the Allen test for collateral circulation to determine the best site for puncture. Sites listed in order of preference are as follows: radial, brachial, and femoral arteries. Palpate and visualize the artery. Apply antiseptic to the sampling site. Palpate the site once again, trying to stabilize the artery. Slight hyperextension of the wrist or elbow can be achieved by placing a rolled up towel under the joint; this can aid palpation and stabilization of the artery. Hold the syringe so the bevel of the needle faces upward, keeping the needle at a 25° to 30° angle to the artery. Insert the needle through the skin into the artery taking care not to puncture the posterior wall of the artery. Arterial pressure should cause the blood to flow into the syringe if the plunger fits properly and the barrel has been lubricated with anticoagulant. Withdraw the needle when an adequate sample has been obtained. Immediately place dry gauze or cotton over the puncture site. Maintain pressure over puncture site for a minimum of 5 minutes (longer if the patient has taken aspirin or anticoagulants). Expel any air bubbles from the sample. Insert needle into a rubber stopper or needle cap. Remove needle/cap assembly and replace with a syringe cap. Mix sample by rolling syringe for 20 seconds immediately prior to analysis. If not analyzed immediately, store the sample in iced water (2°C). Iced samples should be analyzed within 3 hours.

Capillary sampling: Assemble the following equipment: preheparinized capillary sample tubes; capillary tube end caps; mixing wire; magnet; water soluble jelly, if desired; sterile gauze sponges or cotton; skin antiseptic (eg, 70% alcohol). Select the puncture site (typically, the heel on infants, fingertips on adults). Establish increased regional circulation by wrapping the extremity with a warm, moist towel for 5-10 minutes. Loosely mount a capillary tube cap on the end of the capillary tube and insert a mixing wire into the capillary, allowing the mixing wire to slide to the same end of the tube as the loosely mounted capillary cap. Apply antiseptic to the sampling site. Make a skin puncture that forms drops of blood rapidly and fill the capillary with blood from the **middle** of the drop without introducing air into the capillary. Firmly seat both capillary end caps. Mix blood and anticoagulant initially by moving the mixing wire along the full length of the capillary approximately 20 times with a magnet and repeat mixing immediately prior to analysis. If not analyzed immediately, store the sample in iced water.

Storage Instructions Samples not analyzed within 10 minutes should be stored in an ice-slush mixture (approximately 2°C). Syringe barrel plunger assembly should be sufficiently tight to prevent sample dilution with the ice-slush mixture.

Causes for Rejection Large air bubbles will cause all values to be erroneous; the magnitude of the error will be determined by the size of the air bubble, sample and sample air bubble interface, length of time bubble was in contact with sample before analysis and the gradient between sample gas tensions and room air gas tensions. Small bubbles, if immediately expelled, will generally not cause any significant error. Samples with large (more than 0.2 mL) bubbles should be discarded and a new, anaerobic sample obtained.

Normal Findings Normal values (arterial blood), pH: 7.35-7.45; pCO_2: 36-44. The normal partial pressure of oxygen in arterial blood at sea level is generally considered to be >80 mm Hg. Several factors confound interpretation of pO_2 by this simple means, notably altitude of residency, age, hypoventilation, and hyperventilation. Normal ranges of pO_2 are shown in the following table. The arterial pO_2 should be evaluated according to the table of normal ranges shown. The most common causes of hypoxemia are:

- ventilation-perfusion (V/Q) abnormalities in the lungs
- physiologic shunting
- alveolar-capillary diffusion defects
- alveolar hypoventilation
- decreased inspired oxygen concentration

(Continued)

Arterial Blood Gases *(Continued)*

Acceptable Arterial Oxygen Tensions at Sea Level Breathing Room Air (21% oxygen)

	mm Hg
Adult and Child	
Normal	97
Acceptable range	>80
Newborn	
Acceptable range	40-70
Aged	
Acceptable range	
60 y	>80
70 y	>70
80 y	>60
90 y	>50

Interpretation of blood gases should start with the assessment of the ventilatory status by classification of the pCO_2. A low pCO_2 (<30 mm Hg) indicates alveolar hyperventilation. A high pCO_2 (>50 mm Hg) indicates ventilatory failure. A pCO_2 in the range of 30-50 mm Hg represents an acceptable level of alveolar ventilation. Because the lungs and the kidneys work together to achieve acid-base homeostasis, inspection of the arterial pH in conjunction with the pCO_2 will allow determination of the origin of the acid-base disturbance. Acid-base disturbances can be a primary ventilatory problem (respiratory acidosis, respiratory alkalosis) or a primary metabolic problem (metabolic acidosis, metabolic alkalosis). Respiratory acid-base disturbances present for more than 24 hours will result in renal compensation by increasing or decreasing the plasma bicarbonate to normalize pH. Metabolic acid-base disturbances will result in partial or complete compensation by the respiratory system which increases or decreases alveolar ventilation (and thus the pCO_2). The following table lists the seven primary blood gas classifications based on inspection of the arterial pH and pCO_2.

Seven Primary Blood Gas Classifications*

Classification	$PaCO_2$	pH	$p[HCO_3^-]$	BE
Primary Ventilatory				
Acute ventilatory failure	↑	↓	N	N
Chronic ventilatory failure	↑	N	↑	↑
Acute alveolar hyperventilation	↓	↑	N	N
Chronic alveolar hyperventilation	↓	N	↓	↓
Primary Acid-Base				
Uncompensated acidosis	N	↓	↓	↓
Uncompensated alkalosis	N	↑	↑	↑
Partly compensated acidosis	↓	↓	↓	↓
Partly compensated alkalosis	↑	↑	↑	↑
Compensated alkalosis or acidosis	↑ or ↓	N	↑ or ↓	↑ or ↓

*Arrows indicate depressed or elevated values; N = normal; BE = base excess.

Reproduced with permission from Shapiro BA, Harrison RA, and Walton JR, *Clinical Application of Blood Gases,* 2nd ed, Chicago, IL: Year Book Medical Publishers, Inc, 1977, 137.

Critical Values pH values chronically outside of the normal range are a cause for concern. pCO_2 values >50 mm Hg may indicate ventilatory failure. pO_2 values <55 mm Hg while breathing room air may indicate the need for supplemental oxygen therapy.

Limitations Erroneous values can result from improper (aerobic) sample handling, excessive storage at room temperature (more than 10 minutes) before measurement, excessive storage at 2°C (>3 hours) before measurement, improper calibration of the blood gas analyzer, and measurement errors. Potentially hazardous clinical judgments based solely on blood gas values without clinical correlation are discouraged.

Additional Information Heparinized blood is required and may be obtained either from an artery or an "arterialized" capillary. Sodium heparin is generally used as an anticoagulant, it may be used as a powder or a liquid. Errors have been reported from the excessive dilution of the sample with liquid heparin. Disposable kits are available that supply needles with inner cannula that minimize syringe-needle combined dead space, making a minimum sample size of 0.5 mL sufficient. Blood gas analyzers vary, but most can measure capillary samples of as little as 200 μL. Syringes and capillary tubes using powdered heparin obviate the need for concern regarding heparin dilution errors.

References

Hansen JE, "Arterial Blood Gases," *Clin Chest Med*, 1989, 10(2):227-37.

Horne C and Derrico D, "The Art of Arterial Blood Gas Measurement," *Am J Nurs*, 1999, 98(8):26-32.

Zeballos RJ, Weisman IM, and Connery SM, "Comparison of Pulmonary Gas Exchange Measurements Between Incremental and Constant Work Exercise Above the Anaerobic Threshold," *Chest*, 1998, 113(3):602-11.

Arterial Blood Oximetry

Related Information

Arterial Blood Gases *on page 191*

Pulse Oximetry *on page 245*

Synonyms Co-oximetry; Hemoximetry

Applies to Carbon Monoxide Determination

Replaces Calculated Arterial or Venous Oxygen Saturation

Procedure Commonly Includes Total hemoglobin (THb) in g/dL, oxygen saturation (HbO_2Sat) in percent or oxyhemoglobin (HbO_2) in percent, carboxyhemoglobin (HbCO) in percent, methemoglobin (metHb) in percent, and the calculated content of oxygen bound to hemoglobin (cO_2) in volumes percent

Indications Assessment of anemia or polycythemia, assessment of elevated levels of dysfunctional hemoglobins (carboxyhemoglobin, methemoglobin), assessment of oxygen content, correlation of pulse oximetry with blood oximetry (correction for dysfunctional hemoglobins).

Patient Preparation Patient preparation includes assessment of peripheral circulation on both arms, the Allen test. Both the radial and ulnar arteries should be compressed at a level approximately 1 centimeter proximal to the wrist joint while the patient makes a tight fist for approximately 5 seconds. The patient is then instructed to open the fist in a relaxed fashion. The palmar surface of the hand should be blanched. Release compression on the ulnar artery. The palmar surface should flush within 5 seconds. Prolonged delay before flushing indicates decreased ulnar artery flow. Radial arteries lacking collateral ulnar circulation should be avoided as puncture sites if possible. The skin over the puncture site should be swabbed with a Betadine® solution followed by an alcohol swab.

Aftercare The puncture site should be compressed for a minimum of 5 minutes, longer if the patient is taking anticoagulant therapy, aspirin or has a prolonged prothrombin time. After 5 minutes, the puncture site should be inspected for several seconds to ensure that clotting has taken place. During this inspection, palpate the pulse proximal and distal to the puncture site to assess the presence of arterial spasm. A sterile bandage should be placed over the puncture site to keep the puncture site clean while healing. **Warning:** A bandage is **not** a substitute for compression of the puncture site.

Technique Measurement systems use a calibrated system for measurement of the optical absorption and turbidity of blood samples. Absorbancies measured are specific for reduced hemoglobin (RHb), HbO_2, HbCO, and metHb. The values for THb, HbO_2 sat, HbO_2, HbCO, metHb, and O_2 content are calculated from the data obtained from the measured absorbancies.

(Continued)

Arterial Blood Oximetry *(Continued)*

Turnaround Time Measurement of sample takes 1-2 minutes. Report should be available at that time.

Specimen Adequately heparinized (sodium or lithium heparinate) arterial or "arterialized" capillary blood sample. Volume and/or concentration of heparin should be adjusted to yield a final blood concentration of 30-100 units/mL blood in a syringe sample or 50-250 units/mL blood in a capillary sample.

Container Glass or plastic syringes, glass capillary tubes

Sampling Time Samples should be analyzed within 15 minutes (see Storage Instructions).

Collection Syringe sampling: Assemble the following equipment: syringe; needles (20- to 25-gauge (2)); anticoagulant (eg, sodium heparinate - 1000 units/mL); sterile gauze sponges or cotton; skin antiseptic (eg, 70% alcohol and Betadine® swabs); rubber stopper or needle cap; tourniquet; adhesive bandage. Don disposable rubber gloves as an infection control measure. Preheparinized glass or plastic syringes are available in blood gas kits from several manufacturers. Syringes preheparinized with liquid heparin should be held vertically, needle up, and the liquid heparin should be pushed into the dead space of the syringe and needle, expelling all air out of the dead space. If preheparinized syringes are not used, the following procedure should be used. Fit a needle onto the syringe and draw 0.5-1 mL anticoagulant into it. Remove the original needle and replace with a sterile needle. Pull and push syringe plunger several times to coat syringe surface. Holding the syringe with the needle up, expel all liquid heparin into needle cap, taking care not to leave any air bubbles in the dead space of the needle. Perform the Allen test for collateral circulation to determine the best site for puncture (see Arterial Blood Gases *on page 191*). Sites listed in order of preference are as follows: radial, brachial, and femoral arteries. Palpate and visualize the artery. Apply antiseptic to the sampling site. Palpate the site once again, trying to stabilize the artery. Slight hyperextension of the wrist or elbow can be achieved by placing a rolled up towel under the joint; this can aid palpation and stabilization of the artery. Hold the syringe so the bevel of the needle faces upward, keeping the needle at a 25° to 30° angle to the artery. Insert the needle through the skin into the artery taking care not to puncture the posterior wall of the artery. Arterial pressure should cause the blood to flow into the syringe if the plunger fits properly and the barrel has been lubricated with anticoagulant. Withdraw the needle when an adequate sample has been obtained. Immediately place dry gauze or cotton over the puncture site. Maintain pressure over puncture site for a minimum of 5 minutes (longer if the patient has taken aspirin or anticoagulants). Expel any air bubbles from the sample. Insert needle into a rubber stopper or needle cap. Remove needle/cap assembly and replace with a syringe cap. Mix sample by rolling syringe for 20 seconds immediately prior to analysis. If not analyzed immediately, store the sample in iced water (2°C). Iced samples should be analyzed within 3 hours.

Capillary sampling: Assemble the following equipment: preheparinized capillary sample tubes; capillary tube end caps; mixing wire; magnet; water soluble jelly, if desired; sterile gauze sponges or cotton; skin antiseptic (eg, 70% alcohol). Select the puncture site (typically, the heel on infants, fingertips on adults). Establish increased regional circulation by wrapping the extremity with a warm, moist towel for 5-10 minutes. Loosely mount a capillary tube cap on the end of the capillary tube and insert a mixing wire into the capillary, allowing the mixing wire to slide to the same end of the tube as the loosely mounted capillary cap. Apply antiseptic to the sampling site. Make a skin puncture that forms drops of blood rapidly and fill the capillary with blood from the **middle** of the drop without introducing air into the capillary. Firmly seat both capillary end caps. Mix blood and anticoagulant initially by moving the mixing wire along the full length of the capillary approximately 20 times with a magnet and repeat mixing immediately prior to analysis. If not analyzed immediately, store the sample in iced water.

Storage Instructions If not analyzed immediately, samples should be chilled to 2°C in an ice/slush mixture to reduce erythrocyte metabolism. Iced samples should be analyzed within 3 hours after being drawn.

Causes for Rejection Improperly stored samples

Normal Findings The table shows expected values. Elevated levels of HbCO can be secondary to exposure to cigarette, pipe and cigar smoke, faulty gas furnaces, automobile exhaust, or any site of incomplete combustion. Elevated methemoglobin may be hereditary (hemoglobin M disease or enzyme [$NADH_2$-reductase] deficiency) or acquired through exposure to certain drugs or chemicals such as nitrites, nitrates, chlorates, quinones, aminobenzenes, nitrobenzenes, or nitrotoluenes.

Arterial Blood Oximetry

Component	Whole Blood	Expected Values
THb	Newborn	14.0-24.0 g/dL
	Adult male	13.5-18.0 g/dL
	Adult female	12.0-16.0 g/dL
HbO_2 saturation	Arterial	91.9%-98.5%
HbO_2	Arterial	94%-100%
HbCO	Nonsmokers	<1.5% of THb
	Smokers	1.5%-5.0% of THb
	Heavy smokers	5.0%-9.0% of THb
MetHb		<3% of THb or 0-0.24 g/dL
O_2 content	Arterial	15-23 vol %
SHb		0

Critical Values Oxyhemoglobin values <85%; sum of dysfunctional hemoglobins (COHb + MetHb) >15%.

Limitations Oxyhemoglobin or oxygen saturation values from samples that contain air bubbles should be questioned. Bubble size, length of time from obtaining sample, and analysis and gradient of partial pressure of oxygen between sample and atmosphere will determine the magnitude of the error introduced by the bubble. Other values should be unaffected by air contamination. Methylene blue in a concentration of approximately 60 mg/L blood interferes with the measurement of methemoglobin, total hemoglobin, and HbO_2 measurements yielding falsely low values of total hemoglobin and methemoglobin and falsely high values of HbO_2. Excessively high or low pH values will yield erroneously low and high values respectively of methemoglobin. Sulfhemoglobin levels ≥10% will increase $HbCO_2$ and decrease metHb values. Milking or squeezing the area of a capillary puncture will result in mixing of blood and tissue fluids with the liability of erroneous measurements. Inadequate mixing of either a syringe or capillary sample just prior to analysis will result in erroneous total hemoglobin measurements.

References

Hampson NB, "Pulse Oximetry in Severe Carbon Monoxide Poisoning," *Chest*, 1998, 114(4):1036-41.

Mower WR, Sachs C, Nicklin EL, et al, "Pulse Oximetry as a Fifth Pediatric Vital Sign," *Pediatrics*, 1998, 99(5):681-6.

Pierson DJ, "Pulse Oximetry Versus Arterial Blood Gas Specimens in Long-Term Oxygen Therapy," *Lung*, 1990, 168(Suppl):782-8.

Seguin P, Le Rouzo A, Tanguy M, et al, "Evidence for the Need of Bedside Accuracy of Pulse Oximetry in an Intensive Care Unit," *Crit Care Med*, 2000, 28(3):703-6.

♦ **Arterial Lines** *see* Swan-Ganz Catheterization *on page 258*

♦ **Assessment of Pulmonary Disability** *see* Flow Volume Loop *on page 225*

♦ **Assessment of Pulmonary Disability** *see* Spirometry *on page 249*

♦ **Bartlett-Farling-Wimbaly Brush** *see* Protected Catheter Brush *on page 241*

Bedside Spirometry

Related Information

Bronchial Challenge Test *on page 202*

Flow Volume Loop *on page 225*

Spirometry *on page 249*

(Continued)

Bedside Spirometry *(Continued)*

Spirometry, Sitting and Supine *on page 256*

Synonyms Portable Spirometry

Indications Early monitoring of patient with high potential for respiratory problems, monitoring of the acutely ill patient, monitoring recuperating mechanically ventilated patient.

Patient Preparation Avoid heavy meals 3 hours prior to testing. The patient should be conscious and able to follow simple instructions. The patient's height and weight should be measured without shoes. Loose comfortable clothing that does not restrict chest expansion should be worn. Smoking history including last cigarette smoked should be obtained. Current medications should be obtained with particular emphasis on bronchodilators and steroids.

Aftercare Usually none, although patients that complain of lightheadedness and dizziness should not be allowed to walk unobserved until recovery.

Special Instructions Patients that have a tracheostomy stoma may be tested by attaching an infant anesthesia mask to the mouthpiece. Mouthpieces can be adapted directly to most tracheostomy tubes.

Equipment Exhaled sample is collected or passed through a volume or flow measuring device known as a spirometer. Spirometers should meet certain minimum standards defined by the American Thoracic Society. Other equipment needed varies with the type of spirometer being used but should include a disposable mouthpiece and noseclips. Special circumstances may require adaptation of the mouthpiece to a mask, face seal, or tracheostomy adapters.

Technique A spirometer is used to measure exhaled gas and to record the time of collection. Many such devices have recently been miniaturized and advertised as ideal for bedside spirometry. Regardless of whether measurements are made at bedside or in the Pulmonary Function Laboratory, equipment used to measure forced expiratory volumes or flows should meet or exceed equipment standards recommended by the American Thoracic Society (ATS).

Data Acquired Vital capacity (VC), forced vital capacity (FVC), timed forced expiratory volumes; $FEV_{0.5}$, FEV_1, FEV_3, midexpiratory flow rate ($FEF_{25\%-75\%}$), peak expiratory flow rate (PEFR or PF), forced expiratory time (FET, seconds)

Turnaround Time Preliminary results should be available same day. Depending on the facility, an interpreted report may be available in 1-2 days.

Collection Bedside spirometry should be limited to patients on partial or complete bedrest for whom the seated position is contraindicated or for patients whose conditions make frequent serial measurements of pulmonary function desirable. The vital capacity and forced vital capacity maneuvers can be performed in virtually any position. Whenever possible, the patient should be tested in the upright position. Because of postural changes in lung function, it is imperative that the patient's position and angle of elevation of the bed, if any, be kept constant and recorded on the report so that valid comparisons can be made. After applying noseclips, the subject is instructed to take a full inspiration, hold it briefly, then exhale through a mouthpiece into the spirometer as forcefully and completely as possible, keeping the chin slightly elevated throughout the maneuver. Test is repeated a minimum of three times until two reproducible efforts have been obtained. See Causes for Rejection. A maximum number of eight attempts is recommended.

Causes for Rejection Cough, when occurring in the early part of forced expiration, may render all data except total expired volume useless. **Hesitant start:** Peak effort must be applied as close to the start of exhalation as possible or timed forced expiratory volumes may be invalid. The volume exhaled before maximum effort is applied is known as back extrapolated volume and must not exceed 5% of total FVC. **Premature cessation of expiratory effort:** One of the four following conditions defines satisfactory end-of-test.

- Expiratory time is at least 6 seconds and no volume change for at least 1 second.

- If no volume plateau is seen, patient should sustain expiration for a reasonable length of time; "reasonable" in moderately severe obstruction is suggested to be 15 seconds.
- The patient **cannot** or **should** not continue the expiration for medical reasons.
- Tests that consistently exhibit a smooth, curvilinear rise to a volume plateau of at least 1 second duration on a volume-time tracing satisfy end-of-test criteria even if the forced expiratory time is <6 seconds (children, patients with interstitial lung disease).

Early termination of expiration will falsely increase the FEV_1/FVC% and the $FEF_{25\%-75\%}$. **Submaximal effort:** Indicated by a very low, often nonreproducible peak flow. Neuromuscular disease may produce the same pattern. **Nonreproducibility:** The two largest FVCs and the two largest FEV_1s should show <5% variability. Three acceptable tests should be obtained.

Normal Findings Spirometric values are dependent on patient's position during testing. Any position other than seated or standing will generally result in less than maximal values. This should be considered when comparing results with normal values generated by a study whose subjects were tested in an upright posture. Pain, especially thoracic or upper abdominal incisional pain, will further limit inspiratory efforts. One study cites a 40% reduction in vital capacity persisting several days after upper abdominal surgery. Normal range for spirometric indexes is typically ±20% of a reference value based on age, height, and gender, but if available, reference values that allow calculation of or lower limit of normal (LLN) provide a more statistically sound threshold for determining abnormal results.[1] Abnormalities of pulmonary function can be separated into three broad descriptive categories: restrictive, obstructive, and mixed. See Patterns of Spirometric Abnormalities table.

Patterns of Spirometric Abnormalities

	NML* (% of predicted)	Obstructive Diseases	Restrictive Diseases
FVC	≥80*	NML or ↓	↓ to ↓↓↓
FEV_1	≥80*	↓ to ↓↓↓	↓ to ↓↓↓
FEV_1 / FVC %	≥75	↓ to ↓↓↓	NML or ↑
$FEF_{25\%-75\%}$	≥76*	↓↓ to ↓↓↓	↓ to ↓↓↓

*Expressed as actual ratio of FEV_1 / FVC x 100.

↓ mildly reduced.

↓↓ moderately reduced.

↓↓↓ severely reduced.

Restrictive ventilatory defects are characterized by proportional decreases in FVC and FEV_1, leaving the FEV_1/FVC% normal or even slightly elevated. Any lesion affecting the lung, chest wall, or respiratory muscles' ability to take in a normal amount of air yet does not affect the conducting airways' FVC can be classified as a restrictive lung disease. Obstructive diseases are characterized by their involvement of the airways and the resultant reduction in expiratory

Quantification of Impairment by Spirometry (% of predicted)

	FVC	FEV_1	FEV_1 / FVC%*†	$FEF_{25\%-75\%}$
Normal	≥80	≥80	75-85	>76
Minimal (slight)	70-79	70-79	65-74	60-75
Moderate	55-69	55-69	55-64	45-59
Severe	45-54	40-54	45-54	30-44
Very severe	<45	<45	<45	<30

*Expressed as actual ratio of FEV_1 / FVC x 100.

†Female age >40 years.

(Continued)

Bedside Spirometry *(Continued)*

flow. Spirometric studies in the presence of obstructive lung disease generally show a reduced FEV_1, FEV_1/FVC% and flow rates with a relatively normal FVC. In severe obstructive lung disease, the FVC may also be reduced. Asthma, emphysema, and chronic bronchitis are the most common obstructive lung diseases. Mixed disorders generally present with a reduction in all parameters on spirometric examination. While this is a more scientifically sound method, it has not yet gained widespread acceptance. Spirometric values expressed as % of predicted can be used to grade the severity of abnormalities. See table on the previous page.

Critical Values Severe or very severe reductions (see Quantification of Impairment by Spirometry table).

Limitations Spirometry requires a great deal of cooperation and a thorough understanding of expectations on the part of the patient. Poor understanding or lack of motivation will yield falsely low values that may be incorrectly interpreted. Reproducibility of the two best repeat FVCs and FEV_1s within 5% must be demonstrated before a meaningful interpretation can be made. Most portable (handheld) spirometers have severe limitations in their ability to present information necessary to evaluate the acceptability of spirometric efforts according to American Thoracic Society (ATS) standards. A recent evaluation of spirometers found many portable spirometers did **not** meet current ATS performance standards. Whenever possible, spirometry should be performed in the Pulmonary Function Laboratory rather than at the bedside.

Additional Information Patients with asthma may show progressive decline in spirometric values with repeated efforts, yielding excessive variability between the two largest efforts. This may be distinguished from variable effort by noting maximal inspiration on each effort followed by an adequately forceful expiration (sharp peak of expiratory flow volume curve). In such cases, the largest and smallest acceptable efforts should be reported giving the physician a rough assessment of bronchial hyper-reactivity. (See Bronchial Challenge Test *on page 202*.) Patients with neuromuscular disease (myasthenia gravis) may show progressive decline of values with repeated efforts but are seldom able to generate an adequate peak effort and may therefore mimic poor effort or understanding.

Footnotes

1. Morris JF, Koski A, and Johnson LC, "Spirometric Standards for Healthy Nonsmoking Adults," *Am Rev Respir Dis*, 1971, 103(1):57-67.

References

Aaron SD, Dales RE, and Cardinal P, "How Accurate Is Spirometry at Predicting Restrictive Pulmonary Impairment?" *Chest*, 1999, 115(3):869-73.

Celli BR, "The Importance of Spirometry in COPD and Asthma: Effect on Approach to Management," *Chest*, 2000, 117(2 Suppl):15S-9S.

Eaton T, Withy S, Garrett JE, et al, "Spirometry in Primary Care Practice: The Importance of Quality Assurance and the Impact of Spirometry Workshops," *Chest*, 1999, 116(2):416-23.

Enright PL, Arnold A, Manolio TA, et al, "Spirometry Reference Values for Healthy Elderly Blacks. The Cardiovascular Health Study Research Group," *Chest*, 1996, 110(6):1416-24.

Fitzgerald DJ, Speir WA, and Callahan LA, "Office Evaluation of Pulmonary Function: Beyond the Numbers," *Am Fam Physician*, 1996, 56(4):1071.

Hankinson JL, Odencrantz JR, and Fedan KB, "Spirometric Reference Values From a Sample of the General U.S. Population," *Am J Respir Crit Care Med*, 1999, 159(1):179-87.

Johnson BD, Weisman IM, Zeballos RJ, et al, "Emerging Concepts in the Evaluation of Ventilatory Limitation During Exercise: The Exercise Tidal Flow-Volume Loop," *Chest*, 1999, 116(2):488-503.

Linn WS, Solomon JC, Gong H Jr, et al, "Standardization of Multiple Spirometers at Widely Separated Times and Places," *Am J Respir Crit Care Med*, 1996, 153(4 Pt 1):1309-13.

Rebuck DA, Hanania NA, D'Urzo AD, et al, "The Accuracy of a Handheld Portable Spirometer," *Chest*, 1996, 109(1):152-7.

♦ **BFW Brush** *see* Protected Catheter Brush *on page 241*

♦ **Blood Gases, Arterial** *see* Arterial Blood Gases *on page 191*

Bronchial Brush Biopsy

Related Information

Bronchoscopy, Flexible *on page 209*

Procedure Commonly Includes Extending a brush through a flexible fiberoptic bronchoscope and brushing over a lesion for purposes of cytologic examination of cellular material trapped in the bristles of the brush

Indications Aid in the diagnosis of malignancy

Contraindications All are relative contraindications:

- uncooperative patient
- FEV_1 <800-1000 mL
- severe asthma
- hypoxemia uncorrected to an oxygen saturation >90% with supplemental oxygen
- bleeding diathesis
- arrhythmia
- unstable cardiac status
- recent myocardial infarction

Patient Preparation The patient should have no food or drink for 8 hours prior to the procedure (NPO after midnight for AM procedure; early light breakfast for PM procedure). Routine medications may be taken with a small amount of water. Premedication with a narcotic and/or benzodiazepine is given parenterally prior to the procedure. Atropine 0.4 mg I.M. may be given as a vagolytic agent to dry secretions unless contraindicated (ie, arrhythmia, narrow angle glaucoma, urinary retention). Supplemental oxygen is usually administered. The oropharynx is anesthetized with 2% lidocaine via a nebulizer or by gargling. The nares and nasopharynx are anesthetized with 2% lidocaine jelly if the bronchoscope is to be inserted via the nasal route.

Aftercare The patient should be NPO for at least 2 hours after the procedure (until the gag reflex has returned). Outpatients are not allowed to drive until the following day. Mild hemoptysis may be noted for 24 hours.

Complications Hypoxemia and bronchospasm; endobronchial bleeding may occur. It is usually mild and self-limited. Local instillation of epinephrine or iced saline is normally all that is required for treatment.

Equipment Flexible bronchoscope with light source; disposable and reusable, 3 mm and 7 mm size brushes (7 mm size is not commonly used); glass slides; containers with fixative (eg. Carnoy's and Cytolyte® solutions); fluoroscope; syringes; lidocaine; and sedatives

Technique The bronchoscope is passed and the airways are anesthetized in the usual manner. The 3 mm brush is retracted into its teflon catheter so that its distal end is even with the catheter's protective metal tip. The catheter is then passed through the working channel of the bronchoscope and advanced to the lesion (under direct visualization for central lesions and under fluoroscopic guidance for peripheral ones). Once at the site, the brush is extended from its protective catheter and the lesion is brushed back and forth 5-10 times. The brush is then retracted back into the catheter and the whole assembly is withdrawn through the working channel. (The 7 mm brush differs in that it does not have a protective teflon catheter, it is used only for endoscopically visible lesions, and it cannot be withdrawn through the working channel after brushing. Instead the whole bronchoscope must be withdrawn.) The material collected is immediately plated onto glass slides by pressing the brush onto the slide with either a circular or back and forth motion. Generally, two slides can be made per brush. It is imperative that the slides be immersed immediately in a fixative (eg, Carnoy's solution) as any drying will distort cellular morphology. A single brush is used for two separate passes. The brush is then cut and placed in a container with Cytolyte® solution.

The figure on the following page shows a fluoroscopic image of an extended brush in the area of a lung mass.

Data Acquired Cytology

Specimen Cellular material

Collection Cellular material is collected by brushing the area in question with a brush passed through a bronchoscope.

Storage Instructions Glass slides should be placed in fixative (eg, Carnoy's solution). The brush is placed in a container with Cytolyte® solution.

Causes for Rejection Inadequate cellular material, excessive drying of specimen (distorting cellular morphology)

(Continued)

Bronchial Brush Biopsy *(Continued)*

Bronchial Brush Biopsy

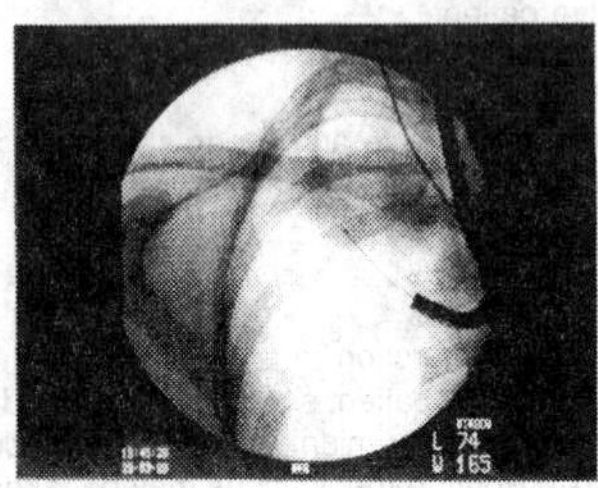

Normal Findings No malignant cells

Limitations It is difficult to sample very peripheral lesions.

Additional Information The diagnostic yield from the combination of bronchial brush biopsy, bronchial washings, and transbronchial biopsy is >90%.

References

Chanez P and Vignola AM, "Bronchial Brushing," *Eur Respir J Suppl*, 1998, 26:26S-9S.

Lee FY and Mehta AC, "Basic Techniques in Flexible Bronchoscopy," Wang KP and Mehta AC, eds, *Flexible Bronchoscopy*, Cambridge, MA: Blackwell Science, Inc, 1995, 95-118.

Wang HH, Sovie S, Trawinski G, et al, "ThinPrep® Processing of Endoscopic Brushing Specimens," *Am J Clin Pathol*, 1996, 105(2):163-7.

Bronchial Challenge Test

Related Information

Allergy Testing, Intracutaneous (Intradermal) *on page 103*

Bedside Spirometry *on page 197*

Flow Volume Loop *on page 225*

Ingestion Challenge Test *on page 125*

Spirometry *on page 249*

Spirometry Before and After Bronchodilators *on page 253*

Synonyms Bronchial Provocation Tests; Histamine Challenge Test; Mecholyl Challenge; Mecholyl Provocation Test; Methacholine Challenge; Methacholine Provocation Test; Provocholine® Challenge

Procedure Commonly Includes $PD_{20}FEV_1$ (provocative dose necessary to cause a 20% reduction from baseline FEV_1). $PD_{35}SG_{aw}$, % change in FEV_1 or SG_{aw} at the end of study, % improvement in FEV_1 or SG_{aw} after administration of bronchodilators.

Indications

- identify and characterize severity of nonspecific bronchial hypersensitivity, especially helpful in the diagnosis of cough-variant asthma or asthma in remission
- evaluate the effectiveness of pharmacological agents in the prevention of provoked bronchospasm
- study the pathophysiology of bronchospasm

Contraindications Relatively contraindicated in the presence of severe restrictive or obstructive lung disease (FEV_1 <1 $liter_{BTPS}$).

Patient Preparation Patients should abstain from the use of: sympathomimetic drugs for 6 hours, metaproterenol for 8 hours, terbutaline or Salbutamol for 12 hours, methylxanthines for 12 hours, sustained release methylxanthines for 48 hours, cromolyn sodium for 48 hours, corticosteroids for 12 hours, smoking for 12 hours, coffee, tea, cola, or chocolate for 6 hours, significant exercise for 2 hours, and exposure to cold air for 2 hours. The patient should be questioned as to these drugs and conditions prior to testing. Record time and nature of recent respiratory illnesses as viral respiratory infections have been shown to leave residual bronchial hyper-reactivity that may linger for months.

Aftercare Administration of an aerosol bronchodilator and measurement of response to bronchodilator should be done on virtually every patient, even those that do not show a clearly positive response to methacholine. Spontaneous reversal of methacholine induced bronchospasm usually takes place within 90 minutes. Methacholine induced bronchospasm is usually readily reversible after inhaled bronchodilator therapy.

Complications Severe bronchospasm may occur, particularly if baseline airway obstruction is present.

Equipment Standard equipment includes a spirometer which meets ATS equipment specifications, mouthpiece, noseclip, 10 compressed gas nebulizers, 20 psi compressed gas source, dosimeter (which delivers a 0.6 second burst of compressed gas to the nebulizer upon actuation) and various doses of methacholine chloride or histamine solution. See table.

Standardized Methacholine Challenge Protocol

Methacholine Concentration (mg/mL)	Cumulative Number of Breaths	Cumulative Dose Units (CDU)
0.025	5	0.125
0.25	10	1.375
2.5	15	13.875
10.0	20	63.875
25.0	25	188.880

Technique Two protocols are widely in use, five breaths per challenge level or 2 minutes of tidal breathing per challenge level. In the 2-minute challenge, the test material is placed in a nebulizer cup attached to a constant output compressor. The patient is instructed to perform tidal breathing for 2 minutes. Measurement of response is done 3 minutes after each exposure. In the 5-breath challenge the patient inhales slowly from FRC to TLC through a dosimeter driven nebulizer cup containing the test material. The dosimeter delivers a 0.6 second nebulization (at 20 psig) of the test material. The breath is held for 3-5 seconds. Both protocols use the same schedules of test material concentrations. Forced expiratory maneuvers are performed before and 3 minutes after inhalation challenge with either a diluent solution or gradually increasing doses of a solution of methacholine. Testing consists of measurement of reproducible FVC and FEV_1 before and after administration of aerosolized diluent solution and aerosolized methacholine chloride/diluent solution. Measurement of spirometry should be done on calibrated spirometers that meet standards recommended by the American Thoracic Society (ATS). Duplicate FEV_1 at each challenge level should be reproducible within 5%.

Data Acquired For clinical use, the PD_{20} FEV_1 (the lowest concentration which produces a 20% reduction in FEV_1 from baseline) is generally reported. Researchers often plot the log of the cumulative dose of methacholine against the FEV_1 response reported as a percentage of the control FEV_1 (FEV_1 after inhalation of the diluent solution).

Turnaround Time Preliminary results are usually available on the day of testing. An interpreted report usually follows in 1-2 days.

Causes for Rejection Nonreproducible forced expiratory maneuvers. FEV_1 should be reproducible to within 5% on any given level of challenge. Drop in FEV_1 should be sustained for 5 minutes to be considered valid. End expiratory coughing may result in nonreproducible FVC values. If the FEV_1 values show reproducibility, efforts that show end-expiratory coughing may be used only if the FEV_1/FVC% and $FEF_{25\%-75\%}$ are ignored and only changes in the FEV_1 are considered.

Normal Findings There is a certain amount of overlap between normal and asthmatic responses to methacholine chloride and histamine toward the end of the challenge procedure. Provocative doses are usually reported as either (Continued)

Bronchial Challenge Test *(Continued)*

the concentration of methacholine in solution or the cumulative dose unit (CDU) necessary to provide a 20% reduction in the baseline FEV_1 or a 35% reduction in the specific conductance (SG_{aw}). A dose unit (DU) is defined as the number of breaths inhaled multiplied by the strength of solution in mg/mL being inhaled. Less than a 20% fall in FEV_1 or 35% fall in SG_{aw} by the end of a challenge, typically, 189 cumulative dose units of methacholine, makes the diagnosis of asthma or nonspecific airway hyper-reactivity unlikely. The table shows suggested guidelines for defining hyper-responsiveness and describing the severity of reaction to a metacholine challenge. A positive methacholine challenge does not always indicate asthma. Recent viral infections and pre-existing obstructive lung disease in the absence of detectable asthma have been shown to cause false-positive reactions to challenge testing.

$PC_{20}FEV_1$ (mg/mL)	Severity
0.03-0.124	Severe
0.125-1.99	Moderate
2.00-7.99	Mild
>8.00	Normal

Limitations While methacholine challenge testing is a sensitive test for bronchial hyper-reactivity, a positive test is not specific for the diagnosis of asthma. Other diseases associated with nonspecific bronchial hyper-reactivity include COPD, bronchiolitis, viral upper respiratory infections, hay fever, cystic fibrosis, sarcoidosis, chemical irritant exposure, and recovery from adult respiratory distress syndromes. Appropriate preparation is imperative for proper interpretation of challenge response. Negative methacholine challenges in patients with positive specific bronchial challenges with chemical agents suspected of causing occupational asthma have been reported.

Additional Information Methacholine chloride is available in ready to mix ampules from Roche Laboratories that are marketed under the name Provocholine®. The following dosage schedule is recommended when using Provocholine®:

- baseline spirometry
- diluent solution spirometry
- 0.025 mg/mL methacholine spirometry
- 0.25 mg/mL methacholine spirometry
- 2.5 mg/mL methacholine spirometry
- 10 mg/mL methacholine spirometry
- 25 mg/mL methacholine spirometry
- aerosolized bronchodilator spirometry

References

Crapo RO, Casaburi R, Coates AL, et al, "Guidelines for Methacholine and Exercise Challenge Testing-1999. This Official Statement of the American Thoracid Society Was Adopted by the ATS Board of Directors, July 1999," *Am J Respir Crit Care Med*, 2000, 161(1):309-29.

Davis BE and Cockcroft DW, "Calculation of Provocative Concentration Causing a 20% Fall in FEV(1): Comparison of Lowest vs Highest Post-Challenge FEV(1)," *Chest*, 2000, 117(3):881-3.

Drotar DE, Davis BE, and Cockcroft DW, "Dose Versus Concentration of Methacholine," *Ann Allergy Asthma Immunol*, 1999, 83(3):229-30.

Elsasser S, Donna E, Demirozu CM, et al, "Metaproterenol Responsiveness After Methacholine- and Histamine-Induced Bronchoconstriction," *Chest*, 1996, 110(3):617-23.

♦ **Bronchial Provocation Tests** *see* Bronchial Challenge Test *on page 202*

Bronchial Washings

Related Information

Bronchoscopy, Flexible *on page 209*

Procedure Commonly Includes Injecting normal saline through the bronchoscope over a radiographically or endoscopically abnormal area of the lung, then suctioning it into a specimen trap

Indications Aid in the diagnosis of malignancy, fungal, and acid-fast infections

Contraindications All are relative contraindications:

- uncooperative patient
- FEV_1 <800-1000 mL
- severe asthma
- hypoxemia uncorrected to an oxygen saturation >90% with supplemental oxygen
- bleeding diathesis
- arrhythmia
- unstable cardiac status
- recent myocardial infarction

Patient Preparation The patient should have no food or drink for 8 hours prior to the procedure (NPO after midnight for AM procedure; early light breakfast for PM procedure). Routine medications may be taken with a small amount of water. Premedication with a narcotic and/or benzodiazepine is given parenterally prior to the procedure. Atropine 0.4 mg I.M. may be given as a vagolytic agent to dry secretions unless contraindicated (ie, arrhythmia, narrow angle glaucoma, urinary retention). Supplemental oxygen is usually administered. The oropharynx is anesthetized with 2% lidocaine via a nebulizer or by gargling. The nares and nasopharynx are anesthetized with 2% lidocaine jelly if the bronchoscope is to be inserted via the nasal route.

Aftercare The patient should be NPO for at least 2 hours after the procedure (until the gag reflex has returned). Outpatients are not allowed to drive until the following day.

Complications Hypoxemia, bronchospasm

Equipment Flexible bronchoscope with light source, 10 mL syringe, normal saline, specimen trap, suction assembly, lidocaine, and sedatives

Technique The bronchoscope is passed and the airways are anesthetized in the usual manner. A specimen trap is connected in series with the suction catheter once the bronchoscope is advanced to the area in question. Normal saline is instilled through the working channel of the bronchoscope and subsequently suctioned into the trap. Usually 2-5 mL aliquots of fluid are instilled with each washing. For endoscopically visible lesions, the fluid is washed directly over the area in question. For lesions which are not visible, the bronchoscope is advanced to the respective segment and washings are taken blindly. For tumors which are diagnosed on sputum cytology but are not radiographically or bronchoscopically visible, washings of each segment can be performed for localization of the tumor.

Data Acquired Cytology, fungal, and AFB studies

Specimen Normal saline with bronchial secretions and cellular material

Container Specimen trap

Collection Through the bronchoscope normal saline is instilled over the area in question, then suctioned into a specimen trap

Causes for Rejection Inadequate volume

Normal Findings No malignant cells, mycobacteria, or fungi

Limitations Unable to perform routine cultures as there is invariably contamination that occurs by passing the bronchoscope through the upper airway. Cultures for *Mycobacterium tuberculosis* may be inhibited by the topical anesthetics.

Additional Information The diagnostic yield from the combination of bronchial washings, bronchial brush biopsy, and transbronchial biopsy is >90% for malignancy.

References

Kumarasinghe P and Jayasundera CI, "Cytological Diagnosis of Bronchial Malignancies Using the Fibreoptic Bronchoscope," *Ceylon Med J*, 1992, 37(2):41-3.

Lee FY and Mehta AC, "Basic Techniques in Flexible Bronchoscopy," *Flexible Bronchoscopy*, Wang KP and Mehta AC, eds, Cambridge, MA: Blackwell Science, Inc, 1995, 95-118.

Bronchoalveolar Lavage (BAL)

Related Information

Bronchoscopy, Flexible *on page 209*

Procedure Commonly Includes Irrigation of a segment or subsegment of the lung through a bronchoscope followed by collection of the aspirate

(Continued)

Bronchoalveolar Lavage (BAL) *(Continued)*

Indications Assist in the diagnosis of both infectious and noninfectious diseases. For infectious diseases it is particularly useful for atypical and opportunistic infections. BAL may aid in diagnosing the following noninfectious diseases: pulmonary alveolar proteinosis, eosinophilic granulomatosis, malignancy, pulmonary hemorrhage, eosinophilic pneumonia, berylliosis, hypersensitivity pneumonitis, asbestosis, silicosis, sarcoidosis, idiopathic pulmonary fibrosis, and collagen vascular diseases.

Contraindications All are relative contraindications:

- uncooperative patient
- FEV_1 <800-1000 mL
- severe asthma
- hypoxemia uncorrected to an oxygen saturation >90% with supplemental oxygen
- bleeding diathesis
- arrhythmia
- unstable cardiac status
- recent myocardial infarction

Patient Preparation The patient should have no food or drink for 8 hours prior to the procedure (NPO after midnight for AM procedure; early light breakfast for PM procedure). Routine medications may be taken with a small amount of water. Premedication with a narcotic and/or benzodiazepine is given parenterally prior to the procedure. Atropine 0.4 mg I.M. may be given as a vagolytic agent to dry secretions unless contraindicated (ie, arrhythmia, narrow angle glaucoma, urinary retention). Supplemental oxygen is usually administered. The oropharynx is anesthetized with 2% lidocaine via a nebulizer or by gargling. The nares and nasopharynx are anesthetized with 2% lidocaine jelly if the bronchoscope is to be inserted via the nasal route.

Aftercare The patient should be NPO for at least 2 hours after the procedure (until the gag reflex has returned). Outpatients are not allowed to drive until the following day. Mild hemoptysis and fever may be noted for 24 hours.

Complications Hypoxemia, bronchospasm, minor bleeding, and pneumothorax (very rare)

Equipment Flexible bronchoscope with light source, sterile specimen cup, syringes with 20-50 mL sterile warmed normal saline, 3-way stopcock, a suction channel adaptor, syringes, lidocaine, and sedatives

Technique The bronchoscope is passed and the airways are anesthetized in the usual manner, without the use of suction. When focal infiltrates are present radiographically, the bronchoscope is advanced to the segmental bronchus that correlates with the infiltrate. If infiltrates are diffused, the lateral segment of the right middle lobe or the superior segment of the lingula is used as it provides the best fluid return. The bronchoscope is "wedged" into a segmental bronchus to completely occlude the lumen. 20-50 mL of sterile, warmed normal saline is slowly injected and then aspirated through the working channel. This is repeated until at least 40 mL total is obtained. The sample obtained is transferred to a sterile specimen cup. The figure shows a bronchoscopic view of subsegments through a wedged bronchoscope as lavage fluid is instilled.

Bronchoalveolar Lavage

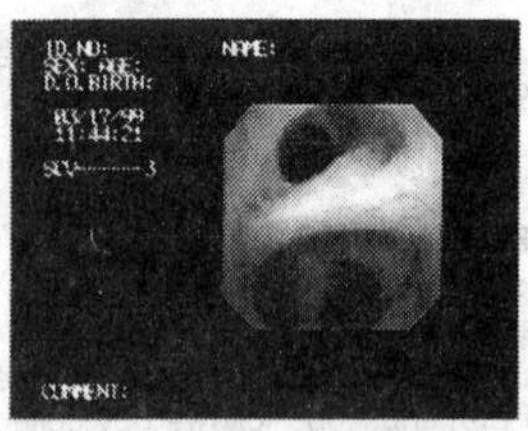

Data Acquired Differential cell count, microbiologic analysis, occasionally cytology and flow cytometry

Turnaround Time 24-48 hours for cell differential, cytology, PCP/fungal/mycobacterial stains, and bacterial culture; up to several weeks for AFB and fungal cultures.

Specimen Aspirated fluid

Container Sterile specimen cup

Collection Sterile, warmed saline is injected and then aspirated from a segmental bronchus through a bronchoscope.

Storage Instructions If delay in transport is more than 1 hour, the specimen should be refrigerated.

Causes for Rejection Invalid results if there are purulent airway secretions, "wedge" is not maintained, or poor fluid return (<40% of that injected)

Normal Findings No evidence of infection or malignancy; normal differential cell counts (approximately 92% macrophages, 7% lymphocytes, and <1% neutrophils, eosinophils, basophils, or mast cells)

Critical Values Differential cell counts vary in many of the diseases listed under Indications.

Limitations Current and recent antibiotic use decreases diagnostic yield of infectious diseases. Differential cell counts may be affected by smoking, chronic bronchitis, and active respiratory infection.

References

Djukanovic R, Dahl R, Jarjour N, et al, "Safety of Biopsies and Bronchoalveolar Lavage," *Eur Respir J Suppl*, 1998, 26:39S-41S.

Helmers RA and Hunninghake GW, "Bronchoalveolar Lavage," *Flexible Bronchoscopy*, Wang KP and Mehta AC, eds, Cambridge, MA: Blackwell Science, Inc, 1995, 160-94.

Kvale PA, "Bronchoscopic Biopsies and Bronchoalveolar Lavage," *Chest Surg Clin N Am*, 1996, 6(2):205-22.

Mares DC and Wilkes DS, "Bronchoscopy in the Diagnosis of Respiratory Infections," *Curr Opin Pulm Med*, 1998, 4(3):123-9.

Rennard SI, Aalbers R, Bleecker E, et al, "Bronchoalveolar Lavage: Performance, Sampling Procedure, Processing, and Assessment," *Eur Respir J Suppl*, 1998, 26:13S-5S.

♦ **Bronchoscopic Lung Biopsy** *see* Bronchoscopy, Endobronchial Biopsy *on page 207*

♦ **Bronchoscopic Lung Biopsy** *see* Bronchoscopy, Transbronchial Biopsy *on page 211*

Bronchoscopy, Endobronchial Biopsy

Related Information

Bronchoscopy, Flexible *on page 209*

Synonyms Bronchoscopic Lung Biopsy; Endobronchial Biopsy Bronchoscopy; Forceps Biopsy

Procedure Commonly Includes Passing biopsy forceps through the bronchoscope and sampling pieces of lung tissue from bronchoscopically visible lesions

Indications Aid in the diagnosis of endobronchial lesions, detected radiographically or on bronchoscopic exam, which are undiagnosed by history, physical exam, and less invasive tests.

Contraindications All are relative contraindications:

- uncooperative patient
- FEV_1 <800-1000 mL
- severe asthma
- hypoxemia uncorrected to an oxygen saturation >90% with supplemental oxygen
- bleeding diathesis
- arrhythmia
- unstable cardiac status
- recent myocardial infarction
- suggestion of a vascular malformation in the biopsy area

Patient Preparation The patient should be NPO for 8 hours prior to the procedure (NPO after midnight for AM procedure; early light breakfast for PM

(Continued)

Bronchoscopy, Endobronchial Biopsy *(Continued)*

procedure). Routine medications may be taken with a small amount of water. Normal coagulation studies and a platelet count >50,000/mm^3 should be documented. Premedication with a narcotic and/or benzodiazepine is given parenterally prior to the procedure. Atropine 0.4 mg I.M. may be given as a vagolytic agent to dry secretions unless contraindicated (eg, arrhythmia, narrow angle glaucoma, urinary retention). Supplemental oxygen is usually administered. The oropharynx is anesthetized with 2% lidocaine via a nebulizer or by gargling. The nares and nasopharynx are anesthetized with 2% lidocaine jelly if the bronchoscope is to be inserted via the nasal route.

Aftercare The patient should be NPO for at least 2 hours after the procedure (until the gag reflex has returned). Outpatients are not allowed to drive until the following day. Mild hemoptysis may be noted for 24 hours.

Complications Hypoxemia and bronchospasm; bleeding risks are increased in patients with coagulopathies, thrombocytopenia (<50,000), and uremia.

Equipment Flexible bronchoscope with light source, biopsy forceps - available as cup forceps (no teeth) or alligator forceps (with teeth) and in various sizes, specimen paper, container with fixative (eg, formalin or Hollande's solution), iced saline, topical epinephrine, syringes, lidocaine, and sedatives

Technique The bronchoscope is passed in the usual manner and directed towards the lesion. The biopsy forceps are inserted into the working channel of the bronchoscope and advanced until they extend beyond the distal tip of the scope. When possible, the scope is wedged in a segmental bronchus prior to the biopsy. The forceps are then opened and applied to the lesion under direct visualization. When as much tissue as possible is engaged the forceps are closed and withdrawn. The biopsy specimen is teased onto specimen paper and placed in a fixative. Although the optimal number of biopsies is not known, multiple pieces should be obtained. Topical epinephrine or iced saline can be useful to control bleeding. The figure shows a bronchoscopic view of biopsy forceps closed on an endobronchial lesion.

Endobronchial Biopsy

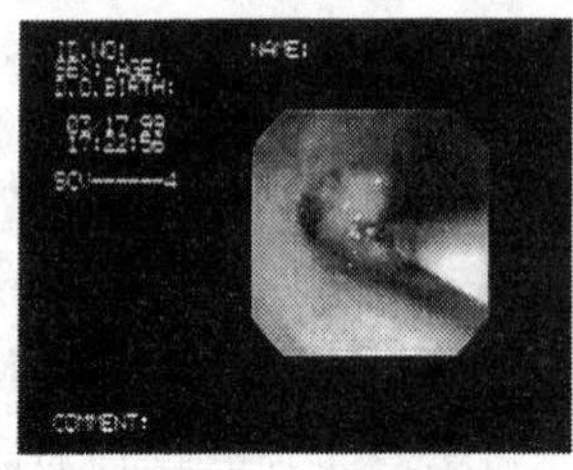

Data Acquired Tissue from endobronchial lesions for staining, histologic examination, and culture

Turnaround Time 24-48 hours; 3-4 days if special stains are performed

Specimen Tissue from endobronchial lesion

Container Jar containing a fixative (eg, formalin or Hollande's) for histologic studies and sterile saline for culture

Collection Tissues samples are obtained by forceps biopsy through a bronchoscope.

Storage Instructions Tissue is placed on specimen paper and submitted in a jar containing a fixative (eg, formalin or Hollande's).

Causes for Rejection Inadequate tissue sample

Normal Findings Normal endobronchial mucosa

Limitations Tissue obtained from the surface of a tumor may be necrotic making histologic exam difficult.

Additional Information The diagnostic yield from the combination of bronchial brush biopsy, bronchial washings, and endobronchial biopsy is >90%.

References

Gasparini S, "Bronchoscopic Biopsy Techniques in the Diagnosis and Staging of Lung Cancer," *Monaldi Arch Chest Dis*, 1997, 52(4):392-8.

Kvale PA, "Bronchoscopic Biopsies and Bronchoalveolar Lavage," *Chest Surg Clin N Am*, 1996, 6(2):205-22.

Robinson DS, Faurschou P, Barnes N, et al, "Biopsies: Bronchoscopic Technique and Sampling," *Eur Respir J Suppl*, 1998, 26:16S-9S.

Saetta M, Jeffery PK, Maestrelli P, et al, "Biopsies: Processing and Assessment," *Eur Respir J Suppl*, 1998, 26:20S-5S.

Shure D, "Transbronchial Biopsy and Needle Aspiration," *Chest*, 1989, 95(5):1130-8.

Bronchoscopy, Flexible

Related Information

Bronchial Brush Biopsy *on page 200*
Bronchial Washings *on page 204*
Bronchoalveolar Lavage (BAL) *on page 205*
Bronchoscopy, Endobronchial Biopsy *on page 207*
Transbronchial Needle Aspiration *on page 267*

Synonyms Fiberoptic Bronchoscopy; Flexible Bronchoscopy

Procedure Commonly Includes Direct visual examination of the upper airway, vocal cords, and tracheobronchial tree. Other procedures may be included (see Related Information) depending on the clinical indications.

Indications There are many diagnostic indications - the confirmation, diagnosis, and staging of bronchogenic and metastatic carcinoma; the assessment of recurrent/unresolved pneumonia, infiltrates in immunocompromised patients, and cavitary lesions; evaluation of interstitial lung diseases, hemoptysis, localized wheezing, stridor, foreign body aspiration, tracheobronchial stricture/stenosis, lung collapse, hoarseness, persistent pneumothorax; suspicion of fistula formation; evaluation postlung transplant, endotracheal intubation; and assessment of postop stump anastomosis.

Contraindications All are relative contraindications:

- uncooperative patient
- FEV_1 <800-1000 mL
- severe asthma
- hypoxemia uncorrected to an oxygen saturation >90% with supplemental oxygen
- bleeding diathesis
- arrhythmia
- unstable cardiac status
- recent myocardial infarction

Patient Preparation The patient should have no food or drink for 8 hours prior to the procedure (NPO after midnight for AM procedure; early light breakfast for PM procedure). Routine medications may be taken with a small amount of water. Premedication with a narcotic and/or benzodiazepine is given parenterally prior to the procedure. Atropine 0.4 mg I.M. may be given as a vagolytic agent to dry secretions unless contraindicated (ie, arrhythmia, narrow angle glaucoma, urinary retention). Supplemental oxygen is usually administered. The oropharynx is anesthetized with 2% lidocaine via a nebulizer or by gargling. The nares and nasopharynx are anesthetized with 2% lidocaine jelly if the bronchoscope is to be inserted via the nasal route.

Aftercare The patient should be NPO for at least 2 hours after the procedure (until the gag reflex has returned). Outpatients are not allowed to drive until the following day. Mild hemoptysis may be noted for 24 hours.

Complications Hypoxemia, bronchospasm, bleeding from the nares (if nasal approach used)

Equipment Flexible bronchoscope, halogen or xenon light source, suction catheter assembly, syringes with 2 mL of 2% lidocaine, and sedatives

Technique Once the patient is prepared (see Patient Preparation) and the bronchoscope tip is lubricated with lidocaine jelly, it is introduced transnasally or transorally (with the use of a bite block) with the patient in the sitting or supine position. The upper airway and vocal cords are thoroughly examined. 2% lidocaine solution is injected through the bronchoscope in 2 mL aliquots

(Continued)

Bronchoscopy, Flexible *(Continued)*

(40 mg per dose) to anesthetize the cords. The bronchoscope is then passed through the cords into the trachea. In the same manner, the tracheobronchial tree is anesthetized with 2% lidocaine (the total dosage should not exceed 400 mg). (If a procedure is to be performed to obtain a sample for microbiologic studies, sterile, methylparaben-free lidocaine is used to avoid the bacteriostatic properties of this preservative.) Once adequate anesthesia has been obtained, a detailed visual examination of the lower airways is performed. If bronchoalveolar lavage or protected catheter brushing is needed, this should occur immediately, prior to the use of suction. Subsequently washings, brush, and other biopsies can be taken as necessary. The figures show a bronchoscopic view of the vocal cords, a bronchoscopic view of the left upper and lower lobe bronchi from the left mainstem bronchus, and a bronchoscopic view of the right upper lobe bronchus and bronchus intermedius from the right mainstem bronchus.

Flexible Bronchoscopy

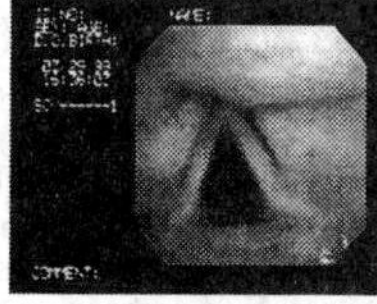

Figure 1

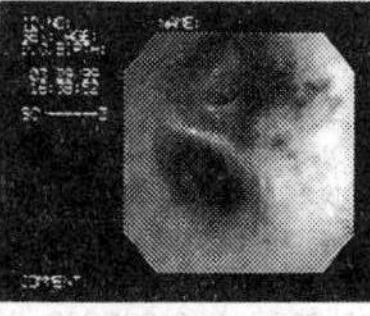

Figure 2

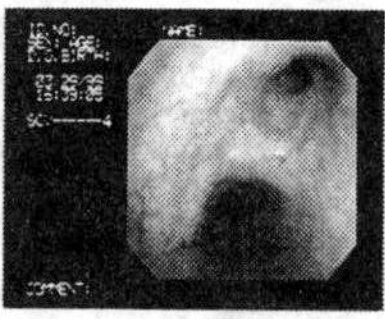

Figure 3

Data Acquired Information regarding the patency and normality of the airways; see entries dealing with procedures listed under Related Information.

Specimen Obtained only if a procedure listed under Related Information is performed (see these listings for further specimen-related information)

Normal Findings Normal endobronchial exam (normal mucosa, no lesions)

Limitations Can only visualize out to the fourth to sixth level bronchi

References

Ahmad M and Dweik RA, "Future of Flexible Bronchoscopy," *Clin Chest Med*, 1999, 20(1):1-17.

Borchers SD and Beamis JF Jr, "Flexible Bronchoscopy," *Chest Surg Clin N Am*, 1996, 6(2):169-92.

Fulkerson WJ, "Current Concepts. Fiberoptic Bronchoscopy," *N Engl J Med*, 1984, 311(8):511-5.

"Medical Investigations. 4:Bronchoscopy," *Br J Nurs*, 1997, 6(10):592-3.

Shennib H and Baslaim G, "Bronchoscopy in the Intensive Care Unit," *Chest Surg Clin N Am*, 1996, 6(2):349-61.

Van Gundy K and Boylen CT, "Fiberoptic Bronchoscopy. Indications, Complications, Contraindications," *Postgrad Med*, 1988, 83(1):289-94.

Bronchoscopy, Rigid

Related Information

Bronchoscopy, Flexible *on page 209*

Synonyms Open Tube Bronchoscope; Open Ventilating Bronchoscopy; Rigid Bronchoscopy

Procedure Commonly Includes Visual examination of trachea and bronchi plus or minus the use of therapeutic modalities under general anesthesia

Indications Current indications are largely therapeutic and often overlap with those of the flexible fiberoptic bronchoscope. These include control of massive hemoptysis, laser therapy, foreign body removal, dilation of tracheobronchial strictures, placement of endotracheal/bronchial stents, cryotherapy, electrocautery, and removal of mucous plugs, blood clots, or necrotic mucosa. Diagnostic modalities similar to those used through the flexible scope are available.

Contraindications

- inability to extend the neck or open the jaw
- typical contraindications to any general anesthesia procedure

All contraindications are relative if the procedure is required for life-threatening reasons.

Patient Preparation Although it is possible to perform rigid bronchoscopy under deep I.V. sedation, it is usually performed under general anesthesia. All preparation given to a surgical procedure applies.

Aftercare Routine postoperative care

Complications Bleeding, ventilatory insufficiency, painful mouth/throat

Equipment Anesthesia equipment, rigid bronchoscope, flexible bronchoscope, many accessories available depending on the indication of the procedure

Technique The procedure is done under general anesthesia with ventilation carried out using the side arm or high frequency jet ventilator. A dental guard is placed to protect the teeth. The neck is hyperextended ("sniff" position) and the lubricated scope is introduced into the trachea (with or without the use of a laryngoscope or previous endotracheal intubation). For visualization of the left bronchial tree, the bronchoscope is moved to the right side of the mouth with the head turned to the right. Although visualization of the right bronchial tree does not require a special position, the best view may be obtained by having the bronchoscope in the left corner of the mouth with the head turned to the left. A flexible bronchoscope and any of a variety of accessories are passed through rigid bronchoscope as needed.

Data Acquired Visual exam of the central airways

Specimen Cellular material, tissue samples, and secretions obtained by washings, brushings, and biopsy, if required

Normal Findings Normal endobronchial exam

Limitations Limited access to the distal and upper airways. Requires general anesthesia.

References

Beamis JF Jr, "Rigid Bronchoscopy," *Interventional Pulmonology*, Beamis JF Jr and Mathur PN, eds, New York, NY: McGraw-Hill Book Co, 1999, 17-28.

Helmers RA and Sanderson DR, "Rigid Bronchoscopy. The Forgotten Art," *Clin Chest Med*, 1995, 16(3):393-9.

Miller JI Jr, "Rigid Bronchoscopy," *Chest Surg Clin N Am*, 1996, 6(2):161-7.

Bronchoscopy, Transbronchial Biopsy

Related Information

Bronchoscopy, Flexible *on page 209*

Synonyms Bronchoscopic Lung Biopsy; Forceps Biopsy; Transbronchoscopic Biopsy Bronchoscopy

Procedure Commonly Includes Passing biopsy forceps through the bronchoscope and sampling pieces of lung tissue from areas of radiographic abnormality

Indications The radiographic presence of any diffuse or focal lung disease undiagnosed by history, physical, and less invasive studies

Contraindications All are relative contraindications:

- uncooperative patient
- FEV_1 <800-1000 mL
- severe asthma
- hypoxemia uncorrected to an oxygen saturation >90% with supplemental oxygen
- bleeding diathesis
- arrhythmia
- unstable cardiac status
- recent myocardial infarction
- radiographic suggestion of vascular malformation in biopsy area

Patient Preparation The patient should have no food or drink for 8 hours prior to the procedure (NPO after midnight for AM procedure; early light breakfast for PM procedure). Routine medications may be taken with a small amount of water. Normal coagulation studies and a platelet count >50,000/mm^3 should be documented. Premedication with a narcotic and/or benzodiazepine is given

(Continued)

Bronchoscopy, Transbronchial Biopsy *(Continued)*

parenterally prior to the procedure. Atropine 0.4 mg I.M. may be given as a vagolytic agent to dry secretions unless contraindicated (ie, arrhythmia, narrow angle glaucoma, urinary retention). Supplemental oxygen is usually administered. The oropharynx is anesthetized with 2% lidocaine via a nebulizer or by gargling. The nares and nasopharynx are anesthetized with 2% lidocaine jelly if the bronchoscope is to be inserted via the nasal route.

Aftercare The patient should be NPO for at least 2 hours after the procedure (until the gag reflex has returned). Outpatients are not allowed to drive until the following day. Mild hemoptysis may be noted for 24 hours.

Complications Hypoxemia and bronchospasm. The risks, of bleeding and pneumothorax are higher than with other bronchoscopic procedures. Bleeding risks are increased in patients with coagulopathies, thrombocytopenia (<50,000/mm^3), uremia, and pulmonary hypertension. The risks of pneumothorax are increased in patients with fibrotic lung disease, those who are coughing, and in those being mechanically ventilated.

Equipment Flexible bronchoscope with light source, biopsy forceps - available as cup forceps (no teeth) or alligator forceps (with teeth) and in various sizes, specimen paper, container with fixative (eg, formalin or Hollande's solution), fluoroscope, syringes, lidocaine, and sedatives

Technique The bronchoscope is passed and the airways are anesthetized in the usual manner. It is directed toward the segment or subsegment where the biopsy is to be taken. The biopsy forceps are inserted into the working channel of the bronchoscope and advanced into the respective segment until the lesion or specific area of the lung to be biopsied is encountered. This is generally performed under fluoroscopic guidance. The patient is then asked to take a deep breath and the forceps are opened. The patient is asked to exhale and the open jawed forceps are advanced (still under fluoroscopic guidance) until resistance is met. The forceps are closed and the patient is asked to indicate if he/she is experiencing pain. If pain is present, the forceps are opened and the procedure is repeated. If there is no pain, the closed jawed forceps are removed, thus obtaining a piece of tissue. Although the optimal number of biopsies is not known, multiple pieces should be obtained. The bronchoscope should remain wedged in the segment for up to 4 minutes to tamponade any potential bleeding. Suction should be used with caution or not at all. Topical epinephrine or iced saline can also be useful to control bleeding. At the end of the procedure, fluoroscopy can be used to check for pneumothorax. The figure shows a fluoroscopic image of open biopsy forceps in the area of a lung mass.

Transbronchial Biopsy

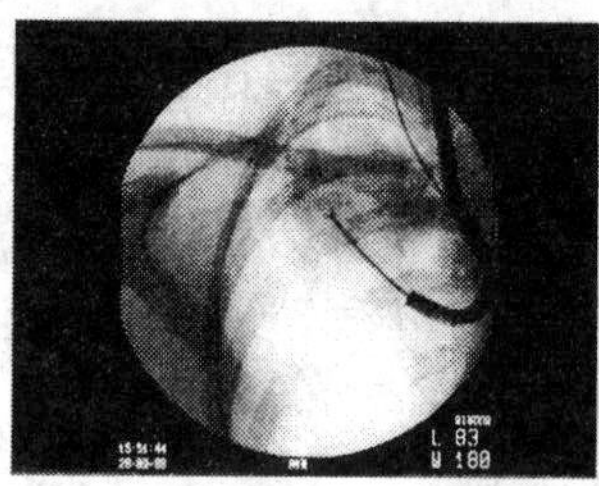

Data Acquired Lung tissue specimens for staining, histological examination, and culture

Turnaround Time 24-48 hours; 3-4 days if special stains are performed

Specimen Lung parenchymal tissue

Container Jaws containing a fixative (eg, formalin or Hollande's) for histologic studies and sterile saline for culture

Collection Tissue samples are obtained by forceps biopsy through a bronchoscope.

Storage Instructions Tissue is placed on specimen paper and placed in the above mentioned container. For culture, the container should be refrigerated if not immediately delivered to the laboratory.

Causes for Rejection Inadequate tissue sample

Normal Findings Normal pulmonary parenchyma

Limitations Due to sampling error and the small size of the samples obtained, the tissue may not reflect the entire pulmonary pathogenic process.

Additional Information The diagnostic yield from the combination of bronchial brush biopsy, bronchial washings, and transbronchial biopsy is >90%.

References

Gasparini S, "Bronchoscopic Biopsy Techniques in the Diagnosis and Staging of Lung Cancer," *Monaldi Arch Chest Dis*, 1997, 52(4):392-8.

Kvale PA, "Bronchoscopic Biopsies and Bronchoalveolar Lavage," *Chest Surg Clin N Am*, 1996, 6(2):205-22.

Robinson DS, Faurschou P, Barnes N, et al, "Biopsies: Bronchoscopic Technique and Sampling," *Eur Respir J Suppl*, 1998, 26:16S-9S.

Saetta M, Jeffery PK, Maestrelli P, et al, "Biopsies: Processing and Assessment," *Eur Respir J Suppl*, 1998, 26:20S-5S.

Shure D, "Transbronchial Biopsy and Needle Aspiration," *Chest*, 1989, 95(5):1130-8.

♦ **Calculated Arterial or Venous Oxygen Saturation** *see* Arterial Blood Oximetry *on page 195*

Carbon Dioxide Challenge Test

Synonyms CO_2 Response Test; Hypercapnic Challenge Test

Procedure Commonly Includes Minute ventilation ($\mathring{V}_E$) in liter$_{BTPS}$/minute, respiratory rate (RR) and tidal volume ($\mathring{V}_E$) at the start and end of the hypercapnic challenge slope of ventilation ($\mathring{V}_E$) plotted against end-tidal carbon dioxide concentration ($P_{ET}CO_2$) or $\mathring{V}_E/P_{ET}CO_2$. **Optional:** Mouth occlusion pressure at 100 msec after occlusion (P_{100}), slope of PO_{100} plotted against $P_{ET}CO_2$.

Indications Quantify the effect of increasing levels of carbon dioxide on the respiratory center of patients suspected of decreased ventilatory drive to carbon dioxide. Quantify the effects of therapeutic agents on respiratory chemosensitivity to carbon dioxide.

Patient Preparation Respiratory stimulants such as caffeine containing beverages (coffee, tea, cola), theophylline preparations, medroxyprogesterone, and protriptyline should be discontinued for at least 12 hours before testing unless the effects of these substances on ventilatory response to CO_2 is desired. Patients should empty their bladder just before testing.

Complications Inhalation of high levels of carbon dioxide during this test can cause generalized vasodilatation which sometimes causes flushing, diaphoresis, and headaches.

Equipment Rebuck describes the construction of a device using materials commonly available in hospitals[1]. The heart of this device is a bag in a box system used to allow the patient to rebreathe the test gas from the bag in the box while ventilation is measured at the other box opening. This unit is shown schematically in the figure on the following page.

Technique The 6-10 L anesthesia bag is filled with a volume equal to the patient's vital capacity plus 1 L of a gas mixture containing 7% CO_2 and 93% O_2. The 7% CO_2 is chosen to approximate average mixed venous concentrations of CO_2, and the 93% O_2 is chosen to eliminate concern for hypoxia during the test. After normal breathing followed by a full expiration, valves are turned that provide the anesthesia bag as a reservoir for ventilation during the test. Exhaled gases are returned to the bag. End-tidal CO_2 is monitored during the test. If occlusion pressures are desired, the inspiratory portion of the circuit is occluded by means of a Starling resistor at random intervals throughout the test. The output of a pressure transducer is then recorded on a high speed (at least 50 mm/second) recorder. The test continues until one of the following occurs:

(Continued)

Carbon Dioxide Challenge Test *(Continued)*

- 4 minutes have elapsed or
- the patient's end-tidal CO_2 concentration equals 9% or
- when the patient complains of dyspnea
- the first 30 seconds of rebreathing are excluded from data analysis.

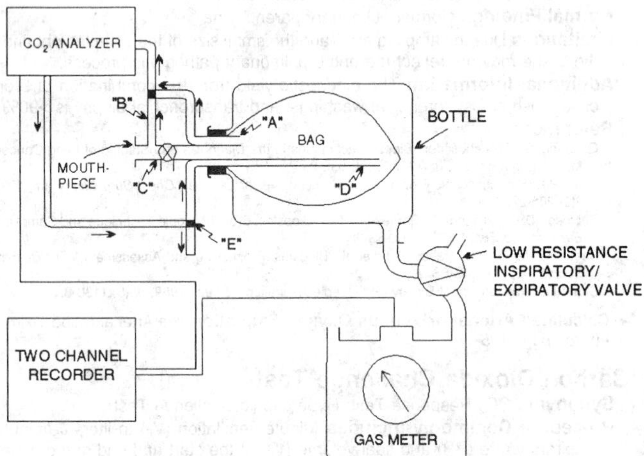

Circuit required for measuring the ventilatory response to CO_2 by rebreathing. The short thick arrows indicate the direction of gas flow to and from the CO_2 analyzer. Reprinted with permission from Rebuck AS, "Measurement of Ventilatory Response to CO_2 by Rebreathing," ***Chest*, 1976, 70(suppl): 118-21.**

Causes for Rejection Hypercapnic patients that exhibit pCO_2 values >55 mm Hg at rest do not usually provide sufficient sample to plot ventilatory response by the end of the test (63 mm Hg). Voluntary erratic breathing caused by malingering will yield misleading data.

Normal Findings In a study of 21 normals by Read, a mean slope of 2.65±1.21 L/minute/mm Hg was found.[2] The range was quite large; 1.16-6.18 L/minute/mm Hg. Similar values were found in a larger study by Irsliger.[3] He studied 126 adults and found a mean slope of 2.6±1.2 with a range of 0.47-6.22 L/minute/mm Hg. When interpreting ventilatory response tests, it is important to know if abnormal pulmonary mechanics (eg, emphysema) are present. This can help distinguish those who cannot breathe (limited by abnormalities in pulmonary mechanics) from those who will not breathe (abnormal sensitivity to carbon dioxide). The occlusion pressure measured at 100 msec is a relatively direct indicator of the output of the respiratory center to the diaphragm and is independent of airflow obstruction. Normal values for a normocapnic P_{100} is 2.6 cm H_2O (range 1.5-5). The occlusion pressure increased at a rate of approximately 0.5-6 cm H_2O for every mm increase in end-tidal CO_2.

Limitations A wide range of normal responses exists, making interpretation difficult.

Footnotes

1. Rebuck AS, "Measurement of Ventilatory Response to CO_2 by Rebreathing," *Chest*, 1976, 70(Suppl):118-21.
2. Read DJ, "A Clinical Method For Assessing the Ventilatory Response to Carbon Dioxide," *Aust Ann Med*, 1967, 16(1):20-32.
3. Irsliger GB, "Carbon Dioxide Response Lines in Young Adults: The Limits of the Normal Response," *Am Rev Respir Dis*, 1976, 114:529-36.

References

Biber B and Alkin T, "Panic Disorder Subtypes: Differential Responses to CO_2 Challenge," *Am J Psychiatry*, 1999, 156(5):739-44.

Hetzel A, Braune S, Guschlbauer B, et al, "CO_2 Reactivity Testing Without Blood Pressure Monitoring?" *Stroke*, 1999, 30(2):398-401.

Maresh CM, Armstrong LE, Kavouras SA, et al, "Physiological and Psychological Effects Associated With High Carbon Dioxide Levels in Healthy Men," *Aviat Space Environ Med*, 1997, 68(1):41-5

♦ **Carbon Monoxide Determination** *see* Arterial Blood Oximetry *on page 195*

Carbon Monoxide Diffusing Capacity, Single Breath

Synonyms DLCO; SB DLCO; Transfer Factor

Procedure Commonly Includes Diffusion capacity of the lung for carbon monoxide (DLCO) reported in mL CO_{STPD}/minute/mm Hg. Alveolar volume (VA), based on dilution of a vital capacity sized breath of test gas by the patient's residual volume, is reported in $liter_{BTPS}$. The "specific diffusing capacity" is the DLCO normalized to lung volume and is reported in mL CO_{STPD}/minute/mm Hg/$liter_{BTPS}$ VA.

Indications

- diagnose or following the course of interstitial lung disease, emphysema, sarcoidosis, pulmonary vascular disease, and intrapulmonary hemorrhage
- distinguish chronic bronchitis (normal DLCO) from emphysema (low DLCO) and interstitial from pleural fibrosis. The specific diffusing capacity (DL/VA) may be useful in separating patients with interstitial lung disease (low DLCO, low DL/VA) from patients with extrapulmonary restrictions such as obesity and diaphragm paralysis (low DLCO, normal or high DL/VA)
- elucidate operative cause of hypoxemia

Reduction of DLCO % of predicted value to <55% has been shown to be predictive of exercise arterial O_2 desaturation. A diffusing capacity ≤50% of predicted is considered to be a criterion for disability in interstitial lung disease.

Patient Preparation The patient should discontinue smoking for 24 hours pretest. Recent hemoglobin and carboxyhemoglobin are desired to allow for correction for high levels of carbon monoxide and high and low levels of hemoglobin. See Spirometry *on page 249.*

Aftercare None usually needed.

Equipment Test is performed on a device which contains a calibrated reservoir of test gas, a helium analyzer, a carbon monoxide analyzer, a timing circuit, an automatic or manually controlled five-way valve, a sample bag, and a sample pump. The testing unit should conform to standards put forth by the ATS. See the figures on the following page.

Turnaround Time Depends on institution, results are usually available on the same day. Interpreted report is usually available the next day.

Specimen Measurement of inspired volume, breath-holding time and inspired and expired concentrations of helium and carbon monoxide before and after respectively, approximately 10 seconds of breath-holding of a vital capacity sized breath of lung diffusion test gas (69% nitrogen, 21% oxygen, 10% helium and 0.3% carbon monoxide).

Collection Test gas is held in reservoir (usually a spirometer). The patient should be sitting. The patient exhales until reaching a maximum end-expiration (residual volume - RV) and then rapidly inspires from test gas reservoir until reaching full inspiration (total lung capacity). The patient exhales rapidly after 10 seconds of breath-holding. A fraction of the exhaled air (usually 750 mL) is allowed to escape to the atmosphere before an exhaled sample (500-1000 mL) is collected to account for anatomical dead space. When testing patients with a VC less than 2 L, reduce the discard volume before sample collection from 750 mL to 500 mL and note this on the report. Exhaled sample is analyzed for helium and carbon monoxide. Test is repeated after a minimum wait of 4 minutes until reproducibility of 5% or 3 mL/minute/mm Hg is achieved.

(Continued)

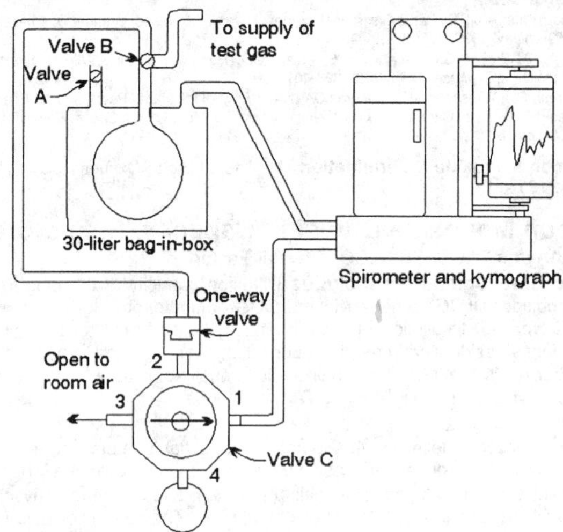

Suggested instrument set-up for single-breath DLCO measurement. Reproduced with permission from Clausen JL, *Pulmonary Function Testing Guidelines and Controversies: Equipment, Methods, and Normal Values*, New York, NY: Academic Press, 1982, 176.

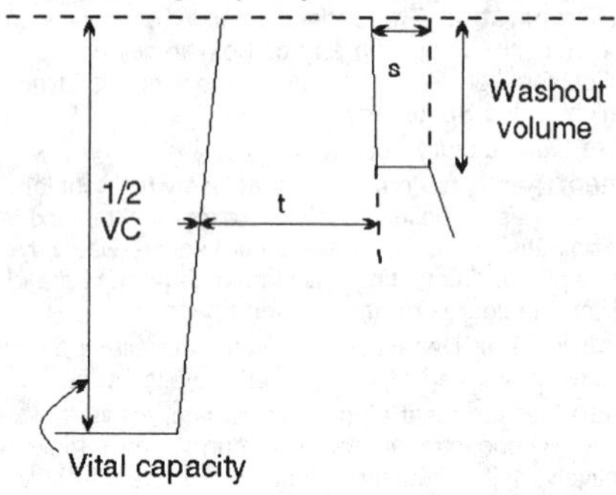

Determination of breath holding time (t) as recommended by Gaensler. The kymograph speed in this example is 160 mm/min or 32 mm/12 sec. The breath holding time is measured from the point of midinspiration (half of vital capacity) to the onset of alveolar gas collection. Washout and sample collection time is designated by (s). Reproduced with permission from Clausen JL, *Pulmonary Function Testing Guidelines and Controversies: Equipment, Methods, and Normal Values*, New York, NY: Academic Press, 1982, 179.

Causes for Rejection Inspiratory vital capacity <90% of the best previously measured vital capacity, breath-holding time <9 seconds or >11 seconds. Slow inspiration or expiration can affect results; inspiratory times should be <4 seconds in patients with obstructive lung disease or 2.5 seconds in the absence of airway obstruction. These represent conditions that fall below ATS standards for performance of a single breath diffusing capacity. They may represent the best performance obtained in spite of repeated efforts and should, therefore, **not** be discarded. They should be reported with a statement on the report which describes which specific standard was not met.

Normal Findings Many prediction equations exist. No one set of prediction equations can be recommended for all labs and patient populations. Appropriate normal regression equations should be chosen by comparing a group of 10 nonsmoking normals free of pulmonary disease with the prediction equation which is being used. Reference equations that result in more than 1 of 10 control subjects showing abnormal results should not be used. The measured DLCO should be corrected for abnormally low or high levels of hemoglobin and carboxyhemoglobin before comparison with predicted value. Values >80% of predicted or >95% confidence interval are considered normal. A **decreased** diffusing capacity is seen in emphysema, idiopathic pulmonary fibrosis, asbestosis, sarcoidosis, scleroderma lung disease, pneumonia, multiple pulmonary emboli, collagen vascular disease, histiocytosis-X, extrathoracic restrictive lung disease, and anemia. The DLCO may be corrected to alveolar volume (DL/VA) to assess nonparenchymal reduction in DLCO, but this practice is controversial and may be inappropriate. Adjustment of the measured DLCO for abnormally high or low levels of hemoglobin may be made. The equation for adjustment to a hemoglobin of 14.6 g/dL (appropriate for adolescent and adult male) is $DLCO_{Hgbadj}$ = (observed DLCO x (10.22 + Hgb)) / (1.7 x Hgb). The equation for the adjustment to a hemoglobin of 13.4 g/dL (appropriate for children younger than 15 years of age and adult female) is $DLCO_{Hgbadj}$ = (observed DLCO x (9.38 + Hgb)) / (1.7 x Hgb)

An **increased** diffusing capacity is seen in polycythemia, asthma, left-to-right shunts, exercise, supine position, intrapulmonary hemorrhage, and increased heart rates.

Limitations Measured values must be corrected for known abnormal hemoglobin and carboxyhemoglobin or methemoglobin values. Overinterpretation of a normal DL/VA in the presence of an abnormal DLCO may decrease the sensitivity of the DLCO to detect early interstitial lung disease.

References

Baylor P and Goebel P, "Clinical Correlates of an Elevated Diffusing Capacity for Carbon Monoxide Corrected for Alveolar Volume," *Am J Med Sci*, 1996, 311(6):266-71.

Borland C, Cox Y, and Higenbottam T, "Reduction of Pulmonary Capillary Blood Volume in Patients With Severe Unexplained Pulmonary Hypertension," *Thorax*, 1996, 51(8):855-6.

Crapo RO and Forster RE, "Carbon Monoxide Diffusing Capacity," *Clin Chest Med*, 1989, 10(2):187-98.

Ljubic S, Metelko Z, Car N, et al, "Reduction of Diffusion Capacity for Carbon Monoxide in Diabetic Patients," *Chest*, 1998, 114(4):1033-5.

Rosenberg E, "The 1995 Update of Recommendations for a Standard Technique for Measuring the Single-Breath Carbon Monoxide Diffusing Capacity," *Am J Respir Crit Care Med*, 1996, 154(3 Pt 1):827-8.

Stam H, Splinter TA, Versprille A, "Evaluation of Diffusing Capacity in Patients With a Restrictive Lung Disease," *Chest*, 2000, 117(3):752-7.

Viegi G, Paoletti P, Prediletto R, et al, "Carbon Monoxide Diffusing Capacity, Other Indices of Lung Function, and Respiratory Symptoms in a General Population Sample," *Am Rev Respir Dis*, 1990, 141(4 Pt 1):1033-9.

Welle I, Eide GE, Bakke P, et al, "Applicability of the Single-Breath Carbon Monoxide Diffusing Capacity in a Norwegian Community Study," *Am J Respir Crit Care Med*, 1998, 158(6):1745-50.

Cardiopulmonary Exercise Testing

Related Information

Cardiopulmonary Stress Test *on page 22*
Maximum Voluntary Ventilation (MVV) *on page 235*
Pulse Oximetry *on page 245*
Spirometry *on page 249*

Synonyms Incremental Exercise Testing

(Continued)

Cardiopulmonary Exercise Testing *(Continued)*

Applies to Disability Assessment; Disability Examination; Exercise Blood Gases; Exercise Oximetry

Procedure Commonly Includes Maximum workload achieved (reported in watts, kilopond meters (kpm), resting energy equivalents (METS), or maximum speed and grade achieved on treadmill), measured or calculated maximum oxygen uptake ($\mathring{V}O_{2max}$), ventilation measured at maximum exercise ($\mathring{V}_{E\ max}$), maximum carbon dioxide output ($\mathring{V}CO_{2max}$), respiratory exchange ratio (R), maximum oxygen pulse, maximum heart rate achieved (HR_{max}), tidal volume (VT), respiratory rate (frequency of breathing or f_b), calculated dead space to tidal volume ratio (VD/VT), oxygen saturation measured by pulse oximetry (O_2 sat %). When necessary, arterial blood gas samples may be obtained during exercise for disability purposes; see Arterial Blood Gases *on page 191*. Some centers obtain noninvasive cardiac output measurements during exercise by CO_2 rebreathing technique.

Indications

- rule out significant cardiopulmonary disease in the presence of normal static pulmonary function (spirometry, lung volumes, diffusion capacity, arterial blood gases)
- detect cardiopulmonary abnormalities when symptoms (generally dyspnea) are out of proportion to findings on tests of static function
- assess cardiopulmonary fitness in disability evaluations
- detect the presence of exercise-induced bronchoconstriction
- assess the presence of peripheral vascular disease
- detect coronary artery disease
- assess the presence of some neuromuscular diseases such as McArdle's syndrome (muscle phosphorylase deficiency)

Contraindications Absolute contraindications include: acute febrile illness, acute EG changes of myocardial ischemia, uncontrolled heart failure, pulmonary edema, unstable angina, acute myocarditis, uncontrolled hypertension (>250 mm Hg systolic, 120 mm Hg diastolic), uncontrolled asthma.

Relative contraindications include: recent (less than 4 weeks previous) myocardial infarction, aortic valve disease, resting tachycardia (heart rate >120 beats/minute), severe electrolyte disturbances, resting electrocardiographic abnormalities, poorly controlled diabetes, epilepsy, cerebrovascular disease, respiratory failure

Patient Preparation The patient should be instructed to wear loose, comfortable clothing and tennis shoes or other comfortable shoes. Heavy meals should be avoided for 2 hours prior to testing.

Aftercare The patient should be allowed to "cool down" gradually rather than allowing abrupt, complete cessation of work. Blood pressures should be taken immediately after reduction in workload and at least once a minute until stabilization at or near baseline value has been reached.

Equipment Volume measuring device (pneumotachometer), O_2 analyzer, CO_2 analyzer, mouthpiece and noseclips (or mask), EKG analyzer, ABG equipment (optional), pulse oximeter, sphygmomanometer, bicycle ergometer or treadmill. Ventilation exhaled or inhaled gas passes through a calibrated volume or flow measuring device (typically, a pneumotach for exhaled flows or a dry gasometer for inhaled volumes). Heart rate is measured by electrocardiogram. Oxygen saturation is measured by electrocardiography. Exhaled concentrations of oxygen and carbon dioxide are measured by calibrated oxygen and carbon dioxide analyzers. Signals from these measuring devices are typically sent to a waveform analyzer or computer for subsequent calculation of reported values. Some systems sample on a breath by breath mode while others will take an average sample representative of conditions during a given workload.

Technique Appropriate medical and medication history must be obtained (see Contraindications). The patient's barefoot height and weight should be measured. Pre-exercise spirometry including MVV should be obtained (see Spirometry *on page 249*). Electrocardiograph leads should be carefully placed at the appropriate sites after adequate skin preparation. Skin preparation includes shaving, if necessary, and rubbing with acetone and a nylon abrader. It may be necessary to secure the electrodes in place with a surgical net vest to avoid excessive noise associated with movement. Baseline electrocardiogram should be obtained. Peripheral circulation should be evaluated and the best site (finger, ear, bridge of nose) for placement of a pulse oximetry probe should be determined. Sphygmomanometer cuff should be taped in place and a baseline blood pressure recorded. The patient should be instructed in the operation of the treadmill or cycle ergometer and appropriate workload incrementations based on the patient's history of physical activity, dyspnea on exertion, spirometry and physical findings. Workload incrementations are designed to achieve patient exhaustion between 8-12 minutes. The mouthpiece/noseclips or mask should be applied. Resting measurements are obtained for 2-3 minutes (until stable). Three minutes of unloaded cycling generally precede application of resistance to ergometer. Thereafter, the workload is increased by the constant, predetermined increment. Incrementation of workload is estimated to yield 8-12 minutes of exercise and is based on the patient's history of activities which cause breathlessness and/or fatigue. This continues until the patient cannot continue because of exhaustion, or should not continue because of medical reasons (eg, hypotensive response, ischemic changes on EKG, severe cardiac arrhythmia, etc).

Turnaround Time Preliminary report is usually available on the same day, interpreted report is available in 1-2 days.

Causes for Rejection Inadequate effort will cause erroneously low values to be reported as maximum. In such cases, no obvious limitation will be seen. Some patients will voluntarily hyperventilate throughout the test, again causing erroneously low values for $\dot{V}O_2$ and workload. Because ventilation during exercise in this case is inappropriately high, it may appear that a ventilatory limitation is present, however, end-tidal CO_2 levels <35 mm Hg should indicate falsely high levels of ventilation.

Normal Findings Normal values for maximum oxygen uptake ($\dot{V}O_2$) usually indicate a normal study. Prediction equations are available. Normally, the heart rate will approach the age-related predicted maximum heart rate (220 - age) at the end of the study. Typically, there will be a ventilatory reserve of 30% to 35% in normals. Predicted maximum ventilation can be calculated by multiplying the FEV_1 by 35 or 40. Normally there is no desaturation associated with exercise. Calculated V_D/V_T generally shows a decline with progressive levels of exercise. A calculated V_D/V_T that remains stable or increases may be

Cardiopulmonary Exercise Test

	Units
Measured Parameters	
Minute ventilation ($\dot{V}E$)	LPM
Respiratory frequency (f_b)	breath/min
Tidal volume (V_T)	mL
Heart rate (HR)	beats/min
Blood pressure (SYS / DIAS)	mm Hg
Oxygen saturation	%
Calculated Parameters	
Oxygen uptake ($\dot{V}O_2$)	mL/min
Oxygen pulse ($\dot{V}O_2$ / HR)	mL/beat
CO_2 production ($\dot{V}CO_2$)	mL/min
Respiratory exchange ratio (R)	
Dead space to tidal volume ratio (V_D / V_T)	
Anaerobic threshold (AT)	mL $\dot{V}O_2$/min

(Continued)

Cardiopulmonary Exercise Testing *(Continued)*

indicative of pulmonary vascular disease. Calculated V_D/V_T values that substitute end-tidal CO_2 for arterial CO_2 values may give misleading results, particularly if obstructive lung disease is present.

Critical Values A maximum $\mathring{V}O_2$ <15 mL/kg (with good patient effort) is generally considered to indicate disability.

Limitations Proper evaluation of exercise performance requires that maximum patient effort be applied during the test. Malingering is possible and may be difficult to evaluate.

Additional Information Postheart or heart-lung transplant patient should be allowed a minimum of 3 minutes between increments in workload to allow for the denervated heart to adjust stroke volume and rate. Measurement of spirometry up to 30 minutes postexercise can aid in detection of exercise induced asthma. A 20% drop in FEV_1 postexercise is indicative of exercise-induced asthma.

Diagnostic Flow Chart for Stress Testing

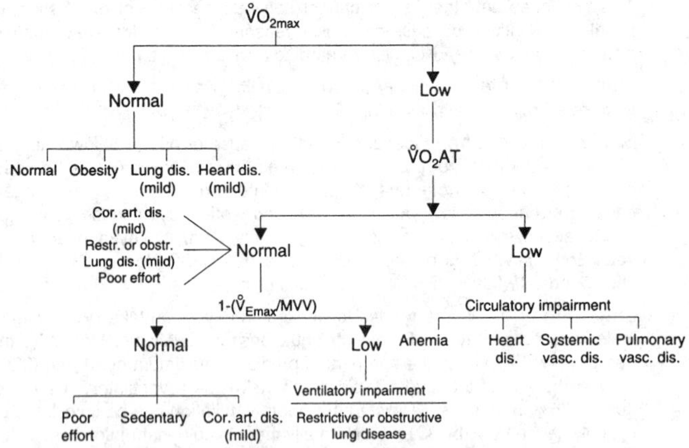

Wasserman's flow chart is especially helpful in the differential diagnosis of dyspnea. The vital relationship of the anaerobic threshold is clearly seen in this schema. The $\mathring{V}O_2$ AT is low if less than 40% of the subject's predicted $\mathring{V}O_{2max}$ and indicates circulatory impairment. The breathing reserve is low if 1-($\mathring{V}_{Emax}$/MVV) is less than 30%.

Printed with permission from Wasserman K, *Principles of Exercise Testing and Interpretation*, Philadelphia, PA: Lea & Febiger, 1987.

References

Bingisser R, Kaplan V, Scherer T, et al, "Effect on Training on Repeatability of Cardiopulmonary Exercise Performance in Normal Men and Women," *Med Sci Sports Exerc*, 1997, 29(11):1499-504.

"Cardiovascular Stress Testing: A Description of the Various Types of Stress Tests and Indications for Their Use," *Mayo Clin Proc*, 1996, 71(1):43-52.

Eschenbacher WL and Mannina A, "An Algorithm for the Interpretation of Cardiopulmonary Exercise Tests," *Chest*, 1990, 97(2):263-7.

Marburger CT, Brubaker PH, Pollock WE, et al, "Reproducibility of Cardiopulmonary Exercise Testing in Elderly Patients With Congestive Heart Failure," *Am J Cardiol*, 1998, 82(7):905-9.

McInnis KJ, Bader DS, Pierce GL, et al, "Comparison of Cardiopulmonary Responses in Obese Women Using Ramp Versus Step Treadmill Protocols," *Am J Cardiol*, 1999, 83(2):289-91, A7.

Metra M, Faggiano P, D'Aloia A, et al, "Use of Cardiopulmonary Exercise Testing With Hemodynamic Monitoring in the Prognostic Assessment of Ambulatory Patients With Chronic Heart Failure," *J Am Coll Cardiol*, 1999, 33(4):943-50.

Morales FJ, Martinez A, Mendez M, et al, "A Shuttle Walk Test for Assessment of Functional Capacity in Chronic Heart Failure," *Am Heart J*, 1999, 138(2 Pt 1):291-8.

Myers J, Gullestad L, Vagelos R, et al, "Clinical, Hemodynamic, and Cardiopulmonary Exercise Test Determinants of Survival in Patients Referred for Evaluation of Heart Failure," *Ann Intern Med*, 1998, 129(4):286-93.

Older P, Hall A, and Hader R, "Cardiopulmonary Exercise Testing as a Screening Test for Perioperative Management of Major Surgery in the Elderly," *Chest*, 1999, 116(2):355-62.

Osada N, Chaitman BR, Miller LW, et al, "Cardiopulmonary Exercise Testing Identifies low Risk Patients With Heart Failure and Severely Impaired Exercise Capacity Considered for Heart Transplantation," *J Am Coll Cardiol*, 1998, 31(3):577-82.

Cardiopulmonary Sleep Study

Related Information

Pulse Oximetry *on page 245*

Synonyms Polysomnography (PSG); Sleep Apnea Study; Sleep Oximetry; Sleep Study; Titration of Oxygen or Nasal CPAP During Sleep

Applies to Respiratory Inductive Plethysmography

Procedure Commonly Includes Sleep studies for the evaluation of cardiopulmonary sleep-related disorders commonly include assessment of the stages of sleep, respiratory airflow, respiratory effort, arterial oxygen saturation by ear oximeter or pulse oximetry, monitoring of body position and periodic leg movements, monitoring of the electrocardiogram.

Indications

- chronic obstructive pulmonary disease (COPD): patients with COPD whose PaO_2 is <55 mm Hg, patients with COPD whose PaO_2 is >55 mm Hg whose illness is complicated by pulmonary hypertension, right heart failure or polycythemia
- restrictive ventilatory disorders: patients with restrictive ventilatory impairment secondary to chest wall and neuromuscular disturbances whose illness is complicated by chronic hypoventilation, polycythemia, pulmonary hypertension, disturbed sleep, morning headaches, daytime somnolence, and fatigue
- disorders of respiratory control: patients with disturbances of respiratory control whose awake $PaCO_2$ is >45 mm Hg or whose illness is complicated by pulmonary hypertension, polycythemia, disturbed sleep, morning headaches, daytime somnolence, and fatigue
- symptoms arising from sleep apnea: patients with excessive daytime sleepiness or sleep maintenance insomnia
- cardiovascular manifestations of sleep apnea: patients with nocturnal cyclic bradyarrhythmias, nocturnal abnormalities of atrioventricular conduction, and ventricular ectopy during sleep that appears increased relative to wakefulness

Contraindications Although they do not represent contraindications, the following represent circumstances in which a cardiopulmonary sleep study is **not** indicated: patients with COPD whose awake PaO_2 is >55 mm Hg and are free of complications; patients with restrictive chest wall, neuromuscular or interstitial lung diseases who are not chronically hypoventilating and who are free of polycythemia, pulmonary hypertension, disturbed sleep, morning headaches or daytime somnolence and fatigue; patients that have the risk factors for sleep apnea of obesity and/or snoring but are free of any symptoms of sleep apnea; patients with systemic hypertension; patients with nocturnal nonspecific cardiac arrhythmias.[1]

Patient Preparation Patients scheduled for sleep studies should continue taking all medications as prescribed. Any medication which is scheduled to be taken before bedtime should be brought with them. Hair should be clean and free of hair care products such as mousse and hairspray.

Equipment Equipment varies with the complexity of the study. Studies may be categorized as simplified (screening) or complete cardiopulmonary sleep study. A full cardiopulmonary sleep study is one in which a full polysomnogram with EEG is performed in which the focus of the study is on cardiac and respiratory parameters. A simplified cardiopulmonary sleep study is one in which only cardiac and respiratory parameters are measured. The role of the simplified study in the diagnosis of sleep apnea has not been definitively established. The following equipment is used to measure the various physiological markers used in a cardiopulmonary sleep study.

(Continued)

Cardiopulmonary Sleep Study *(Continued)*

- Electroencephalogram (EEG): Electrodes are placed at the C3, C4, A1, and A2 positions (International 10-20 system).[2] Sleep staging is recorded using C3/A2; C4/A1 may be used as an alternative if technical difficulties are encountered.
- Electrooculogram (EOG): One electrode is placed on the outer canthus of each eye with the electrode on the right outer canthus being 1 cm above the horizontal and the electrode on the left being 1 cm below the horizontal.
- Electromyogram (EMG): **Chin muscles:** One electrode is applied at the center of the chin with two others beneath the chin (one of these is used as a back-up electrode). **Skeletal muscle EMG:** EMG of the anterior tibialis muscle will allow detection of periodic movements in sleep and assessment of body position.[3] **Respiration:** In a cardiopulmonary sleep study, it is important to measure both actual movement of airflow and the presence of respiratory effort in order to differentiate between obstructive and central sleep apneas. A large number of devices exist which generate either quantitative or semiquantitative assessment of respiratory activity. Semiquantitative techniques that will allow adequate differentiation of central and obstructive events may be used. To detect mouth or nasal airflow, various devices such as CO_2 analyzers, thermistors,[4] laryngeal and tracheal microphones[5,6,7] and impedance pneumography[8,9] have been used successfully. Quantitative techniques such as a pneumotachograph attached to a mask, magnetometers[10,11] and respiratory inductive plethysmography[12,13] have been used successfully. Respiratory inductive plethysmography systems may be used to qualitatively separate central from obstructive apneas. Esophageal balloon/catheter systems or pressure catheters have been used successfully to monitor respiratory effort.[14] **Oxygen saturation:** Ear oximeters and pulse oximeters have proved useful in documenting fluctuations of arterial oxygen saturation. Recent studies have shown that oximeters may underestimate or overestimate the oscillations in arterial oxygen saturation associated with apneic events.[15,16]

Technique The monitoring of the parameters listed may be done during a daytime nap or an overnight sleep study. A recent study concluded that afternoon nap studies may be inadequate for the evaluation of sleep-related breathing disorders.[17] Patients with severe daytime sleepiness and suspected obstructive sleep apnea are best suited for daytime studies because of the ease with which they fall asleep. A minimum of 2-4 hours of sleep should be obtained, including both REM and non-REM sleep and sleep in the supine position. If this is not done, the severity of sleep apnea may be underestimated. A therapeutic trial of nasal CPAP may be done in patients with severe, uncomplicated sleep apnea as a part of the diagnostic study night.

Data Acquired Sleep staging may be performed in fixed intervals (usually 30 seconds) using the criteria proposed by Rechtschaffen and Kales[18] or by other systems which modify the standard sleep scoring system for use in sleep apnea patients.[19] In addition to the scoring of the sleep state, the number of arousals during sleep and the frequency of occurrence of periodic movements in sleep should be tabulated. The total number of movements, the total number of movements associated with arousal or awakenings, and the movement index (number of movements/hour of sleep) should be calculated. Respiratory parameters reported include the number of apneic events and an apnea index (number of apneas/hour of sleep). Recent investigators suggest the reporting of a respiratory disturbance index (number of apneas plus the number of hypoapneas/hour of sleep). Various parameters have been reported using the oxygen saturation as measured by pulse or ear oximetry. Nadir values, mean oxygen saturation, mean oxygen saturation per sleep state, and the number of desaturations >4% have been used. Reporting the percentage of time spent below 90%, 80%, 70%, 60%, and 50% saturation are conveniently expressed by means of a cumulative oxygen saturation histogram plot.

Normal Findings Most investigators agree that the standard definition of apnea is a cessation of airflow for more than 10 seconds. Less agreement is found for the definition of hypoapneas. Proposed definitions include reduction in airflow as measured by thermistors,[20,21] reduction in ventilation measured by a calibrated respiratory inductive plethysmograph,[22] or the combination of reduction in airflow and reduction of oxygen saturation >4%.[23] Such definitions are weakened by the relatively imprecise methods used to measure ventilation. An apnea index <5 apneas/hour of sleep is normal in young to middle-aged adults. An apnea index >5 apneas/hour of sleep is abnormal in this population and confirms the diagnosis of sleep apnea.[24] The older population has a considerably higher incidence of this disorder if an apnea index of 5 is used as the cutoff for normal and abnormal. Therefore, standards for the elderly population need to be established.[25]

Critical Values Saturations measured by pulse oximetry <88% for prolonged periods may indicate the need for continuous and/or nocturnal oxygen therapy, nocturnal nasal continuous positive airway pressure (CPAP) or both.

Limitations Limitations of a cardiopulmonary sleep study are primarily associated with limitations of the methods used for measuring ventilation. Pneumotachography and a mask provide the most accurate method for measuring ventilation, but the use of this set-up is not tolerated well by most patients. Likewise, measurement of esophageal pressure is the best quantitative method for the assessment of respiratory efforts but this may also be poorly tolerated by many patients. Other methods for measuring ventilation (magnetometers, respiratory inductive plethysmography, etc) are at best semiquantitative. Measurements made by respiratory inductive plethysmography may be improved by the use of a body jerkin rather than separate thoracic and abdominal bands which have a tendency to move during sleep. Daytime nap studies may not adequately assess the severity of sleep apnea. If the results of a daytime study do not confirm a clinical suspicion of sleep apnea, an all night sleep study is indicated. A limited sleep study in which only cardiac and respiratory parameters are measured suffers the limitation of being unable to characterize the architecture of REM and non-REM sleep.

Additional Information The Association of Sleep Disorders Centers and the American College of Chest Physicians[1] recommend that sleep study reports contain the following:

- variables measured and methods used to make measurements
- sleep staging - the percentage of each sleep stage and the relationship to age-matched normals; the total sleep time, sleep efficiency, and sleep latency should be noted
- type(s) of respiratory patterns, as well as the total number, number per hour of sleep time, and range and mean duration of patterns, and relationship to sleep stage; the patterns should be defined
- relationship of body position to disordered breathing, if pertinent
- oxygen saturation - the awake baseline level; arterial oxygenation should be described in quantitative terms, using either a continuous saturation versus time technique or discrete intervals
- cardiac rate and rhythm should be described and the relationship of any abnormalities to other cardiopulmonary events noted.
- technician's comments
- interpretation

Footnotes

1. American Thoracic Society, "Indications and Standards for Cardiopulmonary Sleep Studies," *Am Rev Respir Dis*, 1989, 139(2):559-68.
2. Jasper HH, "The Ten Twenty Electrode System of the International Federation," *Electroencephalogr Clin Neurophysiol*, 1985, 10:371-5.
3. Coleman RM, "Periodic Movements in Sleep (Nocturnal Myoclonus) and Restless Legs Syndrome," *Sleeping and Waking Disorders: Indications and Techniques*, Guilleminault C, ed, Menlo Park, CA: Addison-Wesley Publishing Co, 265-95.
4. Fisher JG, Garza G, Flickinger R, et al, "An Alternate Method of Recording Airflow During Sleep," *Sleep*, 1980, 21(4):461-3.
5. Krumpe PE and Cummiskey JM, "Use of Laryngeal Sound Recordings to Monitor Apnea," *Am Rev Respir Dis*, 1980, 122(5):797-801.
6. Cummiskey J, Williams TC, Krumpe PE, et al, "The Detection and Quantification of Sleep Apnea by Tracheal Sound Recordings," *Am Rev Respir Dis*, 1982, 126(2):221-4.

(Continued)

Cardiopulmonary Sleep Study *(Continued)*

7. Peirick J and Shepard JW Jr, "Automated Apnea Detection by Computer: Analysis of Tracheal Breath Sounds," *Med Biol Eng Comput*, 1983, 21(5):632-5.
8. Baker LE and Geddes LA, "The Measurement of Respiratory Volumes in Animals and Man With Use of Electrical Impedance," *Ann N Y Acad Sci*, 1970, 170:667-88.
9. Larsen VH, Christensen PH, Oxhoj, et al, "Impedance Pneumography for Long-Term Monitoring of Respiration During Sleep in Adult Males," *Clin Physiol*, 1984, 4(4):333-42.
10. Mead J, Peterson N, Grimby G, et al, "Pulmonary Ventilation Measured From Body Surface Movements," *Science*, 1967, 156(780):1383-4.
11. Sharp JT, Druz WS, Foster JR, et al, "Use of the Respiratory Magnetometer in Diagnosis and Classification of Sleep Apnea," *Chest*, 1980, 77(3):350-3.
12. Sackner MA, ed, "Monitoring of Ventilation Without a Physical Connection to the Airway," *Diagnostic Techniques in Pulmonary Disease*, New York, NY: Marcel Dekker, 1980, 503-37.
13. Cohn MA, Roa AS, Broudy M, et al, "The Respiratory Inductive Plethysmograph: A New Noninvasive Monitor of Respiration," *Bull Eur Physiopathol Respir*, 1982, 18(4):643-58.
14. Sampson MG, Walsleben JA, Gujavarty KS, et al, "Effect of Esophageal Balloon on Sleep Structure," *Sleep Res*, 1984, 13:211 (abstract).
15. West P, George CF, and Kryger MH, "Dynamic *in vivo* Response Characteristics of Three Oximeters: Hewlett-Packard 47201A, Biox III, and Nellcor N-100," *Sleep*, 1987, 10(3):263-71.
16. Naifeh KH and Severinghaus JW, "How Accurate Are Pulse Oximeters to Profound Brief Hypoxia?" *Sleep Res*, 1987, 161:569 (abstract).
17. Silvestri R, Guilleminault C, Coleman R, et al, "Nocturnal Sleep Versus Daytime Nap Findings in Patients With Breathing Abnormalities During Sleep," *Sleep Res*, 1982, 11:174 (abstract).
18. Rechtschaffen A and Kales A, *A Manual of Standardized Terminology, Techniques and Scoring Systems for Sleep Stages of Human Subjects*, No 204, Washington, DC: National Institute of Health, 1968, 204.
19. Schmidt-Nowara WW, Sano J, and Appel D, "Stage T: A Scoring Modification for Breathing Disturbed Sleep," *Sleep Res*, 1983, 12:356 (abstract).
20. Bliwise D, Bliwise NG, Kraemer HC, et al, "Measurement Error in Visually Scored Electrophysiological Data: Respiration During Sleep," *J Neurosci Methods*, 1984, 12(1):49-56.
21. Catterall JR, Calverley PM, Shapiro CM, et al, "Breathing and Oxygenation During Sleep Are Similar in Normal Men and Normal Women," *Am Rev Respir Dis*, 1985, 132(1):86-8.
22. Bradley TD, Brown IG, Zamel N, et al, "Differences in Pharyngeal Properties Between Snorers With Predominantly Central Sleep Apnea and Those Without Sleep Apnea," *Am Rev Respir Dis*, 1987, 135(2):387-91.
23. Block AJ, Boysen PG, Wynne JW, et al, "Sleep Apnea, Hypoapnea, and Oxygen Desaturation in Normal Subjects: A Strong Male Predominance," *N Engl J Med*, 1979, 300(10):513-7.
24. Guilleminault C, van den Hoed J, and Mitler MM, "Clinical Overview of the Sleep Apnea Syndromes," *Sleep Apnea Syndromes*, Guilleminault C and Dement WC, eds, New York, NY: Alan R Liss, 1978, 1-12.
25. Berry DTR, Webb WB, and Block AJ, "Sleep Apnea Syndrome: A Critical Review of the Apnea Index as a Diagnostic Criterion," *Chest*, 1984, 86:529-31.

References

Ahmed Q, Chung-Park M, and Tomashefski JF Jr, "Cardiopulmonary Pathology in Patients With Sleep Apnea/Obesity Hypoventilation Syndrome," *Hum Pathol*, 1997, 28(3):264-9.

Gupta RM and Gay PC, "Perioperative Cardiopulmonary Evaluation and Management: Are We Ignoring Obstructive Sleep Apnea Syndrome?" *Chest*, 1999, 116(6):1843.

Kingshott RN, Vennelle M, Hoy CJ, et al, "Predictors of Improvements in Daytime Function Outcomes with CPAP Therapy," *Am J Respir Crit Care Med*, 2000, 161(3 Pt 1):866-71.

Newman AB, Enright PL, Manolio TA, et al, "Sleep Disturbance, Psychological Correlates, and Cardiovascular Disease in 5201 Adult: The Cardiovascular Health Study," *J Am Geriatr Soc*, 1997, 45(1):1-7.

Schoem SR, "Oral Appliances for the Treatment of Snoring and Obstructive Sleep Apnea," *Otolaryngol Head Neck Surg*, 2000, 122(2):259-62.

"Standards and Indications for Cardiopulmonary Sleep Studies in Children. American Thoracic Society," *Am J Respir Crit Care Med*, 1996, 153(2):866-78.

- **Chord Compliance** *see* Pulmonary Compliance (Dynamic) *on page 242*
- **Closed Pleural Biopsy** *see* Pleural Biopsy *on page 238*
- **Closing Capacity** *see* Single Breath Nitrogen Elimination *on page 248*
- **Closing Volume** *see* Single Breath Nitrogen Elimination *on page 248*
- **CO_2 Response Test** *see* Carbon Dioxide Challenge Test *on page 213*
- **Conductance** *see* Airway Resistance *on page 187*
- **Conventional Bilateral Bronchography Via a Nasotracheal Catheter** *see* Localized Bronchogram *on page 232*
- **Co-oximetry** *see* Arterial Blood Oximetry *on page 195*
- **CPAP Titration** *see* Pulse Oximetry *on page 245*
- **Density Dependent Spirometry** *see* Volume of Isoflow (V iso $\mathring{V}$) *on page 270*
- **Desaturation Oximetry** *see* Pulse Oximetry *on page 245*

- ♦ **Disability Assessment** *see* Cardiopulmonary Exercise Testing *on page 217*
- ♦ **Disability Examination** *see* Cardiopulmonary Exercise Testing *on page 217*
- ♦ **DLCO** *see* Carbon Monoxide Diffusing Capacity, Single Breath *on page 215*
- ♦ **Ear Oximetry** *see* Pulse Oximetry *on page 245*
- ♦ **Endobronchial Biopsy Bronchoscopy** *see* Bronchoscopy, Endobronchial Biopsy *on page 207*
- ♦ **Exercise ABG** *see* Pulse Oximetry *on page 245*
- ♦ **Exercise Blood Gases** *see* Cardiopulmonary Exercise Testing *on page 217*
- ♦ **Exercise Oximetry** *see* Cardiopulmonary Exercise Testing *on page 217*
- ♦ **Expiratory Reserve Volume** *see* Lung Subdivisions *on page 233*
- ♦ **Fiberoptic Bronchoscopy** *see* Bronchoscopy, Flexible *on page 209*
- ♦ **Finger Oximetry** *see* Pulse Oximetry *on page 245*
- ♦ **Flexible Bronchoscopy** *see* Bronchoscopy, Flexible *on page 209*
- ♦ **Flow Volume Curves** *see* Flow Volume Loop *on page 225*

Flow Volume Loop

Related Information

Bedside Spirometry *on page 197*
Bronchial Challenge Test *on page 202*
Spirometry *on page 249*
Spirometry Before and After Bronchodilators *on page 253*
Spirometry, Sitting and Supine *on page 256*

Synonyms Flow Volume Curves; Spirometry With Flow Volume Loop

Applies to Assessment of Pulmonary Disability; Preoperative Evaluation

Procedure Commonly Includes Forced expiratory vital capacity (FVC), forced inspiratory vital capacity (FIVC), expiratory flow rates at specific percentage of expired vital capacity (eg, $FEF_{25\%}$, $FEF_{50\%}$, $FEF_{75\%}$), inspiratory flow rates at specific percentage of FVC vital ($FIF_{25\%}$, $FIF_{50\%}$, $FIF_{75\%}$), peak flow rates during expiration and inspiration (PEFR, PIFR). Ratio of expiratory and inspiratory flow rates at 50% of vital capacity ($FEF_{50\%}/FIF_{50\%}$) expressed as a percent, and a graphic presentation of the maneuver showing expiratory and inspiratory flow plotted against volume.

Indications Detect upper airway obstructions

Patient Preparation The patient should avoid heavy meals 3 hours prior to testing. The patient should be conscious and able to follow simple instructions. The patient's height and weight should be measured without shoes. Loose comfortable clothing that does not restrict chest expansion should be worn. Smoking history including last cigarette smoked should be obtained. Current medications should be obtained with particular emphasis on bronchodilators and steroids.

Aftercare Usually none, although patients that complain of lightheadedness and dizziness should not be allowed to walk unobserved until recovery.

Equipment Exhaled and inhaled air is collected or passed through a volume or flow measuring device known as a spirometer. Spirometers should meet certain minimum standards defined by the American Thoracic Society (ATS)

Technique A spirometer is used to measure inspiratory and expiratory volumes and flows and record the time of sample collection during a maximal forced exhalation from total lung capacity (TLC) to residual volume (RV) followed by a maximal forced inhalation from RV to TLC. Flow is plotted against volume and instantaneous flows are measured at 25%, 50%, and 75% of exhaled forced vital capacity on both the inspiratory and expiratory limbs. Peak inspiratory and expiratory flows are measured. Reproducibility of the expiratory limb is accomplished using the same criteria as spirometry. Reproducibility of the inspiratory limb is best accomplished by superimposing or visually comparing repeated efforts. (See following figures.)

Test may be performed on adults in a seated or standing position. Children must be tested while seated. After applying a noseclip, the patient is instructed

(Continued)

to take a full inspiration (TLC), hold it briefly, then exhale through a mouthpiece into a spirometer as forcefully and completely as possible. When exhalation has been judged to be complete (patient reaches obvious plateau at RV or 15 seconds of exhalation has occurred), the patient is coached to inhale as forcefully and completely as possible until reaching TLC. Allowing the patient to recover between efforts, the test is repeated a minimum of three times until two reproducible efforts have been recorded. When possible, superimposition of repeated flow volume loops can aid in assessment of reproducibility of data.

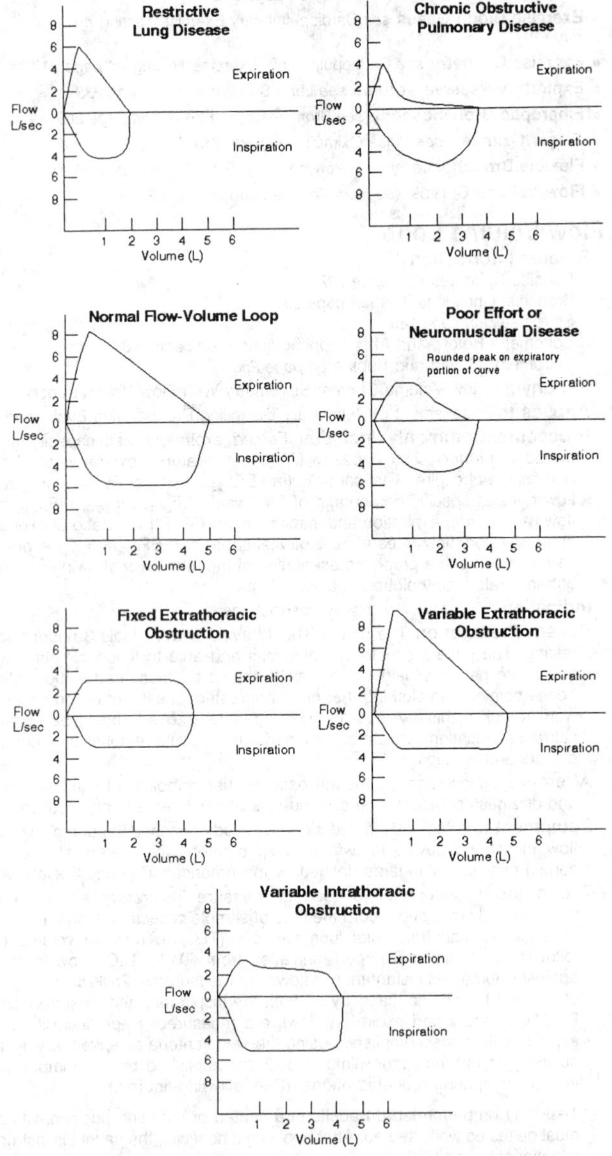

Turnaround Time Preliminary results should be available same day. Depending on the facility, an interpreted report may be available in 1-2 days.

Causes for Rejection The flow volume loop test consists of a forced expiratory maneuver followed by a forced inspiratory maneuver. In addition to the same causes for rejection for spirometry (see Causes for Rejection under Spirometry *on page 249*) poorly performed forced inspiration can limit the usefulness of graphic or numeric data obtained. Many patients perform a low flow stridorous inspiration while attempting to inhale forcefully after a forced exhalation. Have the patient keep an upright posture with an elevated chin to maximize tracheal diameter.

Normal Findings Studies of normal instantaneous inspiratory and expiratory flow rates have been reported by several authors.[1,2,3,4,5] The graphic presentation of the flow volume loop allows for inspection of the shape of the curve and its comparison with a normal loop. Three general types of upper airway obstructions (UAO) which show characteristic configurations are: fixed, variable extrathoracic, variable intrathoracic. These are described as follows.

Fixed UAO refers to the fixed nature of the obstruction with respect to inspiratory and expiratory effort. The expiratory flow plateaus at a high lung volume and peak flow is severely diminished. Inspiratory and expiratory flows are diminished proportional to the degree of obstruction. The inspiratory and expiratory loops may resemble each other quite closely. Causes include goiters, endotracheal neoplasms, stenosis of both main bronchi, postintubation stenosis, and performance of the test through a tracheostomy tube or other fixed orifice device. Estimation of the diameter of a stenotic lesion may be made from ratio of midinspiratory and midexpiratory flows $FIF_{50\%}/FEF_{50\%}$.[6] See the figure on the following page.

Variable extrathoracic lesions cause a reduction in flow rates seen during forced inspiration, the configuration of the expiratory limb of the flow volume loop remains normal (barring coexisting obstructive lung disease). Thus, the obstructive nature of the lesion varies with the phase of respiration. Inspiratory flows are decreased proportional to the degree of obstruction. Causes of variable extrathoracic UAO include unilateral and bilateral vocal cord paralysis, adhesions of the vocal cords, vocal cord constriction, laryngeal edema secondary to burns, and upper airway abnormalities associated with obstructive sleep apnea. See the figure on the following page.

Variable intrathoracic lesions are characterized by an early plateau of expiratory flow followed by a normal inspiratory flow volume curve. Rarely a small peak is seen preceding the expiratory flow plateau, mimicking the picture seen in severe chronic lower airways obstruction. The main cause of variable intrathoracic obstruction is localized noncircumferential tumors of the lower trachea or a mainstem bronchus. Variable intrathoracic obstruction patterns have also been described in polychondritis and tracheomalacis. See the figure on the following page.

The following illustration explains the physiology of variable upper airway obstructions. Figures 1a and 1b show a variable intrathoracic upper airway obstruction. During inspiration (1a) tracheal pressure is negative but greater than pleural pressure. This gradient favors an outward displacement of the tracheal wall. During expiration (1b), however, the driving pressure of expiration falls from pleural pressure at the alveolus along the entire pathway to the mouth. At some point along this path, airway or tracheal pressure falls to a value less than pleural pressure. This pressure gradient favors an inward displacement of airway walls, leading to airway narrowing or collapse. Figures 2a and 2b show a variable extrathoracic (above the manubrium of the sternum) upper airway obstruction. During inspiration (2a), tracheal pressures are less than atmospheric, favoring airway collapse. During expiration (2b), tracheal pressures exceed atmospheric pressures which favors an open airway.

(Continued)

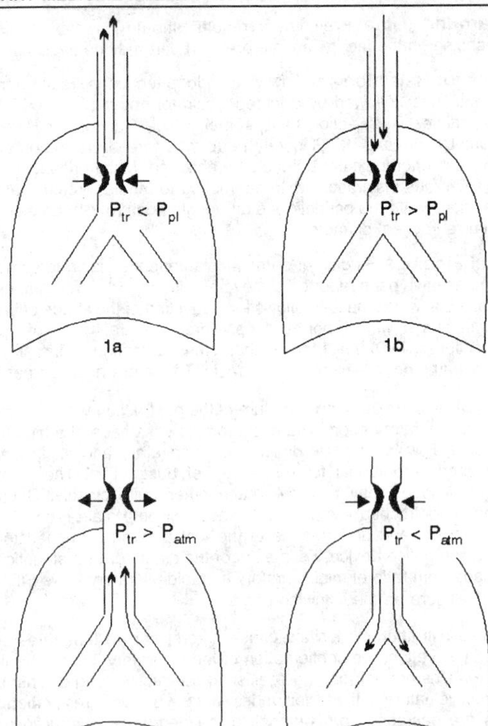

Limitations Requires patient cooperation. Poor effort on inspiration or partial glottis closure may mimic variable extrathoracic obstruction but can usually be distinguished by its lack of reproducibility. Upper airway cross sectional diameter must be reduced to 8 mm or less before the shape of the flow volume loop is affected, making the flow volume loop an unreliable method for **ruling out** clinically suspected UAO.

Additional Information Patients with obstructive sleep apnea may show a characteristic sawtoothing of either the expiratory limb, the inspiratory limb, or both.

Footnotes

1. Bass H, "The Flow Volume Loop: Normal Standards and Abnormalities in Chronic Obstructive Pulmonary Disease," *Chest*, 1973, 63(2):171-6.
2. Cherniack RM and Raber MB, "Normal Standards for Ventilatory Function Using an Automated Wedge Spirometer," *Am Rev Respir Dis*, 1972, 106:38-46.
3. Knudson RJ, Slatin RC, Lebowitz MD, et al, "The Maximal Expiratory Flow-Volume Curve: Normal Standards, Variability and Effects of Age," *Am Rev Respir Dis*, 1976, 113(5):587-600.
4. Schoenberg JB, Beck GJ, and Bouhuys A, "Growth and Decay of Pulmonary Function in Healthy Blacks and Whites," *Respir Physiol*, 1978, 33(3):367-93.
5. Jordanoglory J and Pride NB, "A Comparison of Maximum Inspiratory an Expiratory Flow in Health and in Lung Disease," *Thorax*, 1968, 23:38-45.
6. Gamsu G, Borson DB, Webb WR, et al, "Structure and Function in Tracheal Stenosis," *Am Rev Respir Dis*, 1980, 121(3):519-531.

References

Bollinger CT, "Usefulness of the Flow Volume Loop," *Chest*, 1998, 113(3):847-8.

Clarke DE, Green RJ, Mark JB, et al, "Upper Airway Obstruction Caused by Low-Grade Tracheal Papillary Adenocarcinoma: An Usual Flow-Volume Loop Pattern," *J Thorac Cardiovasc Surg*, 1996, 111(6):1286-8.

Gardner RM, Crapo RO, Nelson SB, "Spirometry and Flow-Volume Curves," *Clin Chest Med*, 1989, 10(2):145-54.

Gardner RM, Hankinson JL, Clausen JL, et al, "ATS Statement on Standardization of Spirometry - 1987 Update," *Am Rev Respir Dis*, 1987, 136:1285-98.

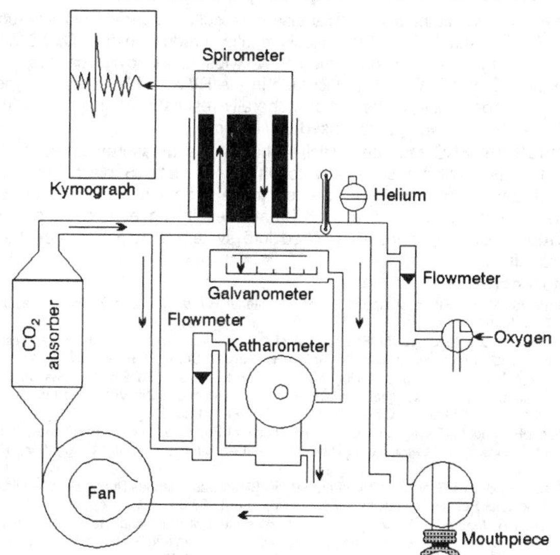

Apparatus for the measurement of FRC by helium dilution. The flowmeter, katharometer, and galvanometer together comprise the helium analyzer. The CO_2 absorber is usually combined with adessicant as well. Reproduced with permission from Cotes JE, *Lung Function*, Oxford, England: Blackwell Scientific Publications, 1979, 112.

Data Acquired Functional residual capacity (FRC) $liter_{BTPS}$, washout or equilibration time in minutes, average tidal volume (Vt) in mL, average respiratory rate (RR)

Turnaround Time Preliminary report is usually available on the same day, interpreted report is usually available the following day.

Causes for Rejection Variation on repeat studies of 500 mL or more, any obvious leaks during the procedure as evidenced (during a N_2 washout) by an increase in expired N_2 not related to a sigh, or (during a helium dilution) by a change in the end expiratory level and/or the amount of O_2 added to keep system volume constant. In a helium dilution test, the total amount of O_2 added to the circuit during the helium dilution test should average the patient's resting O_2 consumption (3.5 mL/kg/minute ±1 mL). Values may be higher in hypermetabolic states, those with significantly lower than ideal body weight, or in those with an increased work of breathing.

Normal Findings Many equations for the prediction of normal lung volumes exist and the range of predictive values is considerable. No one equation can be recommended to apply to all labs and patient populations. Each laboratory should test at least 10 normal individuals and compare their results to the normal values predicted by the equations they wish to use. If more than one individual is shown to be abnormal, those prediction equations may be unsuitable for use in that laboratory and prediction equations more suitable to their population should be sought. Values may be presented as percentage of predicted value or compared with the 95% confidence intervals as has been recently advocated. Alveolar filling diseases, lung resection, and pleural disease result in a decrease in VC, FRC, TLC, and RV. Interstitial lung disease results in a decreased VC and TLC with slightly less reduction in FRC and RV. Inspiratory neuromuscular dysfunction results in a decreased VC and TLC and a normal FRC and RV. Expiratory neuromuscular dysfunction results in a normal FRC and TLC and a reduction in VC with a proportional increase

(Continued)

Functional Residual Capacity *(Continued)*

in RV. Combined neuromuscular disease results in normal FRC with reduction of VC, RV, and TLC. Kyphoscoliosis results in reduction of FRC, VC, and TLC and slightly less reduction of the RV. Ankylosing spondylitis causes reduction in the VC and TLC and an increase in the RV and FRC (pseudohyperinflation). Chronic airway obstruction generally results in an increase in the RV, FRC, and TLC with an increased RV/TLC ratio.

Limitations FRC may be artificially high if the measurement is made at a higher lung volume secondary to pain or anxiety. Subject cooperation is necessary. Erroneous FRC can be made if patient has not established a stable end-expiratory level (4-6 breaths exhibiting end-tidal reproducibility <100 mL) or if patient is switched into system at a point other than end-expiration.

References

Drummond GB, "Effect of Apparatus on Functional Residual Capacity," *Br J Anaesth*, 1996, 76(4):560-2.

Kanengiser LC, Rapoport DM, Epstein H, et al, "Volume Adjustment of Mechanics and Diffusion in Interstitial Lung Disease. Lack of Clinical Relevance," *Chest*, 1989, 96(5):1036-42.

Numa AH, Hammer J, and Newth CJ, "Effect on Prone and Supine Positions on Functional Residual Capacity, Oxygenation, and Respiratory Mechanics in Ventilated Infants and Children," *Am J Respir Crit Care Med*, 1997, 156(4 Pt 1):1185-9.

Pelosi P, Croci M, Ravagnan I, et al, "The Effects of Body Mass on Lung Volumes, Respiratory Mechanics, and Gas Exchange During General Anesthesia," *Anesth Analg*, 1998, 87(3):654-60.

Sasse SA, Berry RB, Nguyen TK, et al, "Arterial Blood Gas Changes During Breath-Holding From Functional Residual Capacity," *Chest*, 1996, 110(4):958-64.

Wauer RR, Maurer T, Nowotny T, et al, "Assessment of Functional Residual Capacity Using Nitrogen Washout and Plethysmographic Techniques in Infants With and Without Bronchopulmonary Dysplasia," *Intensive Care Med*, 1998, 24(5):469-75.

Wrigge H, Sydow M, Zinserling J, et al, "Determination of Functional Residual Capacity (FRC) by Multibreath Nitrogen Washout in a Lung Model and in Mechanically Ventilated Patients. Accuracy Depends on Continuous Dynamic Compensation for Changes of Gas Sampling Delay Time," *Intensive Care Med*, 1998, 24(5):487-93.

♦ **Heliox Spirometry** *see* Volume of Isoflow (V iso $\mathring{V}$) *on page 270*

♦ **Helium Dilution** *see* Functional Residual Capacity *on page 229*

♦ **Hemoximetry** *see* Arterial Blood Oximetry *on page 195*

♦ **Histamine Challenge Test** *see* Bronchial Challenge Test *on page 202*

♦ **Hypercapnic Challenge Test** *see* Carbon Dioxide Challenge Test *on page 213*

♦ **Incremental Exercise Testing** *see* Cardiopulmonary Exercise Testing *on page 217*

♦ **Inspiratory Capacity** *see* Lung Subdivisions *on page 233*

♦ **Inspiratory Reserve Volume** *see* Lung Subdivisions *on page 233*

Localized Bronchogram

Synonyms Localized Bronchography

Replaces Conventional Bilateral Bronchography Via a Nasotracheal Catheter

Indications Document radiographically localized bronchiectasis in patients with recurrent pneumonias or chronic purulent sputum production

Contraindications Same as with bronchoscopy with addition of hypersensitivity to iodine-based dye

Patient Preparation NPO after midnight for a morning bronchoscopy and NPO after light breakfast for afternoon procedures. Routine medications (especially antiasthmatic drugs) may be taken at any time with a small amount of water. Routine lab work including clotting times, BUN, CBC, and platelet count is essential to exclude a coagulopathy - especially if a biopsy is to be performed. Some measure of pulmonary function is useful (spirometry, blood gases) to assess pulmonary reserve and document bronchospasm. Premedication with a narcotic (meperidine 25-75 mg) or minor tranquilizer (diazepam 10 mg) is given parenterally 15-30 minutes before the procedure. Atropine 0.4 mg I.M. is given as a vagolytic agent at the same time unless contraindicated by the presence of arrhythmia, narrow angle glaucoma, or urinary retention.

Aftercare Patients typically experience more coughing after a bronchogram. The patient is returned to floor or clinic for observation. Encourage cough and postural drainage for 1 hour. Nothing by mouth until gag reflex returns; to be determined by physician. Outpatient, NPO for 3 hours.

Special Instructions Procedure is done in fluoroscopy suite.

Complications Hypoxemia may be greater with bronchography than with other bronchoscopic procedures. Therefore, pulse oximetry should be monitored during the procedure, and the oxygen dose should be titrated accordingly.

Equipment 20 mL Dionisol iodine-based dye, bronchoscope

Technique The bronchoscope is inserted in the usual manner. The area of suspected bronchiectasis is either identified on chest x-ray or endobronchially. The bronchoscope is wedged in a lobar or segmental bronchus, or utilizing the bronchoscope, a separate catheter is placed. Dionisol (10-20 mL prewarmed) is rapidly injected through the bronchoscope channel or other tube and monitored fluoroscopically. Still pictures are taken as well.

Data Acquired Radiographs of contrast-filled bronchi in the area of suspected bronchiectasis

Normal Findings Normal endobronchial anatomy

Limitations Unlike complete bronchography, localized bronchoscopy does not show bronchial anatomy throughout the entire tracheobronchial tree, and therefore, if surgical resection is contemplated, an assessment of both lungs is recommended.

Additional Information Although uncommon today due to widespread use of antibiotics, bronchiectasis still occurs. Frequently the bronchiectasis results from endobronchial obstruction (right middle lobe syndrome). Bronchography can help document this disorder and thereby ensure proper treatment. Localized bronchography is tolerated better by the patient than the complete study.

References

Fennessy JJ, "Selective Catheterization of Segmental Bronchi With the Aid of a Flexible Fiberoptic Bronchoscope," *Radiology*, 1970, 95(3):689-91.

Flower CD and Shneerson JM, "Bronchography Via the Fiberoptic Bronchoscope," *Thorax*, 1984, 39(4):260-3.

Jenkins P, Dick R, and Clarke SW, "Selective Bronchography Using the Fiberoptic Bronchoscope," *Br J Dis Chest*, 1982, 76(1):88-90.

Saha SP, Mayo P, Long GA, et al, "Middle Lobe Syndrome: Diagnosis and Management," *Ann Thorac Surg*, 1982, 33(1):28-31.

Taber RE, "Bronchography After Bronchoscopy," *Ann Thorac Surg*, 1984, 37(3):264.

♦ **Localized Bronchography** *see* Localized Bronchogram *on page 232*

♦ **Low Density Gas Spirometry** *see* Volume of Isoflow (V iso $\mathring{V}$) *on page 270*

♦ **Lung Compartments** *see* Lung Subdivisions *on page 233*

Lung Subdivisions

Related Information

Functional Residual Capacity *on page 229*
Spirometry *on page 249*

Synonyms Expiratory Reserve Volume; Inspiratory Capacity; Inspiratory Reserve Volume; Lung Compartments; Static Lung Volumes

Procedure Commonly Includes Expiratory reserve volume (ERV), inspiratory capacity (IC), vital capacity (VC), or slow vital capacity (SVC)

Indications Assessment of severity of disease, diagnostic aid for classification of lung disease into restrictive, obstructive, and mixed disorders. Used with FRC measurement to calculate residual volume (RV), total lung capacity (TLC), and RV/TLC %. The effort which shows the largest vital capacity measurement following a **stable** end-expiratory level should be used for calculating expiratory reserve volume (ERV) and inspiratory capacity (IC). This ERV should be subtracted from the functional residual capacity (FRC) (see Functional Residual Capacity *on page 229*) to obtain a calculated residual volume (RV). The calculated RV is then added to the vital capacity (VC) to obtain a calculated total lung capacity (TLC). The RV is then divided by the TLC to obtain a calculated RV to TLC ratio.

Contraindications Patients who are unable to sit upright, maintain an airtight seal, or perform vital capacity maneuvers

(Continued)

Lung Subdivisions *(Continued)*

Patient Preparation The patient should avoid heavy meals 3 hours prior to testing. The patient should be conscious and able to follow simple instructions. The patient's height and weight should be measured without shoes. Loose comfortable clothing that does not restrict chest expansion should be worn. Smoking history including last cigarette smoked should be obtained. Current medications should be obtained with particular emphasis on bronchodilators and steroids.

Aftercare Usually none

Equipment Exhaled sample is collected or passed through a volume or flow measuring device known as a spirometer. Spirometers should meet certain minimum standards defined by the American Thoracic Society. Other equipment needed varies with the type of spirometer being used but should include a disposable mouthpiece and noseclips. Special circumstances may require adaptation of the mouthpiece to a mask, face seal, or tracheostomy adapters.

Technique The patient should be sitting erect, legs uncrossed, chin slightly elevated. Proper seal should be made with lips on mouthpiece. Noseclips should be applied. The patient should be instructed to relax and breathe in a normal relaxed fashion. An end-expiratory level that remains stable for approximately 10 seconds should be obtained before instructing the patient to inhale as deeply as possible and then exhale slowly and completely for as long as possible or until no volume increment is observed for at least 2 seconds. At this point, the patient should be instructed to return to normal breathing. This procedure is repeated at least in triplicate after visualizing a return to a stable end-expiratory level. Volume displacement spirometers should have a CO_2 absorbent canister, circulating fan, and supplemental O_2 source if repeat measurements without flushing the reservoir with room air are desired.

Turnaround Time Preliminary report is available on the day of the test, interpreted report is given in 1-2 days.

Specimen Inspired and expired volumes versus time are recorded during tidal breathing followed by a vital capacity maneuver.

Causes for Rejection Insufficient tidal breathing sample to determine an average resting end-expiratory level, excessive variation from resting end-expiratory level (variable FRC), poor patient effort, nonreproducibility of SVC and ERV

Normal Findings Numerous reference equations are available and show considerable variability. The following table shows an arbitrary assignment of severity of lung disease based on percentage of predicted value for FRC, TLC, and RV. Values below predicted are suggestive of restrictive lung disease, values above predicted are suggestive of hyperinflation. Conditions associated with increased lung volumes include obstructive lung diseases (asthma, emphysema, chronic bronchitis, bullous lung disease), acromegaly, ankylosing spondylitis. Isolated elevated RV is associated with expiratory muscle weakness and is seen in amyotrophic lateral sclerosis and C_5 spinal cord injuries. Conditions associated with decreased lung volumes include,

Degrees of Severity of Lung Disease Based on % of Predicted Lung Volume

Volume / Capacity	Mild (%)	Moderate (%)	Severe (%)
TLC	70-80	60-70	<60
	120-130	130-150	>150
FRC	55-65	45-55	<45
	135-150	150-200	>200
RV	55-65	45-55	<45
	135-150	150-250	>250

Ries AL and Clausen JL, "Lung Volumes," *Pulmonary Function Testing, Indications and Interpretations,* New York, NY: Grune & Stratton, Inc, 1985, 69-85.

among others, interstitial fibrosis, pleural fibrosis, lung resection, alveolar filling processes, congestive heart failure, thoracoplasty, ALS, and myasthenia gravis. A reduced ERV is commonly seen in obesity.

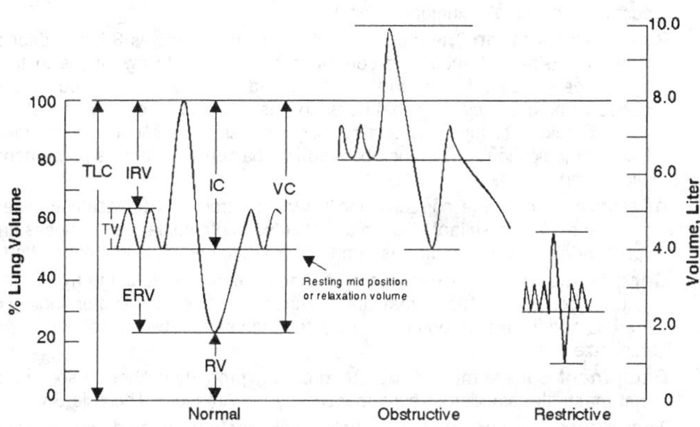

Schematic representation of the subdivisions of the lung in health and disease Each of the basic subdivisions is termed a volume, and combinations of volumes are termed a capacity. FRC, not designated in the figure, is the sum of RV and ERV. Reproduced with permission from Miller WF, *Laboratory Evaluation of Pulmonary Function*, Philadelphia, PA: J.B. Lippincott Co, 1987, 106.

Limitations The total picture of lung compartments can be obscured if the patient is breathing at a higher than normal end-expiratory level (secondary to incisional pain, chest wall pain, or anxiety) or breathing at a lower than normal end-expiratory level (active expiration secondary to anxiety during the measurement of FRC or ERV or both.) Full expiration must be made during the measurement of ERV or the RV will be artificially elevated. Vital capacity and expiratory reserve volume measurements should be duplicated to within 0.2 L reproducibility for the VC and 5% or 60 mL, whichever is larger, for the ERV.

References

Damia G, Mascheroni D, Croci M, et al, "Perioperative Changes in Functional Residual Capacity in Morbidly Obese Patients," *Br J Anaesth*, 1988, 60(5):574-8.

Dillard TA, Rajagopal KR, Slivka WA, et al, "Lung Function During Moderate Hypobaric Hypoxia in Normal Subjects and Patients With Chronic Obstructive Pulmonary Disease," *Aviat Space Environ Med*, 1998, 69(10):979-85.

Giodano A, Calcagni ML, Meduri G, et al, "Perfusion Lung Scintigraphy for the Prediction of Postlobectomy Residual Pulmonary Function," *Chest*, 1997, 111(6):1542-7.

♦ **Maximum Breathing Capacity (MBC)** *see* Maximum Voluntary Ventilation (MVV) *on page 235*

♦ **Maximum Expiratory Flow Rate** *see* Peak Flow *on page 237*

Maximum Voluntary Ventilation (MVV)

Related Information

Cardiopulmonary Exercise Testing *on page 217*
Spirometry *on page 249*

Synonyms Maximum Breathing Capacity (MBC); MBC; MVV

Procedure Commonly Includes Maximum voluntary ventilation (MVV) reported in liter$_{BTPS}$/minute, the mean respiratory rate used during the test and the total test time in seconds.

Indications As a nonspecific assessment of integrative function of the airways, lung parenchyma, thoracic cage, diaphragm and respiratory neuromuscular (Continued)

Maximum Voluntary Ventilation (MVV) *(Continued)*

apparatus; preoperative pulmonary evaluation; prediction of maximum ventilatory reserve for exercise testing; respiratory disability evaluation

Contraindications Patients that are unable to follow instructions or put forth a sustained maximal voluntary respiratory effort.

Patient Preparation The patient should avoid heavy meals 3 hours prior to testing. The patient should be conscious and able to follow simple instructions. The patient's height and weight should be measured without shoes. Loose comfortable clothing that does not restrict chest expansion should be worn. Smoking history including last cigarette smoked should be obtained. Current medications should be obtained with particular emphasis on bronchodilators and steroids.

Aftercare When done correctly, the MVV test produces an acute transient hypocapnia and resultant alkalemia. Patients often complain of dizziness and lightheadedness. Adequate rest, up to 5 minutes, should follow each effort.

Complications Lightheadedness or dizziness secondary to acute hyperventilation is common. Patients may also complain of numbness and/or tingling of the lips and fingers. Adequate rest (up to 5 minutes) between each effort will minimize this.

Equipment Sample may be measured on any properly calibrated spirometer that meets the standards recommended by the American Thoracic Society.

Technique Measurement of exhaled volumes (or inhaled and exhaled volumes) is made over a 10-15 second time increment and a count of the number of respirations during this time period is made. Patients are coached to breathe in and out with maximum respiratory effort with the goal of moving as much air in and out of their lungs during the 10- to 15-second collection time. Respiratory rates of 90-120 breaths/minute generally result in optimal performance. At least three measurements should be made until the two largest calculated MVVs are within 5% of each other. Generally a real time tracing of inspiratory and expiratory volume or accumulated expiratory volume alone is plotted against time.

Turnaround Time Preliminary results are usually available on the day of testing, interpreted results usually follow in 1-2 days.

Causes for Rejection Nonreproducibility of best two efforts (>5% variability). Respiratory rates <90 or >120 breaths/minute may result in less than optimal performance.

Normal Findings Several authors present reference equations for the prediction of a normal MVV. The MVV expressed as a percentage of predicted value may be used along with the standard spirometric measurements VC, FVC, and FEV_1 to grade functional impairment according to the table.

Maximum Voluntary Ventilation (MVV, LPM)

Severity of Impairment	% of Predicted
Mild	65-80
Moderate	50-64
Severe	35-49
Very severe	<35

Limitations The MVV is an extremely effort dependent test. Low values may merely reflect a lack of understanding or effort. Low values do not identify which component of the respiratory apparatus has a deficit. Many laboratories have abandoned the routine use of this test because of this limitation. Some find value in using the MVV to predict potential maximum ventilation during an incremental exercise test. Ventilatory reserve is calculated by subtracting the maximum minute ventilation measured during exercise from the MVV.

Additional Information In the absence of upper airway obstruction, the MVV may be predicted by multiplying the FEV_1 by 35 or 40 (the so-called "indirect MVV.")

References

Rafferty GF, Lou Harris M, Polkey MI, et al, "Effect on Hypercapnia on Maximal Voluntary Ventilation and Diaphragm Fatigue in Normal Humans," *Am J Respir Crit Care Med*, 1999, 160(5 Pt 1):1567-71.

Sahebjami H and Gartside PS, "Pulmonary Function in Obese Subjects With a Normal FEV1/FVC Ratio," *Chest*, 1996, 110(6):1425-9.

Suzuki J, Tanaka R, Yan S, et al, "Assessment of Abdominal Muscle Contractility, Strength, and Fatigue," *Am J Respir Crit Care Med*, 1999, 159(4 Pt 1):1052-60.

♦ **MBC** *see* Maximum Voluntary Ventilation (MVV) *on page 235*
♦ **Mecholyl Challenge** *see* Bronchial Challenge Test *on page 202*
♦ **Mecholyl Provocation Test** *see* Bronchial Challenge Test *on page 202*
♦ **Methacholine Challenge** *see* Bronchial Challenge Test *on page 202*
♦ **Methacholine Provocation Test** *see* Bronchial Challenge Test *on page 202*
♦ **MVV** *see* Maximum Voluntary Ventilation (MVV) *on page 235*
♦ **Nitrogen Washout** *see* Functional Residual Capacity *on page 229*
♦ **Open Tube Bronchoscope** *see* Bronchoscopy, Rigid *on page 210*
♦ **Open Ventilating Bronchoscopy** *see* Bronchoscopy, Rigid *on page 210*
♦ **Oxygen Titration Test** *see* Pulse Oximetry *on page 245*
♦ **P(A-a)O_2** *see* Alveolar to Arterial Oxygen Gradient *on page 188*
♦ **Peak Expiratory Flow** *see* Peak Flow *on page 237*

Peak Flow

Related Information

Spirometry *on page 249*

Synonyms Maximum Expiratory Flow Rate; Peak Expiratory Flow

Procedure Commonly Includes Peak expiratory flow rate is reported in either liter_{BTPS}/second or liters_{BTPS}/minute.

Indications The peak flow measurement is widely used epidemiologically and clinically to follow diurnal variations in airway tone. Peak flow diaries which plot measured peak flow against time of day have been used to investigate occupational asthma and to detect the onset of exacerbations of asthma before clinical symptoms appear. Many clinicians have asthma patients monitor PEF daily and adjust medications or seek medical attention when measured values fall below thresholds that represent percentages of values obtained when clinically stable. The extreme effort of dependence of this measurement diminish its usefulness in these situations. The peak expiratory flow rate has been shown to be one of the most sensitive spirometric indices to decreasing tracheal diameter.

Patient Preparation The patient should avoid heavy meals 3 hours prior to testing. The patient should be conscious and able to follow simple instructions. The patient's height and weight should be measured without shoes. Loose comfortable clothing that does not restrict chest expansion should be worn. Smoking history including last cigarette smoked should be obtained. Current medications history should be obtained with particular emphasis on bronchodilators and steroids.

Aftercare Usually none

Special Instructions Because of the portability and ease of use of the peak flow meter, peak expiratory flow is being used in epidemiology studies and the study of occupational asthma. Because of the effort dependence of this test, interpretation of unsupervised peak flow measurements recorded in a "patient diary" must be looked at with some degree of suspicion.

Technique The patient is asked to inhale to total lung capacity (TLC) and then the mouthpiece of the flow meter or spirometer is inserted in his mouth. Some devices allow mouthpiece to be in place before maximum inhalation. Mouthpiece should be inserted between the teeth or dentures and an airtight seal should be achieved with the lips. A strong, sharp burst of exhalation using maximum available force should be exhaled. Full exhalation is not necessary or desired unless other spirometric indices are being measured. The test is very effort dependent and active coaching is necessary. Peak flow measurements should be repeated until 10% reproducibility is achieved. Careful attention should be placed on orientation of peak meter during measurement. Most peak flow meters should be held horizontally level to measure accurately.

(Continued)

Peak Flow *(Continued)*

Turnaround Time Same day

Specimen The maximum flow rate during a forced expiration is measured by a spirometer or handheld peak flow meter (Wright peak flow meter).

Causes for Rejection Submaximal effort, submaximal inhalation before exhalation, lack of seal around mouthpiece, improper mouthpiece placement.

Normal Findings Numerous prediction equations are available.

Limitations The sensitivity of the peak flow is somewhat tempered by its extreme dependence on effort and lung volume. Malingering should always be considered when peak flow diaries are being used to document occupational asthma. Peak flow studies should be used as an adjunct to, not a replacement for, laboratory spirometry evaluations of airway function. Repeated use of home peak flow meters may render the devices inaccurate after extended use.

References

Boezen M, Schouten J, Rijcken B, et al, "Peak Expiratory Flow Variability, Bronchial Responsiveness, and Susceptibility to Ambient Air Pollution in Adults," *Am J Respir Crit Care Med*, 1998, 158(6):1848-54.

Chan-Yeung M, Chang JH, Manfreda J, et al, "Changes in Peak Flow, Symptom Score, and the Use of Medications During Acute Exacerbations of Asthma," *Am J Respir Crit Care Med*, 1996, 154(4 Pt 1):889-93.

Cote J, Cartier A, Malo JL, et al, "Compliance With Peak Expiratory Flow Monitoring in Home Management of Asthma," *Chest*, 1998, 113(4):968-72.

Doi S, Murayama N, Inoue T, et al, "CD4 T-lymphocyte Activation Is Associated With Peak Expiratory Flow Variability in Childhood Asthma," *J Allergy Clin Immunol*, 1996, 97(4):955-62.

Johns DP, Side E, Kendrick AH, et al, "The Effect of Physiologic and Mechanical Aging on the Performance of Peak Flowmeters," *Chest*, 1998, 113(3):774-9.

Klaustermeyer WB, Kurohara M, and Guerra GA, "Predictive Value of Monitoring Expiratory Peak Flow Rates in Hospitalized Adult Asthma Patients," *Ann Allergy*, 1990, 64(3):281-4.

Leroyer C, Perfetti L, Trudeau C, et al, "Comparison of Serial Monitoring of Peak Expiratory Flow and FEV1 in the Diagnosis of Occupational Asthma," *Am J Respir Crit Care Med*, 1998, 158(3):827-32.

Miller MR, Pedersen OF, and Quanjer PH, "The Rise and Dwell Time for Peak Expiratory Flow in Patients With and Without Airflow Limitation," *Am J Respir Crit Care Med*, 1998, 158(1):23-7.

Nathan RA, Minkwitz MC, and Bonuccelli CM, "Two First-Line Therapies in the Treatment of Mild Asthma: Use of Peak Flow Variability as a Predictor of Effectiveness," *Ann Allergy Asthma Immunol*, 1999, 82(5):497-503.

Pedersen OF, Brackel HJ, Bogaard JM, et al, "Wave-Speed-Determined Flow Limitation at Peak Flow in Normal and Asthmatic Subjects," *J Appl Physiol*, 1997, 83(5):1721-32.

Strayhorn V, Leeper K, Tolley E, et al, "Elevation of Peak Expiratory Flow by a "Spitting" Maneuver: Measured With Five Peak Flowmeters," *Chest*, 1998, 113(4):1134-6.

Tzelepis GE, Zakynthinos S, Vassilakopoulos T, et al, "Inspiratory Maneuver Effects on Peak Expiratory Flow. Role of Lung Elastic Recoil and Expiratory Pressure," *Am J Respir Crit Care Med*, 1997, 156(5):1399-404.

Pleural Biopsy

Related Information

Swan-Ganz Catheterization *on page 258*

Thoracentesis *on page 263*

Synonyms Closed Pleural Biopsy

Procedure Commonly Includes Percutaneous needle biopsy of the pleura under local anesthesia, often performed in conjunction with thoracentesis. A blunt-tipped Cope or Abrams needle is advanced through an intercostal space and several specimens of parietal pleura are obtained. Biopsy samples are sent for histologic and microbiologic analysis, along with pleural fluid. Pleural biopsy has its greatest applicability in the diagnosis of malignant neoplasms involving the pleura and tuberculous pleural effusions.

Indications Pleural biopsy is most useful in the following clinical situations:

- pleural effusion of unclear etiology when a prior thoracentesis has failed to establish a diagnosis
- suspected malignant pleural effusion (eg, bronchogenic carcinoma, breast cancer with pleuropulmonary metastases, mesothelioma, lymphoma, and others)
- Suspected tuberculous pleural effusions; the diagnostic yield from thoracentesis alone is low in pleural infections caused by *Mycobacterium tuberculosis*. This procedure allows direct culture of pleural samples for *M. tuberculosis*, as well as pathologic analysis for caseating granulomas.

Contraindications

- severe, uncorrectable coagulopathy
- platelet count <50,000/mm^3 (in many cases may be temporarily corrected with platelet transfusion)
- inadequate volume of pleural effusion, usually determined radiographically. To perform a pleural biopsy safely, pleural fluid should be present in a large enough volume to physically separate the lung parenchyma from the pleura. The risk of pneumothorax and lung laceration increases with smaller volumes of pleural fluid.
- mechanical ventilation
- emphysema
- infection at the puncture site

Patient Preparation The technique and risks of the procedure are explained to the patient and informed consent is obtained. Pleural biopsy may be safely performed as an outpatient and hospitalization postprocedure is not required in most cases. The patients should be referred to a chest physician. Details regarding procedure scheduling are generally handled by the subspecialist performing the biopsy. In all cases, a recent PA and lateral chest x-ray must be performed and should be readily available for physician review. Decubitus chest radiographs are frequently performed before thoracentesis and pleural biopsy to determine the size of the effusion, degree of fluid loculation, and presence of an underlying lung infiltrate. If coagulopathy is suspected, complete blood count (CBC) and clotting parameters (prothrombin time, partial thromboplastin time) should be drawn and the results are placed on the chart without delay. Bleeding time measurement is optional and not usually necessary. Other studies may be necessary prior to the procedure, at physician discretion (arterial blood gas, pulse oximetry, etc). If a thoracentesis is performed simultaneously with pleural biopsy, the same considerations apply as outlined previously (see Thoracentesis *on page 263*).

Aftercare Following pleural biopsy a "stat" chest x-ray is routinely performed to rule out iatrogenic pneumothorax. Often this film is taken with the patient at end-expiration (ie, an expiratory radiograph) to accentuate a small pneumothorax. Vital signs are usually obtained frequently postbiopsy, depending in part on the patient's baseline cardiopulmonary condition. For example, pulse and blood pressure may be obtained four times at 30-minute intervals for the first 2 hours and then every hour for 4 hours followed by routine measurement. If a large volume of pleural fluid is also removed, some pulmonologists recommend low flow (1-2 L/minute) supplemental oxygen by nasal cannula, but this is probably optional.

Special Instructions If performed in an outpatient setting, patient should contact a physician immediately if dyspnea or severe chest pain should develop after discharge.

Complications

- pneumothorax; probably the single most common adverse outcome. Risk increases with smaller pleural effusions. Pneumothorax is a relatively common complication but is often negligible and only observed with serial chest x-rays. Tension pneumothorax requiring immediate tube thoracostomy has been reported but is unusual.
- hemothorax; secondary to laceration of intercostal vessels. May be potentially life-threatening. Standard biopsy techniques are designed to minimize risk (ie, no pleural samples taken at the "12 o'clock" position when in the intercostal space).
- lung perforation
- vasovagal reactions
- local infection at the needle entrance site (rare)
- implantation of malignant cells along the needle entrance tract with the lung parenchyma (rare, but reported)
- local pain

Equipment The two most popular biopsy needles are the Cope and Abrams needle although others are available. Both needles are blunt-tipped and wide-bore, with an outer trocar, inner cannula, and central stylet. The Abrams needle has a special hook on the outer trocar to grip and cut the pleura. The Cope needle has a similar sharp biopsy chamber in an inner trocar. Pleural

(Continued)

Pleural Biopsy *(Continued)*

fluid can be withdrawn using either needle. The efficacy and safety of both Abrams and Cope needles are similar. Standard thoracentesis equipment is also required.

Technique In most hospitals, pleural biopsies are performed exclusively by pulmonologists or thoracic surgeons, despite it being a "bedside" procedure. Unlike conventional thoracentesis, a procedure commonly performed by internists and resident house staff, pleural biopsy has remained a subspecialty technique. The patient is placed in a comfortable sitting position (as with conventional thoracentesis). The margins of the pleural effusion are located by the physician using physical examination techniques. The appropriate intercostal space is located and the area cleaned with povidone-iodine in a standard sterile fashion. One percent lidocaine is used for cutaneous anesthesia following the sterile prep. Superficial skin incision is made using a scalpel to facilitate needle entry. The Cope or Abrams needle is advanced through the skin incision between ribs and into the pleural space. Pleural fluid may be withdrawn at this time to confirm proper needle positioning and for diagnostic purposes. Following this, the needle is withdrawn slightly until the parietal pleura is engaged. Several passes are made into the pleura using the sharp cutting edge (usually at the 3, 6, and 9 o'clock positions). Once adequate pleural samples have been collected, the remainder of the pleural fluid may be evacuated. The needle is then removed.

Data Acquired In most cases, pleural specimens are sent for:

- acid-fast stain (ie, for *M. tuberculosis*)
- culture for acid-fast bacilli (AFB)
- pathologic analysis; routine light microscopy, H & E stain, silver stain, AFB stain, etc

Less commonly:

- routine Gram's stain, culture and sensitivity
- fungal culture

Specimen Fresh specimens of parietal pleura and any pleural fluid collected separately. Biopsy specimens are usually sent to both the Microbiology and Pathology Laboratories. As with other fresh biopsy specimens, pleural specimens should be hand-carried immediately to the Microbiology Laboratory in a sterile container, with or without sterile saline. No formalin should be added to samples bound for culture. Samples sent to the Pathology Laboratory may be either fresh or placed in fixative (such as formalin).

Normal Findings Normal parietal pleura by microscopy and special staining along with negative results of routine and AFB cultures. Microscopy findings are reported by Pathology Department; culture results per Microbiology Laboratory.

Critical Values Abnormalities as reported. In many cases, the diagnosis of primary bronchogenic or metastatic carcinoma may be established using standard histologic technique. In addition, the finding of caseating granulomas (with or without a positive AFB culture) is suggestive of infection with *M. tuberculosis*.

Limitations Although pleural biopsy is quite specific for both malignancy and tuberculosis, the sensitivity is more limited. The histologic finding of "nonspecific pleural inflammation" is very common, approaching 50% to 70% of biopsies in the published literature. Such a finding may prompt a repeat pleural biopsy since up to 25% of patients with nonspecific inflammatory biopsies may develop malignancy.

Footnotes

1. "Diagnostic Thoracentesis and Pleural Biopsy in Pleural Effusions. Health and Public Policy Committee, American College of Physicians," *Ann Intern Med*, 1985, 103(5):799-802.

References

Chretien J and Danel CJ, "Needle Pleural Biopsy," *The Pleura in Health and Disease*, Chretien J, Bignon J, and Hirsch A, eds, 1985, New York, NY: Marcel Dekker, Inc, 631-42.

Cugell DW, "Thoracentesis and Pleural Biopsy," *Chest Surg Clin N Am*, 1992, 2(3):649-57.

Escudero BC, Garcia CM, Cuesta CB, et al, "Cytologic and Bacteriologic Analysis of Fluid and Pleural Biopsy Specimens With Cope's Needle," *Arch Intern Med*, 1990, 150(6):1190-4.

Kiinasewitz GT and Fishman AP, "Pleural Dynamics and Effusions," *Pulmonary Diseases and Disorders*, 2nd ed, Chapter 135, Fishman AP, ed, New York, NY: McGraw-Hill Book Co, 1988.

Murray JF and Nadel JA, "Bronchoscopy, Lung Biopsy, and Other Procedures," *Textbook of Respiratory Medicine*, Chapter 29, Philadelphia, PA: WB Saunders Co, 1988.

Poe RH, Israel RH, Utell MJ, et al, "Sensitivity, Specificity, and Predictive Values of Closed Pleural Biopsy," *Arch Intern Med*, 1984, 144(2):325-8.

Prakash UB and Reiman HM, "Comparison of Needle Biopsy With Cytologic Analysis for the Evaluation of Pleural Effusion: Analysis of 414 Cases," *Mayo Clin Proc*, 1985, 60(3):158-64.

Scerbo J, Keltz H, Stone DH, "A Prospective Study of Closed Pleural Biopsies," *JAMA*, 1971, 218(3):377-80.

♦ **Pleural Fluid Tap** *see* Thoracentesis *on page 263*

♦ **Polysomnography (PSG)** *see* Cardiopulmonary Sleep Study *on page 221*

♦ **Portable Spirometry** *see* Bedside Spirometry *on page 197*

♦ **Postbronchodilator Spirometry** *see* Spirometry Before and After Bronchodilators *on page 253*

♦ **Preoperative Evaluation** *see* Flow Volume Loop *on page 225*

♦ **Preoperative Evaluation** *see* Spirometry *on page 249*

Protected Catheter Brush

Related Information

Bronchoscopy, Flexible *on page 209*

Synonyms Bartlett-Farling-Wimbaly Brush; BFW Brush

Procedure Commonly Includes Extending a protected brush through a flexible bronchoscope and brushing a potentially infected area for purposes of microbiologic exam of pulmonary secretions trapped in the bristles of the brush

Indications Aid in the diagnosis of patients with clinical or radiographic features suggesting unusual, recurrent, or progressive pulmonary infections

Contraindications All are relative contraindications:

- uncooperative patient
- FEV_1 <800-1000 mL
- severe asthma
- hypoxemia uncorrected to an oxygen saturation >90% with supplemental oxygen
- bleeding diathesis
- arrhythmia
- unstable cardiac status
- recent myocardial infarction

Patient Preparation The patient should have no food or drink for 8 hours prior to the procedure (NPO after midnight for AM procedure; early light breakfast for PM procedure). Routine medications may be taken with a small amount of water. Premedication with a narcotic and/or benzodiazepine is given parenterally prior to the procedure. Atropine 0.4 mg I.M. may be given as a vagolytic agent to dry secretions unless contraindicated (ie, arrhythmia, narrow angle glaucoma, urinary retention). Supplemental oxygen is usually administered. The oropharynx is anesthetized with 2% lidocaine via a nebulizer or by gargling. The nares and nasopharynx are anesthetized with 2% lidocaine jelly if the bronchoscope is to be inserted via the nasal route.

Aftercare The patient should be NPO for at least 2 hours after the procedure (until the gag reflex has returned). Outpatients are not allowed to drive until the following day. Mild hemoptysis may be noted for 24 hours.

Complications Hypoxemia and bronchospasm. Endobronchial bleeding may occur. It is usually mild and self-limited. Local installation of epinephrine or iced saline is normally all that is required for treatment.

Equipment Flexible bronchoscope with light source, protected catheter brush (PCB), sterile container with lactated Ringer's solution, syringes, lidocaine, and sedatives

Technique The bronchoscope is passed and the airways are anesthetized in the usual manner and advanced towards the segmental bronchus of interest without the use of suction. The PCB is advanced until its distal end is visible. The catheter is then directed to a segment proximal to the one of interest and the inner cannula is advanced to dislodge the plug at the distal end that is protecting the brush from contamination. The catheter is then advanced to the segment of interest and the brush is extended from its housing. It is then gently agitated to collect bronchial secretions. The brush is retracted into the

(Continued)

Protected Catheter Brush *(Continued)*

catheter prior to removing it from the bronchoscope. Once removed, the brush is cut from its wire and allowed to fall into a sterile container with a small amount of sterile lactated Ringer's solution in it.

Data Acquired Bronchial secretions for microbiological analysis

Specimen Bronchial secretions

Collection Bronchial secretions are collected by extending the PCB into the area in question.

Storage Instructions The brush is placed in a sterile container with sterile lactated Ringer's and sent immediately to the laboratory.

Causes for Rejection Contaminated specimen, delay in processing

Normal Findings No significant growth of infectious organisms; negative stains for microbiologic organisms

Critical Values Cultures with $>10^3$ colony forming units/mL are considered positive.

Limitations Prior antibiotics, sampling error, requires meticulous technique

References

Chanez P and Vignola AM, "Bronchial Brushing," *Eur Respir J Suppl*, 1998, 26:26S-9S.

Lee FY and Mehta AC, "Basic Techniques in Flexible Bronchoscopy," *Flexible Bronchoscopy*, Wang KP and Mehta AC, eds, Cambridge, MA: Blackwell Science, Inc, 1995, 95-118.

Mertens AH, Nagler JM, Galdermans DI, et al, "Quality Assessment of Protected Specimen Brush Samples by Microscopic Cell Count," *Am J Respir Crit Care Med*, 1998, 157(4 Pt 1):1240-3.

Wang HH, Sovie S, Trawinski G, et al, "ThinPrep Processing of Endoscopic Brushing Specimens," *Am J Clin Pathol*, 1996, 105(2):163-7.

♦ **Provocholine® Challenge** *see* Bronchial Challenge Test *on page 202*

♦ **Pulmonary Artery Catheterization** *see* Swan-Ganz Catheterization *on page 258*

Pulmonary Compliance (Dynamic)

Related Information

Pulmonary Compliance (Static) *on page 243*

Applies to Chord Compliance

Procedure Commonly Includes Pulmonary compliance reported in units of $liter_{BTPS}$/cm H_2O, maximum static elastic recoil pressure reported in units of cm H_2O, dynamic compliance at 60 breaths/minute reported as a percentage of the static compliance measurement ($Cdyn_{60}$).

Indications Assess small airways dysfunction

Contraindications Patients that are unable to follow instructions and relax, patients in whom placement of an esophageal balloon is contraindicated. Transnasal placement of an esophageal balloon is relatively contraindicated in patients with a history of spontaneous nosebleeds. The presence of a large hiatal hernia may render esophageal pressures invalid.

Patient Preparation The patient should not take anything by mouth for 2-3 hours prior to testing. Nasal passage should be treated with a topical Xylocaine®/epinephrine solution to widen nasal passage and minimize discomfort. The patient should take small sips of ice water (if not contraindicated) before and during passage of a nasogastric balloon.

Aftercare Usually none, occasionally patient will experience vagal stimulation during passage of the nasogastric balloon. Placement in a feet up supine position may aid in the treatment of hypotension, dizziness and nausea.

Special Instructions Balloon should be coated with a topical anesthetic treated lubricant to aid in minimizing the gag reflex. Balloon should contain a small amount (usually 0.5 mL) of air. If excessive amounts of air are used esophageal pressures will be overstated resulting in an erroneously low pulmonary compliance.

Technique With the patient in a seated position, an uninflated, 10 cm x 1 cm, thin walled, latex balloon-catheter set-up attached to a pressure transducer is inserted transnasally after topical anesthesia and positioned in the lower one-third of the esophagus. Sips of water will aid in the passage of the balloon. The patient is instructed to perform a Valsalva maneuver with the end of the balloon catheter open to a loose fitting glass syringe. The balloon is then inflated with approximately 0.2-0.5 mL air. Several volume histories are obtained (inhalation to TLC) prior to making any measurement. Measurement of maximal static recoil pressure may be made while holding breath at TLC for several seconds. Peak pressure should be ignored and stable pressure recorded. After several static recoil measurements are made, relaxed shutter interrupted exhalations from TLC to FRC (or RV if the entire pressure volume curve is desired) are made while plotting transpulmonary pressure (pleural pressure minus mouth pressure) against exhaled volume. Compliance measurements (so-called "chord compliance") are made along the exhalation pressure volume curve from points corresponding to FRC and FRC plus 0.5 liter/$_{BTPS}$. Patients are then asked to increase their breathing rate 10 breaths/minute to a maximum rate of 100 breaths/minute. Measurement of transpulmonary pressure and volume are plotted on an X-Y plotter. Dynamic compliance is measured by dividing volume change by pressure change at points of zero flow. Dynamic compliance is typically reported as a percentage of the static compliance or $Cdyn_{60}$ = dynamic compliance measured during 60 breaths/minute panting/static compliance x 100.

Turnaround Time Preliminary report usually available same day, interpreted reports available in 1-2 days.

Specimen Transpulmonary pressures (mouth pressure minus esophageal (**pleural**) pressures) are plotted against volumes obtained from an interrupted, passive, expiratory volume history from TLC to RV. Compliance measurements are made along the recorded pressure lines at points corresponding to FRC and FRC + 1 $liter_{BTPS}$.

Collection Measurement is made by recording mouth pressure and pressures recorded from an esophageal balloon inserted transnasally into the lower one-third of the thorax of an upright seated patient. Volume should be measured from a device that meets standards recommended by the American Thoracic Society (ATS).

Causes for Rejection Wide variations in baseline level of FRC. Active expiratory efforts made against the shutter during interrupted passive exhalation.

Normal Findings Normal value for pulmonary compliance can be derived from the following equation:

C_{st} in $liter_{BTPS}$ = (0.00343 x height in cm) - 0.425

Limitations Technically difficult secondary to correct placement of the balloon and the need for the patient to relax against an obstruction while maintaining an open glottis. Patients often find transnasal passage of the esophageal balloon unpleasant.

References

Bassiri AG, Girgis RE, Doyle RL, et al, "Detection of Small Airway Dysfunction Using Specific Airway Conductance," *Chest*, 1997, 111(6):1533-5.

Guerin C, Le Masson S, de Varax R, et al, "Small Airway Closure and Positive End-Expiratory Pressure in Mechanically Ventilated Patients With Chronic Obstructive Pulmonary Disease," *Am J Respir Crit Care Med*, 1997, 155(6):1949-56.

Khorasani A, Candido KD, Saatee S, et al, "The Relationship Between Dynamic Compliance and Inspiratory Flow," *Anesth Analg*, 1999, 88(2):465.

Liu CH, Niranjan SC, Clark JW Jr, et al, "Airway Mechanics, Gas Exchange, and Blood Flow in a Nonlinear Model of the Normal Human Lung," *J Appl Physiol*, 1998, 84(4):1447-69.

Nikischin W, Gerhardt T, Everett R, et al, "A New Method to Analyze Lung Compliance When Pressure-Volume Relationship Is Nonlinear," *Am J Respir Crit Care Med*, 1999, 159(6):2028.

Officer TM, Pellegrino R, Brusasco V, et al, "Measurement of Pulmonary Resistance and Dynamic Compliance With Airway Obstruction," *J Appl Physiol*, 1998, 85(5):1982-8.

Vollmer WM, McCamant LE, Johnson LR, et al, "Long-Term Reproducibility of Tests of Small Airways Function. Comparisons With Spirometry," *Chest*, 1990, 98(2):303-7.

Pulmonary Compliance (Static)

Related Information

Pulmonary Compliance (Dynamic) *on page 242*

Applies to Frequency Dependence of Compliance

Procedure Commonly Includes Pulmonary compliance reported in units of $liter_{BTPS}/cm\ H_2O$

Indications Characterize the pressure-volume curve of the lung to aid in the diagnosis of emphysema, pulmonary vascular congestion, interstitial lung disease, and pulmonary fibrosis

Contraindications Patients that are unable to follow instructions and relax, patients in whom placement of an esophageal balloon is contraindicated

(Continued)

Pulmonary Compliance (Static) *(Continued)*

Patient Preparation The patient should not take anything by mouth for 2-3 hours prior to testing. The patient should take small sips of ice water (if not contraindicated) before and during passage of a nasogastric balloon.

Aftercare Usually none, occasionally patient will experience vagal stimulation during passage of the nasogastric balloon. Placement in a feet up supine position may aid in the treatment of hypotension, dizziness, and nausea.

Special Instructions Balloon should be coated with a topical anesthetic treated lubricant to aid in minimizing the gag reflex. Balloon should contain a small amount (usually 0.5 mL) of air. If excessive amounts of air are used esophageal pressures will be overstated resulting in an erroneously low pulmonary compliance.

Technique With the patient in a seated position, an uninflated, 10 cm x 1 cm, thin walled, latex balloon-catheter set-up attached to a pressure transducer is inserted transnasally after topical anesthesia and positioned in the lower one-third of the esophagus. Sips of water will aid in the passage of the balloon. The patient is instructed to perform a Valsalva maneuver with the end of the balloon catheter open to a loose fitting glass syringe. The balloon is then inflated with approximately 0.2-0.5 mL air. Several volume histories are obtained (inhalation to TLC) prior to making any measurement. Measurement of maximal static recoil pressure may be made while holding breath at TLC for several seconds. Peak pressure should be ignored and stable pressure recorded. After several static recoil measurements are made, relaxed shutter interrupted exhalations from TLC to FRC (or RV if the entire pressure volume curve is desired) are made while plotting transpulmonary pressure (pleural pressure minus mouth pressure) against exhaled volume. Compliance measurements (so-called "chord compliance") are made along the exhalation pressure volume curve from points corresponding to FRC and FRC plus 0.5 $liter_{BTPS}$.

Turnaround Time Preliminary report usually available same day, interpreted reports available in 1-2 days.

Specimen Transpulmonary pressures (mouth pressure minus esophageal (**pleural**) pressures) are plotted against volumes obtained from an interrupted, passive, expiratory volume history from TLC to RV. Compliance measurements are made along the recorded pressure lines at points corresponding to FRC and FRC + 1 $liter_{BTPS}$.

Collection Measurement is made by recording mouth pressure and pressures recorded from an esophageal balloon inserted transnasally into the lower one-third of the thorax of an upright seated patient. Volume should be measured from a device that meets standards recommended by the American Thoracic Society (ATS).

Causes for Rejection Wide variations in baseline level of FRC. Active expiratory efforts made against the shutter during interrupted passive exhalation.

Normal Findings Normal value for pulmonary compliance can be derived from the following equation:

C_{st} in $liter_{BTPS}$ = (0.00343 x height in cm) - 0.425

Limitations Technically difficult secondary to correct placement of the balloon and the need for the patient to relax against an obstruction while maintaining an open glottis. Patients often find transnasal passage of the esophageal balloon unpleasant.

References

Bittner E, Chendrasekhar A, Pillai S, et al, "Changes in Oxygenation and Compliance as Related to Body Position in Acute Lung Injury," *Am J Surg*, 1996, 62(12):1038-41.

Coast JR, O'Kroy JA, Akers FM 2nd, et al, "Effects of Lower Body Pressure Changes on Pulmonary Function," *Med Sci Sports Exerc*, 1998, 30(7):1035-40.

Gauger PG, Pranikoff T, Schreiner RJ, et al, "Initial Experience With Partial Liquid Ventilation in Pediatric Patients With the Acute Respiratory Distress Syndrome," *Crit Care Med*, 1996, 24(1):16-22.

Hirschl RB, Pranikoff T, Wise C, et al, "Initial Experience With Partial Liquid Ventilation in Adult Patients With the Acute Respiratory Distress Syndrome," *JAMA*, 1996, 275(5):383-9.

Klein U, Karzai W, Zimmermann P, et al, "Changes in Pulmonary Mechanics After Fiberoptic Bronchoalveolar Lavage in Mechanically Ventilated Patients," *Intensive Care Med*, 1998, 24(12):1289-93.

Pulse Oximetry

Related Information

Arterial Blood Gases *on page 191*
Arterial Blood Oximetry *on page 195*
Arterial Cannulation *on page 17*
Cardiopulmonary Exercise Testing *on page 217*
Cardiopulmonary Sleep Study *on page 221*

Synonyms CPAP Titration; Desaturation Oximetry; Oxygen Titration Test

Applies to Ear Oximetry; Finger Oximetry

Replaces Exercise ABG

Procedure Commonly Includes Report generally includes baseline heart rate and functional O_2 saturation, heart rate and lowest functional O_2 saturation during whatever event may be taking place: exercise, sleep or therapeutic intervention such as nasal CPAP or oxygen therapy.

Indications Determine an estimate of the level of arterial oxygenation at rest and in the presence of positive and negative intervention. These include exercise, sleep, and during procedures such as surgery, bronchoscopy, ventilator assist/support therapy, etc.

Contraindications Not to be used in the presence of flammable anesthetics. Contraindications for exercise may be found in the section on cardiopulmonary exercise testing.

Patient Preparation Fingernail polish should be removed with acetone. Permanent or disposable sensors should be applied according to the manufacturer's instructions. When finger probes are used, the patient should be instructed not to grip treadmill rail or handlebars tightly to avoid reduction of circulation to the digits. Preparation depends on the type of test being performed. Exercise patients should wear loose comfortable clothing. Patients should refrain from smoking 24 hours prior to test to avoid the O_2 saturation discrepancy that occurs with elevated carboxyhemoglobin levels. If possible, an arterial blood gas should be drawn and pH, pCO_2, pO_2, Hb, oxyhemoglobin (O_2Hb%), carboxyhemoglobin (COHb%) and methemoglobin (metHb%) should be measured. Draw the heparinized arterial blood sample while the pulse oximetry sensor is in place and the pulse oximetry saturation (SpO_2%) reading is stable. (See Arterial Blood Oximetry *on page 195* and Arterial Blood Gases *on page 191*.) Correlation of oxyhemoglobin (O_2Hb%) (measured by blood oximetry) and SpO_2% (measured by pulse oximetry) should be made. The discrepancy between the O_2Hb% - SpO_2% should be used to determine the endpoint of the maneuver inducing arterial desaturation. For example, if the pulse oximeter displays a SpO_2 reading of 93% and a simultaneously obtained arterial blood sample shows an O_2Hb% of 91%, 2% should be subtracted from subsequent SpO_2 measurements during exercise for a more valid estimate of arterial oxygen saturation. This adjustment should also be made to determine the therapeutic endpoint when titrating supplemental oxygen therapy at rest, during sleep, or exercise.

Aftercare After exercise, allow patient to walk slowly on level treadmill or pedal bicycle ergometer at zero load slowly to allow gradual cool down period. Monitor EKG, blood pressure, and patient status frequently during the first 5 minutes after a maximum exercise test.

Special Instructions Poor collateral circulation may be compensated for by warming the hands with warm towels. Fluctuation ±1% is acceptable. Range of fluctuation should be noted.

Technique Methodology may differ widely depending on the type of challenge or intervention planned. Basic methodology should include correlation with blood oximetry as outlined in Patient Preparation. External EKG should correlate within 5 beats/minute of the pulse oximeter's pulse display. Record baseline functional saturation, external EKG rate and pulse oximeter heart rate along with patient status, workload, and supplemental oxygen given at each stage of the test.

Turnaround Time Preliminary report should be available same day, interpreted report should follow in 1-2 days.

Specimen Spectrophotometric measurement is made by passing light at two specific wavelengths through a pulsing capillary bed (finger, toe, bridge of

(Continued)

Pulse Oximetry *(Continued)*

nose, and ear are the most common sites for sensor placement). Light collection on the other side of the site is proportional to the amount of oxyhemoglobin present in the arterial capillary bed relative to the amount of hemoglobin available for binding with oxygen (exclusive of the dyshemoglobins: carboxyhemoglobin and methemoglobin).

Causes for Rejection Unstable readings secondary to any cause: external light, poor peripheral circulation, or skin pigmentation are common causes.

Normal Findings Normal adult oxyhemoglobin saturation is >95%. Drops in oxyhemoglobin are usually the result of cardiac, pulmonary, or combined cardiopulmonary disease. Significant declines (≥5%) during exercise or sleep are abnormal.

Limitations Test does not measure or take into consideration total hemoglobin or the dyshemoglobins, carboxyhemoglobin, and methemoglobin. May overestimate total oxygen delivery (oxygen content) if not correlated with blood oximetry. Not accurate in the presence of poor peripheral circulation. Accuracy at most units is ±2%, standard deviation is usually 1%.

Additional Information Guidelines for reimbursement of home oxygen therapy state that a resting arterial pO_2 <55 torr or a resting oxygen saturation (SaO_2 or SpO_2%) <88% with evidence of improvement with oxygen therapy qualify a patient for continuous oxygen therapy reimbursement. Guidelines for reimbursement for nocturnal and exercise oxygen therapy state that O_2 saturations during exercise or sleep that fall to <88% that improve with oxygen therapy will be reimbursed. Because of the limitations of pulse oximetry, decisions regarding discontinuing oxygen therapy should **not** be made on the basis of pulse oximetry alone. Assessment of the PaO_2 by arterial blood gas and/or O_2Hb% by arterial blood oximetry should be done before such decisions are made. Carlin et al has shown that patients with PaO_2 ≤55 torr may be denied oxygen therapy if the decision was based on pulse oximetry measurements alone (a significant number of these patients had SpO_2% measurements >88%).

References

Alcain G, Guillen P, Escolar A, et al, "Predictive Factors of Oxygen Desaturation During Upper Gastrointestinal Endoscopy in Nonsedated Patients," *Gastrointest Endosc*, 1998, 48(2):143-7.

Alvarez Lario B, Alonso Valdivielso JL, Alegre Lopez J, et al, "Fibromyalgia Syndrome: Overnight Falls in Arterial Oxygen Saturation," *Am J Med*, 1996, 101(1):54-60.

Bousamra M 2nd, Haasler GB, Lipchik RJ, et al, "Functional and Oximetric Assessment of Patients After Lung Reduction Surgery," *J Thorac Cardiovasc Surg*, 1997, 113(4):675-81.

Carlin BW, Clausen JL, and Ries AL, "The Use of Cutaneous Oximetry in the Prescription of Long-Term Oxygen Therapy," *Chest*, 1988, 94(2):239-41.

Coleman RL, Whitten CW, O'Boyle J, et al, "Unexplained Decrease in Measured Oxygen Saturation by Pulse Oximetry Following Injection of Lymphazurin 1% (Isosulfan Blue) During a Lymphatic Mapping Procedure," *J Surg Oncol*, 1999, 70(2):126-9.

Collins MJ and Bakheit AM, "Does Pulse Oximetry Reliably Detect Aspiration in Dysphagic Stroke Patients?" *Stroke*, 1997, 28(9):1773-5.

Frey B and Butt W, "Pulse Oximetry for Assessment of Pulsus Paradoxus: A Clinical Study in Children," *Intensive Care Med*, 1998, 24(3):242-6.

Hampson NB, "Pulse Oximetry in Severe Carbon Monoxide Poisoning," *Chest*, 1998, 114(4):1036-41.

Hartert TV, Wheeler AP, and Sheller JR, "Use of Pulse Oximetry to Recognize Severity of Airflow Obstruction in Obstructive Airway Disease: Correlation With Pulsus Paradoxus," *Chest*, 1999, 115(2):475-81.

Jensen LA, Onyskiw JE, and Prasad NG, "Meta-analysis of Arterial Oxygen Saturation Monitoring by Pulse Oximetry in Adults," *Heart Lung*, 1998, 27(6):387-408.

Seguin P, Le Rouzo A, Tanguy M, et al, "Evidence for the Need of Bedside Accuracy of Pulse Oximetry in an Intensive Care Unit," *Crit Care Med*, 2000, 28(3):703-6.

Summers RL, Anders RM, Woodward LH, et al, "Effect of Routine Pulse Oximetry Measurements on ED Triage Classification," *Am J Emerg Med*, 1998, 16(1):5-7.

- **Residual Volume** *see* Functional Residual Capacity *on page 229*
- **Respiratory Inductive Plethysmography** *see* Cardiopulmonary Sleep Study *on page 221*
- **Right Heart Catheterization** *see* Swan-Ganz Catheterization *on page 258*
- **Right to Left Shunt Determination** *see* Shunt Determination *on page 247*
- **Rigid Bronchoscopy** *see* Bronchoscopy, Rigid *on page 210*
- **SB DLCO** *see* Carbon Monoxide Diffusing Capacity, Single Breath *on page 215*

Shunt Determination

Related Information

Alveolar to Arterial Oxygen Gradient *on page 188*
Arterial Blood Gases *on page 191*

Synonyms Right to Left Shunt Determination; Shunt Study, 100% O_2

Procedure Commonly Includes Alveolar to arterial gradient of partial pressure of dissolved oxygen while breathing 100% O_2 for a minimum of 20 minutes, reported in mm Hg and the shunt fraction (Q_s/Q_t%) expressed as a percentage of the cardiac output.

Indications Determine the nature of hypoxemia and the nature of a right to left shunt

Patient Preparation As with all arterial puncture procedures, a prothrombin time, if available, can alert one to the need to spend extra time applying direct pressure to the puncture site to allow for coagulation to occur. Test for collateral circulation (Allen test) should be negative before the radial puncture site is used. (See Arterial Blood Gases *on page 191*.)

Aftercare Apply direct pressure to the puncture site until bleeding has stopped and then apply a sterile bandage. Bandaging the puncture site does **not** substitute for the application of direct pressure to the puncture site for at least 5 minutes. Palpate pulse distal to the puncture site to evaluate arterial spasm.

Special Instructions The patient should be instructed to remain in the same position (upright seated posture is standard) throughout the O_2 breathing and obtaining of the ABG. The importance of maintaining an airtight seal on the mouthpiece and the use of noseclips should be stressed.

Technique Provide the patient with a 100% oxygen breathing supply. Typical set-up uses a 100 L Douglas bag (that has been flushed three times to wash the dead space of bag, tubing, and valve dead space) attached to a bidirectional low resistance valve by a 3-way valve and a length of tubing. After flushing the reservoir and measuring the inspired oxygen concentration in the bag, begin the 20-minute oxygen breathing period. The patient is encouraged to take slow, deep breaths during the O_2 breathing. The patient's lips should maintain an airtight seal and noseclips should prevent nasal inspiration. After a minimum of 20 minutes a heparinized, arterial blood gas sample is obtained. If possible, sample end-tidal nitrogen from the breathing valve to ensure an expired N_2 of <1% before obtaining arterial blood sample. Calculate the percentage of right-to-left shunt according to the following equation:

$$Q_s/Q_t\% = \frac{0.0031 \times p(A\text{-}a)O_2}{0.0031 \times p(A\text{-}a)O_2 + 5} \times 100$$

Where:

$Q_s/Q_t\%$ = the fraction of the cardiac output that passes through a right-to-left shunt

$p(A\text{-}a)O_2$ = gradient of alveolar minus arterial oxygen partial pressure after breathing 100% O_2 for a minumum of 20 minutes

Turnaround Time Same day.

Specimen A heparinized arterial blood sample is obtained from the patient after a minimum of 20 minutes of breathing 100% oxygen. Sample can be obtained with patient in any position to evaluate the shunt status of the gravity-dependent portion of lung or lungs. Standard arterial blood gas parameters are measured (pH, pCO_2, and pO_2).

Container Although not studied, it is felt that heparinized glass syringes are preferred over plastic to minimize diffusion of high levels of dissolved oxygen across the walls of the syringe. Sample should be labeled with the patient's name and ID number, position during the 20-minute O_2 breathing and blood draw, and the number of minutes of oxygen breathing.

Causes for Rejection Large air bubbles in sample, excessive (more than 15 minutes) interval between obtaining sample and sample analysis, inspiring room air during 100% O_2 breathing.

Normal Findings Two percent to 5% of the cardiac output passes through a right to left shunt at rest in the normal individual.

(Continued)

Shunt Determination *(Continued)*

Limitations Erroneous results can be obtained if sample is not analyzed immediately, if the patient does not maintain an airtight seal with the O_2 supply, if insufficient (less than 20 minutes) time is allowed for wash-in of oxygen, or if oxygen electrode on the blood gas analyzer is alinear during measurement of high pO_2. Correct sample handling and observation during O_2 breathing can minimize errors. The shunt fraction calculation assumes an arterial to mixed venous oxygen content difference of 5 volume %. Significant variation from this value may occur in some patients resulting in over- or underestimation of percent shunt.

References

Cope JT, Banks D, McDaniel NL, et al, "Is Vertical Vein Ligation Necessary in Repair of Total Anomalous Pulmonary Venous Connection?" *Ann Thorac Surg*, 1997, 64(1):23-8.

Huntington JH, Malviya S, Voepel-Lewis T, et al, "The Effect of a Right-to-Left Intracardiac Shunt on the Rate of Rise of Arterial and End-Tidal Halothane in Children," *Anesth Analg*, 1999, 88(4):759-62.

Jahangiri M, Lincoln C, and Shinebourne EA, "Does the Modified Blalock-Taussig Shunt Cause Growth of the Contralateral Pulmonary Artery?" *Ann Thorac Surg*, 1999, 67(5):1397-9.

Kanterman RY, Darcy MD, Middleton WD, et al, "Doppler Sonography Findings Associated With Transjugular Intrahepatic Portosystemic Shunt Malfunction," *AJR Am J Roentgenol*, 1997, 168(2):467-72.

O'Brien JJ, Butterworth J, Hammon JW, et al, "Cerebral Emboli During Cardiac Surgery in Children," *Anesthesiology*, 1997, 87(5):1063-9.

Rao PS, Chandar JS, and Sideris EB, "Role of Inverted Buttoned Device in Transcatheter Occlusion of Atrial Septal Defects or Patent Foramen Ovale With Right-to-Left Shunting Associated With Previously Operated Complex Congenital Cardiac Anomalies," *Am J Cardiol*, 1997, 80(7):914-21.

Serena J, Segura T, Perez-Ayuso MJ, et al, "The Need to Quantify Right-to-Left Shunt in Acute Ischemic Stroke: A Case-Control Study," *Stroke*, 1998, 29(7):1322-8.

♦ **Shunt Study, 100% O_2** *see* Shunt Determination *on page 247*

Single Breath Nitrogen Elimination

Synonyms Closing Capacity; Closing Volume

Procedure Commonly Includes Closing volume to vital capacity ratio (CV/VC%), closing capacity to total lung capacity ratio (CC/TLC%), slope of phase III (delta $N_{2(750-1250)}$ mL).

Indications Assess distribution of ventilation and presence of small airway dysfunction

Contraindications Patients that are unable to limit inspiratory and expiratory flow rates to <0.5 $liter_{BTPS}$/second, patients with demonstrable airways obstruction

Patient Preparation The patient should avoid heavy meals 3 hours prior to testing. The patient should be conscious and able to follow simple instructions. The patient's height and weight should be measured without shoes. Loose comfortable clothing that does not restrict chest expansion should be worn. Smoking history including last cigarette smoked should be obtained. Current medications should be obtained with particular emphasis on bronchodilators and steroids.

Special Instructions Generally, some sort of feedback circuit that monitors inspiratory and expiratory flow is needed to keep flows ≤0.5 L/second.

Technique The patient is attached to either a spirometer mouthpiece or a mouthpiece attached to a bag-in-box system. The spirometer used should conform to ATS recommended standards. The nitrogen analyzer should have a recent two-point calibration. The O_2 reservoir, either the bag in the box or the spirometer, should be flushed with oxygen until the N_2 measured at the mouthpiece is <0.1%. Initially, the patient valve should be turned to room air and the patient should breathe normally. Instruct the patient to take two deep breaths and then exhale to residual volume (RV). When the patient reaches RV, turn the patient valve so that the next inspiration to total lung capacity (TLC) comes from the 100% O_2 reservoir. Instruct the patient to inhale slowly (<0.5 L/second) to TLC, followed immediately by a slow (<0.5 L/second) exhalation to RV. Flow feedback devices are recommended. Flow, volume and expired nitrogen are continuously measured and recorded during the procedure. They should be repeated two more times. Repeat studies should be delayed until the inspiratory to expiratory nitrogen difference is $<5\%$ during room air breathing. Flow must not exceed 0.7 L/second for more than 300 mL expirate. Vital capacity measurements must show $\leq 10\%$ variation on repeat maneuvers. Inspiratory and expiratory vital capacities must agree within 5%. Three acceptable tracings should be obtained. Mean values obtained from all valid efforts should be reported.

Turnaround Time Preliminary report is available the same day, interpreted report is usually available in 1-2 days.

Specimen Measurement of expired nitrogen after one vital capacity breath of 100% O_2.

Causes for Rejection Excessively high inspiratory or expiratory flow rates (>0.5 L/second), breath-holding at TLC.

Normal Findings The onset of phase IV is not always seen. The normal values for closing volume (CV) are reported in units of [(VC - CV)/VC] x 100. The normal values for closing capacity (CC) are reported as [(VC - CV) + RV/VC] x 100. Closing volumes are age dependent and do not seem to vary with the size of the patient. Normal values range from around 10% at age 20 to around 20% to 25% at age 60. The slope of phase III (delta $N_{2(750-1250)}$) is reported as % nitrogen change/L volume expired and varies from around 1%/liter$_{BTPS}$ at age 20 to around 1.5%/liter$_{BTPS}$ at age 60.

Limitations Although seemingly simple, the test is actually difficult to perform correctly, with emphasis on the need to limit inspiratory and expiratory flows to <0.5 liter$_{BTPS}$/second. Large intraindividual coefficient of variation is noted even when careful attention to flow rates and absence of breath-holding during the procedure. Phase IV may not be evident in healthy young individuals and in patients with a high phase III slope. Poor correlation has been shown between phase IV and an abnormal flow rate $FEF_{25\%-75\%}$ measured on spirometry. A 1973 workshop at the National Heart and Lung Institute stated that the CV and CC are sensitive tests but are probably of low specificity and moderate precision and their validity as a diagnostic test is unknown.

References

Hammer J, Numa A, and Newth CJ, "Total Lung Capacity by N2 Washout From High and low Lung Volumes in Ventilated Infants and Children," *Am J Respir Crit Care Med*, 1998, 158(2):526-31.

Lauzon AM, Elliot AR, Paiva M, et al, "Cardiogenic Oscillation Phase Relationships During Single-Breath Tests Performed in Microgravity," *J Appl Physiol*, 1998, 84(2):661-8.

Manning F, Dean E, Ross J, et al, "Effects of Side Lying on Lung Function in Older Individuals," *Phys Ther*, 1999, 79(5):456-66.

Morris MG, "The Open Circuit Nitrogen Washout Technique for Measuring the Lung Volume in Infants: Methodological Aspects," *Thorax*, 1999, 54(9):790-5.

Vollmer WM, McCamant LE, Johnson LR, et al, "Long-Term Reproducibility of Tests of Small Airways Function. Comparisons With Spirometry," *Chest*, 1990, 98(2):303-7.

♦ **Sleep Apnea Study** *see* Cardiopulmonary Sleep Study *on page 221*
♦ **Sleep Oximetry** *see* Cardiopulmonary Sleep Study *on page 221*
♦ **Sleep Study** *see* Cardiopulmonary Sleep Study *on page 221*
♦ **Specific Airways Resistance** *see* Airway Resistance *on page 187*
♦ **Specific Conductance** *see* Airway Resistance *on page 187*
♦ **Spirogram** *see* Spirometry *on page 249*

Spirometry

Related Information

Bedside Spirometry *on page 197*
Bronchial Challenge Test *on page 202*
Cardiopulmonary Exercise Testing *on page 217*
Flow Volume Loop *on page 225*
Functional Residual Capacity *on page 229*
Lung Subdivisions *on page 233*
Maximum Voluntary Ventilation (MVV) *on page 235*
Peak Flow *on page 237*
Spirometry Before and After Bronchodilators *on page 253*
Spirometry, Sitting and Supine *on page 256*
Volume of Isoflow (V iso $\dot{V}$) *on page 270*

Synonyms Forced Expirogram; Spirogram

Applies to Assessment of Pulmonary Disability; Preoperative Evaluation

(Continued)

Spirometry *(Continued)*

Procedure Commonly Includes Vital capacity (VC); forced vital capacity (FVC); timed forced expiratory volumes, $FEV_{0.5}$, FEV_1, FEV_3; forced expiratory flow between 25% and 75% of the FEV ($FEF_{25\%-75\%}$); peak expiratory flow rate (PEFR or PF); total expiratory time in seconds

Indications

- establish baseline lung function
- detect disease
- follow the course of disease to monitor treatment
- evaluation of impairment
- preoperative evaluation
- identify high risk smokers
- occupational surveys

Patient Preparation The patient should avoid heavy meals 3 hours prior to testing. The patient should be conscious and able to follow simple instructions. The patient's height and weight should be measured without shoes. Loose comfortable clothing that does not restrict chest expansion should be worn. Smoking history including last cigarette smoked should be obtained. Current medications should be obtained with particular emphasis on bronchodilators and steroids.

Aftercare Usually none, although patients that complain of lightheadedness and dizziness should not be allowed to walk unobserved until recovery.

Technique A spirometer is used to measure exhaled gas and to record the time of collection. Two major categories of spirometers exist. Volume displacement spirometers such as the water seal, dry rolling seal, or bellows spirometers record volume change as vertical deflection on a kymograph or a moving stylus on a sheet of paper. The second category of spirometers integrates the measurement of expired flow over time to yield exhaled volume. Pneumotachograms, turbinometers, and hot wire mass flow meters are examples of flow integrating spirometers. Turbinometer type of spirometers have failed to meet current ATS standards of performance. Computer assisted flow integrating spirometers generate a CRT image of volume versus time or flow versus volume which can be inspected during testing and later printed. Graphic representation of spirometric data should be inspected along with numeric data to assess reliability of data (see Causes for Rejection).

Turnaround Time Preliminary results should be available same day. Depending on the facility, an interpreted report may be available in 1-2 days.

Specimen Measurement of exhaled volumes and flow rates during a maximal forced expiratory maneuver from total lung capacity to residual volume.

Collection Exhaled sample is collected or passed through a volume or flow measuring device known as a spirometer. Spirometers should meet certain minimum standards defined by the American Thoracic Society. Test may be performed on adults in a seated or standing position and children in a seated position. After applying noseclips, the subject is instructed to take a full inspiration, hold it briefly, then exhale through a mouthpiece into the spirometer as forcefully and completely as possible. Test is repeated a minimum of three times until two reproducible efforts have been obtained. See following figures.

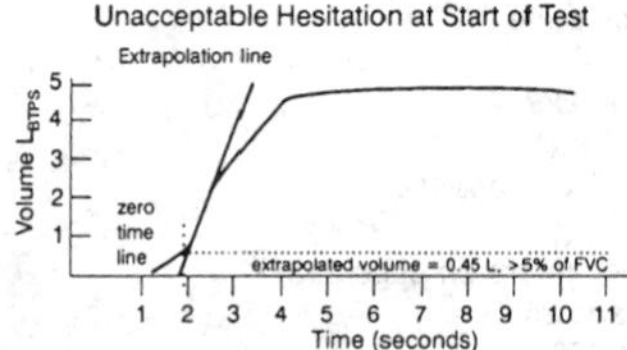

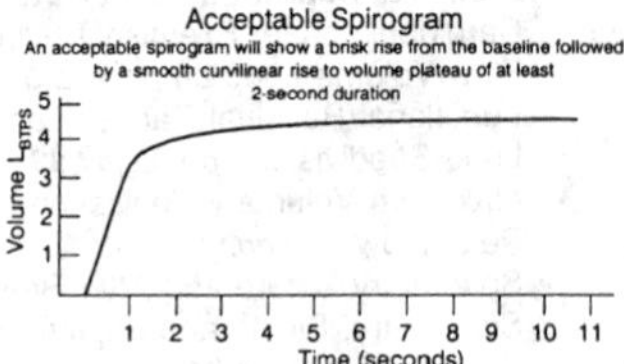

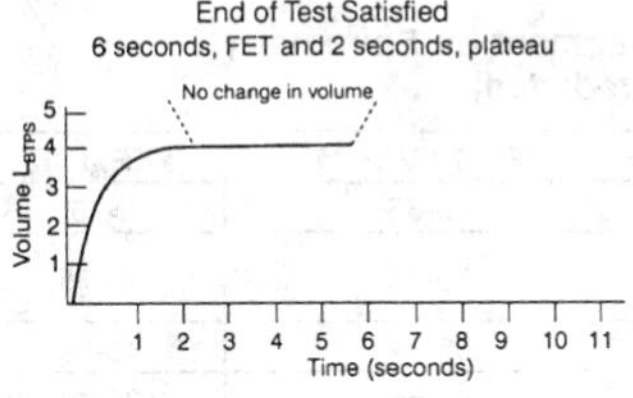

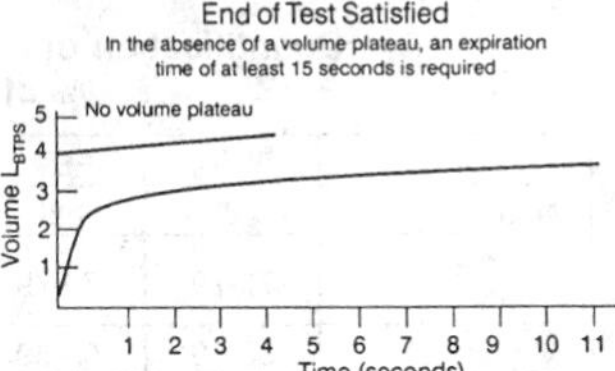

Causes for Rejection **Cough**, especially when it occurs in the early part of forced expiration, may render all data except expired volume useless. **Hesitant start:** Peak effort must be applied before 50% of total volume is exhaled, otherwise measurement of timed forced expiratory volume may be invalid. (Back extrapolated volume.) **Premature cessation of expiratory effort:** Expiratory effort must be maintained until a valid end-of-test has been observed. ATS has defined a valid end-of-test to be:

- when forced exhalation has continued for at least **6** seconds and a volume plateau (**no** volume change) of at least **1** second duration is seen
- in the absence of a volume plateau, a reasonable exhalation time of at least 15 seconds is observed
- when the patient cannot or should not sustain forced exhalation for valid medical reasons
- tests that consistently exhibit a smooth, curvilinear rise to a volume plateau of at least 1 second duration on a volume-time tracing satisfy end-of-test criteria even if the forced expiratory time is <6 seconds (children, patients with interstitial lung disease).

Although difficult to achieve, the first two conditions for a valid end-of-test should be the goal of each testing session.

Early termination falsely increases FEV_1FVC% and increased mean and instantaneous flow rates at middle or low lung volumes. **Submaximal effort:** Indicated by a very low, often nonreproducible peak flow. Neuromuscular disease may produce the same pattern. **Nonreproducibility:** The two largest FVCs and FEV_1s should show <5% variability.

Normal Findings Typically ±20% of a reference value based on age, height, and gender. Some studies advocate the use of 95% confidence limit. Spirometric values expressed as % of predicted can be used to grade the severity of abnormalities.

Limitations Requires patient cooperation. Transient obstruction secondary to cigarette smoking just prior to testing may be observed.

Additional Information Patients with asthma may show progressive decline in spirometric values with repeated efforts yielding excessive variability between two largest efforts. This may be distinguished from variable effort only by a trained pulmonary technologist noting maximal inspiration on each effort followed by an adequately forceful expiration (sharp peak of expiratory flow volume curve). In such cases the largest and smallest acceptable efforts should be reported giving the physician a rough assessment of bronchial hyper-reactivity. (See Bronchial Challenge Test *on page 202.*) Patients with neuromuscular disease (myasthenia gravis) may show progressive decline of values with repeated efforts but are seldom able to generate an adequate peak effort and may therefore mimic poor effort. See the following tables.
(Continued)

Spirometry *(Continued)*

Quantification of Impairment by Spirometry (% of predicted)

	FVC	FEV_1	FEV_1 / FVC%*†	$FEF_{25\%-75\%}$
Normal	≥80	≥80	75-85	>76
Minimal (slight)	70-79	70-79	65-74	60-75
Moderate	55-69	55-69	55-64	45-59
Severe	45-54	40-54	45-54	30-44
Very severe	<45	<45	<45	<30

*Expressed as actual ratio of FEV_1 / FVC x 100.

†Female age >40 years.

Patterns of Spirometric Abnormalities

	NML* (% of predicted)	Obstructive Diseases	Restrictive Diseases
FVC	≥80*	NML or ↓	↓ to ↓↓↓
FEV_1	≥80*	↓ to ↓↓↓	↓ to ↓↓↓
FEV_1 / FVC %	≥75	↓ to ↓↓↓	NML or ↑
$FEF_{25\%-75\%}$	≥76*	↓↓ to ↓↓↓	↓ to ↓↓↓

*Expressed as actual ratio of FEV_1 / FVC x 100.

↓ mildly reduced.

↓↓ moderately reduced.

↓↓↓ severely reduced.

Good understanding of the expectations for maximum performance is the key for obtaining reproducible results. It is often helpful to include a demonstration of a proper forced expiratory maneuver as part of the initial instructions. Subsequent instructions should focus on correcting specific deficits in performance. The three most common deficits are:

- failure to inspire to TLC
- failure to begin exhalation with a prompt, forceful blow
- failure to sustain exhalation until valid end-of-test criteria is met

References

Eaton T, Withy S, Garrett JE, et al, "Spirometry in Primary Care Practice: The Importance of Quality Assurance and the Impact of Spirometry Workshops," *Chest*, 1999, 116(2):416-23.

Enright PL, Arnold A, Manolio TA, et al, "Spirometry Reference Values for Healthy Elderly Blacks. The Cardiovascular Health Study Research Group," *Chest*, 1996, 110(6):1416-24.

Ferguson GT and Petty TL, "Screening and Early Intervention for COPD," *Hosp Pract*, 1998, 33(4):67-72, 79-80.

Finkelstein J, Hripcsak G, and Cabrera MR, "Patients' Acceptance of Internet-Based Home Asthma Telemonitoring," *Proc AMIA Symp*, 1998, 336-40.

Hankinson JL, Odencrantz JR, and Fedan KB, "Spirometric Reference Values From a Sample of the General U.S. Population," *Am J Respir Crit Care Med*, 1999, 159(1):179-87.

Hiebert T, Miles J, and Okeson GC, "Contaminated Aerosol Recovery From Pulmonary Function Testing Equipment," *Am J Respir Crit Care Med*, 1999, 159(2):610-2.

Krieger BP, Isber J, Breitenbucher A, et al, "Serial Measurements of the Rapid-Shallow-Breathing Index as a Predictor of Weaning Outcome in Elderly Medical Patients," *Chest*, 1997, 112(4):1029-34.

Linn WS, Solomon JC, Gong H Jr, et al, "Standardization of Multiple Spirometers at Widely Separated Times and Places," *Am J Respir Crit Care Med*, 1996, 153(4 Pt 1):1309-13.

Rebuck DA, Hanania NA, D'Urzo AD, et al, "The Accuracy of a Handheld Portable Spirometer?" *Chest*, 1996, 109(1):152-7.

Robinson TE, Leung AN, Moss RB, et al, "Standardized High-Resolution CT of the Lung Using a Spirometer-Triggered Electron Beam CT Scanner," *AJR Am J Roentgenol*, 1999, 172(6):1636-8.

Stoller JK, Buist AS, Burrows B, et al, "Quality Control of Spirometry Testing in the Registry for Patients With Severe Alpha1-Antitrypsin Deficiency. Alpha1-Antitrypsin Deficiency Registry Study Group," *Chest*, 1997, 111(4):899-909.

Spirometry Before and After Bronchodilators

Related Information

Bronchial Challenge Test *on page 202*
Flow Volume Loop *on page 225*
Spirometry *on page 249*
Volume of Isoflow (V iso $\dot{V}$) *on page 270*

Synonyms Postbronchodilator Spirometry

Procedure Commonly Includes Vital capacity; forced vital capacity; timed forced expiratory volumes, $FEV_{0.5}$, FEV_1, FEV_3; forced expiratory flows; $FEF_{25\%-75\%}$; peak flow; $FEF_{25\%}$, $FEF_{50\%}$, $FEF_{75\%}$, $\dot{V}_{E\ max\ 25\%}$; $\dot{V}_{E\ max\ 50\%}$; $\dot{V}_{E\ max\ 75\%}$

Indications Assessment of physiologic response to bronchodilator, evaluate the need for additional medication, diagnosis of asthma

Patient Preparation The patient should avoid heavy meals 3 hours prior to testing. Cigarettes should be avoided for 2 hours prior to testing. The patient should be conscious and able to follow simple instructions. The patient's height and weight should be measured without shoes. Loose comfortable clothing that does not restrict chest expansion should be worn. Smoking history including last cigarette smoked should be obtained. Current medication history should be obtained with particular emphasis on bronchodilators and steroids. If assessment of physiologic response to bronchodilator is desired, regularly prescribed bronchodilators should be withheld for 6 hours for inhaled sympathomimetics, 12 hours for short-acting theophylline preparations, and 24 hours for long-acting theophylline preparation. If assessment of the need for additional medication is desired, prebronchodilator and post-bronchodilator testing may be performed while patient continues current bronchodilator therapy without interruption. Resting pulse should be recorded before bronchodilator is given, as administration of a bronchodilator in the presence of resting tachycardia is a relative contraindication.

Aftercare Usually none, although patients that complain of lightheadedness and dizziness should not be allowed to walk unassisted. Some patients, especially those that have not withheld bronchodilators prior to testing may develop tachycardia. Resting pulse rates should be monitored periodically until <100 beats/minute.

Special Instructions Patients that have a tracheostomy stoma may be tested by attaching an infant anesthesia mask to the mouthpiece. Mouthpieces can be adapted directly to most tracheostomy tubes. Effective administration of metered dose bronchodilators may be facilitated by use of a spacing device, especially one that limits inspiratory flow rates. Slow inhalation of the bronchodilator from FRC to RV should be followed by a 5- to 10-second breath-holding period before exhalation.

Technique A spirometer is used to measure exhaled gas and to record the time of collection. Two major categories of spirometers exist. Volume displacement spirometers such as the water seal, dry rolling seal, or bellows spirometers record volume change as vertical deflection on a kymograph or a moving stylus on a sheet of paper. The second category of spirometers integrates the measurement of expired flow over time to yield exhaled volume. Pneumotachograms, turbinometers, and hot wire mass flow meters are examples of flow integrating spirometers. Computer assisted flow integrating spirometers generate a CRT image of volume time or flow volume which can be inspected during testing and later printed. Graphic representation of spirometric data should be inspected along with numeric data to assess reliability of data (see Causes for Rejection). Inhalation of bronchodilator from a metered dose inhaler should occur from FRC to TLC followed by breath-holding for 5-10 seconds. Following a 1-minute waiting period, a second inhalation should be repeated in the same fashion. Repeat testing should be performed when at least 75% of the peak response to the drug is expected (see manufacturer's instructions).

Turnaround Time Preliminary results should be available same day. Depending on the facility, an interpreted report may be available in 1-2 days.

Specimen Measurement of exhaled volumes and flow rates during a maximal forced expiratory maneuver from total lung capacity (TLC) to residual volume

(Continued)

Spirometry Before and After Bronchodilators *(Continued)*

(RV) done before and after administration of an (aerosolized) bronchodilator and an appropriate waiting period suitable for that bronchodilating agent.

Collection Exhaled sample is collected or passed through a volume or flow measuring device known as a spirometer. Spirometers should meet certain minimum standards defined by the American Thoracic Society (ATS). Test may be performed on adults in a seated or standing position and children in a seated position. After applying noseclips the subject is instructed to take a full inspiration, hold it briefly, then exhale through a mouthpiece into the spirometer as forcefully and completely as possible, keeping the chin slightly elevated throughout the maneuver. The test is repeated a minimum of three times until two reproducible efforts have been obtained. Several minutes after baseline spirometry has been obtained and resting pulse shows no tachycardia, an aerosolized bronchodilator is administered via metered dose inhaler, metered dose inhaler and a spacing device, ultrasonic nebulizer, inhaled powder, rubber bulb-type nebulizers, or compressed air-powered nebulizers. Although any bronchodilator may be used, inhaled sympathomimetic amines such as isoproterenol or metaproterenol are usually used. Selective beta-2 agonists should be considered in patients with known cardiac arrhythmias. The timing of postbronchodilator should coincide with the peak response time of the drug being used (5-30 minutes postinhalation with isoproterenol and 10-45 minutes with metaproterenol). The standards for data quality and reproducibility and cause for rejection used for prebronchodilator testing apply to postbronchodilator testing as well. The amount of drug administered and time before performance of postbronchodilator test should be reported.

Causes for Rejection **Cough**, especially when it occurs in the early part of forced expiration, may render all data except expired volume useless. **Hesitant start:** Peak effort must be applied before 50% of total volume is exhaled, otherwise measurement of timed forced expiratory volume may be invalid. (Back extrapolated volume.) **Premature cessation of expiratory effort:** Expiratory effort must be maintained until a valid end-of-test has been observed. ATS has defined a valid end-of-test to be:

- when forced exhalation has continued for at least **6** seconds and a volume plateau (**no** volume change) of at least **1** second duration is seen
- in the absence of a volume plateau, a reasonable exhalation time of at least 15 seconds is observed
- when the patient cannot or should not sustain forced exhalation for valid medical reasons

Although difficult to achieve, the first two conditions for a valid end-of-test should be the goal of each testing session.

Early termination falsely increases $FEV_1/FVC\%$ and increased mean and instantaneous flow rates at middle or low lung volumes (LV). **Submaximal effort:** Indicated by a very low, often nonreproducible peak flow. Neuromuscular disease may produce the same pattern. **Nonreproducibility:** The two largest FVCs and FEV_1s should show <5% variability.

Normal Findings The American Thoracic Society has recommended that increases in the FVC or FEV_1 of at least 20% **and** 0.2 L should be considered significant. Percent change in FVC or FEV_1 should be calculated as follows:

$$\%\ \text{change} = \frac{\text{postbronchodilator value - prebronchodilator value}}{\text{prebronchodilator value}} \times 100$$

Limitations Requires patient cooperation. Poor effort will cause most values reported to be unreliable for evaluative purposes. Transient obstruction secondary to cigarette smoking just prior to testing. Postbronchodilator changes in lung volume may also influence the ratio $FEV_1/FVC\%$. If the FEV_1

and FVC increase equally, or the FVC increases more than FEV_1, the FEV_1/FVC% will show no change or a decline respectively. See figure.

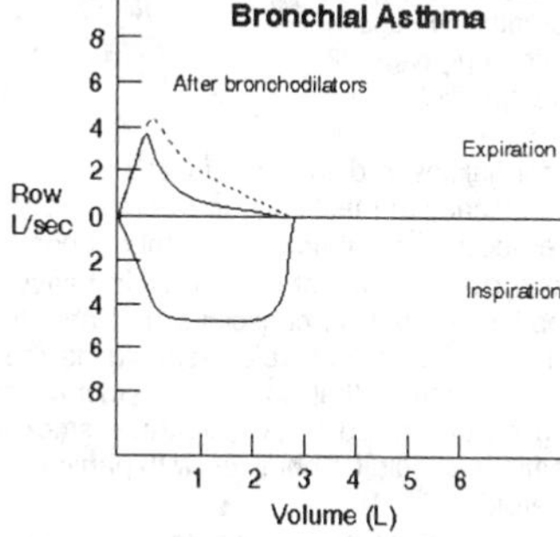

Additional Information Paradoxical decline in spirometric indices have been seen. These may be related to airway sensitivity to metabisulfites used as preservatives in some bronchodilator preparations. Patients with asthma may show progressive decline in spirometric values with repeated efforts yielding excessive variability between two largest efforts. This may be distinguished from variable effort by noting maximal inspiration on each effort followed by an adequately forceful expiration (sharp peak of expiratory flow volume curve). In such cases, the largest and smallest acceptable efforts should be reported giving the physician a rough assessment of bronchial hyper-reactivity. (See Bronchial Challenge Test *on page 202.*) Patients with neuromuscular disease (myasthenia gravis) may show progressive decline of values with repeated efforts but are seldom able to generate an adequate peak effort and may therefore mimic poor effort. Good understanding of the expectations for maximum performance is the key for obtaining reproducible results. It is often helpful to include a demonstration of a proper forced expiratory maneuver as part of the initial instructions. Subsequent instructions should focus on correcting specific deficits in performance. The three most common deficits are:

- failure to inspire to TLC
- failure to begin exhalation with a prompt, forceful blow
- failure to sustain exhalation until valid end-of-test criteria is met

References

Bleecher ER, Tinkelman DG, Ramsdell J, et al, "Proventil® HFA Provides Bronchodilation Comparable to Ventolin® Over 12 Weeks of Regular Use in Asthmatics," *Chest*, 1998, 113(2):283-9.

Crowe JM and Bradley CA, "The Effectiveness of Incentive Spirometry With Physical Therapy for High-Risk Patients After Coronary Artery Bypass Surgery," *Phys Ther*, 1997, 77(3):260-8.

Enright PL, Arnold A, Manolio TA, et al, "Spirometry Reference Values for Healthy Elderly Blacks. The Cardiovascular Health Study Research Group," *Chest*, 1996, 110(6):1416-24.

Hankinson JL, Odencrantz JR, and Fedan KB, "Spirometric Reference Values From a Sample of the General U.S. Population," *Am J Respir Crit Care Med*, 1999, 159(1):179-87.

Linn WS, Solomon JC, Gong H Jr, et al, "Standardization of Multiple Spirometers at Widely Separated Times and Places," *Am J Respir Crit Care Med*, 1996, 153(4 Pt 1):1309-13.

Nelson SB, Gardner RM, Crapo RO, et al, "Performance Evaluation of Contemporary Spirometers," *Chest*, 1990, 97(2):288-97.

O'Donnell DE, "Assessment of Bronchodilator Efficacy in Symptomatic COPD: Is Spirometry Useful?" *Chest*, 2000, 117(2 Suppl):42S-7S.

Rebuck DA, Hanania NA, D'Urzo AD, et al, "The Accuracy of a Handheld Portable Spirometer," *Chest*, 1996, 109(1):152-7.

Sparrow D, O'Connor GT, Weiss ST, et al, "Volume History Effects and Airway Responsiveness in Middle-Aged and Older men. The Normative Aging Study," *Am J Respir Crit Care Med*, 1997, 155(3):888-92.

Stoller JK, Buist AS, Burrows B, et al, "Quality Control of Spirometry Testing in the Registry for Patients With Severe Alpha1-Antitrypsin Deficiency. Alpha1-Antitrypsin Deficiency Registry Study Group," *Chest*, 1997, 111(4):899-909.

Wong HH and Fahy JV, "Safety of one Method of Sputum Induction in Asthmatic Subjects," *Am J Respir Crit Care Med*, 1997, 156(1):299-303.

Spirometry, Sitting and Supine

Related Information

Bedside Spirometry *on page 197*
Flow Volume Loop *on page 225*
Spirometry *on page 249*

Indications

- Detect abnormalities in diaphragm function
- Assess the efficacy of Mestinon® in treatment of myasthenia gravis
- Assess the need for night-time ventilatory support

Patient Preparation The patient should avoid heavy meals 3 hours prior to testing. The patient should be conscious and able to follow simple instructions. The patient's height and weight should be measured without shoes. Loose comfortable clothing that does not restrict chest expansion should be worn. Smoking history including last cigarette smoked should be obtained. Current medications should be obtained with particular emphasis on bronchodilators and steroids.

Aftercare Usually none, although patients that complain of lightheadedness and dizziness should not be allowed to walk unobserved until recovery.

Special Instructions Patients that have a tracheostomy stoma may be tested by attaching an infant anesthesia mask to the mouthpiece. Mouthpieces can be adapted directly to most tracheostomy tubes. Patients with diaphragm dysfunction may find the supine position uncomfortable or intolerable. Every effort should be made to minimize time spent by the patient in the supine position for each effort. Adequate rest in an upright position between efforts is essential. Spirometers that allow patients to inhale from and exhale into the spirometer may require a length of tubing be added to allow testing in the supine position. Only one or two tidal breaths should pass before commencing the vital capacity maneuver, as prolonged breathing of dead space air will increase the patient's sense of panic.

Technique The patient should be treated in the same fashion as a regular spirometry, measuring a vital capacity in the seated position. Repeat testing until two acceptable efforts show <5% variability. (Largest VC - second largest VC/largest VC) x 100 <5%. Allow patient to rest for at least 5 minutes in the seated position. After recovery, have patient lie flat on back and repeat the vital capacity maneuver using the same standards for reproducibility. Allow patient to rest in an upright position after each effort until recovered. Report sitting and supine vital capacity and calculate absolute (mL) and percent decline with change of position. Flow volume loop in sitting and supine position may be done instead of or in addition to vital capacity to obtain additional information.

Turnaround Time Preliminary results should be available same day. Depending on the facility, an interpreted report may be available in 1-2 days.

Specimen Measurement of exhaled volumes and flow rates during a maximal forced expiratory maneuver from total lung capacity to residual volume made while in an upright, seated position and in a supine position.

Collection Exhaled sample is collected or passed through a volume or flow measuring device known as a spirometer while the patient is in a seated position. Spirometers should meet certain minimum standards defined by the American Thoracic Society. After applying noseclips the subject is instructed to take a full inspiration, hold it briefly, then exhale through a mouthpiece into the spirometer as forcefully and completely as possible. Test is repeated a minimum of three times until two reproducible efforts have been obtained. After good results have been obtained in a seated position, the test is repeated with the patient in a supine position. The expiratory maneuver is repeated a minimum of three times until two reproducible efforts have been obtained.

Causes for Rejection Nonreproducibility of test results data is a relative cause for rejection of data. As this test evaluates diaphragm's ability to contract during inspiration, the vital capacity is the most important parameter; the expiratory flow rates (FEV_1, $FEF_{25\%\text{-}75\%}$, $\dot{V}_{E\ max\ 25\%\text{-}50\%,\ and\ 75\%}$) are relatively unimportant. Progressive decline of FVCs or VCs on repeated efforts are often seen in myasthenia gravis and other neuromuscular disorders.

Particular attention should be made to ensure that full inspiration to supine TLC is made, adequate seal is made around mouthpiece without air leakage, full expiration (to RV) is made, and adequate time for the patient's recovery is given between repeat efforts.

Normal Findings Normals show either no decline or very slight decline in vital capacity when tested in a supine position. Although no good studies have been done, a 500 mL decline in VC or FVC is considered evidence of diaphragm dysfunction.

Limitations Requires patient cooperation. Insufficient or inconsistent effort will render sitting vs supine changes in VC unreliable for evaluative purposes.

Additional Information If flow volume loop is done in seated and supine positions, forced expiratory volume in 1 second (FEV_1) in the supine position can be used to predict night-time hypoventilation. If the supine FEV_1 is less than 800-1000 mL, night-time supine hypoventilation is likely. Supine arterial blood gas test during sleep should be done to verify and quantitate degree of alveolar hypoventilation.

References

Aaron SD, Dales RE, and Cardinal P, "How Accurate Is Spirometry at Predicting Restrictive Pulmonary Impairment?" *Chest*, 1999, 115(3):869-73.

Bleecker ER, Tinkelman DG, Ramsdell J, et al, "Proventil® HFA Provides Bronchodilation Comparable to Ventolin® Over 12 Weeks of Regular Use in Asthmatics," *Chest*, 1998, 113(2):283-9.

Crowe JM and Bradley CA, "The Effectiveness of Incentive Spirometry With Physical Therapy for High-Risk Patients After Coronary Artery Bypass Surgery," *Phys Ther*, 1997, 77(3):260-8.

Enright PL, Arnold A, Manolio TA, et al, "Spirometry Reference Values for Healthy Elderly Blacks. The Cardiovascular Health Study Research Group," *Chest*, 1996, 110(6):1416-24.

Hankinson JL, Odencrantz JR, and Fedan KB, "Spirometric Reference Values From a Sample of the General U.S. Population," *Am J Respir Crit Care Med*, 1999, 159(1):179-87.

Linn WS, Solomon JC, Gong H Jr, et al, "Standardization of Multiple Spirometers at Widely Separated Times and Places," *Am J Respir Crit Care Med*, 1996, 153(4 PT 1):1309-13.

Manning F, Dean E, Ross J, et al, "Effects of Side Lying on Lung Function in Older Individuals," *Phys Ther*, 1999, 79(5):456-66.

Meysman M and Vincken W, "Effect of Body Posture on Spirometric Values and Upper Airway Obstruction Indices Derived From the Flow-Volume Loop in Young Nonobese Subjects," *Chest*, 1998, 114(4):1042-7.

O'Donnell DE, "Assessment of Bronchodilator Efficacy in Symptomatic COPD: Is Spirometry Useful?" *Chest*, 2000, 117(2 Suppl):42S-7S.

Pelkonen AS, Hakulinen AL, and Turpeinen M, "Bronchial Lability and Responsiveness in School Children Born Very Preterm," *Am J Respir Crit Care Med*, 1997, 156(4 Pt 1):1178-84.

Rebuck DA, Hanania NA, D'Urzo AD, et al, "The Accuracy of a Handheld Portable Spirometer," *Chest*, 1996, 109(1):152-7.

Stoller JK, Buist AS, Burrows B, et al, "Quality Control of Spirometry Testing in the Registry for Patients With Severe Alpha1-Antitrypsin Deficiency. Alpha1-Antitrypsin Deficiency Registry Study Group," *Chest*, 1997, 111(4):899-909.

Wong HH and Fahy JV, "Safety of One Method of Sputum Induction in Asthmatic Subjects," *Am J Respir Crit Care Med*, 1997, 156(1):299-303.

♦ **Spirometry With Flow Volume Loop** *see* Flow Volume Loop *on page 225*

Sputum Induction

Procedure Commonly Includes Induction of sputum expectoration by inhalation of nebulized pyrogen-free or 3% saline

Indications Aid in the diagnosis of malignancy or infection in patients who are unable to expectorate sputum

Contraindications

- asthma
- bronchospasm
- respiratory distress

Patient Preparation The teeth should be brushed and the oropharynx rinsed to minimize contamination.

Aftercare Monitor for bronchospasm. Beta-agonists may be needed.

Complications Bronchospasm, vigorous coughing

Equipment Ultrasonic nebulizer, pyrogen-free or 3% saline, sputum trap or saline specimen container

Technique Pyrogen-free or 3% saline is administered to the patient by ultrasonic nebulizer for 5-15 minutes, saturating the airways, liquefying thick sputum, and leading to a productive cough. The expectorated sputum is collected in a sputum trap or specimen container. If the patient cannot cough, or oro- or nasotracheal suction catheter may be used to aspirate the specimen.

(Continued)

Sputum Induction *(Continued)*

Data Acquired Sputum for microbiologic and cytologic studies

Turnaround Time Stains yield immediate results, routine cultures in 24-48 hours, mycobacterial and fungal cultures may take weeks.

Specimen Sputum

Container Sputum trap or sterile specimen container

Collection Expectorated sputum is collected after administration of nebulized saline.

Storage Instructions The specimen is collected in a sputum trap or sterile specimen container. It should be immediately stained and plated for culture.

Causes for Rejection >25 squamous epithelial cells/lpf (indicates oropharyngeal contamination)

Normal Findings No malignant cells or pathogenic organisms

Limitations Weak cough, tenacious sputum, or uncooperative patient make retrieval difficult.

References

Kips JC, Fahy JV, Hargreave FE, et al, "Methods for Sputum Induction and Analysis of Induced Sputum: A Method for Assessing Airway Inflammation in Asthma," *Eur Respir J Suppl*, 1998, 26:9S-12S.

Kips JC, Peleman RA, and Pauwels RA, "Methods of Examining Induced Sputum: Do Differences Matter?" *Eur Respir J*, 1998, 11(3):529-33.

♦ **Static Lung Volumes** *see* Functional Residual Capacity *on page 229*

♦ **Static Lung Volumes** *see* Lung Subdivisions *on page 233*

Swan-Ganz Catheterization

Related Information

Arterial Cannulation *on page 17*
Cardiac Catheterization, Adult *on page 21*
Pericardiocentesis *on page 39*
Pleural Biopsy *on page 238*

Synonyms Pulmonary Artery Catheterization; Right Heart Catheterization

Applies to Arterial Lines

Procedure Commonly Includes Insertion of a flexible, balloon-tipped catheter into the pulmonary artery for hemodynamic monitoring of the critically ill patient. Although Swan-Ganz catheterization is considered an invasive procedure, it may be safely performed at the bedside in an intensive care unit setting, using continuous EKG and blood pressure monitoring. In brief, this technique involves cannulation of a large vein, such as the subclavian or internal jugular vein. A flow-directed catheter is advanced through the central venous system into the right atrium (RA), right ventricle (RV), and pulmonary artery (PA). If desired, the catheter may be further "wedged" briefly into a small pulmonary artery branch. Direct pressure measurements are obtained in the respective cardiac chambers and pulmonary artery. An indirect measurement of left atrial filling pressure is obtained when the catheter is "wedged". In addition, other hemodynamic parameters may be easily measured, such as the cardiac output, systemic vascular resistance (SVR), mixed venous oxygen saturation, and intrapulmonary shunt fraction. Swan-Ganz catheterization has become an integral (and sometimes routine) procedure in the modern intensive care unit and has revolutionized the practice of critical care medicine.

Indications Pulmonary artery catheterization is indicated in the following situations:

- acute myocardial infarction with hemodynamic instability
- severe hypotension of unknown etiology, especially if the response to initial therapy is inadequate (eg, volume loading)
- selected cases of septic shock
- adult respiratory distress syndrome, to confirm the diagnosis of noncardiogenic pulmonary edema (normal "wedge" pressure) and to aid in subsequent fluid and ventilator management
- suspected cases of cardiac tamponade, to confirm the diagnosis, monitor hemodynamics during pericardiocentesis, and follow response to therapy
- suspected papillary muscle rupture

- possible ventricular septal defect or atrial septal defect following myocardial infarction
- congestive heart failure responding poorly to diuretics, especially when intravascular volume status is uncertain
- intraoperative monitoring of patients undergoing open heart surgery, particularly coronary artery bypass procedures involving multiple vessels; patients undergoing abdominal aortic aneurysm repair may also benefit from PA catheterization perioperatively

Swan-Ganz catheterization may also be useful in the following scenarios:

- drug overdose, especially when the risk of acute lung damage is high (eg, heroin, aspirin)
- exacerbations of chronic obstructive lung disease requiring intubation; hemodynamic monitoring may detect occult or superimposed causes of respiratory failure not suspected clinically (eg, left ventricular dysfunction)
- end-stage liver failure with deteriorating renal function
- suspected cases of pulmonary hypertension

In general, Swan-Ganz catheterization is indicated when measurement of right atrial, pulmonary artery, and pulmonary artery occlusive pressures will significantly alter patient management. The threshold for performing this procedure varies considerably amongst clinicians; some authorities feel this technique is overutilized and is indicated in only rare circumstances.

Contraindications

- severe, uncorrectable coagulopathy
- presence of a left bundle branch block (LBBB) on EKG; placement of a right heart catheter may lead to complete heart block (A-V dissociation) if an underlying LBBB is present
- local infection at the skin insertion site
- severe hypothermia; in this situation the myocardium is highly irritable and prone to malignant arrhythmias induced by the catheter
- inadequate monitoring equipment; continuous EKG monitoring with blood pressure measurements is necessary during catheter insertion
- patient refusal

Patient Preparation Technique and risks of the procedure are explained to the patient. When patient is comatose or disoriented, the appropriate guardians should be contacted. Catheterization may be safely performed in an intensive care unit, specialized procedure room with telemetry and fluoroscopy, or a formal Cardiac Catheterization Laboratory. A standard emergency room or regular nursing floor is generally not equipped for this procedure. No specific patient preparation is required and often this procedure is performed on an urgent basis. Whenever possible, aspirin and nonsteroidal anti-inflammatory agents should be discontinued in advance, but this is not absolutely necessary. Effects of heparin or warfarin, however, should be reversed prior to catheterization. If an underlying coagulopathy is suspected (eg, disseminated intravascular coagulation, thrombocytopenia), appropriate laboratory studies should be obtained immediately including a platelet count and PT/PTT. In most cases, parenteral sedation is unnecessary; however the use of agents such as meperidine (Demerol®) is at the physician's discretion.

Complications

- balloon rupture
- conduction disturbance (ie, new right bundle branch block 5%)
- arrhythmias (3% ventricular tachycardia, 2% ventricular fibrillation)
- pulmonary infarction/pulmonary hemorrhage
- perforation or rupture of the pulmonary artery
- knotting of the catheter
- thrombosis of a blood vessel (ie, 1% to 2% superior vena cava syndrome)
- pulmonary emboli
- infection (0% to 5%)
- blood loss, including hemothorax, retroperitoneal bleed, etc
- inadvertent arterial puncture (6% femoral)
- pneumothorax and tension pneumothorax (0% to 6%)
- valvular trauma
- disconnection of the introducer apparatus with disappearance into the vein

(Continued)

Swan-Ganz Catheterization *(Continued)*

Equipment

- I.V. pole and pressure monitor manifold, pressure monitor
- normal saline (250-500 mL) with heparin (1000 units) for flush
- pressure bag
- pressure tubing
- stopcocks (3-way)
- cutdown tray (for peripheral approach)
- vein introducer kit
- Swan-Ganz catheter kit
- 1% lidocaine for local anesthesia
- bowl of sterile saline (flush and balloon integrity check)
- suture
- instrument set
- 3 and 5 mL syringes
- 25-gauge needle for anesthesia
- gloves, gowns, masks
- sterile dressing kit (surgical drapes)
- bedside table on which to place instruments
- telemetry monitor for heart rate and rhythm automatic blood pressure cuff, A-line
- Betadine® scrub

Technique Swan-Ganz catheterization can take place via a variety of approaches including internal jugular vein, subclavian vein, femoral vein, or brachial vein. The last of these approaches most commonly entails direct visualization of the brachial vein from a cut-down exposure. The procedure should be performed in a closely monitored setting, enabling constant recording of heart rate, rhythm, and frequent blood pressure readings, usually an intensive care unit. The procedure may be performed at the patient's bedside with or without the assistance of fluoroscopic guidance. Sterile technique is required for catheter insertion. The skin at the site of approach is most commonly prepped with a Betadine® scrub. Often, if the internal jugular or subclavian veins are utilized, the patient is placed in a Trendelenburg position to assist with central venous distension and ease of access. The physician should scrub and wear gown, mask, and gloves. The patient is then draped with sterile sheets (most institutions drape the patient from head to toe, while others require a sterile field only at the site of access). The patient should be cooperative for catheter insertion. If a patient is uncooperative or becomes uncooperative during the procedure, sedation may be given at the discretion of the physician. Upon initiation of the procedure, the skin and subcutaneous tissue are infiltrated with lidocaine (1%) and a small gauge needle. Deeper tissues may then be infiltrated with lidocaine for the comfort of the patient. A thin gauged needle (21-gauge, 1½") is usually attached to a 5 mL syringe and used to localize the vessel of interest for a central venous approach. Once the vessel has been located, a large gauge needle (16- or 18-gauge) is then attached to a syringe and placed into the vessel following the course of the "finder needle." When blood is aspirated easily into the syringe, the syringe is disconnected from the needle and a flexible guidewire is threaded through the needle into the vein. Wire placement can cause a variety of complications, most often ventricular ectopy. If an increase in ectopy is observed, the guidewire should be withdrawn several centimeters. Once the guidewire has been passed into the vessel, the needle is removed from the patient. At no time should the physician lose control of the tip of the guidewire. Failure to control the guidewire can cause serious complications and death if lost in the patient. Once the needle is removed, a dilator is advanced over the guidewire and through the skin, to facilitate passage of a venous introducer. The introducer should be flushed with heparinized saline prior to insertion to avoid air emboli. Once the tract along the guidewire is dilated, the dilator should be slipped off the guidewire (maintaining guidewire position **in** the vein). The introducer and dilator can then be put together as a unit (dilator within introducer) and slid over the guidewire into the vein, again taking care to control the tip of the guidewire outside the patient's body. After the placement of the introducer and guidewire assembly, the guidewire and dilator should be removed from the patient. This leaves only the venous introducer sheath within the patient. At this point, if the introducer has a side port lumen, venous blood should be aspirated and the introducer then flushed. If blood cannot be aspirated via a side-port lumen, the introducer is incorrectly placed and must be reinserted. No blood should come from the center of the introducer since this piece is usually accompanied by a one-way ball valve which does not allow blood leakage. The introducer should then be secured to the patient's skin with sutures. When the venous introducer has been placed, the Swan-Ganz catheter can then be inserted. Prior to catheter insertion, the balloon tip should be checked under sterile water for leaks and the catheter flushed. The catheter should then be connected to the appropriate pressure monitoring lines and flushed again via the pressure tubing to ensure that the catheter is bubble-free and that a column of uninterrupted fluid exists from the tubing through the tip of the catheter. The catheter can then be guided via the introducer, through the central venous system, through the right atrium, right ventricle, pulmonary artery, and into the wedge position. The catheter usually passes smoothly through the circulation, with the aid of the inflated balloon at its tip. The catheter should never be withdrawn with the balloon inflated. Catheter position can be ascertained by pressure wave forms, although fluoroscopy can be quite helpful in guiding the catheter into the wedge position. A chest radiograph is usually obtained after catheter insertion to verify position, as well as to rule out the possibility of pneumothorax if the subclavian or internal jugular approach was utilized.

Normal Findings Normal resting hemodynamic values:

- right atrium → mean: 0-8 mm Hg; A wave: 2-10 mm Hg; V wave: 2-10 mm Hg
- right ventricle → systolic: 15-30 mm Hg; end-diastolic: 0-8 mm Hg
- pulmonary artery → systolic: 15-30 mm Hg; end-diastolic: 3-12 mm Hg
- wedge → A wave: 3-15 mm Hg; V wave: 3-12 mm Hg; mean: 5-12 mm Hg
- AVO_2 difference (mL/L) → 30-50
- cardiac output (L/minute) → 4.0-6.5 (varies with patient size)
- cardiac index (L/minute/m^2) → 2.6-4.6
- pulmonary vascular resistance (dynes - second - cm^{-2}) → 20-130
- systemic vascular resistance (dynes - second - cm^{-2}) → 700-1600

The right atrial waveform normally has two major positive deflections, the A wave and the V wave. The A wave is due to atrial systole and follows the P wave inscribed on the EKG. The X descent follows this initial positive deflection and is often interrupted by a small positive deflection called the C wave, which occurs with tricuspid valve closure. At the nadir of the X descent, full atrial relaxation has occurred and pressure in the right atrium begins to rise again with atrial refilling. Rise in right atrial pressure during ventricular systole is called the V wave and it reaches its peak prior to tricuspid valve opening. The Y descent then occurs as the tricuspid valve opens and the right atrium empties into the right ventricle. The pulmonary artery wedge pressure normally has a waveform similar to left atrial pressure, but is delayed in transmission through the capillary vessels. A normal wedge should show clear A and V waves; however, C waves are most often not visible. X and Y descents should be fairly clear as long as the pressure tracing is not overdamped.

Critical Values Pressure tracings may be virtually diagnostic of certain conditions. For example, mitral stenosis is associated with a pressure gradient in diastole across the mitral valve (wedge or left atrial pressure vs left ventricular pressure). A large V wave in the pulmonary artery wedge tracing may be seen with mitral regurgitation, since the amplitude of the V wave is affected by left atrial filling from the pulmonary veins as well as the regurgitant volume from the left ventricle. Stenotic and regurgitant lesions of the pulmonic and tricuspid valves can also be documented by right sided heart catheterization using simultaneous recordings or by pull back techniques. With regard to the hemodynamic profile rendered by the Swan-Ganz catheter, certain general parameters can be quite useful. Decreases in right atrial pressure, pulmonary capillary wedge pressure, and cardiac index/output can indicate hypovolemia. (Continued)

Swan-Ganz Catheterization *(Continued)*

Waveform Transition As Catheter Is Advanced From RA to Wedge Position

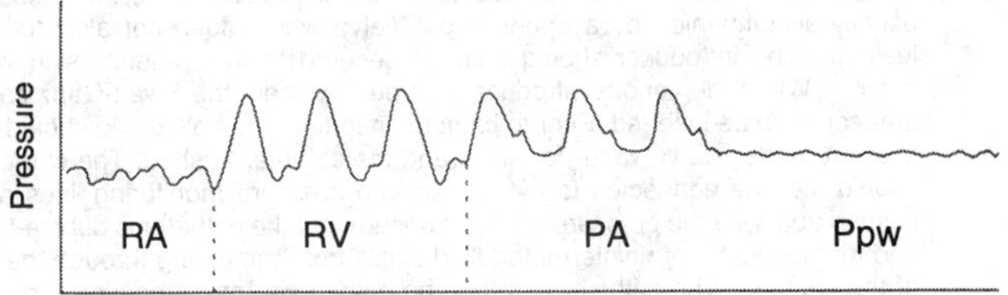

Adapted from Leartherna SW and Marini J, "Clinical Uses of the Pulmonary Artery Catheter," Principles of Critical Care, Chapter 25, New York, NY: McGraw-Hill Book Co, 1992, 327.

In cases of elevated right atrial pressures with concomitant low wedge pressures and low cardiac index/output (especially in the face of an inferior wall myocardial infarction) one may suspect right ventricular involvement and failure. Pulmonary congestion due to left ventricular failure or volume overload will increase the pulmonary artery wedge pressure (ie, congestion usually occurs at a wedge pressure in excess of 18 mm Hg and frank pulmonary edema occurs with a wedge pressure in the upper twenties and above). Cardiogenic shock and pulmonary edema are characterized by signs of hypoperfusion, with hemodynamic data including systemic hypotension, markedly decreased cardiac index (<2.1 L/minute/m^2), and elevated wedge pressures (often well >18 mm Hg). Septic shock is also characterized by clinical signs of hypoperfusion, but may be differentiated from cardiogenic shock by certain hemodynamic data which often include a normal or near normal wedge pressure, an elevated cardiac index/output, and a marked decrease in systemic vascular resistance. Caution should be exercised in that these parameters are only general guidelines, and during the course of a patient's illness, such information may not always be exact. As always, history and physical examination are critical in the diagnostic assessment of each patient. The catheter can aid with diagnostic dilemmas, but is most useful as a management tool. Pulmonary artery catheters can also be useful in the diagnosis of ventricular septal defects by sampling O_2 saturations as the catheter is advanced from the great veins to the right atrium to the right ventricle and out into the pulmonary artery. An oxygen "step-up" from the right atrium to the right ventricle of approximately 10% is indicative of left to right shunting. In the appropriate setting of acute myocardial infarction and sudden deterioration after a stable course, this diagnosis may be a consideration; right heart catheterization is one method to establish the diagnosis. Other causes of an O_2 step-up include coronary fistula draining into the RV, primum atrial septal defects, and pulmonic insufficiency with a patent ductus arteriosus. Cardiac tamponade is another diagnosis which can be documented by pulmonary artery catheter measurements. Rising intrapericardial pressures interfere with diastolic filling of the heart. Marked increases in the end-diastolic pulmonary artery (PA), right ventricular (RV) , and right atrial (RA) pressures to the same value ("equalization of the pressures") strongly suggest tamponade. Somewhat similar findings may be seen with constrictive and restrictive diseases, discussion of which is beyond this outline. Pulmonary hypertension and increased pulmonary vascular resistance can suggest such diagnoses as pulmonary embolism or even mitral stenosis. Care must be taken in the interpretation of all hemodynamic data derived from the catheter.[1]

Footnotes

1. Raper R and Sibbald WJ, "Misled by the Wedge? The Swan-Ganz Catheter and Left Ventricular Preload," *Chest*, 1986, 89(3):427-34.

References

Amin DK and Shah PK, "The Swan-Ganz Catheter," *J Crit Illness*, 1986, 1(4):24-45, 1(5):40-61.

Learthena SW and Marini J, "Clinical Uses of the Pulmonary Artery Catheter," *Principles of Critical Care*, 2nd ed, Chapter 14, Hall JB, Schmidt GA, Wood LDH, et al, eds, New York, NY: McGraw-Hill Book Co, 1998, 155-76.

Matthay MA and Chatterjee K, "Bedside Catheterization of the Pulmonary Artery: Risks Compared With Benefits," *Ann Intern Med*, 1988, 109(10):826-34.

Thoracentesis

Related Information

Pleural Biopsy *on page 238*
Ultrasound, Thoracentesis *on page 506*

Synonyms Pleural Fluid "Tap"

Procedure Commonly Includes Percutaneously inserting a needle and catheter system into the pleural space to withdraw fluid from a patient with radiographically demonstrable pleural fluid for diagnostic and/or therapeutic purposes

Indications The major diagnostic indication is the presence of significant pleural fluid of unclear etiology. The major therapeutic indication is respiratory compromise secondary to a large pleural effusion.

Contraindications

- effusions <10 mm thick or not freely movable on a decubitus radiograph

Relative contraindications:

- platelet count <50,000/mm^3
- uncorrectable coagulopathy
- poor landmarks
- uncooperative patient
- mechanical ventilation with PEEP
- severe emphysema with blebs
- limited respiratory reserve (eg, postpneumonectomy)
- infection at the site of needle entry

Patient Preparation The patient should be sitting, if possible, with crossed arms and head resting on a table. Parenteral pain medications and/or anxiolytics are rarely required.

Aftercare Vital signs are closely monitored. Dyspnea, hypotension, and desaturation suggest a complication. An end-expiratory chest radiograph can be attained to rule out pneumothorax. If asymptomatic with stable vitals and a satisfactory chest radiograph the patient may resume normal activity.

Complications There are many traumatic and nontraumatic potential complications. Traumatic complications include pneumothorax (simple or tension), hemothorax, laceration of an intercostal artery/liver/kidney/spleen, subcutaneous emphysema, infection, air embolism, and tumor seeding of needle tract. Nontraumatic complications include syncope, cough, hypotension, noncardiogenic pulmonary edema, and hypoxemia.

Equipment Complete thoracentesis kits are available. Alternatively, the individual components may be assembled separately. Sterile drapes and gloves, iodine solution/swabs, gauze, a local anesthetic agent (1% lidocaine), four sterile tubes (or two red and two lavender top tubes), syringes, infiltrating needles, and aerobic/anaerobic culture bottles are needed. A heparinized syringe and small bag of ice are needed for pH measurement. A needle and catheter assembly is used. Generally, a 2" 18-gauge angiocatheter is satisfactory, though the 12" 16-gauge catheter that comes in thoracentesis kits may also be used. Liter sized vacuum bottles and connecting tubing are useful for therapeutic procedures. A bandage completes the list.

Technique Once the patient is prepared (see Patient Preparation) the highest level of pleural effusion is determined by physical exam and a mark is placed one intercostal space lower in the posterior axillary line. The area is prepped and draped, and the skin and subcutaneous tissues are infiltrated with local anesthetic. If the pleural space is entered with the infiltrating needle, a note is made of the distance from the skin surface to the fluid. The needle and catheter assembly is then passed, usually attached to a syringe with suction being applied, over the superior aspect of the rib in the anesthetized area (to avoid the neurovascular bundle). Once the parietal pleura is penetrated, the fluid should be easily aspirated into the syringe. The needle and catheter is

(Continued)

Thoracentesis *(Continued)*

supported with the operating hand in contact with the chest wall to avoid inadvertent advancement. If unable to attain fluid, the location may be incorrect, the needle too short, or the fluid too viscous. If the procedure is therapeutic, the catheter is then advanced into the pleural space and the needle withdrawn. Fluid can then be aspirated into large syringes or the catheter can be attached to connecting tubing and the fluid drained into a vacuum bottle. When the needle is removed, or with any disconnection from the catheter, the patient should be asked to exhale or say "eeee" and the operators thumb is placed over the catheter opening so as to avoid drawing air into the pleural space. The initial fluid sample is drawn into or immediately injected into a heparinized syringe which is placed on ice for purposes of pH determination. Subsequent fluid samples are injected into the four sterile tubes and culture bottles. A mL of heparin is added (particularly if bloody) to prevent formation of a coagulum. Once the desired amount of fluid is drained, or when fluid is no longer able to be aspirated, the catheter is withdrawn and pressure is held over the puncture site. Blood should be sent for protein and LDH at around the same time.

Data Acquired Cell counts, chemistries, pH, microbiologic and cytologic studies of pleural fluid

Turnaround Time Immediately for pH; a few hours for chemistries, cell counts, and microbiologic stains; 24-48 hours for routine cultures and cytology; up to weeks for specialized cultures

Specimen Pleural fluid

Container Four sterile tubes (or two red and two lavender top tubes) with 1 mL heparin if effusion is bloody, sterile syringe, culture bottles, vacuum container, heparinized syringe on ice for pH

Collection Pleural fluid is percutaneously aspirated into a syringe or vacuum bottle.

Storage Instructions Heparinized syringe should be placed on ice and immediately transported to the laboratory. If there is delay in transporting other samples, they should be refrigerated. Heparin is added to containers if effusion is bloody.

Causes for Rejection Improper collection and storage technique

Normal Findings No significant pleural fluid

Critical Values The first step is to separate the type of effusion into a transudate (results from imbalances of hydrostatic and osmotic forces in the pleural or pulmonary capillaries) or exudate (results from increased permeability of pleural or pulmonary capillaries). An exudate is present if one or more of three criteria are present:

1. Pleural fluid protein to serum protein ratio >0.5
2. Pleural fluid LDH to serum LDH ratio >0.6
3. Pleural fluid LDH >200 IU or two-thirds the upper limit of normal serum LDH

If none of these criteria are met, the fluid is a transudate.

A hemothorax is indicated by a pleural fluid hematocrit >50% that of peripheral blood while a chylothorax is present if the triglyceride level is >110 mg/dL. Many other values can narrow the differential diagnosis of exudates but are not specific markers of one etiology. Examples include:

- Glucose <60 - parapneumonic, empyema, TB, malignancy, rheumatoid arthritis, hemothorax, paragonimiasis, and Churg-Strauss
- Disease pH <7.2 - complicated parapneumonic, empyema, rheumatoid arthritis, malignancy, TB
- WBC >10,000 - parapneumonic, pancreatitis, pulmonary infarct, collagen-vascular disease, malignancy, TB
- Lymphocytosis >50% - granulomatous disease, malignancy, postoperative
- Eosinophilia >10% - hemo- or pneumothorax, drugs, asbestos, Churg-Strauss, resolving parapneumonic, paragonimiasis
- Protein >6 - parapneumonic, TB
- Pleural fluid amylase: serum amylase, >1 - pancreatic, esophageal rupture, malignancy elevated cholesterol - chyliform, TB, rheumatoid arthritis

- ANA >1:160 - SLE
- Adenosine deaminase >70 units/L - TB
- Interferon gamma >200 pg/mL - TB

Additional Information Pleural fluid cholesterol, bilirubin ratio, albumin gradient, and specific gravity have been used to distinguish transudate from exudate but add little to the above criteria.

References

Bartter T, Santarelli R, Akers SM, et al, "The Evaluation of Pleural Effusion," *Chest*, 1994, 106(4):1209-14.

Grogan DR, Irwin RS, Channick R, et al, "Complications Associated With Thoracentesis. A Prospective, Randomized Study Comparing Three Different Methods," *Arch Intern Med*, 1990, 150(4):873-7.

Norris AM and Burke CM, "Diagnostic Thoracentesis," *Chest*, 1990, 98(5):1251-2.

Ogirala RG and Azrieli FM, "Thoracentesis and Closed Pleural Biopsy," *Interventional Pulmonology*, Beamis JF Jr and Mathur PN, eds, New York, NY: McGraw-Hill Book Co, 1999, 223-40.

Qureshi N, Momin ZA, and Brandstetter RD, "Thoracentesis in Clinical Practice," *Heart Lung*, 1994, 23(5):376-83.

Stogner SW and Campbell GD, "Pleural Effusion. What You Can Learn From the Results of a "Tap"," *Postgrad Med*, 1992, 91(5):439-42, 445-54.

Thoracic Gas Volume

Related Information

Airway Resistance *on page 187*
Functional Residual Capacity *on page 229*

Procedure Commonly Includes Thoracic gas volume (TGV) reported in $liter_{BTPS}$

Indications Used in the calculation of **static lung volumes** in the same fashion as the functional residual capacity. Static lung volumes are used to categorize lung function into obstructive, restrictive, and combined abnormalities. May be used to assess the severity of lung disease. May be compared with FRC measured by helium dilution or nitrogen washout techniques to assess the volume of noncommunicating air spaces within the lungs (cysts or bullae). **Caution**: See Additional Information. Usually measured in conjunction with measurements of airway resistance, which must be standardized to the lung volume at which it is measured to calculate specific airway resistance.

Contraindications Severe claustrophobia may contraindicate this measurement. Patients that cannot follow simple instructions should be excluded.

Patient Preparation The patient should avoid heavy meals 3 hours prior to testing. The patient should be conscious and able to follow simple instructions. The patient's height and weight should be measured without shoes. Loose comfortable clothing that does not restrict chest expansion should be worn. Smoking history including last cigarette smoked should be obtained. Current medications should be obtained with particular emphasis on bronchodilators and steroids.

Aftercare Usually none needed

Special Instructions Patients must often be instructed to press the palms of the hands against their cheeks during occluded airway panting to avoid bowing out of the cheeks. Patients should be instructed to apply gentle effort against the closed shutter, effort should be equal on inspiration and expiration.

Technique Thoracic gas volume is the measurement of all air in the thorax at end expiration (FRC) by plethysmographic technique as opposed to gas dilution technique. (See Functional Residual Capacity *on page 229*.) The patient is placed in a closed chamber which can monitor chamber pressure, mouth pressure (just distal to the mouthpiece), and flow. The patient breathes through a special manifold which contains a shutter for occlusion of the airway. This shutter is closed at end expiration and the subject is asked to pant lightly against the closed shutter, alternately compressing and expanding the volume of air in the lungs and the chamber. During conditions of zero flow (closed shutter) mouth pressure changes reflect alveolar pressure changes. Changes in box pressure secondary to thoracic volume changes are proportional to alveolar gas pressure changes. Because the inverse relationship between mouth (alveolar) and box pressure is linear, Boyle's law, $P_1V_1=P_2V_2$, can be used to solve for the volume of gas being compressed, the thoracic gas volume.

(Continued)

Thoracic Gas Volume *(Continued)*

Turnaround Time Preliminary result usually available same day, interpreted report to follow in 1-2 days.

Specimen Measurement of mouth pressure versus box pressure during end-tidal occluded airway panting in a body plethysmograph.

Causes for Rejection Loops that do not close are usually secondary to compression of gas in the cheeks or varying inspiratory and expiratory effort.

Normal Findings Regression equations derived from studies that used helium dilution technique or nitrogen washout technique for measurement of FRC may be used. No studies used plethysmographic technique to develop normal values for TGV.

Limitations Some patients find being enclosed in a body box uncomfortable, even unacceptable. Some patients find it difficult to pant against a closed shutter.

Additional Information Plethysmographically thoracic gas volume is felt by many to be the "gold standard" for lung volume determination because it measures all gas within the thorax, even gas trapped in pockets that do not communicate with the central airways. Mouth pressures may underestimate alveolar pressures in patients with severe airways obstruction leading to overestimation of thoracic gas volume. Panting with the accessory muscles may compress intra-abdominal gas and lead to erroneously high TGV. This error is insignificant with normal panting technique.

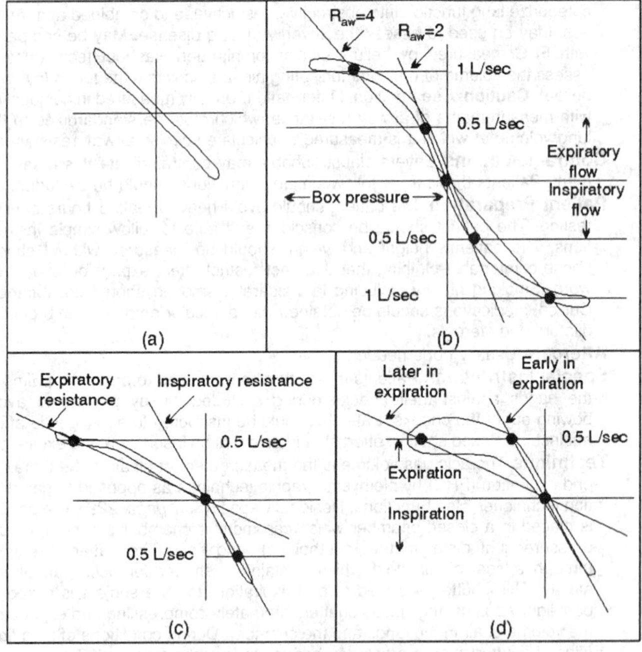

Plethysimographic loops for (a) TGV and (b, c, d) R_{aw}

Reproduced with permission from Clausen, JL, *Pulmonary Function Testing Guidelines and Controversies*, London England: Grund & Stratton, Inc, 1984, 148.

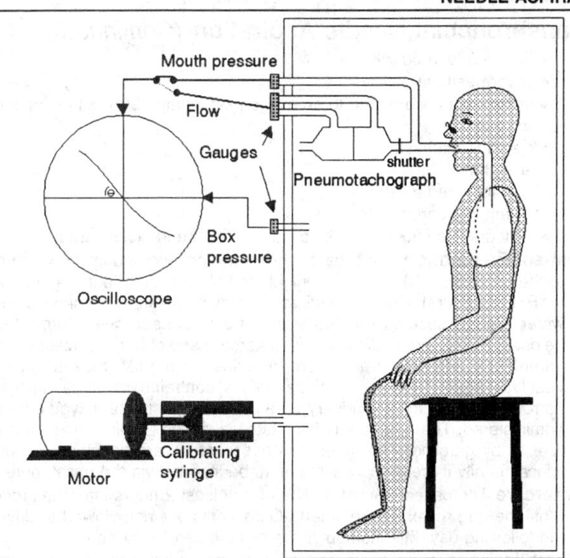

Configuration of a pressure (constant volume) body plethysmograph. Not shown are the large and small ports for pressure relief within the box. Reproduced with permission from Cotes JE, *Lung Function*, Oxford, England: Blackwell, 1979, 116.

References

Agrawal A and Agrawal KP, "Body Plethysmographic Measurement of Thoracic Gas Volume Without Panting Against a Shutter," *J Appl Physiol*, 1996, 81(2):1007-11.

McCrory MA, Mole PA, Gomez TD, et al, "Body Composition by Air-Displacement Plethysmography by Using Predicted and Measured Thoracic Gas Volumes," *J Appl Physiol*, 1998, 84(4):1475-9.

Nikolaizik WH and Schoni MH, "Pilot Study to Assess the Effect of Inhaled Corticosteroids on Lung Function in Patients With Cystic Fibrosis," *J Pediatr*, 1996, 128(2):271-4.

Peslin R and Duvivier C, "Evaluation of a Forced Oscillation Method to Measure Thoracic Gas Volume," *J Appl Physiol*, 1998, 84(3):862-7.

Peslin R and Duvivier C, "Partitioning of Airway and Respiratory Tissue Mechanical Impedances by Body Plethysmography," *J Appl Physiol*, 1998, 84(2):53-61.

Peslin R, Hannhart B, Duvivier C, et al, "Thoracic Gas Volume Measurements in Chronic Obstructive Pulmonary Disease by Low Frequency Ambient Pressure Changes," *Am Rev Respir Dis*, 1988, 137(2):277-80.

Zollinger A, Zaugg M, Weder W, et al, "Video-Assisted Thoracoscopic Volume Reduction Surgery in Patients With Diffuse Pulmonary Emphysema: Gas Exchange and Anesthesiological Management," *Anesth Analg*, 1997, 84(4):845-51.

♦ **Titration of Oxygen or Nasal CPAP During Sleep** *see* Cardiopulmonary Sleep Study *on page 221*

♦ **Total Lung Capacity** *see* Functional Residual Capacity *on page 229*

Transbronchial Needle Aspiration

Related Information

Bronchoscopy, Flexible *on page 209*

Synonyms Wang Needle Aspiration

Procedure Commonly Includes Sampling lymph nodes/masses adjacent to the central airways with a needle extended through a bronchoscope

Indications Aid in the diagnosis and staging of potentially malignant and nonmalignant mediastinal and hilar adenopathy, extrinsic compression of the airway by a peribronchial process, submucosal disease, peripheral nodules, endobronchial lesions, and mediastinal cysts or abscesses

Contraindications All are relative contraindications:

- uncooperative patient

(Continued)

Transbronchial Needle Aspiration *(Continued)*

- FEV_1 <800-1000 mL
- severe asthma
- hypoxemia uncorrected to an oxygen saturation >90% with supplemental oxygen
- bleeding diathesis
- arrhythmia
- unstable cardiac status
- recent myocardial infarction
- radiographic suggestion of vascular structure in biopsy area

Patient Preparation The patient should have no food or drink for 8 hours prior to the procedure (NPO after midnight for AM procedure; early light breakfast for PM procedure). Routine medications may be taken with a small amount of water. Normal coagulation studies and a platelet count >50,000/mm^3 should be documented. Premedication with a narcotic and/or benzodiazepine is given parenterally prior to the procedure. Atropine 0.4 mg I.M. may be given as a vagolytic agent to dry secretions unless contraindicated (ie, arrhythmia, narrow angle glaucoma, urinary retention). Supplemental oxygen is usually administered. The oropharynx is anesthetized with 2% lidocaine via a nebulizer or by gargling. The nares and nasopharynx are anesthetized with 2% lidocaine jelly if the bronchoscope is to be inserted via the nasal route.

Aftercare The patient should be NPO for at least 2 hours after the procedure (until the gag reflex has returned). Outpatients are not allowed to drive until the following day. Mild hemoptysis may be noted for 24 hours.

Complications Hypoxemia and bronchospasm as with all bronchoscopic procedures. Pneumothorax, pneumomediastinum, hemomediastinum, damage to the bronchoscope, and bleeding, though rare, are the major complications of TBNA.

Equipment Flexible bronchoscope with light source, 22- and/or 19-gauge Wang transbronchial needle and assembly, slides, container with preservative (eg, formalin or alcohol-based, eg, Cytolyte®), syringes, lidocaine, and sedatives

Technique The bronchoscope is passed in the usual manner and advanced to the site of interest (usually based on radiographic or bronchoscopic evidence). If a staging procedure is being performed, the highest station is sampled first. For a cytology specimen, the 22-gauge needle is used. It is passed through a straight bronchoscope with the needle retracted into it's protective sheath to avoid damaging the scope. Once the distal metal hub is seen, the scope is advanced to its target and directed in a somewhat perpendicular manner towards the wall of the airway. There are several techniques for penetrating the tracheobronchial wall:

- Hub against the wall: With the needle retracted, the distal metal hub is placed against the tracheobronchial wall and held in place while the needle is extended through.
- Jabbing: An extended needle is directed towards the target and thrust through the intercartilaginous space with the scope fixed proximally
- Piggyback: An extended needle is positioned and the catheter is fixed at the proximal insertion port. The bronchoscope and needle are then pushed forward together until the needle penetrates the wall.
- Cough: The jabbing or piggyback method is used while the patient coughs, assisting needle penetration.

When the needle is inserted, suction is applied proximally to the side port. If there is blood return, the needle is retracted and a different location is chosen. If there is no blood return, the catheter is agitated to assist in sample collection. Suction is then released, the needle is removed from the wall and retracted, the scope straightened, and the catheter is withdrawn from the scope in one smooth motion. The specimen is then blown from the needle onto a slide using air from the syringe. The specimen is then smeared with another slide (smear technique) and immediately placed in a preservative (95% alcohol, Cytolyte®). Alternatively, saline can be used to flush the specimen from the needle (fluid technique) with the fluid and specimen being sent to the Cytology Laboratory. For a histology specimen, the 19-gauge needle is used. The technique for using this needle is very similar to the above described technique. The difference is that there is a 21-gauge needle inside the 19-gauge needle. This 21-gauge needle passes through the tracheobronchial wall first. If there is no blood aspirated through this needle it is retracted and the 19-gauge needle is inserted to the hub. Suction is again applied and, if no blood is aspirated, the needle is partially withdrawn and reinserted several times to obtain the best specimen. As above, suction is then released, the needle retracted, the scope straightened, and the catheter removed. The core of tissue obtained is then flushed into a container with a preservative. The process is repeated until at least two good specimens are obtained. The figures show a bronchoscopic view of a needle that has penetrated the bronchial wall and a fluoroscopic view of a needle extending into a left hilar lesion.

Transbronchial Needle Aspiration

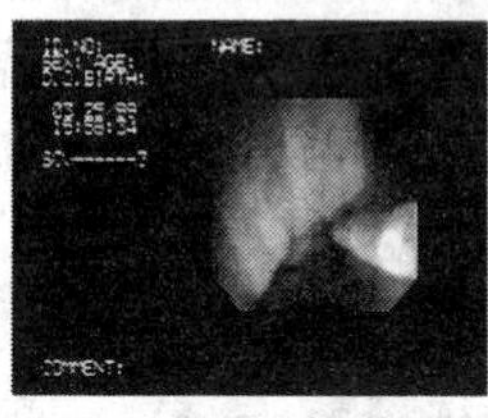

Figure 1

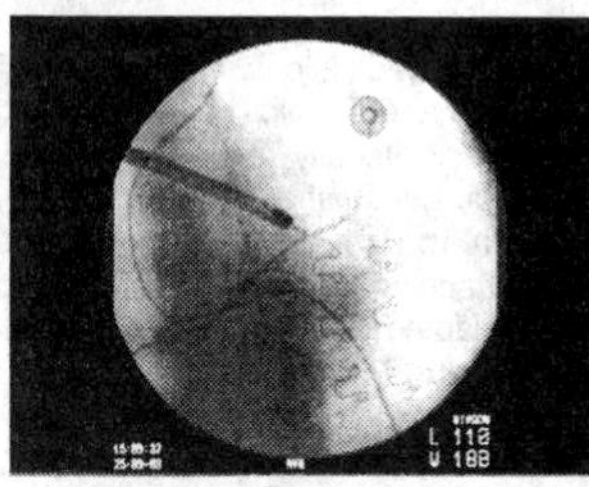

Figure 2

Data Acquired Cytology and/or histology specimens from the areas sampled

Turnaround Time 24-48 hours; 3-4 days if special stains are performed.

Specimen Cellular material or tissue cores from the sampled nodes/lesions

Container Slides or specimen placed in a jar containing a preservative (eg, alcohol, formalin, Cytolyte®)

Collection Through a flexible bronchoscope cells are aspirated into a needle placed through the tracheobronchial wall. Similarly, a core of tissue is cut and aspirated through a larger bore needle.

Storage Instructions Cytology specimens should be immediately placed on slides and immersed in a fixative. Histology specimens should be placed in fixative.

Causes for Rejection Inadequate tissue sample, cells allowed to dry

Normal Findings Nonmalignant cytology and normal histology

Limitations Sampling error; requires experienced cytopathologist

References

Dasgupta A, Mehta AC, and Wang KP, "Transbronchial Needle Aspiration," *Semin Respir Crit Care Med*, 1997, 18(6):571-81.

Gasparini S, "Bronchoscopic Biopsy Techniques in the Diagnosis and Staging of Lung Cancer," *Monaldi Arch Chest Dis*, 1997, 52(4):392-8.

Harrow EM and Wang KP, "The Staging of Lung Cancer by Bronchoscopic Transbronchial Needle Aspiration," *Chest Surg Clin N Am*, 1996, 6(2):223-35.

Kvale PA, "Bronchoscopic Biopsies and Bronchoalveolar Lavage," *Chest Surg Clin N Am*, 1996, 6(2):205-22.

Robinson DS, Faurschou P, Barnes N, et al, "Biopsies: Bronchoscopic Technique and Sampling," *Eur Respir J Suppl*, 1998, 26:16S-9S.

Saetta M, Jeffery PK, Maestrelli P, et al, "Biopsies: Processing and Assessment," *Eur Respir J Suppl*, 1998, 26:20S-5S.

♦ **Transbronchoscopic Biopsy Bronchoscopy** *see* Bronchoscopy, Transbronchial Biopsy *on page 211*

♦ **Transfer Factor** *see* Carbon Monoxide Diffusing Capacity, Single Breath *on page 215*

Volume of Isoflow (V iso $\dot{V}$)

Related Information

Spirometry *on page 249*
Spirometry Before and After Bronchodilators *on page 253*

Synonyms Density Dependent Spirometry; Heliox Spirometry; Low Density Gas Spirometry

Procedure Commonly Includes Volume of isoflow (V iso $\dot{V}$), percent increase in maximum flow measured at 50% of the vital capacity (change $FEF_{50\%}$ or change $\dot{V}_{max\ 50\%}$) and percent increase in maximum flow measured at 25% of the vital capacity measured from residual volumes (change $FEF_{75\%}$ or change $\dot{V}_{max\ 75\%}$).

Patient Preparation The patient should avoid heavy meals 3 hours prior to testing. The patient should be conscious and able to follow simple instructions. The patient's height and weight should be measured without shoes. Loose comfortable clothing that does not restrict chest expansion should be worn. Smoking history including last cigarette smoked should be obtained. Current medications should be obtained with particular emphasis on bronchodilators and steroids. See Spirometry *on page 249.*

Aftercare Usually none, although patients that complain of lightheadedness and dizziness should not be allowed to walk unobserved until recovery.

Special Instructions Patients that have a tracheostomy stoma may be tested by attaching an infant anesthesia mask to the mouthpiece. Mouthpieces can be adapted directly to most tracheostomy tubes.

Technique Forced vital capacity maneuvers are performed at least in triplicate breathing room air and during heliox breathing. The change $\dot{V}_{E\ max\ 50\%}$ value is calculated as follows: Change $\dot{V}_{E\ max\ 50\%} = \dot{V}_{E\ max\ 50\%}(HeO_2) - \dot{V}_{E\ max\ 50\%}(AIR) \times 100 / \dot{V}_{E\ max\ 50\%}$. The change $\dot{V}_{E\ max\ 75\%}$ value is calculated in an identical fashion, measuring flows at 25% of the VC (from RV).

Turnaround Time Preliminary results should be available same day. Depending on the facility, an interpreted report may be available in 1-2 days.

Specimen Measurement of exhaled volumes and flow rates during a maximal forced expiratory maneuver from total lung capacity (TLC) to residual volume (RV). Test is performed during air breathing and low density gas breathing (typically 80% helium, 20% oxygen - heliox). A bag in the box system is interposed between the patient and the spirometer, that is the spirometer measures the room air that is displaced as the patient inhales and exhales from a reservoir (bag) contained in a rigid "box" that is open only to the spirometer. Flow volume curves that represent best $\dot{V}_{E\ max\ 50\%}$ and $\dot{V}_{E\ max\ 75\%}$ are chosen.

Causes for Rejection Cough, especially when it occurs in the early part of forced expiration, may render all data except expired volume useless. **Hesitant start:** Peak effort must be applied before 10% of total volume is exhaled, otherwise measurement of timed forced expiratory volume may be invalid. Back extrapolated volume. **Premature cessation of expiratory effort:** Expiratory effort must be maintained for a minimum of 6 seconds or until the volume-time tracing shows less than 25 mL volume increment for ½ a second. **Early termination** falsely increased FEV_1/FVC% and increased mean and instantaneous flow rates at middle or low lung volume (LV). **Submaximal effort:** Indicated by a very low, often nonreproducible peak flow. Neuromuscular disease may produce the same pattern. **Nonreproducibility:** The second largest FVCs should show 15% variability, the two largest FEV_1 should show <10% variability.

Normal Findings Normal values for the change $\dot{V}_{E\ max\ 50\%}$ and $\dot{V}_{E\ max\ 75\%}$ of 47.3 and 13.7% (mean ±SD) and 29.12 ±23.4% respectively for nonsmokers have been reported. Volume of isoflow is generally reported as a percentage of the vital capacity and shows a significant rise with increasing age. The regression equation, V iso $\dot{V}$ = 0.291 x age + 4.917 ±6.88 SD describes the relationship of V iso $\dot{V}$ and changes in $\dot{V}_{E\ max\ 50\%}$ and V iso $\dot{V}$ following bronchodilators can be interpreted as follows.

Interpretation of Changes in $\mathring{V}_{E\ max}$ and Delta $\mathring{V}_{E\ max\ 50\%}$ After Bronchodilators

$\mathring{V}_{E\ max}$	Delta $\mathring{V}_{E\ max\ 50\%}$	Interpretation
Increased	Increased	Predominant peripheral airways bronchodilation
Increased	Decreased	Predominant central airways bronchodilation
Increased	Unchanged	Proportionally equal peripheral and central airways bronchodilation

Limitations Requires patient cooperation. Transient obstruction secondary to cigarette smoking just prior to testing. FVC of the forced expirations used for comparison of air and heliox flow measurements must be within 25% of each others. Flow rates must be compared isovolumetrically, that is at the same absolute lung volume.

Additional Information A great deal of controversy exists regarding the clinical usefulness of V of iso $\mathring{V}$. Lam and Berend suggest that the test is not very useful for detection of early airways obstruction secondary to its high coefficients of variation. A study by Mink et al has shown that airway geometry differs during air and heliox breathing. Flow comparisons have been made under the assumption that airway geometry was constant.

References

Aaron SD, Dales RE, and Cardinal P, "How Accurate Is Spirometry at Predicting Restrictive Pulmonary Impairment?" *Chest*, 1999, 115(3):869-73.

Davis S, Jones M, Kisling J, et al, "Density Dependence of Forced Expiratory Flows in Healthy Infants and Toddlers," *J Appl Physiol*, 1999, 87(5):1796-801.

Devabhaktuni VG, Torres A Jr, Wilson S, et al, "Effect of Nitric Oxide, Perfluorocarbon, and Heliox on Minute Volume Measurement and Ventilator Volumes," *Crit Care Med*, 1999, 27(8):1603-7.

Eaton T, Withy S, Garrett JE, et al, "Spirometry in Primary Care Practice: The Importance of Quality Assurance and the Impact of Spirometry Workshops," *Chest*, 1999, 116(2):416-23.

Enright PL, Arnold A, Manolio TA, et al, "Spirometry Reference Values for Healthy Elderly Blacks. The Cardiovascular Health Study Research Group," *Chest*, 1996, 110(6):1416-24.

Hankinson JL, Odencrantz JR, and Fedan KB, "Spirometric Reference Values From a Sample of the General U.S. Population," *Am J Respir Crit Care Med*, 1999, 159(1):179-87.

Juniper EF, Buist AS, Cox FM, et al, "Validation of a Standardized Version of the Asthma Quality of Life Questionnaire," *Chest*, 1999, 115(5):1265-70.

Linn WS, Solomon JC, Gong H Jr, et al, "Standardization of Multiple Spirometers at Widely Separated Times and Places," *Am J Respir Crit Care Med*, 1996, 153(4 Pt 1):1309-13.

Vollmer WM, Enright PL, Pedula KL, et al, "Race and Gender Differences in the Effects of Smoking on Lung Function," *Chest*, 2000, 117(3):764-72.

Vollmer WM, McCamant LE, Johnson LR, et al, "Long-Term Reproducibility of Tests of Small Airways Function. Comparisons With Spirometry," *Chest*, 1990, 98(2):303-7.

♦ **Wang Needle Aspiration** *see* Transbronchial Needle Aspiration *on page 267*

UROLOGY

♦ **Arteriogram** *see* Penile Blood Flow *on page 290*
♦ **Bladder Catheterization** *see* Catheterization, Urethral *on page 273*

Catheterization, Urethral

Related Information

Cystoureteroscopy *on page 283*
Cystourethroscopy *on page 285*

Synonyms Bladder Catheterization; Foley Catheterization

Procedure Commonly Includes A catheter is introduced through the urethra into the bladder. Many types of catheters are available for urethral catheterization, and the choice of a specific type of catheter depends upon the reason for catheterization.

Indications Urethral catheterization is performed for both the diagnosis of and therapy for urologic disease. Diagnostic and therapeutic indications include:

- collection of urine for culture (particularly in females)
- measurement of postvoid residuals
- instillation of contrast material for cystourethrography
- urodynamic studies
- relief of infravesical obstruction
- accurate monitoring of urine output
- bladder drainage following surgical procedures
- functional stent following bladder or urethral incisions

Contraindications There are no absolute contraindications to this procedure; however, if more than gentle pressure is necessary during an attempt to pass any catheter into the bladder, the procedure should be aborted before urethral trauma occurs.

Patient Preparation The procedure should be explained to the patient with informed consent obtained. Reasonable expectations should be given in terms of discomfort. Because the urethra is a sterile tract, it should be prepped and draped in a sterile fashion. In the male, it is recommended to give a retrograde injection of 10 cc of 2% lidocaine hydrochloride jelly followed by a urethral clamp for 5 minutes. This will allow the anesthetic to contact the mucosal surfaces. In the female, place the 2% lidocaine hydrochloride jelly on the catheter tip prior to catheterization.

Aftercare No specific aftercare is required. If the catheter is to be left in place, it should be externally secured to the thigh to prevent tension at the bladder neck.

Complications Catheterization is felt to be quite safe. Urethral trauma is associated with urethral pain, spasm, microscopic hematuria, and urinary tract infection.

Equipment There are several types of urethral catheters. The catheter size is usually referred to in terms of the French (Fr) scale (circumference in mL). A straight rubber or latex catheter is often used for one-time catheterization (straight catheterization). These catheters are also available with multiple eyes, making them ideal for irrigating the bladder free of clots. Catheters with a curved tip (coude catheters) are specifically designed to help bypass areas of the male urethra that are difficult to negotiate with a straight catheter. Foley-type catheters are most often used for long-term urethral catheterization. As such, they have a balloon mechanism at the distal end that, when inflated, keeps the catheter from sliding past the bladder neck. Two-way and three-way Foley catheters are available in multiple sizes. Two-way catheters have a

(Continued)

Catheterization, Urethral *(Continued)*

small lumen for inflating the balloon and a larger lumen for urinary drainage. Three-way catheters have a small lumen for inflating the balloon, a lumen for instilling irrigant, and a larger lumen for bladder drainage. One should choose the smallest urethral catheter that will accomplish the purpose of catheterization, because urethral secretions drain more easily around small catheters. Allowing egress of urethral secretions lessens the chance of a clinically significant urethral inflammatory response.

Technique In the male, the penis is placed on stretch perpendicular to the body, pointing slightly toward the umbilicus. Without compressing the urethra, the catheter is placed in the urethral meatus by holding the catheter at the tip. Gentle advancement of the catheter causes the least amount of discomfort. As the bulbomembranous urethra is reached at the level of the external sphincter, one should ask the patient to take slow, deep breaths, which will help relax the patient and often allow easier catheter passage. If resistance is met, one should not attempt forceful catheter insertion but should apply continuous, gentle pressure and ascertain at what level the potential obstruction exists. In the female, spread the labia to identify the urethral meatus. Place the tip of the catheter into the urethral meatus and gently advance the catheter into the bladder.

Data Acquired Urine for analysis

Specimen A complete urinalysis includes both chemical and microscopic analyses. For routine studies, 50-100 mL is adequate. For urinary sediment examination, the first morning urine sample is optimal.

Container Sterile jar

Collection Samples should be hand carried to respective laboratories immediately or quickly refrigerated. Urine sediment should be examined within 1 hour of collection.

Normal Findings The physical examination of the urine includes an evaluation of color, turbidity, specific gravity and osmolality, and pH. The normal color of urine is pale yellow. Abnormal color is most commonly because of concentration, but many foods, medications, metabolic products, and infection may produce abnormal urine color. Freshly voided urine should be clear. Cloudy urine is most commonly a result of phosphaturia or pyuria. The two are readily distinguished by microscopic examination, which demonstrates the presence or absence of leukocytes. Specific gravity (SG) varies from 1.001-1.035. In general, SG reflects the state of hydration but also affords some idea of renal concentrating ability. Conditions that decrease SG include:

- increased fluid intake
- diuretics
- isosthenuria
- diabetes insipidus

Conditions that increase SG include:

- decreased fluid intake
- dehydration caused by fever, sweating, vomiting, and diarrhea
- diabetes mellitus with glucosuria
- inappropriate secretion of antidiuretic hormone
- status postinjection of intravenous iodinated contrast
- dextran infusion

Osmolality is a measure of the amount of material dissolved in the urine and usually varies between 50 and 1200 mOsm/L. Urine osmolality most commonly varies with hydration, and the same factors that affect SG also affect osmolality. Urine pH generally reflects the pH in the serum; however, abnormal alkalinization of the urine occurs with renal tubular acidosis and some urinary tract infections. Abnormal acidification of the urine occurs with uric acid and cystine lithiasis. Chemical examination of urine is performed with a urine dipstick. The abnormal substances commonly tested for with a dipstick are blood, protein, glucose, ketones, urobilinogen and bilirubin, and white blood cells.

Normal urine should contain <3 RBCs/hpf. Healthy adults excrete 80-150 mg of protein in the urine daily, but all cases of dipstick proteinuria should be followed by 24-hour quantitative collection. Glucosuria is abnormal and represents a serum glucose >180 mg/dL. Normal urine does not usually contain ketones or bilirubin and only a small amount of urobilinogen. Normal urine in men and women should contain <2 and <5 leukocytes/hpf, respectively. Urinary sediment should be examined microscopically for cells, casts, crystals, bacteria, yeast, and parasites. A cast is a protein coagulum that is formed in the renal interstitium. Tamm-Horsfall mucoprotein is the basic matrix of all renal casts, and is always present in the urine in the form of hyaline casts. Red blood cell casts are entrapped erythrocytes and are diagnostic of glomerular bleeding. White blood cell casts are observed in acute glomerulonephritis, acute pyelonephritis, and acute tubulointerstitial nephritis. Muddy-brown casts represent sloughed renal tubular epithelial cells, and are indicative of nonspecific renal damage. Normal urine does not contain bacteria, yeast, or parasites.

References

Corujo M, Badlani GH, Regan JB, et al, "A new Temporary Catheter (ContiCath) for the Treatment of Temporary, Reversible, Postoperative Urinary Retension," *Urology*, 1999, 53(6):1104-7.

Cushner HM and Copley JB, "Back to Basics: The Urinalysis: A Selected National Survey and Review," *Am J Med Sci*, 1989, 297(3):193-6.

Parvey HR and Patel BK, "Urethral Complications of Urinary Catheterization Presenting as Primary Scrotal Masses: Sonographic Diagnosis," *J Clin Ultrasound*, 1998, 26(5):261-4.

Shaw ST Jr, Poon SY, and Wong ET, "Routine Urinalysis: Is the Dipstick Enough?" *JAMA*, 1985, 253(11):1596-600.

Teichman JM, Weiss BD, and Solomon D, "Urological Needs Assessment for Primary Care Practice: Implications for Undergraduate Medical Education," *J Urol*, 1999, 161(4):1282-5.

♦ **CMG** *see* Cystometrogram, Complex *on page 275*

♦ **CMG** *see* Cystometrogram, Simple *on page 279*

♦ **Complex Urodynamic Testing of Bladder Function** *see* Cystometrogram, Complex *on page 275*

Cystometrogram, Complex

Related Information

Cystometrogram, Simple *on page 279*

Synonyms CMG; Complex Urodynamic Testing of Bladder Function; Multichannel Cystometrogram

Procedure Commonly Includes Graphic recording of the pressure-volume characteristics of the urinary bladder. Performed in a Urodynamics Laboratory, the bladder is passively filled with water or gas by means of a transurethral catheter. Simultaneous intra-abdominal (rectal) pressure is obtained. Intravesical pressures are measured as the bladder is being filled by means of a microtip transducer or a fluid-filled catheter attached to a transducer. Information regarding bladder sensation, capacity, compliance, tone, and contractility may be obtained along with a cystometrogram (graphic plot of bladder pressure versus volume).

Indications The exact indications are controversial, as with simple cystometry. Most would agree that complex cystometry is useful in evaluating persistent urinary incontinence or retention felt secondary to bladder pathology. Clinical settings include:[1]

- overflow incontinence, to differentiate a flaccid bladder from an obstructed bladder
- urgency incontinence, to document detrusor instability
- bladder sensory or motor dysfunction associated with diabetes, Parkinson disease, multiple sclerosis, or stroke
- postprostatectomy incontinence
- spinal cord injury with voiding disorders
- failed surgery for incontinence

Cystometry is less useful in evaluating:

- stress urinary incontinence
- psychogenic incontinence
- urinary obstruction in the male with retention

Contraindications

- patient refusal
- demented patient with severe cognitive deficits
- inability to pass Foley catheter
- active urinary tract infection

(Continued)

Cystometrogram, Complex *(Continued)*

Patient Preparation Technique and risks are explained to the patient and consent is obtained. The patient should understand that a rectal probe will be inserted. Requisition to the Urodynamics Laboratory should specify current medications. All sedatives, cholinergics, and anticholinergics should be discontinued prior to procedure. No anxiolytics or pain medications are given as premedications. If patient complains of dysuria (along with other voiding problems), obtain urinalysis at physician discretion. In all cases, patient is requested to void immediately prior to procedure. Remove indwelling Foley, if applicable, well in advance.

Aftercare No specific activity restrictions are necessary and previous level of activity may be resumed. At physician discretion, a urinalysis may be ordered 48-72 hours later to exclude procedure-induced infection.

Complications Complex cystometry is felt to be quite safe. Minor complications are similar to those associated with any bladder catheterization and include urethral pain, microscopic hematuria, and urinary tract infection (estimated at <8%).

Equipment Basic equipment includes multilumen catheter for bladder catheterization (or two separate catheters), rectal balloon catheter with transducer, microtip transducers for bladder pressure measurement (or fluid-filled catheter attached to Statham transducer), multichannel recorder, sterile water reservoir (or carbon dioxide gas reservoir), and an adjustable infusion pump.

Technique Complex cystometry may be performed in several ways. The basic procedure is described as follows. After normal voiding, the patient is placed in a supine position. A bladder catheter is inserted transurethrally and residual volume is measured. This catheter may be a triple or double lumen Foley catheter. (Some urologists prefer using two catheters per urethra, one for bladder filling, usually 14F, and a smaller one for pressure measurement.) With the bladder empty, patient is asked to relax completely and avoid all bladder or abdominal contractions. One channel of the catheter is connected with the infusion pump and the other channel is connected with a microtip transducer or fluid-filled catheter/transducer system. The anal probe is inserted and intra-abdominal pressures are continuously recorded. Using the infusion pump, the bladder is filled with sterile, room temperature water through one channel. The rate of filling is clearly documented: whether "slow fill" at 10 mL/minute, "medium fill" at 10-100 mL/minute, or "rapid fill" at >100 mL/minute. In general, the infusion pump allows continuous filling at a constant rate. (If not available, filling may be performed incrementally with gravity drainage.) Intravesical pressures are continuously recorded through the separate channel in the catheter, along with simultaneous anorectal pressures. The patient subjectively reports the first perceived sensation of bladder fullness and the first strong urge to void. Filling is continued until patient reports discomfort or until an involuntary bladder contraction is seen. The described technique is termed "filling cystometry". In some centers, the study is continued past this point and the examiner proceeds with "voiding cystometry". The patient is asked to void as vigorously and completely as possible while the catheter measuring intravesicular pressure is still in place. Pressures within the bladder are recorded as before, throughout bladder emptying. If two separate urethral catheters were used originally, the larger catheter (used for filling) is removed prior to voiding. A number of provocative maneuvers, including the following, may be employed at physician discretion.[2]

- Rapid fill cystometry: After standard cystometry is performed, flow is increased to >100 mL/minute of fluid (or 300 mL CO_2 if gas cystometry used). This is done to provoke detrusor contraction. If these are seen, the diagnosis detrusor areflexia is ruled out.
- Changes in patient position (sitting, standing) and maneuvers such as coughing, heel jouncing. As with rapid fill cystometry, these techniques attempt to overcome the inhibition of the detrusor reflex, which is normally present. If a bladder contraction is recorded, the peripheral nerve supply to the detrusor is intact.
- Saline infusions at temperatures above or below body temperature: This helps in further evaluating bladder sensation in equivocal cases and may also provoke a detrusor contraction.

- Bethanechol (Urecholine®) supersensitivity test: Bethanechol, a parasympathomimetic agent, is injected 2.5 mg subcutaneously and cystometry is repeated 10, 20, and 30 minutes afterwards. In the normal individual, small increases in bladder pressure are seen when cystometry is repeated. A marked increase in bladder pressure 15-20 cm H_2O over baseline indicates a lower motor neuron (LMN) lesion, the "supersensitive bladder". This is based on Cannon's law of denervation - when an end-organ is deprived of its nerve supply it becomes hypersensitive to normal excitatory neurotransmitters. Complete lack of response to bethanechol suggests technical error or myogenic bladder damage.
- Trial of anticholinergics or muscle depressants: If uninhibited detrusor contractions are seen on initial cystometry, the efficacy of specific drugs may be tested by repeating cystometry after drug administration.

In addition, gas cystometry using CO_2 may be used instead of water for filling. Gas cystometry has the advantage of being more convenient and less time-consuming. Disadvantages include inaccuracy of bladder volume measurements (controversial), difficulties reproducing values, and inability to assess voiding cystometry (obviously only fluid may be voided). Tanagho suggests using gas cystometry only as an initial screen, if at all, with equivocal or abnormal results repeated with a liquid medium.[3]

Data Acquired

- residual volume (mL)
- threshold for sensation of bladder fullness (mL)
- maximum cystometric capacity (mL) - volume where patient reports strong urge to void; usually less than true bladder capacity measured during normal, physiologic filling
- bladder contractility
- cystometrogram - bladder pressure (ordinate) plotted against volume (abscissa) on a multichannel recorder
- bladder compliance - Δ volume divided by Δ pressure (ΔV/ΔP) at any point on the cystometrogram
- provocative maneuver results, if performed

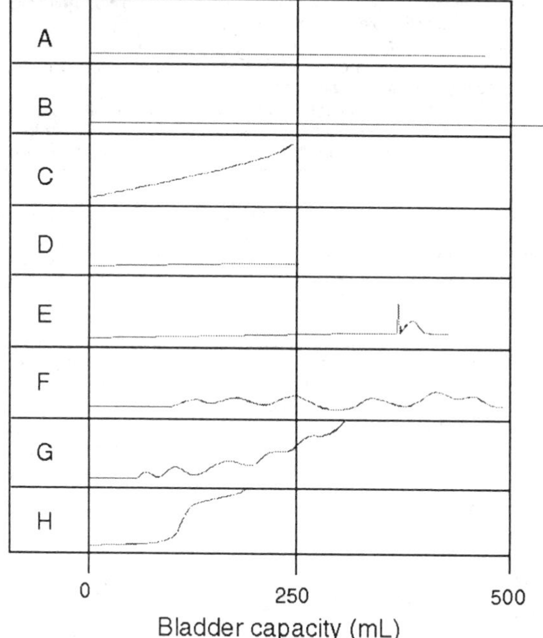

(Continued)

Cystometrogram, Complex *(Continued)*

Normal Findings Official is report issued from the Urodynamics Laboratory. Normal values are identical to those listed for simple cystometry (see Cystometrogram, Simple *on page 279*.) Normal values for provocative testing are described under Technique. With complex cystometry, voluntary or involuntary voiding contractions may be more precisely defined as sustained increases in intravesical pressure, usually 20-40 cm H_2O, with minimal increases in intra-abdominal pressure. The measurement of intra-abdominal pressure serves only as a reference point to ensure that apparent bladder pressure increases are not due to abdominal muscle contraction. This provides an important advantage over simple cystometry.

Critical Values Identical to those listed for simple cystometry (see Cystometrogram, Simple *on page 279*). The graphic recording of pressure-volume characteristics is presumably more accurate than simple cystometry. Direct comparison of the shape of the test curve (as well as the absolute pressure values) may be made with normal CMG tracings and tracings of known pathologic entities. This is depicted in the previous figure.

This chart represents idealized adult cystometrograms for the following conditions:

A. normal filling curve, normal compliance, no contractions
B. large capacity bladder
C. bladder with decreased compliance
D. small-capacity bladder, no involuntary contractions
E. bladder contraction from a cough
F. detrusor contractions, low-amplitude
G. involuntary bladder contractions in a bladder with decreased compliance
H. early onset involuntary bladder contractions (high amplitude)

Limitations

- Complex cystometry is of questionable utility in diagnosis of structural abnormalities, such as prostatic hypertrophy or stress urinary incontinence.
- Passive filling of bladder with water is unphysiologic and with CO_2, is even more unphysiologic.
- Complex cystometry does not measure urine flow, force, urethral function, and myoneural coordination. These parameters require other forms of synchronous urodynamic testing.
- Technical factors may still lead to false-positive or false-negative results. Although considered the "gold standard" for clinical bladder function testing, complex cystometry is far from perfect and more experimental techniques (eg, continuous ambulatory urodynamic monitoring) have been developed.
- Cost and inconvenience are more significant than with simple cystometry. The patient must travel to the Urodynamics Laboratory.

Additional Information The role of complex cystometry in the evaluation of the patient with a voiding disorder (incontinence, retention, bladder discomfort) has not been agreed upon. Clearly, it provides information concerning bladder function which cannot be obtained from cystoscopy or radiographic studies. These latter two procedures examine only structural abnormalities. Some authors rely on the history and physical examination to yield a likely diagnosis and then begin a trial of empiric medical therapy to confirm this diagnosis. Only a small subset of patients undergo complex urodynamic testing. Other experts believe that voiding histories are often inaccurate and cystometry is necessary to identify the neuropathic or unstable bladder. Medical or surgical therapies may then be pursued with confidence.

Footnotes

1. Leach GE and Yip CM, "Urologic and Urodynamic Evaluation of the Elderly Population," *Clin Geriatr Med*, 1986, 2(4):731-55.
2. Wein AJ, English WS, and Whitmore KE, "Office Urodynamics," *Urol Clin North Am*, 1988, 15(4):609-23.
3. Tanagho EA, "Urodynamic Studies," *Smith's General Urology*, 14th ed, Chapter 29, Tanagho EA and McAninch JW, eds, Norwalk, CT: Appleton and Lange, 1995, 514-35.

References

Blaivas J, "Multichannel Urodynamic Studies," *Urology*, 1984, 23(5):421-38.

Gerber GS, Kim JH, Contreras BA, et al, "An Observational Urodynamic Evaluation of Men With Lower Urinary Tract Symptoms Treated With Doxazosin," *Urology*, 1996, 47(6):840-4.
Kraklau DM and Bloom DA, "The Cystometrogram at 70 Years," *J Urol*, 1998, 160(2):316-9.
Massey A and Abrams P, "Urodynamics of the Female Lower Urinary Tract," *Urol Clin North Am*, 1985, 12(2):231-46.
Nigro DA, Wein AJ, Foy M, et al, "Associations Among Cystoscopic and Urodynamic Findings for Women Enrolled in the Interstitial Cystitis Data Base (ICDB) Study," *Urology*, 1997, 49(5A Suppl):86-92.
van Waaljwijk, van Doorn ES, Meier AH, et al, "Ambulatory Urodynamics: Extramural Testing of the Lower and Upper Urinary Tract by Holter Monitoring of Cystometrogram, Uroflowmetry, and Renal Pelvic Pressures," *Urol Clin North Am*, 1996, 23(3):345-71.

Cystometrogram, Simple

Related Information

Cystometrogram, Complex *on page 275*

Synonyms CMG; Cystometry; Filling Cystometrogram; Simple CMG; Urodynamic Testing of Bladder Function

Procedure Commonly Includes Bedside evaluation of urinary bladder function in selected patients with urinary incontinence or retention. The bladder is passively filled with sterile water through a transurethral Foley catheter. Intravesical pressures are measured with an open manometer as bladder volume increases. Information regarding bladder sensation, capacity, and contractility is obtained.

Indications The exact indications for simple cystometry are controversial. Even amongst urologists, considerable debate exists in the medical/surgical literature considering the optimal role of this procedure. Simple cystometry is useful in the patient with persistent urinary incontinence or retention felt to be secondary to impaired bladder filling or storage. Common clinical indications for this test include:

- suspected "neurogenic bladder"
- suspected detrusor motor instability, the hyper-reflexive bladder
- suspected abnormalities in bladder sensation, capacity, or contractility
- the geriatric patient with persistent urinary incontinence of unclear etiology (controversial)

Simple cystometry is less useful in evaluating the following conditions:[1]

- suspected stress urinary incontinence in the female
- suspected psychogenic urinary incontinence in the male
- suspected urinary obstruction in the male

Contraindications

- patient refusal
- the demented patient with severe cognitive impairment; this procedure requires the patient to accurately report sensations of bladder filling
- inability to pass transurethral Foley catheter
- active urinary tract infection

Patient Preparation Technique and risks of the procedure are explained to the patient and consent is obtained. Ideally, patient should be off sedatives, cholinergics, or anticholinergics prior to testing. Indwelling Foley catheters should be removed well in advance so that residual volume may be measured. No pain medications or anxiolytics are routinely necessary. The patient is asked to void, if possible, immediately prior to procedure.

Aftercare No specific postprocedure restrictions are required and previous activity level may be resumed. At physician discretion, a urinalysis (and possibly urine culture) may be ordered on follow-up, 48-72 hours later.

Special Instructions Simple cystometry may be easily performed by a trained nurse or physician assistant and, in most cases, does not require direct physician supervision. This is a considerable advantage over complex cystometry which is usually performed in the Urodynamics Laboratory.

Complications This procedure is considered relatively safe. The vast majority of patients tolerate simple cystometry with minimal problems. Reported complications are similar to those seen with straight catheterization, such as local urethral discomfort, hematuria, and urinary tract infection. The precise complication rate is not known, but in one study involving 171 incontinent geriatric patients, <8% developed new urinary symptoms consistent with infection and <2% required antibiotic therapy.[2]

(Continued)

Cystometrogram, Simple *(Continued)*

Equipment Standard Foley catheter or 14F red rubber catheter required. Alternatively, a 3-channel Foley catheter (often used for bladder irrigation) may be used. Also needed are a urinary catheterization tray (drapes, lubricant, iodine, gloves, syringes, etc), Y-connector, 50 mL syringe, sterile water in graduated container, sterile tubing, nonsterile measuring basin. An open manometer, such as a spinal manometer, is commonly used.

Technique Numerous minor variations in technique have been described with the choice depending on physician preference and patient logistics. In its simplest form, a manometer is not used. After voiding, patient is placed in supine position and a Foley catheter (or 14F red rubber straight catheter) is inserted transurethrally into the bladder. Residual urine volume is measured and the catheter is left in place. With the bladder empty, the patient is requested to relax completely and avoid all bladder or abdominal contractions for the remainder of the procedure. The inner piston of a 50 mL syringe is removed and the syringe tip inserted into the distal (open) end of the catheter. Using the syringe as a funnel, room temperature sterile water is infused through the syringe and catheter in 50 mL increments. The syringe is elevated so the highest level of the fluid column is always 15 cm above the symphysis pubis. Thus, fluid enters the bladder by gravity drainage and not forcibly by syringe pressure. After each 50 mL water, the height of the water column is observed. The patient subjectively reports first perceptible sensation of bladder fullness and first strong urge to void. When patient notes a strong voiding urge, additional volume is added in 25 mL increments until discomfort is reported or an involuntary bladder contraction occurs. A bladder contraction appears as a sharp and sustained rise in the water column despite attempted voluntary bladder relaxation (and may be seen at any time during the procedure). The procedure is terminated at this stage. This brief sequence of maneuvers has been described in several formal studies comparing simple and complex multichannel cystometry.[2,3] A common and time-honored variation of this procedure requires the use of a spinal manometer. Initial steps are identical. After residual volume is measured, a Y-connector is attached to the distal end of the Foley. Through one arm of the Y-connector, sterile water in a calibrated reservoir is instilled by gravity drainage. The other arm is connected to an open spinal manometer via sterile connecting tubing. An anaeroid manometer (Lewis cystometer) may also be used. Pressure within the tubing system is "bled off" into the manometer port. As water incrementally fills the bladder, increasing intravesicular pressure is transmitted back through the tubing and is crudely estimated by the height of the water column in the manometer. A plot of bladder pressure versus volume may be constructed in this manner. Alternatively, a 3-channel Foley may be used. Again, fluid is introduced through 1-catheter channel, but in this technique the spinal manometer is connected to a physically separate channel. This allows more accurate intravesical pressure estimations. When bladder pressure is measured in the fluid in the flow channel (as in the Y-connector arrangement), several confounding variables are introduced, such as the internal resistance to fluid in the catheter. Some of these variables are eliminated by this simple maneuver.

Data Acquired

- residual volume (mL)
- threshold for sensation of bladder fullness (mL) - the volume at which patient reports first sensation of fullness
- maximum cystometric capacity (mL) - the volume at which patient describes a strong urge to void, or the volume just prior to an involuntary contraction
- bladder contractility (presence and number of involuntary bladder contractions, as defined)

If a manometer is used, additional data includes:

- pressure-volume characteristics of the bladder during filling, this is termed the cystometrogram - bladder pressure (ordinate) plotted against volume (abscissa)
- bladder compliance, defined as $\Delta V/\Delta P$ and is derived from the cystometrogram

Normal Findings Approximated as follows:

- residual volume - usually minimal or no urine obtained
- threshold for sensation of bladder fullness, 100-200 mL
- maximum capacity, 400-500 mL
- bladder contractility, no involuntary contractions noted
- cystometrogram[4], normally divided into the following four phases: (see figure)

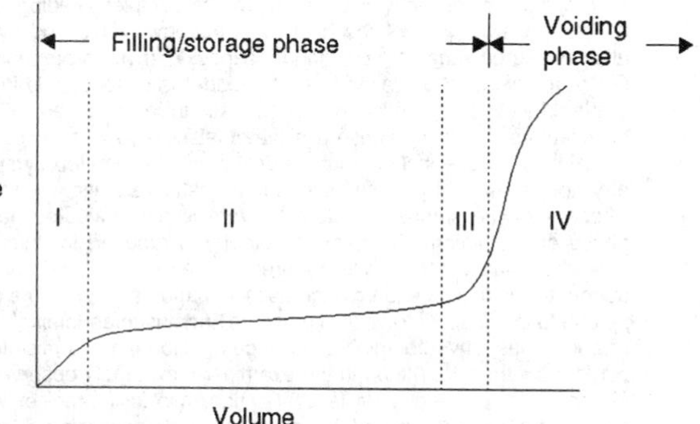

Idealized cystometrogram. Note that the voiding phase is only assessed with complex cystometry. Reproduced with permission from Wein AJ, et al, *Urol Clin North Am,* 1988, 15(4):613.

Phase 1: Initial pressure rise, stabilizes at the initial filling pressure or "resting pressure," normally approximately 10 cm H_2O.

Phase 2: The tonus limb, where compliance is high; pressure normally is low and remains constant as volume increases.

Phase 3: The limit of bladder elastic properties; increasing volume causes marked pressure increases. Normally, the patient can still voluntarily control micturition, even though maximum bladder capacity has almost been reached.

Phase 4: Voluntary voiding (not tested with simple cystometry).

- compliance - normally very high in phase two of the cystometrogram (approaching infinity)

Critical Values Residual volume: Significant postvoid residual may result from sensory neuropathy, lower motor neuron (LMN) disease, or bladder outlet resistance (functional or mechanical).[5]

Threshold of sensation: Decreased sensation (ie, threshold more than 200 mL) is seen with sensory neuropathies such as diabetes mellitus, tabes dorsalis, cauda equina syndrome, or normal variant.

Maximum capacity: Decreased in a variety of disorders including upper motor neuron (UMN) disease, fibrotic bladder (eg, tuberculous interstitial cystitis), dysfunctionalized bladder, etc. Increased capacity (more than 500 mL) is seen with sensory neuropathy, LMN disease, chronic obstruction, bladder "training".

Contractility: Involuntary contractions at volumes less than capacity are abnormal. This condition has been called "detrusor hyper-reflexia" and "uninhibited" or "unstable" bladder. Increased contractility is found in various stroke syndromes, UMN lesions, hypertrophic bladder. Contractility is absent or weak in LMN lesions, sensory neuropathies, or voluntary inhibition.

Cystometrogram: Both the pattern of the tracing (pressure vs volume) and the absolute values should be compared against a standard normal curve. Some cystometrogram patterns may be diagnostic but tracings generated from (Continued)

Cystometrogram, Simple *(Continued)*

simple cystometry are crude and may be difficult to interpret. (See figure in Cystometrogram, Complex *on page 275*.)

Compliance: A noncompliant bladder may result from a variety of disorders, including bladder wall fibrosis, bladder contraction, idiopathic male enuresis.

Limitations Procedure has questionable utility in the diagnosis of voiding disorders due to structural abnormalities, such as stress urinary incontinence or prostatic hypertrophy with retention, or complex voiding disorders. By nature, passive filling of the bladder is nonphysiologic and may potentially alter measured variables (eg, bladder capacity) in yet-to-be-understood ways. Only urologic function related to the bladder is assessed. Urine flow, force, urethral function, and myoneural coordination are not tested. Numerous technical factors may lead to false-positive or false-negative results. As previously mentioned, intravesical pressure is only crudely estimated by spinal manometry and is limited by confounding factors, such as inflow tubing resistance. Phase 4 of the standard cystometrogram is not evaluated (ie, the voiding phase of micturition). Complex cystometry is required for this. Increases in intra-abdominal pressure will alter pressure readings. This is not controlled for adequately in this procedure. Increases in manometric pressure readings may be due to increased intravesical pressure, increased abdominal wall pressure, or both. Thus, any abdominal muscle contraction may be misinterpreted as a bladder contraction. Although the examiner may simply observe the patient's abdomen for signs of muscle contraction, this is imprecise. With complex cystometry this is avoided by simultaneously recording intravesical and anorectal pressures (which estimate intra-abdominal pressure). The cystometrogram generated by manometer readings is discontinuous and crude. Provocative measures (position changes, medications, etc) are not routinely performed. These are usually reserved for complex cystometry.

Additional Information The main advantage of simple cystometry is its convenience and low cost in comparison with more complex urodynamic testing. It may be performed by a trained nurse in less than minutes and need not be done in a hospital setting. Thus, it has been advocated for the evaluation of the nursing home patient or the elderly clinic patient. Several studies have compared simple and complex cystometry directly. Sutherst and Brown (1984) found that simple cystometry achieved a sensitivity of 100% for bladder instability with 89% specificity (when compared with complex cystometry as a gold standard). Ouslander (1988) also showed a high degree of correlation between the two tests in terms of bladder capacity and stability. However, the role of cystometry has not been clearly defined. Some authorities believe that only a small percentage of patients with voiding disorders need to undergo cystometry. This subpopulation may be identified using statistically derived algorithms based primarily on historical and physical examination findings.[6] Others feel that the urologic history is misleading often enough (or inaccurate in the demented geriatric patient) to justify frequent use of simple cystometry. In many cases, it is argued, management of a voiding disorder will be influenced by the objective results from cystometry. In all cases, test results must be interpreted in conjunction with the clinical suspicion.

Footnotes

1. Hinman F Jr, "Office Evaluation of Urodynamic Problems," *Urol Clin North Am*, 1979, 6(1):149-54.
2. Ouslander J, Leach G, Abelson S, et al, "Simple Versus Multichannel Cystometry in the Evaluation of Bladder Function in an Incontinent Geriatric Population," *J Urol*, 1988, 140(6):1482-6.
3. Sutherst JR and Brown MC, "Comparison of Single and Multichannel Cystometry in Diagnosing Bladder Instability," *Br Med J [Clin Res]*, 1984, 288(6432):1720-2.
4. Wein AJ, English WS, and Whitmore KE, "Office Urodynamics," *Urol Clin North Am*, 1988, 15(4):609-23.
5. Tanagho EA, "Urodynamic Studies," *Smith's General Urology*, 14th ed, Chapter 29, Tanagho EA and McAninch JW, eds, Norwalk, CT: Appleton and Lange, 1995, 514-35.
6. Hilton P and Stanton SL, "Algorithmic Method for Assessing Urinary Incontinence in Elderly Women," *Br Med J [Clin Res]*, 1981, 282(6268):940-2.

References

Blaivas J, "Multichannel Urodynamic Studies," *Urology*, 1984, 23(5):421-38.

Gerber GS, Kim JH, Contreras BA, et al, "An Observational Urodynamic Evaluation of Men With Lower Urinary Tract Symptoms Treated With Doxazosin," *Urology*, 1996, 47(6):840-4.

Kraklau DM and Bloom DA, "The Cystometrogram at 70 Years," *J Urol*, 1998, 160(2):316-9.
Massey A and Abrams P, "Urodynamics of the Female Lower Urinary Tract," *Urol Clin North Am*, 1985, 12(2):231-46.
Nigro DA, Wein AJ, Foy M, et al, "Associations Among Cystoscopic and Urodynamic Findings for Women Enrolled in the Interstitial Cystitis Data Base (ICDB) Study," *Urology*, 1997, 49(5A Suppl):86-92.
van Waaljwijk, van Doorn ES, Meier AH, et al, "Ambulatory Urodynamics: Extramural Testing of the Lower and Upper Urinary Tract by Holter Monitoring of Cystometrogram, Uroflowmetry, and Renal Pelvic Pressures," *Urol Clin North Am*, 1996, 23(3):345-71.

♦ **Cystometry** *see* Cystometrogram, Simple *on page 279*
♦ **Cystoscopy** *see* Cystourethroscopy *on page 285*

Cystoureteroscopy

Related Information

Catheterization, Urethral *on page 273*
Cystourethroscopy *on page 285*

Synonyms Ureteroscopy

Procedure Commonly Includes Direct visualization of the upper urinary tract, including dilatation and inspection of the ureters and the intrarenal collecting system. Flexible ureteroscopes are of small enough caliber to extend into the upper urinary tract combined with an instrument channel that accepts wires, baskets, and flexible lithotripsy probes.

Indications Indications for ureteroscopy include calculi removal, diagnosis, and therapeutic procedure other than calculi removal:

- lower ureteral calculi
- upper ureteral calculi, failed lithotripsy
- renal calculi, failed lithotripsy
- calculi associated with obstruction
- calculi plus suspicion of urothelial carcinoma
- evaluation of radiographic filling defects or obstruction
- evaluation of unilateral gross hematuria
- evaluation of unilateral malignant cytology
- surveillance after conservative treatment of an upper urinary tract tumor
- passage of a ureteral catheter for obstruction of fistula
- removal of a foreign body
- resection/fulguration of selected rumors
- dilation/incision of strictures

Contraindications Patients should be evaluated for active urinary tract infection, as instrumentation may exacerbate the condition and increase the risk for bacteremia and sepsis.

Patient Preparation The procedure and risks should be explained to the patient with informed consent obtained. The patient should be NPO after midnight for a morning procedure and NPO after a light breakfast for an afternoon procedure. Perioperative antibiotics are required. Generally, patients are given a broad-spectrum antibiotic immediately before the procedure (ampicillin and gentamicin) and this is continued for several dosages after the procedure. A general or regional anesthetic is normally required because of pain created when passing a rigid instrument or dilating the lower ureter.

Aftercare No specific aftercare is required. After the procedure, the patient is observed in a recovery area. Vital signs are recorded once, and prn in the "high-risk" patient. If no complications have occurred and sedation has worn off, the patient may be discharged from the testing area.

Complications In general, cystourethroscopy with ureteroscopy is considered a safe procedure. However, there is a smaller margin of safety for endoscopic surgery in the ureter and kidney, mainly because of the smaller anatomic size of the ureter as compared to the lower urinary tract. Risks are minimized with careful patient selection, complete urologic work-up, availability of essential instruments, and availability of fluoroscopy. The majority of serious complications are rare but include urethral perforation, false passage, and avulsion. Microscopic hematuria is common and self-limited.

Equipment Cystourethroscopy with ureteroscopy can be performed with either rigid or flexible endoscopes. Flexible ureteroscopes have become the preferred endoscope, with small enough caliber to extend into the upper

(Continued)

Cystoureteroscopy *(Continued)*

urinary tract combined with an instrument channel that accepts wires, baskets, biopsy forceps, and lithotripsy probes. Many smaller flexible instruments may be passed into the ureter without prior dilation depending on the ureter size. Because the size is not predictable, most authorities routinely dilate the ureter before a ureteroscopic procedure. Dilation expands the safety margin as the ureteroscopes are passed, and it allows potentially larger fragments of calculi to be removed. There are many acceptable methods of acute cystoscopic dilation for ureteroscopy, however, a dilating method over a prepositioned guidewire has been safest and most satisfactory. Although somewhat more cumbersome than passing a dilator directly, there are fewer false passages and intramural ureteral perforations with this method.

Technique The technique of balloon dilation involves passing a standard cystoscope into the bladder (see Cystourethroscopy for Method and Technique). The ureteral orifice is identified, and the floppy end of the balloon guidewire is inserted through the orifice and positioned into the renal pelvis. The position of the guidewire is monitored fluoroscopically throughout the dilatation process. Once the guidewire is in place, the balloon catheter is passed over the guidewire and its radiopaque markers positioned across the intramural ureteral tunnel and orifice. Once the dilating balloon is in proper position, the balloon is inflated. Generally, a 50% solution radiographic contrast agent is used to inflate the balloon for it to be visible fluoroscopically. Inflation is carried out slowly at a rate of 2 ATM/minute until all waisting of the balloon is removed. After the balloon is removed, the guidewire is left in place for the ureteroscope. The flexible ureteroscope is passed over the guidewire, which is back-loaded through its working channel. Fluoroscopic monitoring ensures proper positioning in the ureter. Once the ureteroscope is in the ureter, the irrigating fluid (0.9% normal saline or sorbitol) is attached to the irrigation channel of the instrument and direct visual advancement is performed. At this point, the guidewire is removed. Full examination of the upper urinary tract is performed with visual inspection and fluoroscopic guidance.

Data Acquired This examination provides information regarding the patency and normality of the upper urinary tract, and the renal collecting system. It is also used as a vehicle for sampling the ureter and renal pelvis via brushing and biopsy techniques.

Specimen Ureteral and intrarenal biopsies

Container Formulin jars, slides in 95% alcohol

Normal Findings Normal examination of the upper urinary tract

References

Bagley DH, "Ureteropyeloscopy With Flexible Fiberoptic Instruments," *Ureteroscopy*, Huffman JL, Bagley DH, and Lyon ES, eds, Philadelphia, PA: WB Saunders Co, 1988, 131-55.

Batter SJ and Dretler SP, "Ureterorenoscopic Approach to the Symptomatic Caliceal Diverticulum," *J Urol*, 1997, 158(3 Pt 1):709-13.

Biester R and Gillenwater JY, "Complications Following Ureteroscopy," *J Urol*, 1986, 136(2):380-2.

Blute ML, Segura JW, and Patterson DE, "Ureteroscopy," *J Urol*, 1988, 139(3):510-2.

Conlin MJ, Marberger M, and Bagley DH, "Ureteroscopy. Development and Instrumentation," *Urol Clin North Am*, 1997, 24(1):25-42.

Elashry OM, Elbahnasy AM, Rao GS, et al, "Flexible Ureteroscopy: Washington University Experience With the 9.3F and 7.5F Flexible Ureteroscopes," *J Urol*, 1997, 157(6):2084.

Erhard M, Salwen J, and Bagley DH, "Ureteroscopic Removal of Mid and Proximal Ureteral Calculi," *J Urol*, 1996, 155(1):56-7.

Hernandez D, Larrea Masvidal E, Castillo M, et al, "Ureteroscopy: Our Results and Complications," *Arch Esp Urol*, 1993, 46(5):405-9.

Huffman JL and Bagley DH, "Balloon Dilation of the Ureter for Ureteroscopy," *J Urol*, 1988, 140(5):954-6.

Keeley FX Jr, Bibbo M, and Bagley DH, "Ureteroscopic Treatment and Surveillance of Upper Urinary Tract Transitional Cell Carcinoma," *J Urol*, 1997, 157(5):1560-5.

Kim HL and Gerber GS, "Performing Flexible Ureteroscopy Through a Cystoscopy Introducer Sheath," *Urology*, 1999, 54(3):557-8.

Rozanski TA, Salazar F, and Thompson IM, "Direct Visual Bladder Catheterization Using a Short Rigid Ureteroscope," *Urology*, 1998, 51(5):827-8.

Scarpa RM, De Lisa A, and Usai E, "Diagnosis and Treatment of Ureteral Calculi During Pregnancy With Rigid Ureteroscopes," *J Urol*, 1996, 155(3):875-7.

Tawfiek ER and Bagley DH, "Management of Upper Urinary Tract Calculi With Ureteroscopic Techniques," *Urology*, 1999, 53(1):25-31.

Cystourethroscopy

Related Information

Catheterization, Urethral *on page 273*
Cystoureteroscopy *on page 283*

Synonyms Cystoscopy

Procedure Commonly Includes Direct visualization of the anterior and posterior urethra, bladder neck, and bladder. Material for both cytologic and histologic examination can be obtained. With local urethral anesthesia, biopsy and cauterization of the urethral and bladder mucosa can be accomplished with light sedation. In addition, upper tract instrumentation can be performed.

Indications The primary indication for cystourethroscopy is the diagnosis of lower urinary tract disease. The most common indication is in the evaluation of microscopic and gross hematuria. Additional indications involving the lower urinary tract include evaluation of voiding symptoms, both obstructive and irritative, which may be the result of neurologic, inflammatory, neoplastic, or congenital abnormalities. Access to the upper urinary tract can also be obtained cystoscopically.

Contraindications Patients should be evaluated for active urinary tract infection, as instrumentation may exacerbate the condition and increase the risk for bacteremia and sepsis.

Patient Preparation The procedure should be explained to the patient with informed consent obtained. Reasonable expectations should be given in terms of discomfort. Because the urethra is a sterile tract, it should be prepped and draped in a sterile fashion. In the male, it is recommended to give a retrograde injection of 10 cc of 2% lidocaine hydrochloride jelly followed by a urethral clamp for 5 minutes. This will allow the anesthetic to contact the mucosal surfaces. In the female, 10 cc of 2% lidocaine hydrochloride jelly should be instilled into the urethra prior to the procedure.

Aftercare No specific aftercare is required. After the procedure, the patient is observed in a recovery area. Vital signs are recorded once, and prn in the "high-risk" patient. If no complications have occurred and sedation has worn off, the patient may be discharged from the testing area.

Complications In general, cystourethroscopy is considered a low-risk procedure. The majority of serious complications are rare, and include urethral or bladder perforation, false passage, and avulsion. Microscopic hematuria is common and self-limited.

Equipment Cystourethroscopy can be performed with either rigid or flexible endoscopes. Rigid endoscopes allow better optics, a larger working chamber for accessory instruments, a larger lumen for water flow, and easier manipulation for maintaining bladder orientation. The advantages of flexible endoscopes include greater comfort for the patient, ability to perform the procedure in the supine position, ease of introduction over an elevated bladder neck, and the ability to inspect at any angle with deflection of the instrument tip. A variety of endoscope sizes are available. In general, the choice of an endoscope with respect to size should be the smallest outer circumference to accomplish the task. If diagnostic cystourethroscopy is being performed, a small instrument is adequate. If a larger working channel is needed for accessory equipment, a larger endoscope is chosen.

Technique Procedure may be performed with the patient in the supine or sitting position depending on the catheter used. Prior to insertion of the instrument, the urethral meatus should be inspected. If the meatal size appears inadequate to accept the endoscope, it should be dilated first. The endoscope sheath should be generously lubricated with 2% lidocaine hydrochloride jelly. In the male, the penis should be grasped and straightened at a right angle to the abdomen. The endoscope is inserted into the meatus and the anterior urethra is inspected. As the endoscope is gently advanced into the bulbar urethra, the endoscope and penis are lowered until parallel with the floor. This allows passage of the instrument through the membranous urethra. The endoscope is continually advanced into the bladder with careful inspection of the prostatic urethra. In the female, inspection of the urethra is easily performed by inserting the endoscope under direct vision into the urethral meatus and by

(Continued)

Cystourethroscopy *(Continued)*

directing the instrument cephalad toward the umbilicus. Once inside the bladder, a systematic evaluation of the entire bladder surface is performed.

Data Acquired This examination provides information regarding the patency and normality of the lower urinary tract and the bladder mucosa. It is also used as a vehicle for sampling the urethral and bladder mucosa via brushing and biopsy techniques.

Specimen Urethral or bladder mucosa washings, brushings, or biopsy

Container Formulin jars, slides in 95% alcohol

Normal Findings Normal examination of the lower urinary tract

♦ **Filling Cystometrogram** *see* Cystometrogram, Simple *on page 279*
♦ **Foley Catheterization** *see* Catheterization, Urethral *on page 273*

Injection of the Corpora Cavernosa With Pharmacologic Agents (Papaverine, Phentolamine)

Related Information

Nocturnal Penile Tumescence Test *on page 287*
Penile Blood Flow *on page 290*

Synonyms Intracavernous Injection of Papaverine; Papaverine Test

Procedure Commonly Includes Injection of a vasoactive compound such as papaverine into the corpora cavernosa of the penis in order to produce an erection. Papaverine is a phosphodiesterase inhibitor which relaxes smooth muscle (both vascular and nonvascular) and stimulates venous congestion. The cavernous tissue of the penis becomes filled with blood and a pharmacologic erection is induced. This procedure is useful in evaluating men with erectile dysfunction. It has been used to differentiate organic (biologic) impotence from psychogenic impotence. Papaverine injection produces a full erection in healthy males as well as individuals with psychogenic impotence. In patients with vasculogenic impotence, however, papaverine injection is unlikely to produce an erection. Thus, if a full erection results from papaverine injection, vascular insufficiency is probably excluded as the cause of impotence.

Indications The Papaverine Test is useful in identifying patients whose erectile dysfunction is secondary to vascular insufficiency. It may also be used to confirm results obtained from nocturnal penile tumescence testing, particularly when unsupervised home testing is performed (see Nocturnal Penile Tumescence Test *on page 287*).

Contraindications Relative contraindications to testing include:

- prior adverse reaction to papaverine
- uncorrectable coagulopathy
- orthostatic hypotension
- hemoglobinopathies (sickle cell trait, sickle cell disease, etc)

Patient Preparation A medical history and physical examination is required for all patients with erectile failure. Screening laboratory studies such as prolactin, follicle stimulating hormone (FSH), luteinizing hormone (LH), and testosterone are often ordered prior to any procedures. If the patient is a good candidate, the technique of papaverine injection is discussed with the patient along with potential complications. Informed consent is obtained. Special scheduling for this procedure is not necessary since injection is performed quickly in a physician's office.

Aftercare All patients should remain in the testing center until the erection has completely subsided. In the majority of patients this occurs spontaneously within hours or minutes, but a few may require pharmacologic reversal. Reversal is performed either by aspiration alone or by injection of epinephrine plus aspiration.

Complications Intracavernous injection is a safe procedure. Minor adverse reactions include priapism, lightheadedness, and penile hematoma. As noted above, priapism can be reversed if necessary.

Technique Papaverine injection may be carried out in conjunction with objective measurements of penile tumescence, such as Snap-Gauge or Rigiscan (see Nocturnal Penile Tumescence Test *on page 287*). These devices are optional. The penis is examined immediately prior to testing. The flaccid penis is injected with papaverine hydrochloride and, if desired, phentolamine mesylate also. Phentolamine decreases adrenergic tone and facilitates smooth muscle relaxation. A fine hypodermic needle is commonly used, such as a 26-gauge, 3/8" needle. No local anesthesia is required. A tourniquet is not necessary and the injection is made directly into the corpora cavernosa. Usual doses employed are 50 mg of papaverine and 1-6 mg of phentolamine in a volume of 2 mL. After injection, the patient is asked to stand next to the examination table and penile response is then observed.

Data Acquired

- time elapsed from injection to maximal penile response
- observer's subjective rating of erection quality: absent, partially rigid, full tumescence, and rigidity
- objective measurement of penile tumescence (in millimeters) and/or rigidity (from 0% to 100%) if formal monitoring devices are used
- duration of erection

Normal Findings Healthy individuals with normal sexual function achieve full erections after papaverine injection. Studies also suggest that men with psychogenic impotence also respond with full erections after papaverine. Most erections are produced within 10 minutes of injection and may last several hours.

Critical Values Absent or partial erections after papaverine injection suggest a vascular cause for impotence. An incomplete erectile response may also be secondary to other factors such as excessive patient anxiety, incorrect technique, etc. Thus, some authors regard an incomplete response as "inconclusive" and not diagnostic of vascular insufficiency. A normal erectile response makes vasculogenic impotence unlikely.

Additional Information Intracavernous injection with papaverine was first introduced in the early 1980s. Since then it has grown in popularity, due to its safety, convenience, and speed. It is easier to perform than formal, overnight nocturnal penile tumescence monitoring. It also is a dynamic assessment of erectile function, unlike the penile brachial index (PBI) which measures blood flow in the flaccid penis. More research is required for this promising technique.

References

Abber JC, Lue TF, and Orvis BR, et al, "Diagnostic Tests for Impotence: A Comparison of Papaverine Injection With the Penile-Brachial Index and Nocturnal Penile Tumescence Monitoring," *J Urol*, 1986, 135(5):923-5.

Vardi Y, Sprecher E, and Gruenwald I, "Logistic Regression and Survival Analysis of 450 Impotent Patients Treated With Injection Therapy: Long-Term Dropout Parameters," *J Urol*, 2000, 163(2):471.

Virag R, Frydman D, Legman M, et al, "Intracavernous Injection of Papaverine as a Diagnostic and Therapeutic Method in Erectile Failure," *Angiology*, 1984, 35(2):79-87.

♦ **Intracavernous Injection of Papaverine** *see* Injection of the Corpora Cavernosa With Pharmacologic Agents (Papaverine, Phentolamine) *on page 286*

♦ **Multichannel Cystometrogram** *see* Cystometrogram, Complex *on page 275*

♦ **Nocturnal Erection Monitoring** *see* Nocturnal Penile Tumescence Test *on page 287*

Nocturnal Penile Tumescence Test

Related Information

Injection of the Corpora Cavernosa With Pharmacologic Agents (Papaverine, Phentolamine) *on page 286*

Penile Blood Flow *on page 290*

Synonyms Nocturnal Erection Monitoring; NPT; Sleep Erection Monitoring

Procedure Commonly Includes Objective measurement of penile tumescence and/or rigidity during sleep to document the presence of sleep-associated erections. Nocturnal penile tumescence (NPT) testing may be performed in a formal Sleep Laboratory under electroencephalographic monitoring or at the patient's home using inexpensive portable devices. A variety of these screening devices are available, such as the mercury-filled strain gauge (records maximal changes in penile circumference), the Snap-Gauge (records

(Continued)

Nocturnal Penile Tumescence Test *(Continued)*

penile rigidity), and the Rigiscan (records continuous rigidity and tumescence). NPT monitoring is a frequently used ancillary test of erectile dysfunction and is based on the assumption that men with psychogenic impotence have normal erections during sleep, whereas men with organic impotence have impaired erections during sleep.

Indications NPT testing is indicated when the etiology of erectile failure is unclear after a complete medical history and physical. This procedure may be useful in differentiating organic impotence (ie, from diabetes, medications) from psychogenic impotence. It should be noted that NPT testing is based on a number of assumptions which have recently come under some scrutiny. Important limitations exist.

Contraindications There are no absolute contraindications to NPT testing. However, the following are several situations where home NPT monitoring may be inappropriate. In these instances, the results of unsupervised home NPT monitoring are unreliable. Formal sleep monitoring in a laboratory may be more accurate and reliable.

- patient with dementia
- patient with poor vision or poor hand coordination who is unable to apply penile loops
- patient with suspected malingering behavior

Patient Preparation The details of NPT testing are discussed with the patient and consent is obtained. If the procedure is to be performed at home, several guidelines are useful. The patient should maintain his normal sleeping hours as much as possible. Interruptions should be minimized. Heavy alcohol or narcotic use should be avoided due to the potential suppressive effects on erectile function. Similarly, sleeping medications should be avoided unless under a physician's specific instructions. The patient should take his usual prescription medications unless otherwise directed by physician. In certain cases, NPT testing is best performed in a Sleep Laboratory with all night polygraphic sleep monitoring. This form of testing is valid, reliable, and expensive. Testing may need to be repeated on a second night (and sometimes a third night) if there is evidence of erectile dysfunction on the first night. Similar caveats regarding alcohol and narcotic use also apply. The details of scheduling are handled by the referring physician in conjunction with the Sleep Laboratory.

Aftercare No specific activity restrictions are necessary.

Complications None. NPT testing is a safe, noninvasive procedure.

Technique Several devices are available for home NPT monitoring and are briefly described below. Other similar devices are also available.

- NPT stamp test: This simple screening test uses adhesive paper stamps 1¹/₄" x 1" similar to postage stamps. A strip of four stamps is snugly wrapped around the penis with the overlying stamp wetted and sealed. The following morning the stamp ring is examined for breaks along the perforations. This may be repeated over a three night period.
- Strain-Gauge: This device measures changes in penile circumference. An elastic loop is placed around the shaft of the penis. The loop contains a conductive medium such as mercury. An increase in penile circumference causes a stretching of the loop and a change in electrical signal. This is recorded on a portable monitor.
- Snap-Gauge (Dacomed Corp, Minneapolis, MN): This measures penile rigidity, unlike the previous techniques which measure only penile circumference. Three plastic elements are arranged in parallel on a Velcro fastener which is wrapped around the penis. Each plastic film breaks at a predetermined rigidity of the penis (ie, 10 oz, 15 oz, 20 oz).
- Rigiscan (Dacomed Corp, Minneapolis, MN): This device consists of two loops surrounding the penis, attached to a small computer with memory capacity. The Rigiscan measures both penile tumescence and rigidity on a continuous basis.

Normal Findings Data acquired by home NPT testing is reviewed by physician. The definition of a positive or normal test is highly dependent on the type of monitoring technique employed. For example, a normal Stamp Test consists of a stamp ring broken at the perforations. This indicates that at least one nocturnal erection has occurred, but it provides no data regarding rigidity of erection, movement artifact, frequency, and duration of erections. For the Snap-Gauge, a normal test is defined as rupture of all three plastic elements. Again, this device does not assess erection duration or frequency. More complex instruments such as the mercury-filled Strain-Gauge and the Rigiscan provide continuous data over an extended time period. Normal values for penile tumescence and rigidity have been generated from healthy individuals. For the Rigiscan, penile tumescence is measured in millimeters at the base and the tip of the penis and penile rigidity is reported on a relative scale (0% to 100%) and is also measured at the base and tip. A 60% rigidity value by Rigiscan corresponds to the lowest intracorporeal pressure necessary for an erection. Although normative values have been established, the criteria for diagnosing organic impotence are variable and not well established. The precise cut-points for diagnosing organic impotence have not been agreed upon.

Limitations

- basic assumptions underlying NPT have been challenged by some
- home NPT devices have a significant false-positive and false-negative rate
- supervised NPT testing with polysomnogram recording is expensive and labor intensive
- specific criteria used to diagnose organic impotence has not been standardized
- few studies have addressed the diagnostic accuracy of home NPT devices
- patients with the penile-steal syndrome may have normal NPT results
- motion artifact may be misleading and significant

Additional Information As reviewed by Schiavi,[1] NPT testing is based on several assumptions:

- NPT is normal in men with psychogenic impotence
- normal NPT excludes organic impotence
- NPT is abnormal in men with organic impotence

The weight of the data available supports these three assumptions. However, each has been challenged and it is likely that exceptions exist to each of these "rules." Thus, if NPT testing is normal in a patient in whom vasculogenic impotence is strongly suspected, further diagnostic evaluation may be warranted. Nevertheless, this procedure is safe, well-tolerated and often valid. Effective therapeutic interventions are available for men with either vasculogenic or psychogenic impotence, and thus this differentiation becomes important clinically. An abnormal NPT result often prompts further investigative studies of a more invasive nature. Formal NPT testing in a Sleep Laboratory is considered by some experts to be the best (and perhaps the only) test capable of differentiating organic from psychogenic impotence.

Footnotes

1. Schiavi RC, "Nocturnal Penile Tumescence in the Evaluation of Erectile Disorders: A Critical Review," *J Sex Marital Ther*, 1988, 14(2):83-97.

References

Bradley WE, "New Techniques in Evaluation of Impotence," *Urology*, 1987, 29(4):383-8.

De Wire DM, "Evaluation and Treatment of Erectile Dysfunction," *Am Fam Physician*, 1996, 53(6):2101-8.

Guay AT, Heatley GJ, and Murray FT, "Comparison of Results of Nocturnal Penile Tumescence and Rigidity in a Sleep Laboratory Versus a Portable Home Monitor," *Urology*, 1996, 48(6):912-6.

Guldner GT and Morrell MJ, "Nocturnal Penile Tumescence and Rigidity Evaluation in Men With Epilepsy," *Epilepsia*, 1996, 37(12):1211-4.

Hatzichristou DG, Hatzimouratidis K, Ioannides E, et al, "Nocturnal Penile Tumescence and Rigidity Monitoring in Young Potent Volunteers: Reproducibility, Evaluation Criteria and the Effect of Sexual Intercourse," *J Urol*, 1998, 159(6):1921-6.

Hirshkowitz M and Moore CA, "Sleep-Related Erectile Activity," *Neurol Clin*, 1996, 14(4):721-37.

Knoll LD and Abrams JH, "Application of Nocturnal Electrobioimpedance Volumetric Assessment: A Feasibility Study in Men Without Erectile Dysfunction," *J Urol*, 1999, 161(4):1137-40.

Sattar AA, Wery D, Golzarian J, et al, "Correlation of Nocturnal Penile Tumescence Monitoring Duplex Ultrasonography and Infusion Cavernosometry for the Diagnosis of Erectile Dysfunction," *J Urol*, 1996, 155(4):1274-6.

Schiavi RC, "Nocturnal Penile Tumescence in the Evaluation of Erectile Disorders: A Critical Review," *J Sex Marital Ther*, 1988, 14(2):83-97.

Veldhuis JD, Iranmanesh A, Mulligan T, et al, "Disruption of the Young-Adult Synchrony Between Luteinizing Hormone Release and Oscillations in Follicle-Stimulating Hormone, Prolactin, and

(Continued)

Nocturnal Penile Tumescence Test *(Continued)*

Nocturnal Penile Tumescence (NPT) in Healthy Older Men," *J Clin Endocrinol Metab*, 1999, 84(10):3498-505.

♦ **NPT** *see* Nocturnal Penile Tumescence Test *on page 287*

♦ **Papaverine Test** *see* Injection of the Corpora Cavernosa With Pharmacologic Agents (Papaverine, Phentolamine) *on page 286*

Penile Blood Flow

Related Information

Injection of the Corpora Cavernosa With Pharmacologic Agents (Papaverine, Phentolamine) *on page 286*

Nocturnal Penile Tumescence Test *on page 287*

Ultrasound, Penile Duplex *on page 500*

Synonyms Penile Doppler Studies

Applies to Penile Blood Pressure as Compared to Brachial Blood Pressure

Replaces Arteriogram

Procedure Commonly Includes Compression of penis with pneumatic cuff and measurement of systolic blood pressure. Brachial blood pressure is also recorded.

Indications To determine if the cause of impotence is vasculogenic. It is also used in postoperative evaluation of penile blood flow following lower abdominal and pelvic surgeries.

Equipment A 9.5 MHz directional ultrasound volcimeter is used to locate the cavernous artery. If this cannot be accomplished, the dorsalis penis or the frenucar artery may be used. A 1-2.5 cm pneumatic cuff attached to an aneroid manometer is placed around the base of the penis and inflated to suprasystolic pressure. The cuff is then slowly deflated until the Doppler shifted arterial signal is resumed. This pressure is recorded. The steps listed are repeated three times and the average penile blood pressure is calculated. Obtain a brachial systolic pressure three times and calculate the mean systolic blood pressure. Calculate the ratio of the penile systolic blood pressure to the brachial systolic blood pressure to yield the penile-brachial index (PBI) or penile flow index. If the PBI is normal, this procedure should be repeated following a 3-minute exercise of the buttocks and legs such as running in place or bicycling. If the difference between the exercise PBI (EPBI) and the resting PBI (RPBI) is >0.15, this is consistent with pelvic steal syndrome.

Turnaround Time Immediate

Sampling Time 1-2 hours

Causes for Rejection Patient with Texas catheter

Normal Findings Penile-brachial index <0.8

Limitations It may be technically difficult to detect the cavernous artery pulse because it is not a superficial artery. It is adequate blood flow to this artery, not the dorsalis penis, that is necessary for erection. Also, these studies are performed on the flaccid not the the erect penis. The test may be found to be objectionable to patient or technician.

Additional Information In the work-up of impotence, one should obviously start with a good sexual as well as medical history (including medication) and physical. Such clues as a slow onset of symptoms, evidence of claudication, and the presence of decreased pulses and bruits suggest a vascular etiology. In addition, baseline blood work should be done before any procedures are performed. This should include electrolytes, blood glucose, urinalysis, CBC, liver, renal and thyroid functions, serum FSH, LH prolactin, and testosterone. Penile Doppler studies are commonly performed following nocturnal penile tumescence monitoring (NPTM) that is suggestive of organic disease. It should be remembered that normal NPTM do not necessarily mean that impotence is psychogenic as only changes in penile circumference are measured not necessarily the degree of rigidity or duration of erection. In addition, patients with penile steal syndrome may have completely normal NPTMs. Therefore Doppler studies should probably be performed even if NPTMs are normal and there is suspicion of vasculogenic impotence. If the preliminary H & P suggests diffuse vascular disease, abdominal x-ray, and

Bone Density

Synonyms DEXA; Dual Energy X-ray Absorptiometry; DXA

Procedure Commonly Includes The gold standard for measuring bone density is dual energy x-ray absorptiometry (DEXA) measuring central sites (spine and hip). The technique involves passage of a pencil beam or fan beam x-ray through the bone to be measured. X-ray is collected at a detector, the x-ray energy is changed to electrical signal and sent to a computer for analysis and display. The amount of x-ray which passes through the bone is proportional to the amount of calcium in the bone (based on cadaver studies ashing bone for calcium content).

Indications HCFA has published guidelines, the Bone Mass Measurement Act (BMMA) on July 1, 1998 for measurement of bone density (by many techniques) in Medicare beneficiaries. The indications are as follows.

- An estrogen-deficient woman at clinical risk of osteoporosis as determined by a physician or qualified nonphysician practitioner based on her medical history and other findings.
- A person with vertebral abnormalities as demonstrated by x-ray to be indicative of osteoporosis, osteopenia, or vertebral fracture.
- A person receiving or expecting to receive long-term glucocorticoid (steroid) therapy (equivalent to ≥7.5 mg of prednisone per day for longer than 3 months).
- A person with primary hyperparathyroidism.
- A person being monitored to assess the response to or efficacy of an FDA-approved osteoporosis drug therapy.

Other insurers vary in their coverage and indications for bone density, generally requiring multiple risk factors for coverage. These risk factors may include amenorrhea, anticonvulsant therapy, height loss >1½ inches, any previous fracture, eating disorders, low body weight (<127 lb), smoking family history, early menopause, and rheumatoid arthritis to name a few.

Patient Preparation Barium in the small or large intestines will obscure measurement. The patient should remove all metal in the path of the x-ray.

Special Instructions The patient needs to lay on back for the procedure. Any movement will interfere with the scanning procedure.

Turnaround Time 5-10 minutes if only one site is measured; 10-15 minutes for two sites; 20-30 minutes if total body is measured.

Limitations Lumbar spine density is often falsely elevated in older patients who have extra vertebral calcium deposits such as in osteophytes from degenerative disk disease and facet arthritis or aortic calcification. Hip density and peripheral sites are preferred in these patients. The machines have a weight limit, which varies from 260-300 lb.

Additional Information The World Health Organization has established definitions of normal/abnormal based on T-scores (standard deviation units below peak bone mass - bone mass in young normals 20-40 years of age).

T-score: greater than or equal to -1: normal; between -1 and -2.5: osteopenia; less than -2.5: osteoporosis

The National Osteoporosis Foundation (NOF) has published treatment guidelines based on bone mineral density and risk factors. The NOF recommends treatment if the T-score is less than -1.5 if risk factors are present (previous fracture, positive family history of osteoporosis, body weight less than 127 lb, or current smoker). Treatment is recommended without risk factors if the T-score is less than -2.0.

Breast Examination

Synonyms CBE; Clinical Breast Examination

Procedure Commonly Includes Examination of the breast

Indications Screening for malignancy of the breast or work-up of symptomatic breast disease

Patient Preparation The patient should unclothe the upper half of the body and may be provided with a gown that does not interfere with inspection and palpation. Good lighting is essential.

(Continued)

Breast Examination *(Continued)*

Special Instructions In premenopausal women, the ideal breast examination is performed 3-10 days after the period begins, when the breasts are the least tender and the least dense.

Technique Inspection begins with the patient erect with her arms relaxed. The breasts are compared for asymmetry, skin lesions, skin changes, and nipple-areola abnormalities. Examination continues with the patient raising her arms over her head, with her hands on her hips, and with her arms relaxed as she leans forward. Palpation is performed with the patient lying on her back, with the ipsilateral arm raised above the head. The breast is then systematically palpated. The examination should extend superiorly to the clavicle, inferiorly to the lower rib cage, medially to the sternal border, and laterally to the midaxillary line. The vertical strip method of covering the area is most effective. Palpation is performed with the pads of the index, middle, and fourth fingers. A dime-sized rotary motion facilitates the palpation of a small movable mass. Pressure is varied in order to palpate the various depths within the breast. Palpation of the subareolar area is important. Gently compressing the areola and nipple completes the palpation of the area. Finally, the arms are elevated and supported and the axillary area is palpated with the patient erect. Palpation of the supra- and infraclavicular areas concludes the clinical breast examination.

Data Acquired All clinically significant abnormalities and anatomic variations should be documented in the patient's medical record. The physical findings should be described in clear, concise, descriptive terms, such as diffuse, discrete, distinct, firm, full, hard, localized, lumpy, nodular, red, soft, tender, uniform, and vague. The exact location of any finding is given. Superficially located tumors may cause bulges in the breast contour or retraction of the overlying skin. Tumors deeper within the breast that involve the fibrous septa may also cause retraction. Edema of the skin of the breast (peau d'orange) is usually extensive and readily apparent. Erythema is another sign of pathology that is evident on inspection. Erythema may be due to cellulitis or abscess in the breast, but a diagnosis of inflammatory carcinoma should always be considered. The new onset of nipple retraction should be regarded with a high index of suspicion. Ulceration and eczematous changes of the nipple may be the first signs of Paget disease. Spontaneous nipple discharge is abnormal and requires investigation. Ductograms of the single duct can demonstrate intraluminal lesions. All discrete masses should be further evaluated with diagnostic mammography and ultrasound. Depending on the findings, FNA-B, excisional biopsy, or ultrasound-guided biopsy may be warranted.

References

Marchant DJ, "Clinical Breast Examination Technique," *Breast Disease*, Marchant DJ, ed, Philadelphia, PA: WB Saunders Co, 1997.

Morrow M, "Physical Examination of the Breast," *Diseases of the Breast*, Harris JR, Lippman MD, Morrow M, et al, eds, Philadelphia, PA: Lippincott Williams & Wilkins, 1996.

♦ **CBE** *see* Breast Examination *on page 295*

Cervical Polypectomy

Related Information

Colposcopy *on page 298*
Endocervical Curettage *on page 305*
Endometrial Biopsy *on page 307*
Papanicolaou Smear *on page 316*

Synonyms Biopsy, Cervix; Polypectomy, Cervix

Procedure Commonly Includes Removal of an endocervical polyp

Indications Cervical polypectomy is indicated:

- in patients with visible cervical polyp
- in patients with postmenopausal bleeding and cervical polyp present (in conjunction with endometrial biopsy). **Note:** It may be desirable to perform endometrial biopsy at the same time as a cervical polypectomy, even in asymptomatic women. In addition, endocervical curettage may be done in conjunction with colposcopy if there is an abnormal Pap smear.

Contraindications

- pregnancy

- active cervicitis

Care should be exercised when removing a large cervical polyp and/or in patients who have a history of bleeding disorders. Patients should be observed closely for bleeding at the site of biopsy of cervical polyp removal.

Patient Preparation Cervical polypectomy is performed as an outpatient procedure. Most cervical polyps are incidentally noted during routine pelvic exam and Pap smear and are, therefore, removed at the time of these procedures in the outpatient setting. Anesthesia or premedication with pain medicines is not indicated. The cervix does not have pain receptors but rather stretch and pressure receptors.

Aftercare Occasionally patients will experience mild vasovagal symptoms during or after the procedure. The patient should be allowed time to sit or lie on the examining table before sending them home. Minor cramping may occur after the procedure, particularly if the cervical canal was manipulated. The patient may experience some light vaginal spotting for 1-3 days after the procedure. If Monsel's paste is applied to the polyp stalk site, a brownish black discharge will be noted. Menstrual pads are preferred over tampons for management of discharge.

Technique After informed consent is obtained, the patient is placed in the dorsal lithotomy position on an examination table with stirrups. A vaginal speculum is inserted gently and adjusted to expose the entire cervix. A Pap smear is obtained, if it has not previously been done. The cervix is gently cleansed with a cotton-tipped applicator soaked in Betadine® or other cleansing solution (if iodine allergy). The base of the polyp is grasped with a tissue cervical biopsy forceps, Kevorkian cervical biopsy forceps, or a ringed forceps. Care is taken to remove the polyp at the base of the stalk. Hemostasis is then generally obtained with silver nitrate-impregnated sticks. If bleeding is brisk, occasionally Monsel's solution (ferric subsulfate) is needed. Rarely, the application of a single absorbable 3-0 suture is required to stop bleeding.

Specimen The polyp removed is placed in a fixative solution (formalin, Bouin, Holland, etc). The specimen should be clearly labeled for pathology review. The clinician should provide all pertinent clinical information relative to specimen interpretation.

Normal Findings Cervical polyps are invariably benign, however, they are submitted to the laboratory for confirmation.

Additional Information Cervical polyps will recur particularly if the stalk is left in place.

References

Robboy SJ, Kraus FT, and Kurman RJ, "Gross Description, Processing, and Reporting of Gynecologic and Obstetric Specimens," *Blaustein's Pathology of the Female Genital Tract*, 4th ed, Kurman RJ, ed, New York, NY: Springer-Verlag, 1994, 1225-45.

Chorionic Villus Sampling

Related Information

Amniocentesis *on page 293*

Synonyms CVS

Procedure Commonly Includes Under ultrasound guidance, the transcervical or transabdominal procurement of placental tissue for genetic analysis at 10-12 weeks of gestation

Indications Advanced maternal age (age 35 or older at the time of delivery) or any other indication for early prenatal genetic screening

Contraindications Active cervical infection. The transcervical approach is difficult when the placenta is fundal.

Patient Preparation The patient should have a full bladder. Patient should drink 1 quart of fluid 1 hour prior to the procedure.

Aftercare No intercourse for several days after the procedure.

Special Instructions **Duration of Procedure:** 30-60 minutes

Complications A pregnancy loss rate of 0.6% to 2%.

Equipment Standard ultrasound and chorionic villus sampling equipment including a soft 5.7 French, 27 cm cannula, a syringe, and tissue growth media

(Continued)

Chorionic Villus Sampling *(Continued)*

Technique A speculum is placed into the vagina. The cervix is cleansed with antiseptic solution and sometimes grasped with a tenaculum. Under direct visualization by ultrasound, the cannula is then advanced into the uterus and a small amount of placental tissue is aspirated. Growth and analysis are performed at a certified Genetic Laboratory.

Data Acquired Karyotype of the fetus

Turnaround Time 1-3 weeks

Specimen Placental tissue

Causes for Rejection Inadequate amount of specimen, bacterial contamination

Normal Findings Normal chromosomes (or normal genes if gene probes are to be used)

Critical Values Any karyotype other than normal 46,XX or 46,XY

Limitations On rare occasions, the placenta may exhibit some mosaicism which is not present in the fetus (a 46,XX reading may be from maternal tissue being cultured in 1% of procedures with the risk of maternal cells being accidentally cultured with amniocentesis is 0.3%)

References

"Chorionic Villus Sampling," *ACOG Committee Opinion 560*, Washington, DC: American College of Obstetrics and Gynecology, 1995.

Wapner RJ, "Chorionic Villus Sampling," *Obstet Gynecol Clin North Am*, 1997, 24(1):83-110.

♦ **Clinical Breast Examination** *see* Breast Examination *on page 295*

Colposcopy

Related Information

Cervical Polypectomy *on page 296*
Endocervical Curettage *on page 305*
Flexible Fiberoptic Sigmoidoscopy *on page 76*
Loop Electrosurgical Excisional Procedure (LEEP) *on page 311*
Papanicolaou Smear *on page 316*

Procedure Commonly Includes Colposcopy is a clinical procedure that allows examination of the epithelium and underlying vasculature of the uterine cervix and surrounding anogenital area. Characteristic tissue images, composed of epithelial cell morphology and vascular patterns, enable the clinical recognition of pathology. The procedure is enhanced by the use of chemical solutions (acetic acid and Lugol's iodine) applied to the epithelium as contrasting agents to assist in differentiating normal from abnormal tissue.

Indications Diagnostic evaluation of patients with abnormal cervical cytology or evaluation of an observed cervical, vaginal, vulvar, or perianal lesion

Contraindications There are no contraindications to colposcopic examination. Great care, however, should be taken if biopsy is necessary in patients who are pregnant or are in their early postpartum period, and in patients who are receiving anticoagulation therapy or who have bleeding disorders. If possible, it is best to defer biopsy in pregnant patients or patients in their early postpartum period until approximately 4-6 weeks postpartum. If deferment is not reasonable, then biopsy should be performed in a controlled setting by experienced personnel.

Patient Preparation Patient education with regard to the significance of an abnormal Pap smear, the objectives of colposcopy, and the importance of follow-up should be part of the informed consent process. Colposcopy is performed as an outpatient evaluation. The procedure is generally well tolerated, however, premedication with an analgesic may be administered after informed consent is obtained.

Aftercare Occasionally, patients will experience mild vasovagal symptoms during or after their procedure. Patients should be allowed time to sit or lie on the examination table before sending them home. Patients should be advised to expect mild vaginal spotting for 1-3 days after the procedure, if a biopsy is obtained. If Monsel's paste is applied to a biopsy site, a brownish black discharge will also noted. Menstrual pads are preferred over tampons for management of discharge. Minor cramping pain may occur after the procedure; ibuprofen or acetaminophen should be sufficient for analgesia.

Special Instructions The clinician should correlate the clinical history with both the Pap smear results, colposcopy findings, and the cervical biopsy results. All specimens should clearly be labeled at the time they are obtained.

Equipment The colposcope is a stereoscopic magnifying instrument with a powerful light source that provides a three-dimensional image of the surface epithelium and the underlying vasculature of the cervix, vagina, and external anogenital area. The magnification range is from 5x to 40x, however, 5x and 16x are generally most useful for diagnostic evaluation. The colposcope is equipped with a green filter which enhances the visualization of the vascular bed of the cervix. This filter absorbs red light, and the transmitted visual image of the vasculature is perceived as black. The relative merits of the commercially available colposcopes are discussed in a thorough review[1].

A wide array of punch biopsy-type instruments are used for obtaining cervical biopsy specimens. Kevorkian and Tischler-Morgan biopsy forceps are most commonly used for cervical biopsy. When concerns for bleeding exist, or biopsy of an endocervical lesion in a narrow canal is desired, the smaller Mini-Townsend biopsy forceps may be useful. Endocervical curettage is best performed using a Kevorkian curette (to be distinguished from the Kevorkian biopsy forceps). The Keyes punch biopsy instrument is useful for vulvar or perianal biopsy. This instrument bores a small plug of skin of varying depth, depending on the pressure employed during the biopsy.

Technique It has been known for many years that cervical, vaginal, vulvar, and perianal diseases are linked by the human papilloma virus. Thus, when screening for dysplastic processes, it is wise to inspect the entire anogenital area, in addition to evaluation of the cervix.

After informed consent is obtained, the patient is placed in dorsal lithotomy position on an examination table with stirrups. The vaginal speculum is inserted gently and adjusted to expose as much of the cervix and vagina as possible. The colposcope and table height are then positioned to optimize visualization of the cervix and vagina. If a Papanicolaou smear or cervicovaginal cultures are desired, it is best to obtain them at this time. Cervical smears taken after the application of acetic acid are less reliable. The cervix is then gently cleansed with a cotton-tipped applicator.

Prior to application of any solution, systematic evaluation of the ectocervix, the accessible portion of the endocervix, the vaginal fornices, and the vaginal walls is performed. The transformation zone should be visualized to its most cranial extent. Greater exposure to the endocervical canal may be achieved in several ways:

1. placing pressure behind either the anterior or posterior cervical lip with a cotton-tipped applicator
2. using gentle traction on the cervix itself with a cotton-tipped applicator
3. placement of an endocervical speculum into the endocervical canal.

After inspection of the cervix, examine the vaginal fornices and vaginal walls in a systematic manner by rotation and withdrawal of the speculum.

After thorough inspection of all tissues, 2% acetic acid is applied generously to the cervix using a large cotton swab. This assists in differentiating normal squamous epithelium from dysplastic epithelium by coagulating the cytoplasmic and nuclear proteins of the squamous epithelium, making them opaque and white. Dysplastic epithelium will generally appear whiter than normal epithelium. The action of acetic acid is short-lived and reapplication is often necessary during the colposcopic procedure.

After completion of cervical and vaginal colposcopy, remove the speculum and inspect the vulva and perianal region in a similar manner. Inspect systematically and thoroughly both prior to and after the application of acetic acid. When applying acetic acid, it should be noted that vulvar and perianal epithelium requires longer exposure time to before characteristic acetowhitening appears.

Tissue sampling: If biopsy is performed, patients may experience brief cramping pain, however, local anesthetic is seldom necessary. Any lesion identified as suspicious for a dysplastic or neoplastic process should be biopsied. Colposcopic findings that may indicate a need for biopsy are discussed

(Continued)

Colposcopy *(Continued)*

in the table. As a general guideline, however, the following findings may warrant biopsy:

- areas of leukoplakia
- acetowhite lesions with a suspect appearance on colposcopic examination
- lesions with abnormal vascular patterns
- lesions which are unusual and difficult to interpret

As invasive processes are often surrounded by areas of dysplasia, the biopsy should be obtained in the central portion of an identified lesion to accurately determine the full depth extent of a lesion.

Endocervical curettage is performed when there is uncertainty as to the existence of an unsuspected abnormality within the endocervical canal, when an identified lesion extends into the canal, or when visualization of the SC junction is difficult, as well as when the Pap smear reveals AGCUE (atypical glandular cells of unknown etiology). It is most often carried out with the Kevorkian curette. The curette is gently introduced deep into the endocervical canal and, with firm pressure applied to the endocervical tissue, the curette is withdrawn to obtain the specimen.

Vulvar and perianal biopsies may be obtained with either Tischler or Kevorkian biopsy instruments. These tissues, however, are much more sensitive than those of the cervix and vagina, and biopsy with these instruments may be painful. Punch biopsy with a 3-5 mm Keyes instrument is usually adequate for diagnosis and much better tolerated. It is best to infiltrate the underlying subepithelial or subepidermal papillary dermis tissue with 1-3 mL 1% lidocaine prior to biopsy. The Keyes instrument is placed on the lesion and simultaneous pressure and rotation is applied until the dermis is entered (a loss of resistance is noted at this point). A biopsy depth of at least 5 mm is desirable. The instrument is removed and the core of tissue is elevated with a fine-toothed forceps. Then the underlying dermis is cut with small scissors or a scalpel. After obtaining the specimen, pressure at the biopsy site should be maintained with a cotton-tipped applicator until bleeding stops. If excessive bleeding is encountered, the application of a small amount of Monsel's solution (ferric subsulfate) is often helpful. Rarely, the application of a single absorbable 3-0 suture is required to stop bleeding.

Data Acquired Document all findings on a colposcopic diagram. The preferred colposcopic terminology is described in the table. Drawings should clearly indicate the location of the TZ. If it is not visible, this should be documented. Notation of the epithelial surface contour, color, degree of opacity, appearance of the subepithelial capillary system, and presence of acetowhitening is made. The location and extent of visible lesions and the location of each biopsy site should also be documented.

Specimen Submit all biopsy specimens in a fixative solution (formalin, Bouin, Hollande, etc). The location of each biopsy should be clearly labeled for pathology review. Preferably, the specimen should be oriented upright to assist in identification of the specimen surface. This reduces the possibility of "tangential" sectioning, which may obscure analysis (ie, of depth of invasion, if a neoplastic process is present). In addition, it is the responsibility of the clinician to provide all pertinent clinical information relevant to specimen interpretation. Thus, the inclusion of clinical data such as age, date of last menstrual period, whether pregnant, postpartum or postmenopausal, history of prior abnormal Pap smears, or treatment must be communicated to improve the accuracy of specimen interpretation.

Additional Information Colposcopy permits precise definition of the site, size, and characteristics of cervical and anogenital lesions. Some operational definitions which assist in colposcopic evaluation of the **cervix** are necessary. The **ectocervix** is defined as the portion of the cervix that is visible during clinical examination. The **endocervix** is that part of the cervix which can no longer be seen without using a special instrument in order to open the canal. The **squamocolumnar (SC)** junction is the point where the stratified squamous epithelium meets the glandular epithelium of the cervix. The location of the SC junction changes throughout life in a metaplastic process in which columnar epithelium differentiates into squamous epithelium. This junction tends to be in a more ectocervical location at younger ages and endocervical location after menopause. The **transformation zone (TZ)** is the area of metaplasia in which columnar epithelium has differentiated into squamous epithelium. **Note:** A great majority of the dysplastic processes occur at the TZ, therefore, visualization of this zone is an essential aspect of the colposcopic evaluation. If it is not possible to visualize the TZ in its entirety, the colposcopic evaluation is considered unreliable for diagnostic purposes.

Pattern recognition in colposcopic diagnosis of dysplastic or neoplastic processes is based on evaluation of the surface contour, color, degree of opacity, and visualization of the subepithelial capillary system. The table is a summary of colposcopic terminology and histologic correlation. Accurate interpretation of colposcopic findings, however, requires considerable experience with colposcopic-histologic correlation. The following is intended to be merely an introduction to the subject; colposcopic atlases are available to further assist in the interpretation of normal and abnormal findings.[2] **Colposcopic reporting:** The International Federation of Cervical Pathology and Colposcopy (IFCPC) recently approved a modified version of the basic colposcopic terminology at its Seventh World Congress[3] and the terms discussed in this section are derived from the recommendations of the IFCPC. **Histologic reporting:** Over the years, several classification systems have been used for specimen reporting (see table in Papanicolaou Smear *on page 318*). While the Bethesda system is the preferred classification system for cervical cytology, the CIN classification system, cervical intraepithelial neoplasia I-III, is most commonly used for the histologic reporting of cervical lesions. A familiarity with the classification system used by your pathologist, however, is necessary for proper patient management.

Colposcopic Terminology and Histologic Correlation

Normal colposcopic findings

1. Original (native) squamous epithelium

   Smooth, pink epithelium that has originally been established on the cervix and vagina during development. There is no evidence of columnar epithelium underlying the native squamous epithelium (ie, mucus-secreting epithelial glands or clefts, nabothian cysts). Vascular patterns are not conspicuous.

2. Columnar epithelium

   A single layer of mucus-producing epithelium extending from the endometrium to the squamous epithelium of the ectocervix or vagina. Anatomically, columnar epithelium may be present in the endocervix, on the portio, or even in the vagina. It has an irregular surface with long stromal papillae and deep clefts. Underlying stromal vessels give it a dark red color. After application of acetic acid, columnar epithelium will have a grape-like appearance.

3. Transformation zone

   The area between the original squamous epithelium and columnar epithelium in which metaplastic squamous epithelium has replaced previously everted columnar epithelium. Nests of columnar epithelium are surrounded by acquired squamous epithelium, gland openings, and nabothian cysts. Stromal vessels will have appropriate tree-like branching patterns.

Abnormal colposcopic findings and potential significance

1. Within the transformation zone

   Acetowhite epithelium: A focal area that is seen only after application of acetic acid. The white epithelium is a transient phenomenon that is seen in areas of increased nuclear density.
   - May represent condyloma or cervical intraepithelial neoplasia (CIN I-III)

   Punctuation: A focal area in which the capillaries have a stippled pattern produced by end-on view of intraepithelial capillaries, increased vessel diameter, and spacing.
   - May represent condyloma or CIN I-III

   Mosaic: A focal area in which the epithelium has been compartmentalized into a mosaic or tile-like pattern by blood vessels containing stromal papillae.
   - May represent condyloma or CIN I-III

(Continued)

Colposcopy *(Continued)*

Leukoplakia (keratosis): Appears as whitened epithelium seen before the application of acetic acid.

- May represent hyperkeratosis, parakeratosis, condyloma or CIN I-III

Iodine-negative epithelium: Epithelium that does not stain with Lugol's or Schiller's iodine. **Note:** Fully differentiated normal squamous epithelium is glycogen-containing and will stain brown.

- May represent metaplastic epithelium or CIN I-III

Atypical vessels: Blood vessel patterns which are irregular, with bizarre branching patterns, often appearing as commas, corkscrews, or course untapering branching patterns.

- May represent CIN III or invasive cancer

2. Outside the transformation zone (ectocervix, vagina, vulva)
   Colposcopic findings are similar to above.

Colposcopically suspect invasive carcinoma: Often seen as irregular, raised or ulcerated lesions with atypical blood vessels.

Unsatisfactory colposcopy: Any colposcopy in which at-risk tissue cannot be adequately visualized for evaluation for the following reasons:
Squamocolumnar junction not visible
Severe inflammation or atrophy
Cervix not visible

Miscellaneous findings: Nonacetowhite micropapillary surface

- Often normal or associated with mild inflammation or chemical irritants.

Condyloma: Human papillomavirus effects are variable in appearance. On the cervix, these may be irregular, with flat or raised acetowhite areas; they may be hyperkeratotic, or have a micropapillary character. Vaginal, vulvar, and perianal condyloma may be hyperkeratotic or acetowhite, papillary and exophytic or flat, and vascular. Satellite lesions are common.

Inflammation: Diffuse hyperemia that may lead to punctuation and mosaicism, however, with normal intercapillary distance. Discharge and ulceration may be present.

- May represent infection with organisms such as *Trichomonas vaginalis*, gonorrhea, *Chlamydia*, herpes, etc

Atrophy: Thin epithelium

- Characteristic of low estrogen states

Ulcer: Denuded epithelium and stroma

Other: Polyps, nabothian cysts, etc

Sources of error:

If the TZ zone is not visualized in its entirety, tissue at greatest risk for dysplasia or neoplasia will not be adequately evaluated. For proper diagnostic evaluation, endocervical curettage and cervical conization or LEEP conization may be performed. In some cases, patients with cervical smears suggestive of a severe dysplastic process have a colposcopically normal appearing cervix. Random biopsy is not sufficient to rule out a dysplastic process. Again, in these cases, patients will require endocervical curettage or, possibly, conization or LEEP conization for diagnostic purposes; however, the clinician needs to take care to review the clinical history and perhaps repeat the colposcopy prior to cervical conization. Inexperience with colposcopic-histologic correlation may lead to failures in diagnosis.

Footnotes

1. Ferris DG, Willner WA, and Ho JJ, "Colposcopes: A Critical Review," *J Fam Pract*, 1991, 33(5):506-15.
2. Singer A and Monaghan JM, "Lower Genital Tract Precancer," *Colposcopy, Pathology and Treatment*, Boston, MA: Blackwell Scientific Publications, 1994.
3. Stafl A and Wilbanks G, "An International Terminology of Colposcopy: Report of the Nomenclature Committee of the International Federation of Cervical Pathology and Colposcopy," *Obstet Gynecol*, 1991, 77(2):313.

References

Robboy SJ, Kraus FT, and Kurman RJ, "Gross Description, Processing, and Reporting of Gynecologic and Obstetric Specimens," *Blaustein's Pathology of the Female Genital Tract*, 4th ed, Kurman RJ, ed, New York, NY: Springer-Verlag, 1994, 1225-45.

Wright VC, "Contemporary Colposcopy," *Obstet Gynecol Clin North Am*, 1993.

Contraction Stress Test for Confirming Fetal Well-Being

Related Information

Biophysical Profile *on page 294*
Nonstress Test (NST) for Evaluation of Fetal Well-Being *on page 315*
Ultrasound for Obstetrics - 2nd and 3rd Trimester *on page 321*

Procedure Commonly Includes The administration of I.V. oxytocin or stimulation of the patient's nipples (for intrinsic oxytocin release) in order to produce three uterine contractions in 10 minutes while the patient's fetus is monitored by electronic means.

Indications If fetal compromise is suspected or if a previous nonstress test was abnormal

Contraindications Relative contraindications include women at risk for preterm labor or those women with placenta previa or previous classical uterine scar.

Patient Preparation The patient should be instructed not to eat or drink anything in case surgical intervention is necessary (cesarean section).

Special Instructions **Duration of Procedure:** Up to 2 hours

Complications Occasionally uterine contractions can cause fetal bradycardias which may require surgical intervention.

Equipment Electronic fetal monitor/tocodynamometer

Technique The patient is placed on a fetal monitor as described in the nonstress test. If the breast stimulation method is chosen, the patient places warm cloths on her nipples for approximately 5 minutes. Then she reaches under her hospital gown and takes one or both nipples between the forefinger and thumb and rolls them continuously one way and then the other. If the intravenous (I.V.) oxytocin method is chosen, an I.V. is started with lactated Ringer's or D_5 lactated Ringer's solution at 125 mL/hour. Pitocin®, 1-2 milliunits/minute I.V. is then administered. After 30 minutes, if there is no response from the uterus, the dose is increased by 1-2 milliunits/minute.

Data Acquired An adequate test requires at least three uterine contractions in 10 minutes for interpretation. The fetal heart should be traced continuously throughout this period.

Normal Findings No decelerations of the fetal heart tones are seen. Repeated decelerations after the uterine contractions ("late decelerations") mandate further evaluation and possible delivery for fetal indications.

Critical Values Repeated late decelerations and deep decelerations that occur with no temporal relation to the contraction termed "variable decelerations" are of clinical concern.

Limitations Maternal habitus or early gestational age may limit the ability of the monitor to pick up fetal heart tones or uterine contractions. Uteri remote from term often do not respond to oxytocin and so larger doses and more time may be needed. As many as half of fetuses that have abnormal responses to the contraction stress test subsequently have no demonstrable abnormality.

References

"Antepartum Fetal Surveillance. ACOG Technical Bulletin Number 188," *Int J Gynaecol Obstet*, 1994, 44(3):289-94.

♦ **CVS** *see* Chorionic Villus Sampling *on page 297*

♦ **DEXA** *see* Bone Density *on page 295*

Diaphragm Fitting

Synonyms Diaphragm, Vaginal Fitting

Procedure Commonly Includes Examination of the vagina and cervix to fit a shallow rubber dome that is used with a spermicide to cover the cervix.

Indications Provide a barrier method of contraception by stopping sperm from entering the cervical canal for the prevention of pregnancy and protection against sexually transmitted diseases.

Contraindications

- hypersensitivity to rubber, latex, or spermicides
- active vaginal infection or a history of toxic shock syndrome

(Continued)

Diaphragm Fitting *(Continued)*

Patient Preparation Scheduled as outpatient visit lasting approximately 30 minutes. Counseling regarding diaphragm use, advantages, and disadvantages should be provided. The patient's history is necessary to assess if diaphragm barrier contraceptive method is an appropriate choice. The patient should have a complete pelvic examination to determine pelvic abnormalities.

Special Instructions Emphasis on fact that effectiveness depends on the patient's motivation and correct use. Follow-up visit needed about 2 weeks after fitting to assess correct placement by patient and discuss her concerns.

Equipment Set of diaphragm rings or diaphragms in arching, coil, and flat spring types; (sizes range from 50-100 mm in diameter in 5 mm increments); nonsterile gloves

Technique Place patient in dorsal lithotomy position. Measure for diaphragm size by inserting gloved index and middle fingers together into vagina up to posterior fornix. With tip of thumb, mark point directly beneath inferior margin of pubic bone and withdraw fingers in this position. Determine diaphragm size by placing one end of fitting diaphragm or ring on the tip of the middle finger with opposite end lying just in front of thumb tip. This equals approximate diameter of diaphragm needed. Insert fitting diaphragm or ring of measured size into the vagina by holding the diaphragm with the dome down (convex) and press the opposite sides of the rim together between the thumb and third finger. Spread the vagina with the opposite hand. Hold compressed diaphragm dome down and advance it inward along rear wall of vagina as far as it will go. With the index finger, push the front rim of the diaphragm up and simultaneously open the third finger and thumb until diaphragm locked in place just above pubic bone. Try both larger and smaller size to determine best fit where cervix is covered by diaphragm and locked in place between upper edge of pubic bone and posterior wall of vagina.

Data Acquired Size of diaphragm that fits in millimeter diameter

Normal Findings Diaphragm or ring remains in place without discomfort after patient walks around room.

Additional Information Correct size selected when cervix is completely covered and one finger only fits between pubic bone and anterior rim of diaphragm. Sides of diaphragm held firmly by vaginal walls without buckling. The patient should demonstrate insertion and removal of diaphragm after washing her hands. A prescription for selected diaphragm by rim type and size is given to patients with instruction on insertion and use of diaphragm.

References

Ortho-McNeil, "Ortho Diaphragm Kits," *Physicians' Desk Reference*, 53rd ed, Montvale, NJ: Medical Economics Company, 1999, 2211-2.

Romero CM, "Procedure: Diaphragm Fitting," *Saunders Manual of Medical Practice*, Rakel RE, ed, Philadelphia, PA: WB Saunders Co, 1996, 463-5.

♦ **Diaphragm, Vaginal Fitting** *see* Diaphragm Fitting *on page 303*

Doppler Utilization for Finding Fetal Heart Tones in Pregnant Patients

Procedure Commonly Includes The use of a 2-3 MHz Doppler for hearing fetal heart tones in the maternal uterus

Indications Determining fetal viability acutely as long as the patient is over 12 weeks gestational age

Special Instructions Procedure usually takes less than 1 minute, if fetal heart tones are found.

Equipment A 2-3 MHz Doppler listening device which has a focal length of at least 3 cm. Most likely this is labeled for "early fetal heart tones or vascular very deep vessels". **Do not attempt to use the superficial vascular Doppler for this purpose. A false-negative may result.**

Technique The Doppler probe is placed on the maternal bare abdomen. Ultrasonic gel, surgical lubricant, or common vegetable oils have been used as coupling agents. If the patient is 3 months pregnant, place the probe at the top of the pubic bone, angling down toward the rectum. A full bladder may increase your chance of hearing the heart tones depending on the maternal habitus. If the patient appears to be 4 or 5 months pregnant, the midline half way between the umbilicus and pubic bone should be the optimal listening spot. From that position, sweep the Doppler probe slowly around until fetal heart tones are heard. In a morbidly obese patient, the pannus may have to be lifted in order to hear fetal heart tones. Another good window in morbidly obese patients is right through the umbilicus and angled down. If the patient is in her third trimester, the fetal heart tones are best heard at McBurney's point or its mirror image on the left. It is helpful to have one hand on the maternal pulse while searching for the fetal pulse in order to differentiate between the two pulses.

Data Acquired Fetal heart tones should be heard separately from the mother's vascular pulsations in the range of 120-160 beats/minute. These may be heard as a whooshing sound, which is the placenta, or as a clicking sound, which is the actual fetal heart valves. Either one will indicate the fetal heart rate and viability.

Normal Findings Normal fetal heart tones are between 120-160 beats/minute (bpm). In cases of acute hemorrhage or fever, fetal heart tones may be up to 200 beats/minute. In cases of fetal distress, they may be significantly lower than 120 beats/minute. These must be distinguished from the maternal pulse. Either of these abnormalities may require obstetrical intervention.

Critical Values If the fetal heart tones are not heard and viability needs to be assessed, an obstetrical ultrasound is the next step. If fetal heart tones are clearly heard to be <120 beats/minute, obstetrical medical consultation should be obtained. Hydration of the mother, left lateral displacement of the uterus (lying the mother on her left side) and administration of oxygen through nasal cannula are immediate steps to resolve a presumed fetal bradycardia. If the fetal heart tones are clearly heard to be >170 beats/minute, obstetrical medical consultation should be obtained. The practitioner should look for signs of infection or hypovolemia in the mother, such as placental abruption with associated sequestered hemorrhage or other source of hypotension. These should be corrected while fetal compromise is being assessed by the obstetrical provider.

Limitations Early gestational age or location of the fetal heart outside of the focal length of a Doppler device will result in false-negative findings (a fetal heart tone will not be found even though the heart is beating). Maternal weight or a retroverted uterus may make it difficult for smaller fetal hearts to be heard. An anterior placenta may make it hard to find the exact fetal heart location, but the rate should be audible from the pulsations within the placenta. Lack of coupling agent will limit audibility.

References

Parer JT, "Fetal Heart Rate," *Maternal-Fetal Medicine Principles and Practice*, 3rd ed, Creasy R and Resnick R, eds, Philadelphia, PA: WB Saunders Co, 1994, 306-7.

♦ **Dual Energy X-ray Absorptiometry** *see* Bone Density *on page 295*
♦ **DXA** *see* Bone Density *on page 295*
♦ **ECC** *see* Endocervical Curettage *on page 305*
♦ **Echohysteroscopy** *see* Saline Infusion Sonography *on page 319*

Endocervical Curettage

Related Information

Cervical Polypectomy *on page 296*
Colposcopy *on page 298*
Endometrial Biopsy *on page 307*
Loop Electrosurgical Excisional Procedure (LEEP) *on page 311*
Papanicolaou Smear *on page 316*

Synonyms ECC

Procedure Commonly Includes Endocervical curettage allows tissue sampling from the cervical canal for subsequent histologic evaluation.

Indications Endocervical curettage is indicated:

1. In patients with atypical glandular cells (AGUS) identified at cervical cytologic screening
2. In patients with dysplasia involving the endocervical canal
3. In patients whose transformation zone extends into the endocervical canal and/or is not fully visualized.

(Continued)

Endocervical Curettage *(Continued)*

Note: It may also be desirable to perform endocervical curettage at the time of endometrial biopsy in patients with abnormal uterine bleeding to evaluate for cervical stromal involvement of an endometrial cancer, although with the adoption of surgical staging for endometrial carcinoma, this indication has been questioned.

Contraindications

- pregnancy
- active cervicitis

Care should be exercised when sampling the endometrium of patients on anticoagulation therapy or who have bleeding disorders, although generally endometrial biopsy may be performed safely in these patients without intervention or discontinuation of anticoagulation agents.

Patient Preparation Endocervical curettage is performed as an outpatient procedure, usually at the time of colposcopic evaluation or endometrial biopsy. Patients may experience slight cramping during and shortly after curettage. Premedication with an nonsteroidal anti-inflammatory 1 hour prior to the procedure may be advisable in some patients.

Aftercare Occasionally, patients will experience mild vasovagal symptoms during or after their procedure. Patients should be allowed time to sit or lie on the examination table before sending them home. They otherwise need not restrict their activities at home. Minor cramping pain may occur after the procedure. Ibuprofen or acetaminophen should be sufficient for analgesia. Patients may also briefly experience light vaginal spotting after the procedure.

Equipment The procedure is most often carried out with a Kevorkian curette.

Technique The patient is placed in the dorsal lithotomy position with speculum placement to allow adequate visualization of the cervix. The curette is gently introduced deep into the endocervical canal. If the catheter does not pass easily, a single-toothed tenaculum may be applied to grasp the cervix for countertraction. Firm pressure is then applied to the endocervical tissue, and the curette is withdrawn to obtain the specimen. This motion is repeated several times until a representative circumferential endocervical sampling is obtained.

Specimen The tissue obtained at aspiration or curettage is then placed on a Telfa pad or in normal saline for inspection. Multiple passes may be made if it is felt that the tissue obtained is inadequate for pathology review. After the sampling is complete, the tissue is transferred to a fixative solution (formalin, Bouin's, Hollande, etc) for pathology review. It should be clearly labeled and the all pertinent clinical information relevant to specimen interpretation, including indications for the endocervical curettage, should be provided. This includes clinical data such as age, date of last menstrual period, whether postpartum or postmenopausal, history of prior abnormal Pap smears or treatment, and any hormonal therapy.

Causes for Rejection Specimens with scant tissue may be nondiagnostic. A large portion of the material retrieved by this method will be cervical mucous. It is, therefore, important to inspect the material prior to submitting the specimen in order to ensure that adequate tissue has been retrieved for histologic examination. In addition, a curette placed too deeply into the endocervical canal may inadvertently sample endometrial, rather than endocervical tissue, and may lead to misleading or nondiagnostic results.

Normal Findings Pathology reporting may describe lesions as:

- fragments of normal endocervix
- condylomatous
- atypical epithelium
- neoplastic

Limitations Because epithelial and stromal tissue is often disrupted during endocervical curettage, the depth of involvement of a dysplastic or neoplastic process cannot be determined in many cases. Follow-up diagnostic evaluation with biopsy or LEEP conization is often necessary if the endocervical curettage reveals an abnormality.

References

Ferenczy A and Wright TC, "Anatomy and Histology of the Cervix," *Blaustein's Pathology of the Female Genital Tract*, 4th ed, Kurman RJ, ed, New York, NY: Springer-Verlag, 1994, 185-202.
Singer A and Monaghan JM, "Lower Genital Tract Precancer," *Colposcopy, Pathology and Treatment*, Boston, MA: Blackwell Scientific Publications, 1994.

Endometrial Biopsy

Related Information

Cervical Polypectomy *on page 296*
Endocervical Curettage *on page 305*
Office Hysteroscopy *on page 315*
Saline Infusion Sonography *on page 319*

Synonyms Endometrial Curettages; Endometrial Suction Aspiration

Procedure Commonly Includes Curetting/aspiration of endometrial tissue for biopsy via a thin plastic catheter or curette inserted via the cervical canal. May include endocervical curettage for specific indications.

Indications

- determine the cause of abnormal uterine bleeding (dysfunctional uterine bleeding versus hyperplasia versus neoplasia versus endometritis)
- prior to hormone replacement therapy in women at high risk of uterine cancer
- infertility evaluation
- follow-up of previous diagnosis of atypia or adenomatous hyperplasia
- evaluation of enlarged uterus (along with pelvic ultrasound)
- monitoring the uterine safety of hormonal therapy such as tamoxifen
- screening postmenopausal women with endometrial cells on Pap smear
- included as part of the evaluation of AGCUS (atypical glandular cells on Pap screening)

Contraindications

- pregnancy
- severe pelvic inflammatory disease or cervicitis
- cervical stenosis (relative)
- anticoagulant therapy
- coagulation disorders (relative)

Patient Preparation Procedure and risks (see Complications) are explained and consent is obtained. No anesthesia is used, although a woman may take an oral nonprescription pain medication prior to procedure. This is an outpatient procedure.

Aftercare The patient is to remain supine for a few moments following the procedure. The patient is assessed for vasovagal reaction and uterine cramps (both of which usually subside rapidly). If no heavy bleeding is noted and vasovagal reaction (if it occurred) has subsided, the patient may be discharged. The patient may resume normal activities.

Complications The main complications which can occur are mild pain during the procedure and cramping afterwards for 1-2 days and bleeding. The extent to which a woman tolerates the procedure depends upon the ability of the endocervical canal to yield to the biopsy instruments. In general, parous women tolerate this procedure well. Other problems which can occur include need for a dilation and curettage (D&C) if the tissue obtained at endometrial biopsy is not diagnostic, missed abnormality by biopsy, infection, and perforation of the uterus (rare).

Equipment A 3 mm Pipelle endometrial suction curette, vaginal speculum, formalin specimen bottles with labels, antiseptic solution for cleansing cervix, tenaculum (often not needed), uterine sound (often not needed), endocervical Novak curette (for certain indications)

Technique First, perform a bimanual examination with the patient in the dorsal lithotomy position, to determine the position and size of the uterus. A vaginal speculum is then gently inserted to visualize the cervix. The cervix is cleansed with antiseptic solution, like Betadine®, (subsequent instrumentation is done without touching the vulva or vaginal walls). The Pipelle or GynoSampler 3 mm plastic endometrial suction curette is first inserted through the cervical os to the fundus, with the piston fully inserted. (Use of the single-toothed tenaculum may be required to stabilize the cervix and/or to straighten the angle of the internal os; sounding the uterus is often not done in parous women, as the

(Continued)

Endometrial Biopsy *(Continued)*

depth of the uterus can normally be gauged with the Pipelle itself). If the internal os is stenosed, an "os dilator set" can be used prior to the endometrial suction curette. Document the depth of the uterus. Stabilize the sheath of the Pipelle with one hand, and draw the piston back completely in one continuous motion to create negative pressure within the lumen of the Pipelle. Rotate the sheath between the thumb and index finger and move it in and out between the fundus and internal os about four times (which samples all quadrants of the endometrium). During this passage, the negative pressure within the sheath draws endometrial tissue into the curette opening, where it is sheared away and carried into the sheath lumen. Withdraw the device. Expel the sample into the appropriately labeled formalin specimen bottle(s) by advancing the piston into the sheath. Remove the vaginal speculum. Endocervical curettage (may be done if the endometrial biopsy is being performed to rule out neoplasm): a Novak endocervical curette is introduced into the external os, up to the internal os; the endocervical canal is curetted 360° twice, and the sample is placed in a specimen bottle containing formalin and appropriately labeled. Because the Novak curette is metal, care must be taken not to exert too much force upon entry into the endometrial cavity as uterus perforation can occur. The Novak curette is associated with more patient discomfort and is thus reserved when adequate endometrial tissue is, otherwise, not obtained with the Pipelle.

Specimen Endometrial tissue

Container Sterile specimen bottles containing formalin, labeled appropriately with relevant clinical information such as menopause status and hormone use

Normal Findings Categories for pathologic interpretation include:

Insufficient for diagnosis (scant tissue or menstrual blood only)

Normal:

- atrophic endometrium
- proliferative endometrium
- secretory endometrium

Abnormal:

- polyp (**Note**: The endometrial aspiration biopsy does not always reliably remove all endometrial polyps)
- hyperplasia (simple or complex, with or without atypia)

Cancer:

- endometrial adenocarcinoma
  Papillary villoglandular
  Secretory
  Ciliated cell
  Adenocarcinoma with squamous differentiation
- mucinous carcinoma
- serous carcinoma
- clear-cell carcinoma
- squamous carcinoma
- undifferentiated carcinoma
- mixed types
- miscellaneous carcinoma
- metastatic carcinoma

Limitations The Pipelle (Unimar, Inc, Wilton, CT) and Novak curette have demonstrated >90% accuracy overall when compared to hysterectomy specimens.[1] The accuracy of this instrument in detecting more focal lesions, is somewhat less. Moreover, 15% to 43% of patients diagnosed with atypical hyperplasia may actually harbor a concurrent adenocarcinoma not detected by biopsy.[2] Therefore, if the clinical suspicion for endometrial carcinoma is high and endometrial biopsy is not definitive, further evaluation with saline infusion sonography (SIS), operative hysteroscopy with biopsy, or formal operative fractional dilation and curettage (D&C) is recommended.

Additional Information Endometrial biopsy has become a reliable office tool for evaluating postmenopausal women with abnormal uterine bleeding. A Pap smear should be obtained. When the specimen obtained by endometrial biopsy is sufficient for diagnosis, D&C is rarely needed. Use of pelvic ultrasound, often combined with endometrial biopsy, increases diagnostic sensitivity. Saline infusion (hystero-)sonography may further increase diagnostic yield particularly in women with abnormal bleeding thought to be of focal origin and for patients in which inadequate tissue was obtained by aspiration method. The specimen can be submitted for evaluation of infection and thus the tissue can be placed in a sterile specimen container containing a small amount of sterile saline and promptly sent to the laboratory for aerobic and anaerobic cultures. Depending on the clinical situation, special request can be submitted for acid-fast bacilli (AFB), *Mycoplasma*, or viral culture.

Footnotes

1. Stovall TG, Ling FW, and Morgan PL, "A Prospective, Randomized Comparison of the Pipelle Endometrial Sampling Device With the Novak Curette," *Am J Obstet Gynecol*, 1991, 165 (5 Part 1):1287-90.
2. Janicek MF and Rosenshine NB, "Invasive Endometrial Cancer *in utero* Resected for Atypical Endometrial Hyperplasia," *Gynecol Oncol*, 1994, 52(3):373-8.

References

Apgar BS, "Endometrial Biopsy," *Procedures for Primary Care Physician*, Chapter 73, Pfenninger JL and Fowler GC, eds, St Louis, MO: CV Mosby Co, 1994.

Thacker HL, "Osteoporosis and Menopause," *Clinical Preventive Medicine*, Matzen RN and Lang RS, eds, St Louis, MO: CV Mosby Co, 1993.

- **Endometrial Curettages** *see* Endometrial Biopsy *on page 307*
- **Endometrial Suction Aspiration** *see* Endometrial Biopsy *on page 307*

Estimation of Gestational Age by Measuring Fundal Height

Procedure Commonly Includes The use of a tape measure in centimeters to measure from the top of the pubic bone to the top of the uterine fundus for estimation of gestational age.

Indications Unknown gestational age or estimation of adequate fetal growth

Equipment A measuring tape marked in centimeters

Technique With the patient lying in the supine position, locate the top of the pubic bone. Place the "0" of the tape measure under a finger on the top of the pubic bone. From the patient's xiphoid process, using a wave-like rolling motion with your fingers, serially come down the abdomen until the top of the fundus is palpated. This is a soft area but harder than the other abdominal contents. (Do not continue to roll down until you feel the actual hard parts of the fetus as this will give you an underestimation of gestational age.) When the top of the fundus is located, place the tape measure loosely under your finger and record the length.

Data Acquired The number of centimeters from the top of the pubic symphysis to the uterine fundus should be approximately equal to the gestational age in weeks for a singleton pregnancy.

Normal Findings A fundal height within 2 cm of the expected gestational age in **menstrual** weeks. A discrepancy >2 cm should be evaluated by ultrasonography and obstetrical consultation.

Critical Values 3 cm above or below the expected value

Limitations Gestational ages below 17 weeks cannot be measured using an abdominal approach. (They must be estimated using a bimanual approach with one hand in the vagina and one on the abdomen.)

References

Johnson TR, Walker MA, and Niebyl JR, "Preconception and Prenatal Care," *Obstetrics: Normal and Problem Pregnancies*, 3rd ed, Chapter 7, Gabbe SG, Niebyl JR, and Simpson JL, eds, New York, NY: Churchill Livingstone, 1996, 161-84.

"Prenatal Care" *Williams Obstetrics*, 20th ed, Chapter 9, Cunningham FG, et al, eds, Stamford, CT: Appleton & Lange, 1997, 227-50.

Fine Needle Aspiration Biopsy of the Breast

Synonyms FNA-B, Breast; Needle Biopsy, Breast

Procedure Commonly Includes Needle biopsy of a palpable breast mass

Indications Palpable, dominant breast mass

Contraindications Bleeding diathesis

(Continued)

Fine Needle Aspiration Biopsy of the Breast *(Continued)*

Patient Preparation The procedure can be done in the office at the time of evaluation. Mammography should be performed prior to any invasive procedure.

Complications Ecchymosis and hematoma formation, bleeding, infection, pneumothorax

Equipment Skin antiseptic (eg, alcohol skin wipe), 10 mL syringe, 21- to 22-gauge 1 inch needle with a transparent hub, a sterile 4 x 4 gauze pad, and an adhesive bandage Optional equipment includes a sterile tuberculin syringe with 1% lidocaine for local anesthesia.

Technique Using universal precautions, the mass is localized and fixed with the fingers of the nonaspirating hand. A movable mass is pushed over a rib and compressed against it. Then, while maintaining pressure on the surrounding tissue, the fingers are spread open, stabilizing and trapping the mass under the tightened skin. The fingers are not moved from this position during the entire FNA. Because taut skin is less sensitive, the patient's discomfort is reduced if the pressure is maintained. The skin over the mass is then cleansed with antiseptic, such as an alcohol skin wipe. A local anesthetic is optional, as is brief application of ethyl chloride spray if available. The needle is inserted at an angle almost perpendicular to the mass. Apply 3-4 mL of negative pressure only when the needle tip is within the mass. Then 20 short, thrusting, jack-hammerlike strokes each no longer than the diameter of the mass usually produce an abundant cell sample. Negative pressure in the syringe is released before removing the needle from the breast. A sterile gauze is placed over the aspiration site, and firm pressure is applied for at least 2 minutes. Then a bandage is placed over the RNA-B site. When blood collects in the hub of the needle, cellular elements are difficult to identify. Another RNA-B may be performed at a different angle into the mass in an attempt to avoid aspiration of blood.

Data Acquired Differentiation of cyst from solid

Specimen Cellular material

Container Glass bottle containing 95% ethyl alcohol, sterile slides, Cytolyte® (alcohol and buffered saline). The needle is disconnected from the syringe. Then air is drawn up into the syringe, the needle is reattached, and the aspirate is ejected through the needle, touching a slide at a 45° angle. The drop of tissue juice is then gently smeared with a second slide (as in preparing a hematologic smear). As soon as the slide is smeared, it is fixed is the same manner as a Pap smear (in a jar of ethyl alcohol), and Cytolyte® is then drawn up into the syringe and reinjected into the Cytolyte® bottle.

Storage Instructions Samples should immediately be sent to the Cytology Laboratory.

Causes for Rejection Insufficient cells, grossly bloody sample

Limitations The physician should not rely on a negative aspiration, unless the primary care physician performs FNA-B frequently and the Cytology Laboratory has considerable experience evaluating this material. False-negatives range from 0% to 4%. Most false-negatives are due to sampling errors, which tend to be associated with small tumor size.

Additional Information When a skilled cytopathologist is available for interpretation of the specimen, FNA-B has many advantages including simplicity, accuracy, low morbidity, minimal patient discomfort, and relatively low cost. It is immediately available as an office procedure that can be done at the time the patient is first seen in the office.

References

Foster R, "Techniques for Diagnosis of Palpable Breast Masses," *Diseases of the Breast*, Harris JR, Lippman MC, Morrow M, et al, eds, Philadelphia, PA: Lippincott Williams & Wilkins, 1996.

Marchant DJ, "Fine Needle Aspiration Technique," *Breast Disease*, Marchant DJ, ed, Philadelphia, PA: WB Saunders Co, 1997.

Fine Needle Aspiration of the Breast

Synonyms FNA, Breast

Procedure Commonly Includes Needle aspiration of a palpable breast mass

Indications Palpable, dominant breast mass

Contraindications Bleeding diathesis

Patient Preparation The procedure can be done in the office at the time of evaluation. Mammography should be performed prior to any invasive procedure.

Complications Ecchymosis and hematoma formation, bleeding, infection, pneumothorax

Equipment Skin antiseptic (eg, alcohol skin wipe), 10 mL syringe, 21- to 22-gauge 1 inch needle with a transparent hub, a sterile 4 x 4 gauze pad, and an adhesive bandage. Optional equipment includes a sterile tuberculin syringe with 1% lidocaine for local anesthesia.

Technique Using universal precautions, the mass is localized and fixed with the fingers of the nonaspirating hand. A movable mass is pushed over a rib and compressed against it. Then, while maintaining pressure on the surrounding tissue, the fingers are spread open, stabilizing and trapping the mass under the tightened skin. The fingers are not moved from this position during the entire FNA. Because taut skin is less sensitive, the patient's discomfort is reduced if the pressure is maintained. The skin over the mass is then cleansed with antiseptic, such as an alcohol skin wipe. A local anesthetic is optional, as is brief application of ethyl chloride spray if available. The needle is inserted at an angle almost perpendicular to the mass. Apply 3-4 mL of negative pressure only when the needle tip is within the mass. Then, the fluid from the cyst is withdrawn, and the needle is removed from the breast.

Data Acquired Differentiation of cyst from solid

Specimen Cyst fluid. Typical cyst fluid is thin and slightly opalescent and varies from light tan to dark green.

Container For bloody cyst fluid, cytology may be obtained by putting the fluid immediately in a container of Cytolyte® (a mixture of alcohol and buffered saline).

Storage Instructions Samples should immediately be sent to the Cytology Laboratory.

Limitations Cytologic examination of cyst fluid is not cost-effective and is rarely of clinical value in the management of a patient with a cyst. Intracystic carcinomas are rare. Even when there is intracystic carcinoma, the fluid is rarely cytologically diagnostic.

Additional Information Clinical suspicion for an intracystic neoplasm and further investigation is needed if there is grossly bloody cyst fluid, as well as the presence of a residual mass after aspiration. A persistent residual mass, multiple recurrences after aspiration of the same cyst, and a bloody aspirate are all indications to obtain tissue for pathologic examination.

FNA of a gross breast cyst is both diagnostic and therapeutic.

References

Foster R, "Techniques for Diagnosis of Palpable Breast Masses," *Diseases of the Breast*, Harris JR, Lippman MC, Morrow M, et al, eds, Philadelphia, PA: Lippincott Williams & Wilkins, 1996.

Marchant DJ, "Fine Needle Aspiration Technique," *Breast Disease*, Marchant DJ, ed, Philadelphia, PA: WB Saunders Co, 1997.

♦ **FNA-B, Breast** *see* Fine Needle Aspiration Biopsy of the Breast *on page 309*

♦ **FNA, Breast** *see* Fine Needle Aspiration of the Breast *on page 310*

♦ **Heel Ultrasound** *see* Quantitative Ultrasound *on page 318*

♦ **Hydrosonography** *see* Saline Infusion Sonography *on page 319*

♦ **Hysteroscopy, Office** *see* Office Hysteroscopy *on page 315*

♦ **Large Loop Excision of Transformation Zone (LLETZ)** *see* Loop Electrosurgical Excisional Procedure (LEEP) *on page 311*

♦ **LEEP** *see* Loop Electrosurgical Excisional Procedure (LEEP) *on page 311*

♦ **LETZ** *see* Loop Electrosurgical Excisional Procedure (LEEP) *on page 311*

♦ **LLETZ** *see* Loop Electrosurgical Excisional Procedure (LEEP) *on page 311*

Loop Electrosurgical Excisional Procedure (LEEP)

Related Information

Colposcopy *on page 298*

(Continued)

Loop Electrosurgical Excisional Procedure (LEEP) *(Continued)*

Endocervical Curettage *on page 305*

Synonyms Large Loop Excision of Transformation Zone (LLETZ); LEEP; LETZ; LLETZ; Loop Excision of Transformation Zone (LETZ)

Procedure Commonly Includes Removal of cervical tissue, including the transformation zone, for diagnostic or therapeutic purposes.

Indications

Diagnostic indications for LEEP conization:

- when cervical cytology reveals high grade squamous intraepithelial lesion (HGSIL) and follow-up colposcopy is normal or deemed inadequate for diagnosis (usually due to inability to visualize the entire transformation zone during colposcopic examination)
- when endocervical curettage is positive for dysplasia/neoplasia
- exclude invasion when colposcopically identified lesions extend into the cervical canal
- when adenocarcinoma *in situ* is diagnosed by biopsy or with endocervical curettage

Therapeutic indications for LEEP or LEEP conniption:

- any biopsy-proven CIN (cervical intraepithelial neoplasia) ectocervical lesion may be treated with LEEP
- therapeutic LEEP conniption may also be performed for treatment of lesions that extend into the cervical canal

Contraindications LEEP should not be performed in patients with an obvious invasive cervical cancer. Great care should be taken if LEEP is necessary in patients who are receiving anticoagulation therapy or who have bleeding disorders.

The safety of LEEP in pregnancy has not been established. If possible, it is best to defer the procedure in pregnant patients or patients in their early postpartum period until the approximately 4-6 weeks postpartum. If LEEP must be performed under these circumstances, then the procedure should be performed in a controlled setting (operating room) by experienced personnel.

Patient Preparation Patient education with regard to the significance of the cervical disease, treatment objectives, and the importance of follow-up should be part of the informed consent process. LEEP is usually performed as an elective, outpatient procedure. The procedure is generally well tolerated with only local anesthetic, however, premedication with an analgesic and/or an anxiolytic may be administered after informed consent is obtained. Scheduling LEEP within 1 week of the completion of menses minimizes the likelihood that the patient is pregnant.

Aftercare Occasionally patients will experience mild vasovagal symptoms during or after their procedure. Patients should be allowed time to sit or lie on the examination table before sending them home. Patients are advised to restrict their activities for 24-48 hours and refrain from intercourse for 3-4 weeks after the procedure. Showers or tub baths are allowed. Patients should also be advised to expect vaginal drainage or spotting for 1-3 weeks after the procedure. If Monsel's paste (ferric subsulfate) is applied, a particulate brownish black discharge will also noted. Menstrual pads are preferred over tampons for management of discharge. Minor cramping pain may occur after the procedure; ibuprofen or acetaminophen should be sufficient for analgesia.

Complications Thermal injury is one of the most common complications of this procedure. Excess thermal damage to the cervix occurs most often when contact with tissue is made before the electric current is applied, or the current is stopped and restarted within the cervical tissue. Vaginal burns occur most often when the cervix is poorly visualized. Vaginal sidewall retractors help to minimize this risk. Failures in the grounding system may account for burns at distant sites. Perioperative bleeding is an unusual complication when Monsel's solution and ball electrode fulguration is available. Late bleeding complications have been reported in <15% of cases[1,2] and may require reapplication of Monsel's, fulguration, or the suture ligation. Patients with bleeding disorders or who are on anticoagulation therapy, pregnant or newly postpartum patients, and patients with obvious (vascular) invasive cancer are at greatest risk for bleeding complications. Infection occurs uncommonly after this procedure. Cervical stenosis has been reported in 1% to 4% of patients after a LEEP procedure.[3] This condition may lead to pelvic endometriosis, hematometra, or pyometra. There are no published clinical data to suggest an increased risk of cervical incompetence or sterility after LEEP.

Equipment Electrosurgical generators used for LEEP are identical to those used in laparoscopic and urologic surgery. LEEP makes use of low voltage and relatively high frequency alternating electric current for tissue excision. Output is monopolar and patients require a gel-adhesive electrode pad (usually placed on the patient's thigh) for grounding. The pad wire should be connected to the generator and the circuit should be tested prior to starting the procedure. Most generators allow a choice of cutting, coagulation, or blend modes. Blend modes allow concurrent surgical excision and coagulation for hemostasis. Several loops, with an insulated shaft to prevent accidental thermal injury, are available. Tungsten or stainless steel wires approximately 0.2 mm thick are used for excision. Round and square loops are available in a variety of sizes (common sizes range from 1.0 x 1.0 cm to 2.0 x 1.5 cm). Ball electrodes ranging from 3-5 mm are useful for fulguration of a bleeding excision bed. Smoke evacuators are necessary to eliminate smoke and steam generated during the procedure and submicron particle masks are worn for protection against live virus particles.

Technique After informed consent is obtained, the patient is placed in dorsal lithotomy position on an examination table with stirrups. The vaginal speculum is inserted gently and adjusted to expose as much of the cervix and vagina as possible. Lateral vaginal wall retractors may also be used for improved exposure. The cervix is first evaluated colposcopically with a 5% acetic acid solution. Lugol's iodine solution may also be used for identification of areas of dysplasia. Anesthesia is then obtained with 5-10 mL of 2% lidocaine containing 1:200,000 epinephrine. This may be applied with a 26- to 32-gauge spinal needle as a paracervical block at the 3 o'clock and 9 o'clock positions immediately lateral to the cervix (taking care to avoid intravascular injection) or superficially infiltrated into the cervix in a circumferential pattern.

The loop is then attached to the current source, which is usually controlled with a foot pedal. A blend mode is most effective. The amount of current will depend, in part, on the loop size used (larger loops require greater power, usually 35-55 watts). To avoid significant thermal injury, it is important to always apply the current prior to making contact with the cervical tissue and perform the excision in one smooth motion, without stopping within the tissue. Place the loop 5 mm lateral to the lesion or to the transformation zone and, with the current applied, slowly press the loop perpendicularly into the cervical tissue to a depth of 5-8 mm. The loop is then slowly drawn through the cervical tissue, applying current the entire time, and then withdrawn perpendicularly when approximately 5 mm lateral to the lesion or the transformation zone. For larger lesions or a wide transformation zone, two or more passes may be required for complete excision.

LEEP conization may be performed for lesions that extend into the endocervical canal. While several techniques are described, one technique that effectively maximizes the depth of endocervical excision is as follows. The transformation zone is first excised as described above. This allows a second, deeper pass to be made (usually with a 1.0 x 1.0 cm loop) to target the cervical canal more caudally.

When LEEP conization is applied for diagnostic purposes, the remaining endocervical tissue should be sampled with endocervical curettage. The curette is gently introduced deep into the endocervical canal. If the catheter does not pass easily, a single-toothed tenaculum may be applied to grasp the cervix for countertraction. Firm pressure is then applied to the endocervical tissue and the curette is withdrawn to obtain the specimen. This motion is repeated several times until a representative circumferential endocervical sampling is obtained.

(Continued)

Loop Electrosurgical Excisional Procedure (LEEP) *(Continued)*

For hemostasis, the entire excision bed is fulgurated with the ball electrode (coagulation setting of 40-55 watts). Pressure and Monsel's solution may then be applied to this area for continued hemostasis.

Container Submit all specimens in a fixative solution (formalin, Bouin, Hollande, etc)

Collection Because margins of dysplasia or neoplasia are of interest, the specimen should be oriented and clearly labeled for accurate pathology review. This is most easily accomplished by likening the cervix to a clock and placing a simple suture at the anatomical "12 o'clock position" on the excised specimen. If two or more passes are made with the loop, the relative orientation of one specimen with respect to the other should be communicated to the pathologist (ie, sample #1 = ectocervical sample, sample #2 = endocervical sample). In addition, the clinician should provide all pertinent clinical information relevant to specimen interpretation, including indication for the procedure. The inclusion of clinical data such as age, date of last menstrual period, whether pregnant, postpartum or postmenopausal, history of prior abnormal Pap smears, or treatment must be communicated to improve the accuracy of specimen interpretation.

Additional Information

Histologic reporting: Over the years, several classification systems have been used for specimen reporting (see table in Papanicolaou Smear *on page 318*). While the Bethesda system is the preferred classification system for cervical cytology, the CIN classification system, cervical intraepithelial neoplasia I-III, is most commonly used for the histologic reporting of cervical lesions. A familiarity with the classification system used by your pathologist, however, is necessary for proper patient management.

Specimen margins and depth of invasion: Particular attention is paid to LEEP specimen margins. Patients with a preneoplastic lesion and histologically negative specimen margins may be followed with surveillance Pap smears and/or colposcopy at 4- to 6-month intervals for 2 years. Any signs of recurrence requires re-evaluation with colposcopy and possible treatment. Of note, there is always a possibility to skip lesions in patients with negative specimen margins, particularly with glandular lesions of the cervix.

Management of patients with histologically positive margins must be individualized. Reported recurrence/persistence rates for histologically positive margins vary between 10% to 75%.[3,4] Follow-up colposcopy and Pap smear may be adequate in some patients. Re-excision, however, may be appropriate for other patients if sufficient concern regarding the possibility of invasive cancer remains.

When an invasive cancer is identified, the submitted LEEP specimen should allow for accurate determination of depth of invasion.

Footnotes

1. Leusley DM, Cullimore J, Redman CW, et al, "Loop Diathermy Excision of the Cervical Transformation Zone in Patients With Abnormal Cervical Smears," *Br Med J [Clin Res]*, 1990, 300(6741):1690-3.
2. Prendiville W, Cullimore J, and Norman S, "Large Loop Excision of the Transformation Zone (LLETZ). A New Method of Management for Women With Cervical Intraepithelial Neoplasia," *Br J Obstet Gynaecol*, 1989, 96(9):1054-60.
3. Spitzer M, Chernys AE, and Seltzer VL, "The Use of Large-Loop Excision of the Transformation Zone in an Inner-City Population," *Obstet Gynecol*, 1993, 82(5):731-5.
4. Murdoch JB, Morgan PR, Lopes A, et al, "Histological Incomplete Excision of CIN After Large Loop Excision of the Transformation Zone (LLETZ) Merits Careful Follow-up, not Retreatment," *Br J Obstet Gynaecol*, 1992, 99(12):990-3.

References

Singer A and Monaghan JM, *Lower Genital Tract Precancer: Colposcopy, Pathology and Treatment*, Boston, MA: Blackwell Scientific Publications, 1994.

♦ **Loop Excision of Transformation Zone (LETZ)** *see* Loop Electrosurgical Excisional Procedure (LEEP) *on page 311*

♦ **Needle Biopsy, Breast** *see* Fine Needle Aspiration Biopsy of the Breast *on page 309*

Nonstress Test (NST) for Evaluation of Fetal Well-Being

Related Information

Biophysical Profile *on page 294*
Contraction Stress Test for Confirming Fetal Well-Being *on page 303*

Synonyms NST for Fetal Well-Being

Procedure Commonly Includes Use of a tocodynamometer placed on the maternal abdomen for detection of uterine contractions and a Doppler device trained on the fetal heart. A strip is obtained which shows the fetal heart rate varying from second to second.

Indications Assess fetal well-being after 32 weeks gestational age

Patient Preparation If fetal distress is suspected and cesarean section may be necessary, an empty stomach is preferred.

Special Instructions **Duration of Procedure:** 30 minutes to several hours

Equipment A fetal monitor (usually obtained from the Labor & Delivery unit)

Technique The patient is placed in the semirecumbent position and the monitors are applied using adjustable straps. The fetal heart is identified with a Doppler. Coupling gel is used to improve transmission. The placement of the contraction monitor is usually in the upper part of the fundus in an area that does not overlie a hard part of the fetus such as back or hips.

Data Acquired A strip is generated which repeats the frequency and pattern of uterine contractions as well as the fetal heart rate and its variations.

Normal Findings Contractions may be present or absent. If the patient is remote from term but has frequent contractions, obstetrical consultation should be obtained.

Fetal heart rate should be between 120-160 beats/minute. A "reactive" tracing reveals a fetal heart rate acceleration of at least 15 beats/minute lasting at least 15 seconds at least twice in a 20-minute period. Failure to detect fetal heart rate accelerations in a 40-minute period represents a "nonreactive" tracing and further testing may be required. Fetal decelerations may reflect significant fetal distress.

Critical Values If the fetal heart tone is >190 beats/minute or <100 beats/minute, urgent obstetrical consultation should be obtained. If regular or profound decelerations of the heartbeat are seen, urgent obstetrical consultation should be sought.

Limitations Early gestational age and maternal habitus may limit the ability of both the Doppler to detect fetal heart tones and the tocotonometer to register uterine contractions.

References

Druzin ML, "Antepartum Fetal Heart Rate Monitoring. State of the Art," *Clin Perinatol*, 1989, 16(3):627-42.

"Fetal Heart Rate Patterns: Monitoring, Interpretation, and Management," *ACOG Technical Bulletin 207*, Washington, DC: American College of Gynecology and Obstetrics, July, 1997.

"Interpretation of Fetal Heart Rate Records: Baseline Heart Rate and Variability," *Management of Common Problems in Obstetrics and Gynecology*, 3rd ed, Chapter 49, Mishell DR Jr and Brenner PF, eds, Boston, MA: Blackwell Scientific Publications, 1994.

♦ **NST for Fetal Well-Being** *see* Nonstress Test (NST) for Evaluation of Fetal Well-Being *on page 315*

Office Hysteroscopy

Related Information

Endometrial Biopsy *on page 307*

Synonyms Hysteroscopy, Office

Procedure Commonly Includes Direct visualization of the endocervical canal and endometrial cavity by means of a flexible or rigid diagnostic hysteroscope. This procedure permits rapid and direct visual inspection of the endometrium that is inaccessible by pelvic examination. Office hysteroscopy is performed by a trained and skilled gynecologist in an office setting. It is safe and rapid (2-5 minutes) means of evaluating abnormal uterine bleeding, infertility, recurrent miscarriages, and postmenopausal bleeding.

(Continued)

Office Hysteroscopy *(Continued)*

Indications Performed in response to several conditions: Abnormal bleeding from the uterus/cervix, localization of "lost IUD", evaluation of abnormal endometrial cells on Pap test, hyperplasia, infertility, evaluation of abnormal/indeterminate endometrial echo on transvaginal ultrasound, and evaluation of postmenopausal bleeding

Contraindications

Absolute contraindications:

- pelvic inflammatory disease
- pregnancy
- cervical cancer
- uncooperative patient
- inadequate operator experience or inadequate instrumentation

Relative contraindications:

- active uterine bleeding
- severe cervical stenosis severe cardiorespiratory disease and/or metabolic acidosis

Patient Preparation Procedure is most optimally performed when the patient is not menstruating. In menstruating women, the procedure is scheduled 2-7 days after the period has ended (proliferative phase). Hysteroscopy can be attempted in the presence of heavy bleeding, however, clarity of visualization may hamper its performance. If the last menses is unknown, pregnancy testing is mandatory before instrumentation. The patient is placed in the dorsal lithotomy position. Visual inspection of the cervix and bimanual examination is performed to exclude the presence of pelvic inflammatory disease or mucopurulent discharge. Other than scheduling the exam around the period, no special preparations are needed for office hysteroscopy. Patients may eat and take any prescribed medications before the procedure. To minimize pain, patients may take Tylenol® or any over-the-counter nonsteroidal. A paracervical block may be used by some practitioners. Patients with artificial heart valve or artificial joints may need prophylactic antibiotics.

Aftercare Vasovagal reactions are rare but can occur. The patient may resume all activities including work, exercise, and intercourse. Patients should notify office for persistent pain, fever, or abdominal discomfort.

Equipment Choice of the type of hysteroscope used is left to the discretion of the physician. Either a small, 3.6-5.0 mm flexible hysteroscope or rigid hysteroscope is used. The distending medium can be CO_2 channeled through a hysteroinsufflator or liquid distending medium (normal saline, lactated Ringer's, or glycine). Additional equipment needed includes fiber optic cable, light source, video monitor, and camera.

Specimen Directed endometrial biopsies can be obtained by hysteroscopy. If a global endometrial process exists, then Pipelle biopsy can be performed.

Limitations Endometrial abnormalities including endometrial polyps, submucosal fibroids, intrauterine synechiae, endometrial hyperplasia, adenomyosis, septate uterus, endocervical polyps, endometrial cancer, foreign bodies, retained products of conception, and normal anatomy (proliferative, secretory, and atrophic endometrium) can be visualized by a skilled hysteroscopist. Operator inexperience will lead to faulty diagnosis.

References

Bradley LD and Widrich T, "State-of-the-Art Flexible Hysteroscopy for Office Gynecologic Evaluation," *J Am Assoc Gynecol Laparosc*, 1995, 2(3):263-7.

Finikiotis G, "Hysteroscopy: A Review," *Obstet Gynecol Surv*, 1994, 49(4):273-83.

Papanicolaou Smear

Related Information

Cervical Polypectomy *on page 296*
Colposcopy *on page 298*
Endocervical Curettage *on page 305*

Synonyms Pap Smear

Procedure Commonly Includes Sampling of exfoliated ectocervical and endocervical cells by gentle scraping and brushing of the uterine cervix for the purposes of detection of cervical disease.

Indications Cervical cytology screening is the mainstay of early detection for cervical carcinoma. Since the introduction of Pap screening in the United States, the incidence and mortality of cervical cancer has declined by more than 40%.[1] In 1988, a consensus recommendation was developed by several organizations, including the American College of Obstetrics and Gynecology, recommending that annual cervical cancer screening commence in all women who are or have been sexually active or who have reached 18 years of age.[2] It was further recommended that after a woman had three or more consecutive, satisfactory, normal annual Pap smears, the screening could be performed less frequently, at the discretion of her physician. In addition, patients reporting abnormal uterine bleeding or discharge of uncertain etiology should undergo cervical cytologic examination at the time of their evaluation to exclude the presence of cervical dysplasia or neoplasia. The Pap smear, however, is a screening tool and is not intended to be diagnostic. When cervical cytology is abnormal, or a gross cervical lesion is identified at visual inspection, colposcopy and/or biopsy of this lesion is indicated for histologic diagnosis.

Contraindications Pregnancy is not considered a contraindication, however, care should be exercised when obtaining the endocervical component of the specimen. At later gestational ages, a cotton-tipped applicator, rather than an endocervical brush, is used for endocervical cell collection.

Patient Preparation The patient should be instructed to avoid intravaginal placement of lubricants, medications, or other potentially obscuring factors prior to the examination. Ideally, cervical cytology should be not be obtained during menses, as the presence of blood may obscure significant cytologic findings. Irregular vaginal bleeding, however, is a symptom of cervical cancer and, under these circumstances, evaluation should not be deferred.

Aftercare Essentially none. Occasionally patients may experience light vaginal bleeding after the examination, particularly during pregnancy.

Equipment To facilitate vaginal examination, a table equipped with foot rests (stirrups) and a bivalve vaginal speculum is required. An Ayer's or other similar spatula is used to obtain the ectocervical sample. An endocervical brush or cotton-tipped applicator is used for endocervical sampling. For specimen processing, a glass slide, fixative spray, and items necessary for proper patient identification of the specimen are required. Alternatively, for the ThinPrep® system, the specimen is suspended in solution.

Technique Sampling errors account for a high proportion of false-negative smears in cervical cancer screening and adherence to proper technique is important in minimizing these errors.

To avoid contaminating the specimen with lubricant, the Pap smear should be obtained prior to bimanual examination. The patient is placed in the dorsal lithotomy position with speculum placement to allow visualization of the entire cervix. Gently remove vaginal discharge or blood with large cotton swabs prior to sampling. A scraping of the portio, including the entire transformation zone, is obtained with a spatula. Next, the endocervical brush is inserted into the cervical canal, gently rotated 90°, and then withdrawn.

Specimen Exfoliated cervical cells are acquired for cytologic examination

Collection For conventionally processed smears, proper fixation is essential. The collected material should be applied uniformly to a slide by rotation of the smear of the spatula and then the endocervical brush onto the glass slide. To avoid air drying, the specimen should be fixed within seconds of specimen retrieval. The spray fixative should be held at least 10 inches away to avoid cell damage during this process.

In an effort to optimize the collection and preparation of cells for cytologic evaluation, fluid-based processing of cervical cytology has recently been introduced. The specimen is collected in the same manner as described above and the cells are then rinsed from the collection device into a vial of preservative solution for further processing by the Cytology Laboratory. This facilitates cytology screening by increasing the yield of cells available for inspection, improving their distribution onto glass slides, and reducing obscuring debris. One system, the ThinPrep® (Cytyc Corporation, Boxborough, MA), has been approved by the Food and Drug Administration for this purpose.

(Continued)

Papanicolaou Smear *(Continued)*

When submitting specimens for cytologic evaluation, it is the responsibility of the clinician to provide all pertinent clinical information relevant to specimen interpretation. Thus, to improve the accuracy of specimen interpretation, clinical data such as age, date of last menstrual period, whether pregnant, postpartum or postmenopausal, history of prior abnormal Pap smears, or treatment must be communicated.

Normal Findings In past years, several classification systems have been suggested for cervical cytologic and histologic reporting. The Bethesda System for reporting cervical/vaginal cytologic diagnoses, revised in 1991, is now the predominant reporting system used in the majority of Cytology Laboratories throughout the country.[3] The table describes the Bethesda System in comparison to prior classification systems.

Comparison of Classification Systems for Cervical Specimen Reporting

WHO System	CIN System	Bethesda System*
Normal	Normal	Normal
Atypical	—	Infection / reactive / ASCUS
Dysplasia		
Mild	CIN 1	LGSIL
Moderate	CIN 2	HGSIL
Severe	CIN 3	HGSIL
Carcinoma	Carcinoma	HGSIL
In situ	*In situ*	
Invasive carcinoma	Invasive carcinoma	Invasive carcinoma

*Preferred reporting system.

CIN = cervical intraepithelial neoplasia
LGSIL = low grade squamous intraepithelial lesion
HGSIL = high grade squamous intraepithelial lesion

Limitations While enthusiasm for the screening tool is well deserved, no test is perfect. False-negative smear rates of 3% to 30% have been reported.[4] A significantly higher rate of false-negative Pap smears are observed when the transformation zone, the metaplastic cervical epithelium at greatest risk for dysplasia, is not adequately sampled. Notation of an "absence of endocervical cells" on a Cytology report indicates that the transformation zone may not have been adequately sampled. The presence of blood or inflammatory elements will also be noted on Cytology reporting if it has the potential to obscure significant findings.

Footnotes

1. Ries LA, Kosary CL, Hankey BF, et al, *SEER Cancer Statistics Review, 1973-1995*, Bethesda, MD: National Cancer Institute, 1998.
2. *Cervical Cytology: Evaluation and Management of Abnormalities, ACOG Technical Bulletin, No 183*, August, 1993.
3. Broder S, "From the National Institutes of Health," *JAMA*, 1992, 267(14):1892.
4. Sprenger E, Schwarzmann P, Kirkpatrick M, et al, "The False-Negative Rate in Cervical Cytology. Comparison of Monolayers to Conventional Smears," *Acta Cytol*, 1996, 40(1):81-9.

♦ **Pap Smear** *see* Papanicolaou Smear *on page 316*

♦ **Polypectomy, Cervix** *see* Cervical Polypectomy *on page 296*

Quantitative Ultrasound

Synonyms Heel Ultrasound; QUS; Ultrasound, Quantitative

Procedure Commonly Includes This procedure measures transmission of high frequency sound waves through bone, usually the heel. The procedure is less expensive than DEXA, it does not use ionizing radiation, and the equipment is portable and simple to use. QUS can be performed at multiple sites such as the calcaneus, ulna, patella, phalanges, and tibia, but the calcaneous is the most accepted site. Three prospective studies have shown calcaneal ultrasound performed similarly to DEXA in predicting the risk of fractures in elderly women. QUS has a high correlation (r=0.8) with DEXA at the same site, but only a moderate correlation with the spine or femur (r=0.4-0.6). Precision appears to be less (2% to 8%) than with central DEXA (1.5% to 3%).

QUS is an approved technique for Medicare reimbursement. However, it is not approved to monitor bone mineral density (BMD) in patients on therapies since longitudinal data has not been evaluated and published.

Patient Preparation The patient must remove hose, stocking, or socks for heel measurement. The actual measurement takes only minutes.

Equipment Numerous companies make ultrasound devices. For the heel, two basic systems exist, a "wet" system in which the heel is immersed in a body temperature water bath and a "dry" system using a gel to transmit the sound wave. Most systems combine velocity of transmission (speed of sound) with attenuation of sound waves (broadband ultrasound attenuation) to develop a stiffness index. This combination appears to correlate better with DEXA than either measure alone and has a proven fracture prediction.

Additional Information Values for lunar Achilles are reported as a stiffness index, a percent of peak bone mass. T-scores (standard deviation units below peak bone mass) and Z-scores (compared to age-matched controls) are also reported. As with DEXA, osteopenia is defined as a T-score between -1 and -2.5 and osteoporosis is less than -2.5. The T-scores cannot be assumed equivalent to T-scores reported for DEXA and some units have substantially higher (less negative or more positive) scores than DEXA. Thus, a conservative approach is to recommend central DEXA for anyone with a QUS T-score of less than -1.0.

♦ **QUS** *see* Quantitative Ultrasound *on page 318*

Saline Infusion Sonography

Related Information

Endometrial Biopsy *on page 307*

Synonyms Echohysteroscopy; Hydrosonography; Saline Solution-enhanced Endovaginal Ultrasonography; SIS; Sonoendovaginal Ultrasonography; Sonohysterography; Sonohysterosalpinogography

Procedure Commonly Includes Assessment of the uterine cavity for menstrual disorders has changed tremendously with the introduction of saline infusion sonography (SIS). Saline injected intracervically enhances the view of the endometrium and myometrium and also provides an acoustic view that allows for three-dimensional investigation of the uterine cavity and ovaries. This method is superior to TVUS (transvaginal ultrasound) because indistinct images and difficult localization of lesions occur.

Indications Evaluation of abnormal uterine bleeding refractory to medical therapy, postmenopausal bleeding, evaluation of bizarre sonolucencies in patients on tamoxifen observed by conventional TVUS, evaluation of thickened endometrium by conventional TVUS, evaluation of myometrium and adnexa, preoperative assessment of uterine fibroids

Patient Preparation SIS requires minimal preparation and no anesthesia. Since this is an invasive procedure, pelvic infection must be ruled out prior to performing this test. The procedure is best scheduled in the early proliferative phase in menstruating women. The risk of interrupting a viable intrauterine pregnancy is lowest at this time, and there are fewer artifacts thereby improving visualization of endometrial polyps and uterine fibroids. Prophylactic antibiotics are recommended for patients with prosthetic heart valves/joint. Preprocedure administration of nonsteroidal anti-inflammatory drugs (NSAIDs) is optional. Voiding before SIS is important. Bladder distention is not required and may make the evaluation with a transvaginal probe onerous.

A bimanual examination is performed with the patient in the dorsal lithotomy position. Conventional TVUS is performed using a transvaginal probe covered with a condom and gel. The uterine size, endometrial echo, and measurement of the adnexal structures is obtained. After completing the TVUS, the cervix is visualized by placing an open-sided speculum in the vagina to facilitate introduction of the intrauterine catheter. The cervix is visualized and cleansed with an antiseptic solution, and the intrauterine catheter is inserted. Sterile saline, lactated Ringer's, or glycine is infused slowly at a rate of 5-30 mL/minute, while the physician/sonographer views the TVUS monitor. Anterior and

(Continued)

Saline Infusion Sonography *(Continued)*

posterior endometrial echo measurements are recalculated, as well as any intracavitary masses. Both procedures take 5-20 minutes.

Aftercare None needed except for usual precautions for possible vasovagal resection.

Equipment Standard transvaginal ultrasound imager with high frequency transducer (7.5 MHz) covered by a condom and gel, open-sided vaginal speculum, any commercial intrauterine catheter, sterile saline, lactated Ringer's, or glycine

Specimen An endometrial Pipelle can be performed following the procedure if a global endometrial process exists. A directed biopsy, best performed by operative hysteroscopy, is indicated when focal lesions are detected.

Limitations SIS allows the clinician to evaluate the uterus for intracavitary lesions. It also provides for differentiation of the causes of increased endometrial thickness on conventional TVUS. Representative features of uterine polyps, fibroids, synechiae, and endometrial thickening associated with endometrial hyperplasia/malignancy are noted. Patients with markedly retroverted uterus, multiple uterine fibroids, uterine enlargement greater than 12- to 14-week size are imaged less well with SIS. An experienced sonographer is necessary for optimal SIS images.

Additional Information This test is most useful for preoperative assessment of intracavitary lesions and evaluation and triage of abnormal uterine bleeding.

References

Widrich T, Bradley LD, Mitchinson AR, et al, "Comparison of Saline Infusion Sonography With Office Hysteroscopy for the Evaluation of the Endometrium," *Am J Obstet Gynecol*, 1996, 174(2):1327-34.

- ♦ **Saline Solution-enhanced Endovaginal Ultrasonography** *see* Saline Infusion Sonography *on page 319*
- ♦ **SIS** *see* Saline Infusion Sonography *on page 319*
- ♦ **Sonoendovaginal Ultrasonography** *see* Saline Infusion Sonography *on page 319*
- ♦ **Sonohysterography** *see* Saline Infusion Sonography *on page 319*
- ♦ **Sonohysterosalpinogography** *see* Saline Infusion Sonography *on page 319*

Ultrasound for Obstetrics - 1st Trimester

Procedure Commonly Includes Abdominal scanning with an ultrasound machine to look for a viable fetus in the uterus. May also be done with a vaginal probe.

Indications When fetal viability needs to be confirmed

Patient Preparation In the very early pregnancy, usually only a transvaginal probe scan is done. However, if an abdominal scan is needed to confirm or corroborate findings, a full bladder is best. A patient should drink approximately 1 quart water 1 hour before the procedure.

Special Instructions Procedure takes approximately 15 minutes.

Equipment Ultrasound imaging methods are based on insonating target tissues with low energy (<100 mW/cm^2), high frequency (3.5-7.5 MHz) sound waves and recording the reflected echoes. Emitting crystals may be sequentially activated (linear array), or a single crystal may be swept through a prescribed arc (a sector array), or a hybrid curvilinear array may be used.

Technique Ultrasound gel, surgical lubricant, or vegetable oil may be used as a coupling agent and spread on the maternal abdomen. The transducer is applied to the maternal abdomen just cephalad to the pubic bone and angled down toward the rectum. Sweeping up and down and changing to a right angle and sweeping back and forth is the surest way to visualize everything in the lower pelvis. If the goal is to find an intrauterine gestation, this should be easily seen abdominally from about 8 weeks past the last menstrual period and vaginally about 5 weeks past the last menstrual period. Usually a dark sac is seen with a small lighter bean-shaped area, which represents the fetal pole. Pulsations seen within the fetal pole represent the fetal heartbeat.

Data Acquired While most internists and family practitioners will use this only to check for viability, nomograms do exist for measuring both the gestational sac and the crown rump length (CRL) of the fetus to estimate gestational age. If the nomogram is not available, a rough estimate may be made by adding the number 6.5 to the CRL in centimeters (ie, CRL (in cm) + 6.5 = weeks of gestation).

Normal Findings After the 5th week after the last menstrual period, a gestational sac of some sort should be seen within the uterine cavity. A blush of lighter colored endometrium is often seen around the sac. Sometimes the layers of the sac are visible separately from each other. A fetal pole should also be seen. If the patient is more than 5 weeks past the last menstrual period and nothing is seen in the uterus, one must suspect an ectopic pregnancy. Another explanation for absence of a fetal pulse is a pregnancy earlier than what would be expected from the patient's last menstrual period. If a blood pregnancy test is higher than 3000 mIU/mL and nothing is seen within the uterus, ectopic pregnancy must be suspected.

Critical Values If the gestational sac is >3.0 cm and there is no fetal pole or if the fetus measures 1.5 cm and there is no heartbeat, a spontaneous abortion is probable. If the woman is 6-8 weeks past the last menstrual period and nothing is seen in the uterus, an ectopic pregnancy must be suspected. If the serum hCG is >3000 mIU/mL and nothing is seen in the uterus, again ectopic pregnancy must be considered.

Limitations Maternal habitus may sometimes limit what can be seen by ultrasound. Bowel gas, an empty bladder, and uterine fibroid tumors may also interfere with first trimester obstetrical ultrasound. A retroverted uterus may be difficult to evaluate transabdominally.

References

Guidelines for the Performance of the Antepartum Obstetrical Ultrasound Examination, Laurel, MD: American Institute of Ultrasound in Medicine, 1994.

"Ultrasonography in Pregnancy. ACOG Technical Bulletin Number 187," *Int J Gynaecol Obstet*, 1994, 44(2):173-83.

Ultrasound for Obstetrics - 2nd and 3rd Trimester

Related Information

Amniocentesis *on page 293*
Biophysical Profile *on page 294*
Contraction Stress Test for Confirming Fetal Well-Being *on page 303*

Procedure Commonly Includes Passing high frequency sound waves into the body. The reflected echoes are detected and analyzed to form an image of the fetus.

Indications Evaluate fetal well-being; scan for birth defects; detect multiple pregnancies; guide amniocentesis; determine the position of the fetus; determine the position of the placenta; look for abruption of the placenta; look for masses and tumors of the uterus, ovaries, and fallopian tubes; evaluate fetal growth; establish gestational age

Patient Preparation Full bladder is desirable. Have patient drink 1 quart of water 1 hour before procedure.

Special Instructions Duration of Procedure: 30 minutes

Equipment Low energy (<100 mW/cm^2), high frequency (3.5-7.5 MHz) sound waves are used to evaluate fetal anatomy. The reflected echo signals are interpreted by a digital computer. The emitting crystals may be activated sequentially (linear array), or a single crystal may be swept through an arch (a sector array) or a combination may be used (curvilinear array). In some machines, continuous wave Doppler is used to evaluate the umbilical cord. Coloring of the Doppler images may add some definition. Cine-loops automatically store several seconds worth of images. These can be played back later and analyzed. Three-dimensional imaging is available at some centers.

Technique The transducer most often used is the curvilinear display. Oil, gel, or other coupling agent is spread liberally over the patient's abdomen. Extensive training is usually required for a full interpretation of the scan, but some useful information can be obtained by most practitioners. The exact type of data to be obtained depends on the indications for the obstetrical ultrasound.

Data Acquired Looking for the fetal head usually yields the most information. The fetal head appears as an oval shape, echogenic all the way around with

(Continued)

Ultrasound for Obstetrics - 2nd and 3rd Trimester *(Continued)*

hypoechoic areas inside. The biparietal diameter is most accurate measurement and is measured transversely at the level of the thalami, a small hypoechoic butterfly-shaped midline structure. However, any measurement across the fetal skull will allow an approximate estimate of gestational age. To estimate gestational age in weeks, multiply the diameter in centimeters by 4.

Specimen None (unless amniocentesis) obtained in conjunction with obstetrical ultrasound

Normal Findings Complete evaluation should be performed by an ultrasonographer or obstetrician trained in ultrasonography. In the acute setting, fetal viability and estimated gestational age of the fetus can be determined. Fetal lie may also be determined (whether the fetus is cephalic, breech, or transverse). Occasionally, one will be able to tell if the placenta is near the cervical os or detached. The placenta has a medium gray appearance. If there is a large hypo- or hyperechoic region between the placenta and the uterus, the possibility of abruption should be entertained. However, most abruptions cannot be diagnosed by ultrasound.

Critical Values Any reported abnormality by the ultrasonographer necessitates obstetrical consultation.

Limitations Interpretation will be limited by the experience of the operator, the resolution of the equipment, and the maternal habitus. Abdominal scarring and bowel gas can also obscure the information obtained.

References

Guidelines for the Performance of the Antepartum Obstetrical Ultrasound Examination, Laurel, MD: American Institute of Ultrasound in Medicine, 1994.

"Ultrasonography in Pregnancy. ACOG Technical Bulletin Number 187," *Int J Gynaecol Obstet*, 1994, 44(2):173-83.

♦ **Ultrasound, Quantitative** *see* Quantitative Ultrasound *on page 318*

Vaginal Wet Prep

Synonyms Wet Prep

Procedure Commonly Includes A pelvic examination and obtaining a sample of vaginal secretions. Examination of cells under the microscope.

Indications Differentiate yeast from clue cells and trichomonads

Patient Preparation The complete examination may take approximately 30 minutes. The patient will need a complete pelvic exam. The patient should be undressed from the waist down. The patient should not be menstruating at the time of the exam. A complete gynecologic history should be obtained including sexual history. Current medications should be obtained with particular emphasis on recent antibiotic use, and last menstrual period should be documented.

Technique The patient should be in the dorsal lithotomy position for a pelvic exam with feet in stirrups and sheet draped over legs. The lamp should be used for visualization. A speculum should be used according to the patient's size. The examiner wears nonsterile gloves and inserts the speculum into the vagina.

Obtain secretions from the vaginal wall with a cotton swab. Place the swab in a test tube or specimen container prepared with 1-2 mL sterile normal saline and transport to the microscope. Test tube placement minimizes contamination risk.

Measure the acid of the discharge by touching the swab to pH paper. The normal acidity of the vagina is between 4 and 4.5.

Prepare a slide with two separate pools of discharge. Place a coverslip over one pool. Drop 10% KOH on the uncovered sample. Assess sample for a fishy odor which is common for bacterial vaginosis. This is documented as a "positive whiff test". Next, place a coverslip over this sample. Examine each area under the microscope using low power (10x). Check 10 fields on each side and then switch to 40x and check 10 more fields.

Normal Findings Normal findings include epithelial cells, lactobacilli, an occasional white blood cell, and a few red blood cells if the women is menstruating and sperm if recent unprotected intercourse. Normal pH is between 4 and 4.5. A more alkaline pH level, >4.5, may indicate bacterial vaginosis or trichomoniasis. A negative whiff test should be present.

Limitations An unclean microscope, menstruation, contamination at collection

Additional Information Abnormal findings include:

- >20% clue cells (bacterial vaginosis)
- many WBCs and cocci bacteria
- reduced lactobacilli
- hyphae (yeast)
- trichomonads (usually motile)
- pH >4.5
- positive whiff (bacterial vaginosis)

References

Davies J, "Common Vaginal Infections." *Adv Nurs Pract*, 1998, 6(11):35-8, 47, 93.

♦ **Wet Prep** *see* Vaginal Wet Prep *on page 322*

DIAGNOSTIC RADIOLOGY

COMPUTED TOMOGRAPHY

- ♦ **Abdomen, CT** *see* Computed Transaxial Tomography, Abdomen Studies *on page 327*
- ♦ **Arthrography, CT** *see* Computed Transaxial Tomography, Arthrography *on page 329*
- ♦ **Bone Densitometry, CT** *see* Computed Transaxial Tomography, Bone Densitometry *on page 329*
- ♦ **Brain, CT** *see* Computed Transaxial Tomography, Head Studies *on page 332*
- ♦ **Cervical Spine, CT** *see* Computed Transaxial Tomography, Spine *on page 340*

Computed Transaxial Tomography, Abdomen Studies

Related Information

Computed Transaxial Tomography, Pelvis *on page 338*
Magnetic Resonance Scan, Abdomen *on page 393*

Synonyms Abdomen, CT; CT, Lower Abdomen; CT, Total Abdomen; CT, Upper Abdomen

Procedure Commonly Includes CT scan of liver, spleen, kidneys, pancreas, aorta, retroperitoneum, gastrointestinal tract, pelvis. **Note:** In some departments, a request for a CT study of the abdomen will yield a study extending inferiorly to the pubic symphysis. In others, the study will extend only to the pelvic brim. See Computed Transaxial Tomography, Pelvis *on page 338.*

Indications Diagnosis and/or evaluation of cysts, tumors, masses, aneurysm, metastases, abscesses, and trauma. The modality is also often used for staging of known tumors. Suspected pancreatic or adrenal pathology may be a good indication for a spiral/helical examination. The evaluation of the liver may benefit from a dynamic CT exam. These decisions are best made by the radiologist when he/she is familiar with the clinical data.

Contraindications Patient cooperation is of the utmost importance as the examination requires the patient to remain motionless for the duration of the study. The time of the study will vary from 20-40 minutes depending on the equipment being used. Children and uncooperative adults may require sedation.

Patient Preparation The patient's oral intake is restricted to fluid only for 4 hours prior to the examination. Medication schedule should not be interrupted. Should the patient have recently undergone a barium examination of the gastrointestinal tract, a digital radiograph obtained with the scanner prior to commencement of the procedure may be helpful in excluding the presence of barium within the bowel. The latter may produce significant artifact and thus render the study nondiagnostic. Where possible, all CT scan studies of the abdomen should be performed prior to normal GI barium studies. A recent serum creatinine is requested on all patients 60 years of age and older, patients with known significant atherosclerotic disease, diabetes mellitus, or with pre-existing renal disease. Intravenous contrast material is routinely administered for this examination. Physician may opt to omit intravenous contrast. Patients undergoing a CT study of the abdomen are requested to drink approximately 450 mL of a dilute barium solution (approximately 1% barium) commencing 1 hour prior to the examination. Inclusion of the pelvis in

(Continued)

Computed Transaxial Tomography, Abdomen Studies *(Continued)*

this examination requires further patient preparation. See Computed Transaxial Tomography, Pelvis *on page 338*.

Special Instructions CT scan of the abdomen may be requested by a practicing physician. The abdominal area of interest should be specified along with pertinent clinical history. This will allow the diagnostic radiologist to tailor the examination for maximum diagnostic yield. For example, studies being performed for detection of renal calculi should be performed without contrast material, as the contrast, when excreted from the kidney, will mask the presence of small calculi within the collecting system. Adequate evaluation of small structures within the abdomen may require modification of technique such as thin slices or overlapping slices. A further example would be in the evaluation of the liver for primary or metastatic tumor. Maximum yield in the demonstration of such abnormalities requires examination both with and without contrast material.

Equipment This examination may be performed on any one of many commercially available computerized tomography scanners.

Technique Standard examination of the abdomen consists of 1 cm contiguous slices obtained from the dome of the diaphragm to the pelvic brim or pubic symphysis depending upon whether one groups the pelvis with the abdomen or treats it separately.

Turnaround Time A verbal telephone report of the scan will be given to the referring physician if specified. A written report will be available.

Causes for Rejection Patients with residual barium within the GI tract from a prior conventional barium study - this nondilute barium produces considerable artifact rendering the examination suboptimal and often nondiagnostic, uncooperative patients who are not candidates for sedation/anesthesia

Additional Information Patients should be informed that the examination may take 45 minutes to 1 hour and that oral contrast and intravenous contrast are commonly required. If the pelvis is included with the abdominal CT study, rectal contrast material and placement of a vaginal tampon in the case of females may also be required. The patient's medical record should accompany the patient. This will furnish the radiologist with sufficient information to tailor the examination as he/she deems appropriate. For example, patients suspected of an adrenal adenoma may require thin (2 mm) slices through the adrenal glands for the detection of such an abnormality; if spiral/helical CT were available, this would be a good application.

References

Byun JY, Ha HK, Yu SY, et al, "CT Features of Systemic Lupus Erythematosus in Patients With Acute Abdominal Pain: Emphasis on Ischemic Bowel Disease," *Radiology*, 1999, 211(1):203-9.

Daly B, Sukumar SA, Krebs TL, et al, "Nonbiliary Laparoscopic Gastrointestinal Surgery: Role of CT in Diagnosis and Management of Complication," *AJR Am J Roentgenol*, 1996, 167(2):455-9.

Federle MP, Yagan N, Peitzman AB, et al, "Abdominal Trauma: Use of Oral Contrast Material for CT Is Safe," *Radiology*, 1997, 205(1):91-3.

Fishman EK, "Spiral CT: Clinical Applications in the Gastrointestinal Tract," *Clin Imaging*, 1997, 21(2):111-21.

Ginzburg E, Carrillo EH, Kopelman T, et al, "The Role of Computed Tomography in Selective Management of Gunshot Wounds to the Abdomen and Flank," *J Trauma*, 1998, 45(6):1005-9.

Halvorsen RA Jr and Thompson WM, "Computed Tomographic Staging of Gastrointestinal Tract Malignancies, Part I. Esophagus and Stomach," *Invest Radiol*, 1987, 22(1):2-16.

Hopper KD, Keeton NC, Kasales CJ, et al, "Utility of Low mA 1.5 Pitch Helical Versus Conventional High mA Abdominal CT," *Clin Imaging*, 1998, 22(1):54-9.

Kim TK, Chung JW, Han JK, et al, "Hepatic Changes in Benign Obstruction of the Hepatic Inferior Vena Cava: CT Findings," *AJR Am J Roentgenol*, 1999, 173(5):1235-42.

Larson RE, Semelka RC, Bagley AS, et al, "Hypervascular Malignant Liver Lesions: Comparison of Various MR Imaging Pulse Sequences and Dynamic CT," *Radiology*, 1994, 192(2):393-9.

Rencken IO, Sola A, al-Ali F, et al, "Necrotizing Enterocolitis: Diagnosis With CT Examination of Urine After Enteral Administration of Iodinated Water-Soluble Contrast Material," *Radiology*, 1997, 205(1):87-90.

Stafford RE, McGonigal MD, Weigelt JA, et al, "Oral Contrast Solution and Computed Tomography for Blunt Abdominal Trauma: A Randomized Study," *Arch Surg*, 1999, 134(6):622-6; discussion 626-7.

Thompson WM and Halvorsen RA Jr, "Computed Tomographic Staging of Gastrointestinal Tract Malignancies, Part II," *Invest Radiol*, 1987, 22(2):96-105.

Winter TC, Ager JD, Ngheim HV, et al, "Upper Gastrointestinal Tact and Abdomen: Water as an Orally Administered Contrast Agent for Helical CT," *Radiology*, 1996, 201(2):365-70.

Computed Transaxial Tomography, Arthrography

Synonyms Arthrography, CT

Procedure Commonly Includes CT scanning of any joint subsequent to instillation of air and/or contrast material under fluoroscopic guidance to obtain thin, overlapping slices through the joint in question are obtained.

Indications CT arthrography of the shoulder is often undertaken to evaluate the unstable shoulder for an abnormality involving the glenoid labrum or in search of an abnormal joint capsule. When performed in the ankle, elbow, and knee joints, it is more frequently done for osteochondritis dissecans and confirmation/localization of a loose body.

Contraindications Uncooperative patient

Patient Preparation No intravenous contrast material is administered for this procedure, therefore no preliminary laboratory work is required. No dietary restrictions.

Aftercare Physical exertion should be restricted until the air and contrast material have been reabsorbed through the joint capsule. This is usually complete within 24-36 hours.

Equipment This examination can be performed on any of the commercially available CT scanners.

Technique In the case of the shoulder examinations, a slice thickness of 4 mm with the table incrementing at 3 mm prior to each slice is generally satisfactory. A 2 mm slice with equal or slightly greater table increments may be required in the elbow.

Additional Information The improved spatial resolution afforded by magnetic resonance imaging coupled with the natural contrast that this modality provides may soon supersede CT arthrography in the knee and should advances continue in MR, the CT procedure may be totally replaced.

References

Brossmann J, Preidler KW, Daenen B, et al, "Imaging of Osseous and Cartilaginous Intraarticular Bodies in the Knee: Comparison of MR Imaging and MR Arthrography With CT and CT Arthrography in Cadavers," *Radiology*, 1996, 200(2):509-17.

Farin PU, Kaukanen E, Jaroma H, et al, "Site and Size of Rotator-Cuff Tear. Findings at Ultrasound, Double-Contrast Arthrography, and Computed Tomography Arthrography With Surgical Correlation," *Invest Radiol*, 1996, 31(7):387-94.

Hauger O, Moinard M, Lasalarie JC, et al, "Anterolateral Compartment of the Ankle in the Lateral Impingement Syndrome: Appearance on CT Arthrography," *AJR Am J Roentgenol*, 1999, 173(3):685-90.

Rafii M and Minkoff J, "Advanced Arthrography of the Shoulder With CT and MR Imaging," *Radiol Clin North Am*, 1998, 36(4):609-33.

Resnick D, "Arthrography, Tenography, and Bursography," *Diagnosis of Bone and Joint Disorders*, 3rd ed, Chapter 13, Resnick D, ed, Philadelphia, PA: WB Saunders Co, 1995, 277.

Steinbach LS and Schwartz M, "Elbow Arthrography," *Radiol Clin North Am*, 1998, 36(4):635-49.

Tung GA and Brody JM, "Contemporary Imaging of Athletic Injuries," *Clin Sports Med*, 1997, 16(3):393-417.

Yu JS, Greenway G, and Resnick D, "Osteochondral Defect of the Glenoid Fossa: Cross-Sectional Imaging Features," *Radiology*, 1998, 206(1):35-40.

Computed Transaxial Tomography, Bone Densitometry

Synonyms Bone Densitometry, CT; Single and Dual Energy Quantitative Computed Tomography

Procedure Commonly Includes A noninvasive, quantitative bone mineral determination. The technique's usefulness lies in its ability to give a quantitative image. It can be used to measure trabecular, cortical, or integral bone, centrally or peripherally.

Indications The quantitative CT technique for vertebral mineral determination has been used to study skeletal changes in osteoporosis and other metabolic bone diseases.

Contraindications Patient cooperation is of the utmost importance as the examination requires the patient to remain motionless for the duration of the study. The time of the study will vary from 10-20 minutes depending on the equipment being used.

(Continued)

Computed Transaxial Tomography, Bone Densitometry *(Continued)*

Patient Preparation This examination does not require the use of intravenous contrast material. Because of this, there are no dietary restrictions prior to the examination. Medication schedules should not be interrupted.

Special Instructions The use of computed tomographic scanners for quantitative purposes requires great attention to detail to ensure accurate and precise measurements. The use of a calibration phantom measured simultaneously with the patient is helpful in assuring quality and accuracy.

Equipment This examination may be performed on most commercially available computed tomography scanners.

Technique Generally, a total of four vertebral bodies between T-12 and L-4 are measured. Vertebral bodies with compression deformities are to be avoided. T-12 should also be avoided if the lungs are hyperinflated and the vertebral body remains in the lung field. An 8 or 10 mm thick slice is obtained through the center of each vertebral body. The slice should be obtained with the gantry tilted so that it lies parallel to the end plates of the vertebral body. Baseline and final measurement are to be performed in dual energy mode. Thus, two scans must be obtained through each vertebral body. One of these with a low kilo voltage per (kVp) setting and the second with a high kVp setting. It is important that these two scans are obtained back to back with a minimal time lapse between the acquisitions.

Turnaround Time A verbal telephone report of the scan will be given to the referring physician if specified. A written report will be available.

Causes for Rejection Residual barium in the gastrointestinal tract may produce beam hardening artifact thus negating the value of the study.

Additional Information It should be noted that table height influences the results. The standard table height should be selected for each commercially available CT scanner. Care should be taken not to include portions of the end plates within the thickness of the scan.

References

Grampp S, Majumdar S, Jergas M, et al, "Distal Radius: *In vivo* Assessment With Quantitative MR Imaging, Peripheral Quantitative CT, and Dual X-ray Absorptiometry," *Radiology*, 1996, 198(1):213-8.

Harcourt JP, Lennox P, Phelps PD, et al, "CT Screening for Temporal Bone Abnormalities in Idiopathic Bilateral Sensorineural Hearing Loss," *J Laryngol Otol*, 1997, 111(2):117-21.

Jergas M and Genant HK, "Quantitative Bone Mineral Analysis," *Diagnosis of Bone and Joint Disorders*, Chapter 52, 3rd ed, Resnick D, ed, Philadelphia, PA: WB Saunders Co, 1995.

Lang TF, Augat P, Lane NE, et al, "Trochanteric Hip Fracture: Strong Association With Spinal Trabecular Bone Mineral Density Measured With Quantitative CT," *Radiology*, 1998, 209(2):525-30.

Computed Transaxial Tomography, Dynamic Study

Synonyms Dynamic Study, CT

Procedure Commonly Includes Dynamic CT refers to rapid sequential imaging of an anatomic area of interest subsequent to delivery (usually intravenously, rarely intra-arterially) of a bolus of contrast material. While it is possible to extract some physiologic information utilizing this technique, this is not a major indication.

Indications The examination is most commonly utilized to highlight vasculature thus improving ability to demonstrate thrombosis, aneurysmal dilatation, or differential rate of flow in the case of aortic dissection. The technique may be used for evaluation of vascularity of abnormal masses. The latter may be helpful in the characterization of hepatic lesions such as hemangiomas which commonly demonstrate initial peripheral enhancement with later central enhancement and eventual equalization with the surrounding hepatic parenchyma.

Contraindications Patient cooperation is of the utmost importance.

Patient Preparation The reader is referred to Patient Preparation for the area of anatomic interest (eg, for liver, see Computed Transaxial Tomography, Abdomen Studies *on page 327*).

Special Instructions The reader is referred to the special instructions for the anatomic area of interest (eg, dynamic CT of the chest, see Computed Transaxial Tomography, Thorax *on page 342*).

Equipment Standard commercially available CT scanners

Technique The volume of the bolus of contrast material, the slice thickness, and the delay between administration of the bolus and commencement of scanning will vary depending upon the anatomic area of interest and the information required. Most commercially available CT scanners include software that permits a rapid scanning technique to facilitate a dynamic examination.

References

Bader TR, Herneth AM, Blaicher W, et al, "Hepatic Perfusion After Liver Transplantation: Noninvasive Measurement With Dynamic Single-Section CT," *Radiology*, 1998, 209(1):129-34.

Chen JH, Chai JW, Huang CL, et al, "Proximal Arterioportal Shunting Associated With Hepatocellular Carcinoma: Features Revealed by Dynamic Helical CT," *AJR Am J Roentgenol*, 1999, 172(2):403-7.

Foley WD, "Dynamic Hepatic CT," *Radiology*, 1989, 170(3 Pt 1):617-22.

Frederick MG, McElaney BL, Singer A, et al, "Timing of Parenchymal Enhancement on Dual-Phase Dynamic Helical CT of the Liver: How Long Does the Hepatic Arterial Phase Predominate?" *AJR Am J Roentgenol*, 1996, 166(6):1305-10.

Ito K, Awaya H, Mitchell DG, et al, "Gallbladder Disease: Appearance of Associated Transient Increased Attenuation in the Liver at Biphasic, Contrast-Enhanced Dynamic CT," *Radiology*, 1997, 204(3):723-8.

Nagata K, Murata T, Shiga T, et al, "Dynamic Computed Tomography Predicts Tumor Temperature and Response to Thermoradiotherapy in Superficial and Subsurface Tumors," *Cancer*, 1999, 86(1):177-85.

Tsushima Y, Blomley JK, Kusano S, et al, "The Portal Component of Hepatic Perfusion Measured by Dynamic CT: An Indicator of Hepatic Parenchymal Damage," *Dig Dis Sci*, 1999, 44(8):1632-8.

Tsushima Y, Koizumi J, Yokoyama H, et al, "Evaluation of Portal Pressure by Splenic Perfusion Measurement Using Dynamic CT," *AJR Am J Roentgenol*, 1998, 170(1):153-5.

Tsushima Y, Unno Y, Koizumi J, et al, "Hepatic Perfusion Changes After Transcatheter Arterial Embolization (TAE) of Hepatocellular Carcinoma: Measurement by Dynamic Computed Tomography (CT)," *Dig Dis Sci*, 1998, 43(2):317-22.

Ueda K, Matsui O, Kawamori Y, et al, "Hypervascular Hepatocellular Carcinoma: Evaluation of Hemodynamics With Dynamic CT During Hepatic Arteriography," *Radiology*, 1998, 206(1):161-6.

Computed Transaxial Tomography, Extremities

Synonyms Extremities, CT

Procedure Commonly Includes Intravenous administration of contrast material with subsequent CT scans of the portion of the extremity in question. Both extremities are usually included in the field of view. In the majority of cases, this provides a normal side for comparative purposes.

Indications The modality has been employed primarily to evaluate bone and soft tissue neoplasms. Occasionally, the modality may be used in inflammatory conditions for localization of an abscess or evaluation of the extent of the abnormality. The cross-sectional display afforded by this modality is useful in localizing abnormalities of the extremities and in determining the intramedullary and extraosseous extent of such abnormalities. The modality is used infrequently for the evaluation of trauma involving the extremities; however, it has been found most useful in evaluating trauma involving the hip joints and shoulder joints.

Contraindications Uncooperative patient. Patients with extremities in traction are not good candidates for this examination. The presence of a cast on the extremity will produce some significant artifact thus degrading the image somewhat.

Patient Preparation Diet should be restricted to liquids only for 4 hours prior to the examination. Medication schedule should not be interrupted. Intravenous contrast material may be administered at the discretion of the radiologist. Because of this, a recent serum creatinine is also requested on patients 60 years of age or older, those with significant atherosclerotic disease, those with a known diagnosis of diabetes mellitus, or with pre-existing renal disease.

Equipment Examination may be performed on any of the commercially available CT scanners.

Technique Examination usually consists of 1 cm contiguous slices obtained throughout the area of interest subsequent to the intravenous administration

(Continued)

Computed Transaxial Tomography, Extremities *(Continued)*

of contrast material. The size and location of the lesion may require modification of the examination technique by the radiologist.

Turnaround Time Written report available.

Limitations The patient's weight should be <300 lb. This is the table limitation on most commercially available CT scanners.

Additional Information This method of imaging the extremities has, to a large degree, been superseded by magnetic resonance imaging in the recent past. Unfortunately, computed tomography lacks both the spatial resolution and the soft tissue contrast necessary for the evaluation of many different pathologic conditions involving bone. The inherent contrast of MRI is a major advantage when imaging the appendicular skeleton. The ever increasing array of surface coils now available coupled with the excellent spatial resolution provided by magnetic resonance has superseded computed tomography for the evaluation of the extremities.

References

Cole RJ, Bindra RR, Evanoff BA, et al, "Radiographic Evaluation of Osseous Displacement Following Intra-Articular Fractures of the Distal Radius: Reliability of Plain Radiography Versus Computed Tomography," *J Hand Surg [Am]*, 1997, 22(5):792-800.

Conway WF, Totty WG, and McEnery KW, "CT and MR Imaging of the Hip," *Radiology*, 1996, 198(2):297-307.

Demas BE, Heelan RT, Lane J, et al, "Soft-Tissue Sarcomas of the Extremities: Comparison of MR and CT in Determining the Extent of Disease," *AJR Am J Roentgenol*, 1988, 150(3):615-20.

Kuszyk BS and Fishman EK, "Direct Coronal CT of the Wrist: Helical Acquisition With Simplified Patient Positioning," *AJR Am J Roentgenol*, 1996, 166(2):419-20.

Preidler KW, Brossmann J, Daenen B, et al, "Measurements of Cortical Thickness in Experimentally Created Endosteal Bone Lesions: A Comparison of Radiography, CT, MR Imaging, and Anatomic Sections," *AJR Am J Roentgenol*, 1997, 168(6):1501-5.

Preidler KW, Peicha G, Lajtai G, et al, "Conventional Radiography, CT, and MR Imaging in Patients With Hyperflexion Injuries of the Foot: Diagnostic Accuracy in the Detection of Bony and Ligamentous Changes," *AJR Am J Roentgenol*, 1999, 173(6):1673-7.

Roolker W, Teil-van Buul MM, Ritt MJ, et al, "Experimental Evaluation of Scaphoid X-Series, Carpal Box Radiographs, Planar Tomography, Computed Tomography, and Magnetic Resonance Imaging in the Diagnosis of Scaphoid Fracture," *J Trauma*, 1997, 42(2):247-53.

Computed Transaxial Tomography, Head Studies

Related Information

Magnetic Resonance Angiography, Brain *on page 391*

Magnetic Resonance Scan, Brain *on page 401*

Synonyms Brain, CT; Head Studies, CT

Procedure Commonly Includes CT scan of the brain

Indications Evaluation of known/suspected primary or secondary neoplasm, cystic lesions, hydrocephalus, head trauma, seizure disorder, multiple sclerosis, atrophy, Alzheimer disease, normal pressure hydrocephalus, Parkinson disease, dementia, depression, organic brain syndrome, etc.

Contraindications Assuming a cooperative or quiescent patient, there are no absolute contraindications to a CT scan of the head. A decision must be taken, however, as to whether the study is to be done with or without intravenous contrast material. While each case must be assessed individually, the following broad guidelines may be helpful. Those studies indicated by virtue of a recent infarct, cerebrovascular accident or stroke, or those being done for assessment of atrophy, Alzheimer disease, normal pressure hydrocephalus, Parkinson's disease, hydrocephalus, evaluation of an intraventricular shunt, assessment of ventricular size, subdural hematoma, or suspected dementia are examined without contrast material. Patients for whom the indication is headache, psychiatric condition (such as anorexia or bulimia), tumor follow-up, rule out tumor, rule out metastasis, multiple sclerosis, seizure disorders, depression, and organic brain syndrome are generally studied with contrast material. Patients in whom the indication is one of infection, abscess, meningitis, transient ischemic attack, arteriovenous malformation, remote subdural hematoma, or who have recently undergone a craniotomy and are being studied for postoperative evaluation are best studied with and without contrast material. Patients with a known diagnosis of plasmacytoma or multiple myeloma should not receive intravenous contrast material. Patients with compromised renal function may or may not benefit from intravenous contrast material. A recent serum creatinine and BUN will be helpful in deciding whether or not the latter group of patients receive contrast material.

Patient Preparation The examination should be ordered and a requisition with information pertaining to the reason for the request and the clinical history should be completed by the referring physician. If there is the slightest possibility that intravenous contrast material will be administered, the patient's oral intake should be limited to liquids for at least 4 hours prior to the examination. Care must be taken to ensure the patient does not become dehydrated and medications should not be interrupted. A recent serum creatinine is requested on patients with pre-existing renal disease, diabetes mellitus, significant atherosclerotic disease, and advancing age (60 years and older). Agitated patients and children may require sedation prior to the examination. In these cases, an order for the appropriate sedative and dose should be recently recorded within the patient's chart. Sedatives should be administered by a physician within the Radiology Department.

Equipment Any commercially available computed tomographic scanner

Technique CT scans of the head are usually obtained at 15° angulation to the orbitomeatal line, a line connecting the lateral canthus of the eye with the external auditory canal. Contiguous slices 8 or 10 mm in thickness are obtained from the vertex of the skull to the foramen magnum. The orbital roof should be included. The patient is positioned supine for the examination. The head is placed securely in a head holder. The chin is flexed comfortably towards the chest. The appropriate 15° angulation can be obtained by angulation of the gantry if necessary.

References

Servadei F, Murray GD, Penny K, et al, "The Value of the "Worst" Computed Tomographic Scan in Clinical Studies of Moderate and Severe Head Injury," *Neurosurgery*, 2000, 46(1):70-5; discussion: 75-7.

Stodilka RZ, Kemp BJ, Prato FS, et al, "Importance of Bone Attenuation in Brain SPECT Quantification," *J Nucl Med*, 1998, 39(1):190-7.

Tsukamoto Y, "CT Study of Closure of the Hemipharynx With Head Rotation in a Case of Lateral Medullary Syndrome," *Dysphagia*, 2000, 15(1):17-8.

van der Naalt J, Hew JM, van Zomeren AH, et al, "Computed Tomography and Magnetic Resonance Imaging in Mild to Moderate Head Injury: Early and Late Imaging Related to Outcome," *Ann Neurol*, 1999, 46(1):70-8.

Computed Transaxial Tomography, Larynx

Related Information

Magnetic Resonance Scan, Nasopharynx, Oropharynx, and Hypopharynx *on page 422*

Synonyms Larynx, CT; Neck, CT

Procedure Commonly Includes Routine neck CT (see neck CT) with subsequent 3 x 3 mm scans and breath holding or a spiral/helical CT (if available) with single breath hold acquisition. In the latter case, coronal reconstructions are helpful in assessment of tumor extent.

Indications Evaluate laryngeal tumors (squamous cell carcinoma). Imaging of laryngocele, thyroglossal duct cyst, complications after intubation and trauma or other indications.

Contraindications Uncooperative patient

Patient Preparation Intravenous contrast agent will usually be used to identify the relationship of tumor mass to vessels or to differentiate small lymph nodes from vessels. The patient should be limited to a liquid diet for at least 4 hours prior to the CT examination. A medication schedule should be maintained. The use of intravenous contrast material will be at the discretion of the diagnostic radiologist. Because of this, a recent serum creatine is requested in all patients 60 years of age or older and those patients with known significant atherosclerotic disease, diabetes mellitus, or pre-existing renal disease.

Special Instructions When interest is primarily focused on the larynx, the examination can be tailored to extend from the inferior aspect of the tongue or the superior aspect of the epiglottis inferiorly to just below the cricoid cartilage or upper trachea. Patients who have a metal tracheostomy tube should have this replaced with a plastic tube prior to the examination as the metallic tube

(Continued)

Computed Transaxial Tomography, Larynx *(Continued)*

will produce significant artifact. Spiral/helical CT allows for data acquisition over the entire larynx during a single breath hold. Phonation may be used to determine vocal cord mobility as well as distend the piriform sinuses. Phonation may also be valuable in evaluating the extent of supraglottic tumors around the piriform sinuses and aryepiglottic folds. MRI may provide additional information regarding laryngeal cartilage invasion and transglottic tumor extension.

Equipment This examination may be performed on any one of many commercially available computerized tomographic scanners.

Technique Two data sets are acquired, the first is contiguous 5 mm slices from the base of the tongue to the clavicles in quiet respiration, the second comprises thin sections through the larynx with suspended respiration.

Turnaround Time A verbal telephone report of the scan will be given to the referring physician if specified. A written report will be available.

References

Alexander AE Jr, Lyons GD, Fazekas-May MA, et al, "Utility of Helical Computed Tomography in the Study of Arytenoid Dislocation and Arytenoid Subluxation," *Ann Otol Rhinol Laryngol*, 1997, 106(12):1020-3.

Becker M, "Larynx and Hypopharynx," *Radiol Clin North Am*, 1998, 36(5):891-920, vi.

Curtin HD, "Imaging of the Larynx: Current Concepts," *Radiology*, 1989, 173(1):1-11.

Harnsberger HR, "The Larynx and Hypopharynx," *Handbook of Head and Neck Imaging*, 2nd ed, Chapter 11, St Louis, MO: CV Mosby Co, 1995.

Thabet HM, Sessions DB, Gado MH, et al, "Comparison of Clinical Evaluation and Computed Tomographic Diagnostic Accuracy for Tumors of the Larynx and Hypopharynx," *Laryngoscope*, 1996, 106(5 Pt 1):589-94.

Wang SJ, Borges A, Lufkin RB, et al, "Chondroid Tumors of the Larynx: Computed Tomography Findings," *Am J Otolaryngol*, 1999, 20(6):379-82.

Williams DW 3rd, "Imaging of Laryngeal Cancer," *Otolaryngol Clin North Am*, 1997, 30(1):35-58.

Yumoto E, Sanuki T, and Hyodo M, "Three-Dimensional Endoscopic Images of Vocal Fold Paralysis by Computed Tomography," *Arch Otolaryngol Head Neck Surg*, 1999, 125(8):883-90.

Zbaren P, Becker M, and Lang H, "Pretherapeutic Staging of Laryngeal Carcinoma. Clinical Findings, Computed Tomography, and Magnetic Resonance Imaging Compared With Histopathology," *Cancer*, 1996, 77(7):1263-73.

Computed Transaxial Tomography, Multiplanar Reconstruction and Display

Synonyms Multiplanar Reconstruction and Display, CT; Sagittal and Coronal Reconstruction. CT

Procedure Commonly Includes A standard CT examination of particular body part (eg, lumbar spine). These images are obtained in the axial projection. Subsequent to this, computer software may be programmed to reformat the acquired data into the sagittal and coronal projections.

Indications Helpful in the evaluation of pituitary tumor, spinal canal size, disc configuration. Also helpful in the evaluation of comminuted fractures of the spine, pelvis, and face.

Patient Preparation The reader is referred to Patient Preparation listed under the specific anatomic area to be studied.

Special Instructions The reader is referred to Special Instructions listed under specific anatomic areas to be studied.

Equipment This examination may be performed on most commercially available computerized homographic scanners.

Technique Generally speaking, thin contiguous or overlapping slices produce the best results.

Turnaround Time A verbal telephone report of the scan will be given to the referring physician if specified. A written report will be available.

Causes for Rejection Scan slices not in sequence, scan slices not all in same plane

Additional Information Computed tomographic multiplanner reconstructions have been demonstrated to have several applications. These include but are not limited to evaluation of aortic aneurysms, evaluation of renal and hepatic blood supply prior to surgical intervention, evaluation of the pituitary gland, imaging of complex pelvic fractures, spinal injuries, etc. Software packages are also available to allow 3-D reformatting.

References

Achenbach S, Moshage W, Ropers D, et al, "Curved Multiplanar Reconstructions for the Evaluation of Contrast-Enhanced Electron Beam CT of the Coronary Arteries," *AJR Am J Roentgenol*, 1998, 170(4):895-9.

Herman GT, "Three-Dimensional Imaging on a CT or MR Scanner," *J Comput Assist Tomogr*, 1988, 12(3):450-8.

Hopper KD, Huber SJ, Kasales CJ, et al, "The Clinical Usefulness of Routine Stacked Multiplanar Reconstruction in Helical Abdominal Computed Tomography," *Invest Radiol*, 1997, 32(9):550-6.

Lakits A, Prokesch R, Scholda C, et al, "Multiplanar Imaging in the Preoperative Assessment of Metallic Intraocular Foreign Bodies. Helical Computed Tomography Versus Conventional Computed Tomography," *Ophthalmology*, 1998, 105(9):1679-85.

Lakits A, Steiner E, Scholda C, et al, "Evaluation of Intraocular Foreign Bodies by Spiral Computed Tomography and Multiplanar Reconstruction," *Ophthalmology*, 1998, 105(2):307-12.

Lo Cicero J 3rd, Costello P, Campos CT, et al, "Spiral CT With Multiplanar and Three-Dimensional Reconstructions Accurately Predicts Tracheobronchial Pathology," *Ann Thorac Surg*, 1996, 62(3):811-7.

Ogata I, Komohara Y, Yamashita Y, et al, "CT Evaluation of Gastric Lesions With Three-Dimensional Display and Interactive Virtual Endoscopy: Comparison With Conventional Barium Study and Endoscopy," *AJR Am J Roentgenol*, 1999, 172(5):1263-70.

Computed Transaxial Tomography, Neck

Related Information

Magnetic Resonance Scan, Nasopharynx, Oropharynx, and Hypopharynx *on page 422*

Procedure Commonly Includes 5 mm sequential sections through the neck extending from base of tongue to the lung apices

Indications Assessment of lymphadenopathy

Contraindications Uncooperative patient

Patient Preparation Intravenous contrast agent will usually be used to identify the relationship of tumor mass to vessels or to differentiate small lymph nodes from vessels. The patient should be limited to a liquid diet for at least 4 hours prior to the CT examination. A medication schedule should be maintained. The use of intravenous contrast material will be at the discretion of the diagnostic radiologist. Because of this, a recent serum creatine is requested in all patients 60 years of age or older and those patients with known significant atherosclerotic disease, diabetes mellitus, or pre-existing renal disease.

Special Instructions Additional thin slices may be obtained at the discretion of the radiologist. A spiral/helical data is desirable to facilitate sagittal or coronal reconstruction.

Equipment Any commercially available CT scanner

Technique See Procedure Commonly Includes and special instructions.

Turnaround Time A verbal telephone report of the scan will be given to the referring physician if specified. A written report will be available.

References

Davis BT, Bagg A, and Milmoe GJ, "CT and MR Appearance of Castleman's Disease of the Neck," *AJR Am J Roentgenol*, 1999, 173(3):861-2.

Hanasono MM, Kunda LD, Segall GM, et al, "Uses and Limitations of FDG Positron Emission Tomography in Patients With Head and Neck Cancer," *Laryngoscope*, 1999, 109(6):880-5.

Harnsberger HR, *Handbook of Head and Neck Imaging*, 2nd ed, St Louis, MO: CV Mosby Co, 1995.

Kinoshita T, Ishii K, Mori Y, et al, "Castleman Disease in the Anterior Neck: The Role of Ga-67 Scintigraphy," *Clin Nucl Med*, 1996, 21(8):626-8.

Lo Cicero J 3rd, Costello P, Campos CT, et al, "Spiral CT With Multiplanar and Three-Dimensional Reconstructions Accurately Predicts Tracheobronchial Pathology," *Ann Thorac Surg*, 1996, 62(3):818-22.

Nagy M and Backstrom J, "Comparison of the Sensitivity of Lateral Neck Radiographs and Computed Tomography Scanning in Pediatric Deep-Neck Infections," *Laryngoscope*, 1999, 109(5):775-9.

Som PM, Curtin HD, and Mancuso AA, "Imaging-Based Nodal Classification for Evaluation of Neck Metastatic Adenopathy," *AJR Am J Roentgenol*, 2000, 174(3):837-44.

Umeda M, Nishimatsu N, Teranobu O, et al, "Criteria for Diagnosing Lymph Node Metastasis From Squamous Cell Carcinoma of the Oral Cavity: A Study of the Relationship Between Computed Tomographic and Histologic Findings and Outcome," *J Oral Maxillofac Surg*, 1998, 56(5):585-93.

Computed Transaxial Tomography, Orbits

Related Information

Magnetic Resonance Scan, Orbit *on page 426*

Synonyms Orbits, CT

Procedure Commonly Includes CT study of orbits

Indications Tumor, foreign body, trauma, ophthalmologic conditions that threaten vision

Contraindications Assuming a cooperative or quiescent patient, there are no absolute contraindications to a CT study of the orbits. Administration of intravenous contrast material is variable depending upon the patient's suspected diagnosis. Intravenous contrast material is generally indicated in suspected tumor, pseudotumor, arteriovenous malformation, or vascular abnormality. The search for a foreign body is not an indication for contrast material.

Patient Preparation The examination should be ordered and a requisition with pertinent information pertaining to the reason for the request and the clinical history should be completed by the referring physician. If there is the slightest possibility that intravenous contrast material will be administered, the patient's oral intake should be limited to liquids for at least 4 hours prior to the examination. Care must be taken to ensure the patient does not become dehydrated and medications should not be interrupted. A recent serum creatinine is requested on patients with pre-existing renal disease, diabetes mellitus, significant atherosclerotic disease, and advancing age (60 years of age and older). Agitated patients and children may require sedation prior to the examination. In these cases, an order for the appropriate sedative and dose should be recently recorded within the patient's chart. Sedatives, when necessary, should be administered by a physician within the Radiology Department.

Equipment Commercially available CT scanners

Technique Contiguous 2 mm slices extending from the infraorbital margin to slightly above the supraorbital rim. The study may be extended if pathology indicates. A spiral examination will facilitate sagittal/coronal reconstruction for optimal visualization of the optic nerve, superior ophthalmic vein, etc. A negative angulation -20° to the orbitomeatal baseline while the eyes are maintained in the upward gaze position will facilitate optimum visualization of the optic nerve. If a blow-out fracture of the orbit is suspected, the study should be continued inferiorly for visualization of the maxillary sinuses and nasal cavity.

Additional Information CT remains the imaging modality of choice in many cases of ocular pathology due to the excellent natural contrast afforded by retro-orbital fat. MR is also extremely sensitive to globe and lid motion. MR however can demonstrate associated intra-axial pathology, sella and parasellar lesions and intraorbital lesions equally well.

References

Ainbinder DJ, Haik BG, and Mazzoli RA, "Anophthalmic Socket and Orbital Implants. Role of CT and MR Imaging," *Radiol Clin North Am*, 1998, 36(6):1133-47.

Harnsberger HR, "The Normal and Diseased Orbit," *Handbook of Head and Neck Imaging*, 2nd ed, St Louis, MO: CV Mosby Co, 1995.

Hidayat AA, Mafee MF, Laver NV, et al, "Langerhans' Cell Histiocytosis and Juvenile Xanthogranuloma of the Orbit. Clinicopathologic, CT, and MR Imaging Features," *Radiol Clin North Am*, 1998, 36(6):1229-40.

Lakits A, Prokesch R, Scholda C, et al, "Orbital Helical Computed Tomography in the Diagnosis and Management of eye Trauma," *Ophthalmology*, 1999, 106(12):2330-5.

Mafee MF, Pai E, and Philip B, "Rhabdomyosarcoma of the Orbit. Evaluation With MR Imaging and CT," *Radiol Clin North Am*, 1998, 36(6):1215-27.

Mauriello JA Jr, Lee HJ, and Nguyen L, "CT of Soft Tissue Injury and Orbital Fractures," *Radiol Clin North Am*, 1999, 37(1):241-52.

Ozgen A and Ariyurek M, "Normative Measurements of Orbital Structures Using CT," *AJR Am J Roentgenol*, 1998, 170(4):1093-6.

Rhea JT, Rao PM, and Novelline RA, "Helical CT and Three-Dimensional CT of Facial and Orbital Injury," *Radiol Clin North Am*, 1999, 37(3):489-513.

Rubin PA and Remulla HD, "Orbital Venous Anomalies Demonstrated by Spiral Computed Tomography," *Ophthalmology*, 1997, 104(9):1463-70.

Rubin PA, Watkins LM, Rumelt S, et al, "Orbital Computed Tomographic Characteristics of Globe Subluxation in Thyroid Orbitopathy," *Ophthalmology*, 1998, 105(11):2061-4.

Wenig BM, Mafee MF, and Ghosh L, "Fibro-Osseous, Osseous, and Cartilaginous Lesions of the Orbit and Paraorbital Region. Correlative Clinicopathologic and Radiographic Features,

Including the Diagnostic Role of CT and MR Imaging," *Radiol Clin North Am*, 1998, 36(6):1241-59.

Computed Transaxial Tomography, Paranasal Sinuses

Related Information

Magnetic Resonance Scan, Sinuses *on page 431*
Paranasal Sinuses *on page 363*

Synonyms Paranasal Sinuses, CT; Sinuses, CT

Procedure Commonly Includes The examination is composed of contiguous 3-5 mm slices obtained from the inferior portion of the maxillary sinuses, cephalad to the superior extent of the frontal sinuses.

Indications Diagnose and/or evaluate tumors, masses, metastases, inflammatory conditions, and traumatic involvement. The modality is commonly used for staging of tumors.

Contraindications Patients who are not candidates for sedation/anesthesia, uncooperative patient; patient cooperation is of the utmost importance as the examination requires the patient to remain motionless for the duration of the study.

Patient Preparation Patients oral intake should be restricted to fluid for 4 hours prior to the examination. Medication schedule should not be interrupted. Administration of intravenous contrast material is at the discretion of the diagnostic radiologist. If a patient is being evaluated for trauma or inflammatory disease of the paranasal sinuses, no intravenous contrast material is usually administered. If a mass is identified in the course of the examination, or if a patient is known to have a tumor, then intravenous contrast material is usually given. Because of this, a recent serum creatinine is requested in all patients 60 years of age and older and those patients with known significant atherosclerotic disease, diabetes mellitus, or pre-existing renal disease. Children and uncooperative adults may require sedation.

Special Instructions If the nasopharynx is to be included in the examination, the study should be extended inferiorly to the hard palate or slightly below. The oral pharynx may be included by continuing to the base of the tongue. If there is a question of tumor invasion of the orbit from a sinus then coronal sections are very helpful.

Technique This examination may be performed in any one of many commercially available computerized tomographic scanners. Standard examination of the paranasal sinuses consist of 3-5 mm contiguous slices as previously described.

Turnaround Time Verbal telephone report of the scan will be given to the referring physician if specified. A written report will be available.

Additional Information Some departments offer a limited CT study of the paranasal sinuses which is competitive with plain film radiographs of the sinus in terms of pricing. This consists of 5 or 6 transaxial images through the sinus obtained parallel to Reid's baseline. The examination is achieved by obtaining a lateral digital image of the skull. From this the distance between the hard palate and the superior aspect of the frontal sinuses is measured. The distance is then divided by 5 or 6 to get the interslice distance. The slice thickness is 3-5 mm.

References

Baroody FM, Suh SH, and Naclerio RM, "Total IgE Serum Levels Correlate With Sinus Mucosal Thickness on Computerized Tomography Scans," *J Allergy Clin Immunol*, 1997, 100(4):563-8.

Bhattacharyya N, "Test-Retest Reliability of Computed Tomography in the Assessment of Chronic Rhinosinusitis," *Laryngoscope*, 1999, 109(7 Pt 1):1055-8.

Bhattacharyya T, Piccirillo J, and Wippold FJ 2nd, "Relationship Between Patient-Based Descriptions of Sinusitis and Paranasal Sinus Computed Tomographic Findings," *Arch Otolaryngol Head Neck Surg*, 1997, 123(11):1189-92.

Cartelliere M and Vorbeck F, "Endoscopic Sinus Surgery Using Intraoperative Computed Tomography Imaging for Updating a Three-Dimensional Navigation System," *Laryngoscope*, 2000, 110(2 Pt 1):292-6.

Damilakis J, Prassopoulas P, Mazonakis M, et al, "Tailored Low Dose Three-Dimensional CT of Paranasal Sinuses," *Clin Imaging*, 1998, 22(4):235-9.

Dammann F, Pereira P, Laniado M, et al, "Inverted Papilloma of the Nasal Cavity and the Paranasal Sinuses: Using CT for Primary Diagnosis and Follow-up," *AJR Am J Roentgenol*, 1999, 172(2):543-8.

(Continued)

Computed Transaxial Tomography, Paranasal Sinuses *(Continued)*

Hahnel S, Ertl-Wagner B, Tasman AJ, "Relative Value of MR Imaging as Compared With CT in the Diagnosis of Inflammatory Paranasal Sinus Disease," *Radiology*, 1999, 210(1):171-6.

Harnsberger HR, "Sinonasal Imaging: Imaging Issues in Sinusitis," *Handbook of Head and Neck Imaging*, 2nd ed, Chapter 15, St Louis, MO: CV Mosby Co, 1995.

Kim HJ, Friedman EM, Sulek M, et al, "Paranasal Sinus Development in Chronic Sinusitis, Cystic Fibrosis, and Normal Comparison Population: A Computerized Tomography Correlation Study," *Am J Rhinol*, 1997, 11(4):275-81.

Metson R, Gliklich RE, Stankiewicz JA, et al, "Comparison of Sinus Computed Tomography Staging Systems," *Otolaryngol Head Neck Surg*, 1997, 117(4):372-9.

Witte RJ, Heurter JV, Orton DF, et al, "Limited Axial CT of the Paranasal Sinuses in Screening for Sinusitis," *AJR Am J Roentgenol*, 1996, 167(5):1313-5.

Computed Transaxial Tomography, Pelvis

Related Information

Computed Transaxial Tomography, Abdomen Studies *on page 327*

Synonyms Lower Abdomen, CT; Pelvis, CT

Procedure Commonly Includes CT scan pelvic area includes bladder, prostate, ovaries, uterus, lower retroperitoneum, and iliac lymph node chains

Indications Evaluation of cysts, tumors, masses, metastasis, inflammatory processes, and lymphadenopathy

Contraindications Uncooperative patient

Patient Preparation Dietary restrictions include fluids only for 4 hours prior to the examination. Medication schedule should not be interrupted. Intravenous contrast material may be administered. This is at the discretion of the radiologist. A recent serum creatinine is requested in all patients 60 years of age and older and those patients with known significant atherosclerotic disease, diabetes mellitus, or pre-existing renal disease, in case intravenous contrast administration is necessary. 450 mL dilute barium (1%) is administrated orally commencing at least 1 hour prior to the examination. This facilitates good opacification of the small bowel. A small volume (4-8 oz) of dilute contrast material is given per rectum to facilitate opacification of the distal large bowel. In the case of females, placement of a vaginal tampon may be helpful in further defining the anatomy.

Special Instructions A CT study of the pelvis may be requested by a practicing physician. The patient's medical record should accompany them to furnish the radiologist with adequate clinical information thus facilitating tailoring of the examination to ensure maximum diagnostic benefit.

Technique Study may be performed on any one of the many commercially available computed tomographic scanners. Traditionally, sequential 1 cm slices are obtained from the pelvic brim through the pubic symphysis. If spiral capability is available it is recommended as it facilitates higher quality multiplanar reconstructions. Intravenous administration of contrast material facilitates opacification of the major vascular structures in addition to the ureters and urinary bladder. Oral contrast, rectal contrast, and a vaginal tampon aid in defining the anatomy within the pelvis.

Turnaround Time A verbal telephone report of the scan will be given to the referring physician if specified. A written report will be available.

Causes for Rejection The presence of residual concentrated barium deposits within the large bowel secondary to a prior gastrointestinal exam, creates artifacts which usually detracts from diagnostic usefulness of the study. Where possible, CT studies of the abdomen and pelvis should be completed before conventional gastrointestinal barium examinations. Should these studies be performed in the reverse order, laxative use or cleansing enema may aid in elimination of the concentrated barium.

Additional Information The patient should be informed the examination may take 30-45 minutes and that oral, rectal, and intravenous contrast media may be necessary for the examination.

References

Fielding JR, Aliabadi N, Renshaw AA, et al, "Staging of 119 Patients With Renal Cell Carcinoma: The Yield and Cost-Effectiveness of Pelvic CT," *AJR Am J Roentgenol*, 1999, 172(1):23-5.

Hamilton RJ, Blend MJ, Pelizzari CA, et al, "Using Vascular Structure for CT-SPECT Registration in the Pelvis," *J Nucl Med*, 1999, 40(2):347-51.

Meyer JI, Herts BR, Einstein DM, et al, "Pelvic Computed Tomography of Breast Carcinoma Patients. Should it Routinely Be Added to Abdominal Computed Tomography?" *Cancer*, 1997, 79(3):500-4.

Oh YK, Ha CS, Samuels BI, et al, "Stages I-II Follicular Lymphoma: Role of CT of the Abdomen and Pelvis in Follow-up Studies," *Radiology*, 1999, 210(2):483-6.

Quillin SP, Brink JA, Heiken JP, et al, "Helical (Spiral) CT Angiography for Indentification of Crossing Vessels at the Ureteropelvic Junction," *AJR Am J Roentgenol*, 1996, 166(5):1125-30.

Scoutt LM, McCarthy SM, and Moss AA, "The Pelvis," *Computed Tomography of the Body*, Moss AA, ed, Philadelphia, PA: WB Saunders Co, 1992.

Shah AA, Buckshee N, Yankelevitz DF, et al, "Assessment of Deep Venous Thrombosis Using Routine Pelvic CT," *AJR Am J Roentgenol*, 1999, 173(3):659-63.

Takebayashi S, Hosaka M, Takase K, et al, "Computerized Tomography Nephroscopic Images of Renal Pelvic Carcinoma," *J Urol*, 1999, 162(2):315-8.

Yazici M, Sozubir S, Kilicoglu G, et al, "Three-Dimensional Anatomy of the Pelvis in Bladder Exstrophy: Description of Bone Pathology by Using Three-Dimensional Computed Tomography and its Clinical Relevance," *J Pediatr Orthop*, 1998, 18(1):132-5.

Computed Transaxial Tomography, Sella Turcica

Synonyms Sella Turcica, CT

Procedure Commonly Includes Thin slices through the anatomic area of sella turcica for evaluation of suspected pathology

Indications MR is an ideal method for evaluation of the sella turcica and its contents and has replaced thin slice high resolution CT. CT use is now limited to those patients who cannot be imaged with MR due to claustrophobia, pacemaker, aneurysm clip, etc. Evaluation of patients suspected of having intrasella or extrasella abnormalities including those that present with amenorrhea, galactorrhea, or increased prolactin levels.

Contraindications In the absence of a history of allergy to iodine, intravenous contrast material is administered in almost all cases. The exceptions include patients with known compromised renal function, patients with plasmacytoma, and multiple myeloma.

Patient Preparation The examination should be ordered and a requisition stating pertinent information pertaining to the reason for the request and the clinical history should be completed by the referring physician. If there is the slightest possibility that intravenous contrast material will be administered, the patient's oral intake should be limited to liquids for at least 4 hours prior to the examination. Care must be taken to ensure the patient does not become dehydrated and medications should not be interrupted. A recent serum creatinine is requested on patients with pre-existing renal disease, diabetes mellitus, significant atherosclerotic disease and advancing age (60 years of age and older). Agitated patients and children may require sedation prior to the examination. In these cases, an order for the appropriate sedative and dose should be recently recorded within the patient's chart. Sedatives should be administered by a physician within the Radiology Department.

Equipment This examination can be performed on any commercially available CT scanner.

Technique A slice thickness of 2-3 mm is suggested. Slices should be contiguous. Spiral examination is preferred if available.

Additional Information Instant oblique reconstruction or sagittal/coronal reconstruction can be utilized for additional evaluation. A slight overlapping of slices optimizes the sagittal/coronal reconstruction if the slice thickness is >2 mm and conventional rather than spiral technique is employed. Optimum visualization of the sella turcica is best achieved with coronal sections. Axial sections are usually reserved for those patients in which it is difficult or impossible to achieve coronal scans. For coronal positioning the patient is positioned supine. The optimal position for coronal scanning is 90° from Reid's baseline. To achieve this position, the patient is supine with the upper torso elevated by supports 10" to 12" above the table. Hyperextend the head and neck and secure the head holder. Alternatively, the patient may be scanned in the prone position. Here a vertical submental position is utilized. The head and neck are extended and secured in the head holder to provide a scanning plain at 90° to Reid's baseline. If the coronal position is impossible, then obtain axial images and reformat these in the sagittal and coronal projections utilizing instant oblique reconstruction. The coronal position is difficult to

(Continued)

Computed Transaxial Tomography, Sella Turcica *(Continued)*

maintain and when utilized, rapid sequence scanning may be implemented to facilitate rapid completion of the study.

References

Fitz Patrick M, Tartaglino LM, Hollander MD, et al, "Imaging of Sellar and Parasellar Pathology," *Radiol Clin North Am*, 1999, 37(1):101-21.

Freda PU and Post KD, "Differential Diagnosis of Sellar Masses," *Endocrinol Metab Clin North Am*, 1999, 28(1):81-117.

Gsponer J, De Tribolet N, Deruaz JP, et al, "Diagnosis, Treatment, and Outcome of Pituitary Tumors and Other Abnormal Intrasellar Masses. Restrospective Analysis of 353 Patients," *Medicine*, 1999, 78(4):236-69.

Nasseri SS, McCafferty TV, Kasperbauer JL, et al, "A Combined, Minimally Invasive Transnasal Approach to the Sella Turcica," *Am J Rhinol*, 1998, 12(6):409-16.

Sutton LN, Wang ZJ, Wehrli SL, et al, "Proton Spectroscopy of Suprasellar Tumors in Pediatric Patients," *Neurosurgery*, 1997, 41(2):388-94.

Tzen KY, Yen TC, and Lin KJ, "Value of Ga-67 SPECT in Monitoring the Effects of Therapy in Invasive Aspergillosis of the Sphenoid Sinus," *Clin Nucl Med*, 1999, 24(12):938-41.

Computed Transaxial Tomography, Spine

Related Information

Magnetic Resonance Scan, Cervical and Thoracic Spine *on page 406*

Synonyms Cervical Spine, CT; Dorsal Spine, CT; Lumbar Spine, CT; Spine, CT

Replaces Discogram

Procedure Commonly Includes CT scan of cervical, dorsal, lumbar, and/or sacral spine

Indications

- diagnosis of disc herniation
- evaluation of spinal canal stenosis
- evaluation of facet disease
- evaluation of spondylolysis
- evaluation of infectious disease involving an intervertebral disc or a vertebral body

Patient Preparation No preparation by nursing personnel is required. Intravenous contrast material is generally not indicated. Intrathecal contrast material may be administered at the discretion of the radiologist depending upon the reason for the examination. There should be no barium present within the gastrointestinal tract as this will produce considerable artifacts when the lower thoracic, lumbar, or lumbosacral spine is being evaluated. Examination of the cervical spine is best performed when the patient suspends respiration and swallowing during the exposures. Slice thickness utilized may be 2-5 mm. A spiral study or slight overlap is recommended if sagittal and coronal reconstructions are to be performed. When the primary area of interest is the upper cervical spine, the chin should be extended to eliminate artifacts created from dental hardware. When scanning patients with a history of cervical trauma, movement of the patient should be done with extreme care. When the thoracic spine is to be examined, the examination is usually tailored to a specific portion of the thoracic spine depending on the patient's symptomatology. Again, slice thickness of 2-5 mm may be employed at the discretion of the radiologist. Evaluation of the lumbar spine is not infrequently performed subsequent to myelography. In these cases, the thecal sac is opacified by water soluble contrast material. A slice thickness of 4-5 mm is utilized and the table moves in increments of 3-5 mm at the discretion of the radiologist.

Special Instructions The exam may be requested by a practicing physician. The area of interest must be specified along with pertinent clinical history and reason for the CT scan. To achieve optimal postscanning reconstruction, complete immobilization and patient cooperation is imperative. Coronal, sagittal, or instant oblique reconstruction is of definite value in assessing the neural canal and foramina. Isodensity and gray scale reversal may also be of value in visualizing herniated disc material.

Equipment Examinations may be performed on all commercially available CT scanners.

Technique Slice thickness and table incrementation are at the discretion of the radiologist. The parameters mentioned serve only as rough guidelines.

Turnaround Time A verbal telephone report of the scan will be given to the referring physician if specified. A written report will be available.

Causes for Rejection Inability of the patient to remain motionless, presence of barium within the bowel when lower thoracic, lumbar, and sacral spines are to be examined

Additional Information High resolution computed tomography has had a major impact on the neuroradiologic diagnosis of lumbar disc herniation. The modality facilitates noninvasive diagnoses with an accuracy approaching 93%. The modality is more accurate than myelography alone as it facilitates a diagnosis of lateral disc herniation. Magnetic resonance however has certain advantages over computed tomography of the spine. This modality allows direct multiplanar imaging, utilizes nonionizing radiation, and facilitates imaging of the entire lumbar spine and conus medullaris.

References

Berne JD, Velmahos GC, El-Tawil Q, et al, "Value of Complete Cervical Helical Computed Tomographic Scanning in Identifying Cervical Spine Injury in the Unevaluable Blunt Trauma Patient With Multiple Injuries: A Prospective Study," *J Trauma*, 1999, 47(5):896-902.

Blackmore CC, Ramsey SD, Mann FA, et al, "Cervical Spine Screening With CT in Trauma Patients: A Cost-Effectiveness Analysis," *Radiology*, 1999, 212(1):117-25.

Chafetz NI, Rothman SLG, Genant HK, et al, "The Spine," *Computed Tomography of the Body*, Moss AA, Gamsu G, and Genant HK, eds, Philadelphia, PA: WB Saunders Co, 1992.

Daffner RH, "CT of the Craniovertebral Junction," *AJR Am J Roentgenol*, 1996, 167(2):365-6.

Hanson JA, Blackmore CC, Mann FA, et al, "Cervical Spine Injury: A Clinical Decision Rule to Identify High-Risk Patients for Helical CT Screening," *AJR Am J Roentgenol*, 2000, 174(3):595.

Le Blang SD and Nunez DB Jr, "Helical CT of Cervical Spine and Soft Tissue Injuries of the Neck," *Radiol Clin North Am*, 1999, 37(3):515-32.

Nunez DB Jr and Quencer RM, "The Role of Helical CT in the Assessment of Cervical Spine Injuries," *AJR Am J Roentgenol*, 1998, 171(4):951-7.

Ross JS, "The Cervical Spine," *Neuroimaging Clin N Am*, 1995, 5(3).

Computed Transaxial Tomography, Spiral/Helical Examination

Special Instructions This entry describes a technique rather than a specific examination; thus, it is applicable to many anatomic areas and the appropriate CPT code should be selected.

References

Silverman PM, Cooper CJ, Waltman DI, et al, "Helical CT: Practical Considerations and Potential Pitfalls," *Radiographics*, 1995, 15(1):25-36.

Computed Transaxial Tomography, Temporal Bone

Synonyms Middle and Inner Ear, CT; Temporal Bone, CT

Replaces Polytomography of the Temporal Bone

Procedure Commonly Includes Thin sections through the temporal bone for evaluation of the middle and inner ear and the jugular fossa; contiguous thin slices through the temporal bone for evaluation of suspected pathology

Indications CT is most valuable is assessing the temporal bone in cases of trauma, tumors, inflammatory processes, genetic or other abnormalities.

Contraindications Patient cooperation is most important. The examination requires the patient to remain motionless for the duration of the study. The time of the study will vary from 10-20 minutes depending on the equipment being used. Children and uncooperative adults may require sedation.

Patient Preparation The patient should be limited to a liquid diet for at least 4 hours prior to the CT examination. Medication schedules should be maintained. The use of intravenous contrast material is at the discretion of the diagnostic radiologist. Generally speaking, no intravenous contrast material is administered unless the presence of tumor is suspected. In all patients 60 years of age and older and those patients with known significant atherosclerotic disease, diabetes mellitus, or pre-existing renal disease, a recent serum creatinine is required prior to administration of contrast material.

Equipment The examination may be performed on all commercially available CT scanners.

Technique The examination should extend from the petrous ridges superiorly to slightly below the external auditory meatus. The tilt line should be parallel

(Continued)

Computed Transaxial Tomography, Temporal Bone *(Continued)*

with the orbitomeatal line. Consecutive 2 mm slices are suggested for evaluation of the temporal bone and ideally these should overlap slightly. Alternatively a spiral exam can be utilized to facilitate multiplanar reconstruction.

Turnaround Time A verbal telephone report of the scan will be given to the referring physician if specified. A written report will be available.

Additional Information In cases of trauma where cerebrospinal fluid leak is to be excluded, intrathecal contrast material is helpful. An adequate study is dependent upon knowledge of pertinent, specific clinical information.

References

Caldemeyer KS, Sandrasegaran K, Shinaver CN, et al, "Temporal Bone: Comparison of Isotropic Helical CT and Conventional Direct Axial and Coronal CT," *AJR Am J Roentgenol*, 1999, 172(6):1675-82.

Harnsberger HR, "The Temporal Bone: External, Middle, and Inner Ear Segments," *Handbook of Head and Neck Imaging*, 2nd ed, St Louis, MO: CV Mosby Co, 1995.

Lemmerling MM, Mancuso AA, Antonelli PJ, et al, "Normal Modiolus: CT Appearance in Patients With a Large Vestibular Aqueduct," *Radiology*, 1997, 204(1):213-9.

Lemmerling MM, Stambuck HE, Mancuso AA, et al, "Normal and Opacified Middle Ears: CT Appearance of the Stapes and Incudostapedial Joint," *Radiology*, 1997, 203(1):251-6.

Maassen MM, Lehner R, Ludtke R, et al, "Preoperative Assessment of the Implantable Middle Ear Pump System Using CT Scans and Conventional X-rays of the Temporal Bone," *Ear Nose Throat J*, 1997, 76(7):457-63.

Reisser C, Schubert O, Forsting M, et al, "Anatomy of the Temporal Bone: Detailed Three-Dimensional Display Based on Image Data From High-Resolution Helcial CT: A Preliminary Report," *Am J Otol*, 1996, 17(3):473-9.

Swartz JD, "Current Imaging Approach to the Temporal Bone," *Radiology*, 1989, 171(2):309-17.

Computed Transaxial Tomography, Thorax

Procedure Commonly Includes CT study of the chest extending from the lung apices to the posterior costophrenic sulci. The study may extend inferiorly to image the adrenal glands because they are a relatively frequent site of metastasis from primary lung carcinoma.

Indications The examination facilitates evaluation of abnormalities of the lungs, mediastinum, pleura, and chest wall. Conventional PA and lateral views of the chest represent the basic screening tool in the identification of abnormalities involving the thorax. The axial anatomic display and superior density discrimination of computed tomography provides information pertaining to the extent of disease and more precise characterization of abnormalities initially noted on physical examination, chest films or on the barium swallow.

Contraindications Patient cooperation is of utmost importance as the examination requires the patient to remain motionless for the duration of the study. The time of the study will vary from 10-30 minutes depending on the equipment being used. Children and uncooperative adults may require sedation.

Patient Preparation The patients should be limited to a liquid diet for at least 4 hours prior to the CT examination. Medication schedules should be maintained. The use of intravenous contrast material may be required at the discretion of the diagnostic radiologist. Because of this, a recent serum creatinine is requested in all patients 60 years of age and older, and those patients with known significant atherosclerotic disease, diabetes mellitus, or pre-existing renal disease. In the case of children who need sedation, a recent (within 30 days) recording of the child's weight and a written order by the child's physician must be in the patient's medical record. All children should be accompanied by a responsible adult. Opacification of the esophagus with thick barium paste may be of value in some cases and administration should be at the discretion of the diagnostic radiologist.

Special Instructions The exam may be requested by a practicing physician. The area of interest must be specified along with pertinent clinical history and reason for the CT scan. The test should be complete in 10-30 minutes. Intravenous contrast material may be administered.

Equipment The examination may be performed on any number of commercially available CT scanners.

Technique A routine CT study of the chest consists of sequential 1 cm slices obtained from the apices through the posterior costophrenic sulci. The study may be extended to include the adrenal glands if a diagnosis of primary bronchogenic carcinoma is known or suspected. The technique may vary depending upon the indications for the study. A spiral examination is used routinely in chest CT where possible. This technique allows the acquisition of a large volume of data on a single breath hold facilitating multiplanar reconstruction and ensuring the entire area is visualized. The examination may be tailored by the diagnostic radiologist to answer specific questions. Recently, spiral CT has been effectively employed in the diagnosis of pulmonary thromboembolic disease. When utilized for this purpose a bolus of 100-150 mL of contrast material is required. More recently, the technique is being used to screen for lung cancer in patients at increased risk. In this situation, no contrast material is required. High resolution CT (HRCT) refers to studies done employing very thin slices (1 or 2 mm thick) and reconstructed using the high spatial frequency algorithm (bone algorithm). A third step sometimes employed to further increase resolution is retargeting the area of interest to decrease the pixel size. This technique is useful when assessing the parenchyma for bronchiectasis or characterizing early signs of interstitial lung disease. The patient's medical record should accompany the patient to the department in order to ensure that the radiologist is furnished with sufficient information to tailor the examination appropriately.

Turnaround Time A verbal telephone report of the scan will be given to the referring physician if specified. A written report will be available.

Causes for Rejection Inability of the patient to cooperate is the major problem. Should the uncooperative patient not be a candidate for sedation and/or anesthesia, the study cannot be performed.

References

Akira M, Hamada H, Sakatani M, et al, "CT Findings During Phase of Accelerated Deterioration in Patients With Idiopathic Pulmonary Fibrosis," *AJR Am J Roentgenol*, 1997, 168(1):79-83.

Lee KN, Levin DL, Webb WR, et al, "Pulmonary Alveolar Proteinosis: High-Resolution CT, Chest Radiographic, and Functional Correlations," *Chest*, 1997, 111(4):989-95.

Miller WT Jr, Tino G, and Friedburg JS, "Thoracic CT in the Intensive Care Unit: Assessment of Clinical Usefulness," *Radiology*, 1998, 209(2):491-8.

Naidich DP, Zerhouni EA, Hutchins GM, et al, "Computed Tomography of the Pulmonary Parenchyma, Part 1: Distal Air-Space Disease," *J Thorac Imaging*, 1985, 1(1):39-53.

Reittner P and Müller NL, "Spiral CT in the Diagnosis of Pulmonary Embolism," *Appl Radiol*, 1999, December:32-6.

Remy-Jardin M, Doyen J, Remy J, et al, "Functional Anatomy of the Thoracic Outlet: Evaluation With Spiral CT," *Radiology*, 1997, 205(3):843-51.

Takahashi M, Maguire WM, Ashtari M, et al, "Low-Dose Spiral Computed Tomography of the Thorax: Comparison With the Standard-Dose Technique," *Invest Radiol*, 1998, 33(2):68-73.

Zerhouni EA, Naidich DP, Stitik FP, et al, "Computed Tomography of the Pulmonary Parenchyma, Part 2: Interstitial Disease," *J Thorac Imaging*, 1985, 1(1):54-64.

Computed Transaxial Tomography, Treatment Planning

Synonyms Radiotherapy Treatment Planning; Treatment Planning, CT

Procedure Commonly Includes The area of the tumor is scanned while the patient reclines on a flat table top during quiet respiration. Care must be taken to ensure that the patient is in the treatment position. The CT study will allow accurate localization of tumor. Single transaxial imaging method provides multilevel accurate body contours. The modality provides accurate density detail formerly not available. Three-dimensional treatment planning can now be performed with the accurate anatomical data available from computed tomographic scans. In addition to this, computed tomography can be utilized to monitor the response of a tumor to treatment. Scans through the proximal portion of the field, the central axis of the radiation field, and the distal portion of the field should be obtained. Should there be a marked distortion of anatomy, further scans between these landmarks may be required. The use of contrast material is at the discretion of the radiologist and radiotherapist and will be influenced by location and characteristics of tumor.

Indications Procedure indicated in those patients with a known tumor that is to be treated with radiotherapy. The purpose of the examination is to ensure that the radiotherapy administered is appropriately distributed throughout tumor volume and to minimize radiation to normal structures.

(Continued)

Computed Transaxial Tomography, Treatment Planning *(Continued)*

Contraindications Patient cooperation is of utmost importance. The patient must be able to assume the treatment position and to remain motionless but without suspending respiration during the course of the study which generally can be completed in less than 15 minutes.

Patient Preparation Limitation to a liquid diet for a 4-hour period prior to the CT examination is not required unless the intravenous administration of contrast material is necessary. Medication schedules should be maintained. In patients 60 years of age and older, or those with known significant atherosclerotic disease, diabetes mellitus, or pre-existing renal disease, a recent serum creatinine will be required if the patient is to receive intravenous contrast material.

Special Instructions Scan may be requested by a radiation therapy physician who is in the process of planning therapy or assessing therapeutic results.

Equipment The examination may be performed on any number of commercially available CT scanners.

Technique The patient is scanned on a flat table top during quiet respiration while in the treatment position. Scans are obtained through the central axis of the tumor and through the upper and lower extent of tumor. Further images between these scans may be required depending on anatomical considerations. The use of intravenous contrast material is at the discretion of the radiologist and radiation therapist.

Turnaround Time A verbal telephone report of the scan will be given to the referring physician if specified. A written report will be available.

Additional Information Scan passes will be marked on the patient with radiopaque material by the Radiation Therapy Department personnel who will position the patient within the scanner.

References

Adamietz IA, Baum RP, Schemman F, et al, "Improvement of Radiation Treatment Planning in Squamous-Cell Head and Neck Cancer by Immuno-SPECT," *J Nucl Med*, 1996, 37(12):1942-6.

Bahner ML, Debus J, Zabel A, et al, "Digitally Reconstructed Radiographs From Abdominal CT Scans as a New Tool for Radiotherapy Planning," *Invest Radiol*, 1999, 34(10):643-7.

Fielding JR, Silverman SG, Samuel S, et al, "Unenhanced Helical CT of Ureteral Stones: A Replacement for Excretory Urography in Planning Treatment," *AJR Am J Roentgenol*, 1998, 171(4):1051-3.

Hopper KD, Singapuri K, and Finkel A, "Body CT and Oncologic Imaging," *Radiology*, 2000, 215(1):27-40.

Martinez-Monge R, Fernandes PS, Gupta N, et al, "Cross-Sectional Nodal Atlas: A Tool for the Definition of Clinical Target Volumes in Three-Dimensional Radiation Therapy Planning," *Radiology*, 1999, 211(3):815-28.

Miller JS, Puckett ML, and Johnstone PA, "Frequency of Coexistent Disease at CT in Patients With Prostate Carcinoma Selected for Definitive Radiation Therapy: Is Limited Treatment-Planning CT Adequate?" *Radiology*, 2000, 215(1):41-4.

Vijayakumar S, Chen GT, Low NN, et al, "Beam's Eye View - Based Radiation Therapy: Description of Methods," *Radiographics*, 1992, 12(5):961-8.

♦ **CT, Lower Abdomen** *see* Computed Transaxial Tomography, Abdomen Studies *on page 327*

♦ **CT, Total Abdomen** *see* Computed Transaxial Tomography, Abdomen Studies *on page 327*

♦ **CT, Upper Abdomen** *see* Computed Transaxial Tomography, Abdomen Studies *on page 327*

♦ **Discogram** *see* Computed Transaxial Tomography, Spine *on page 340*

♦ **Dorsal Spine, CT** *see* Computed Transaxial Tomography, Spine *on page 340*

♦ **Dynamic Study, CT** *see* Computed Transaxial Tomography, Dynamic Study *on page 330*

♦ **Extremities, CT** *see* Computed Transaxial Tomography, Extremities *on page 331*

♦ **Head Studies, CT** *see* Computed Transaxial Tomography, Head Studies *on page 332*

♦ **Larynx, CT** *see* Computed Transaxial Tomography, Larynx *on page 333*

- ♦ **Lower Abdomen, CT** *see* Computed Transaxial Tomography, Pelvis *on page 338*
- ♦ **Lumbar Spine, CT** *see* Computed Transaxial Tomography, Spine *on page 340*
- ♦ **Middle and Inner Ear, CT** *see* Computed Transaxial Tomography, Temporal Bone *on page 341*
- ♦ **Multiplanar Reconstruction and Display, CT** *see* Computed Transaxial Tomography, Multiplanar Reconstruction and Display *on page 334*
- ♦ **Neck, CT** *see* Computed Transaxial Tomography, Larynx *on page 333*
- ♦ **Orbits, CT** *see* Computed Transaxial Tomography, Orbits *on page 336*
- ♦ **Paranasal Sinuses, CT** *see* Computed Transaxial Tomography, Paranasal Sinuses *on page 337*
- ♦ **Pelvis, CT** *see* Computed Transaxial Tomography, Pelvis *on page 338*
- ♦ **Polytomography of the Temporal Bone** *see* Computed Transaxial Tomography, Temporal Bone *on page 341*
- ♦ **Radiotherapy Treatment Planning** *see* Computed Transaxial Tomography, Treatment Planning *on page 343*
- ♦ **Sagittal and Coronal Reconstruction. CT** *see* Computed Transaxial Tomography, Multiplanar Reconstruction and Display *on page 334*
- ♦ **Sella Turcica, CT** *see* Computed Transaxial Tomography, Sella Turcica *on page 339*
- ♦ **Single and Dual Energy Quantitative Computed Tomography** *see* Computed Transaxial Tomography, Bone Densitometry *on page 329*
- ♦ **Sinuses, CT** *see* Computed Transaxial Tomography, Paranasal Sinuses *on page 337*
- ♦ **Spine, CT** *see* Computed Transaxial Tomography, Spine *on page 340*
- ♦ **Temporal Bone, CT** *see* Computed Transaxial Tomography, Temporal Bone *on page 341*
- ♦ **Treatment Planning, CT** *see* Computed Transaxial Tomography, Treatment Planning *on page 343*

GENERAL RADIOLOGY

♦ **Abdomen for Fetal Age** *see* Abdomen X-ray *on page 347*

Abdomen X-ray

Synonyms KUB

Applies to Abdomen for Fetal Age; Decubitus Abdomen

Procedure Commonly Includes Abdomen series includes AP and upright abdomen and PA chest on patients who are able to stand. Lateral decubitus abdomen and supine chest on patients who cannot stand. Abdomen for kidney stones involves an AP abdomen and a coned-down view over the bladder area. Abdomen for gallstones involves the abdomen series and one coned-down view of the right upper quadrant. Abdomen for aneurysm or aortic calcification includes an AP and lateral. Abdomen for IUD placement includes an AP and lateral abdomen. Abdomen for multiple pregnancy, breech presentation, fetal age, position or death, or to rule out pregnancy includes AP abdomen only. Please see Ultrasound listings.

Indications

- assessment of intestinal obstruction
- location of foreign bodies, tubes, free peritoneal or retroperitoneal air
- displacement of the gastric air bubble
- elevation of the diaphragm
- displacement of the lateral and pelvic fat lines
- disturbances of normal bowel patterns and renal shadow
- fetal age in late pregnancy
- detection and localization of calcifications

Contraindications Plain films of the abdomen are contraindicated in early pregnancy and ultrasound is the method of choice for evaluation of the abdomen under these circumstances.

Patient Preparation Consult physician in charge before giving any medication. Physician should write orders in cases of bleeding or obstruction. For a usual adult routine, some radiologists prefer not to use any cathartics prior to this examination. Cathartics are used in many cases when a plain film of the abdomen is obtained prior to excretory urography. In these cases, on the evening before the examination, a cathartic such as castor oil or a bowel cleansing preparation such as GoLYTELY® may be administered. The patient should omit breakfast for morning appointments and omit lunch for afternoon appointments. Since preparation of abdomen in pediatric patients is so dependent on age and clinical problem, it is left to the judgment of a referring physician. In special cases, consult pediatric radiologist.

Special Instructions Requisition **must** state type of pills patient is receiving and if patient can stand.

Technique AP film of the abdomen. This film is obtained in the recumbent position and is often referred to as a KUB as it is commonly employed in examinations of the urinary tract. The letters stand for kidneys, ureters, and bladder. The AP film of the abdomen obtained in the erect position will allow demonstration of gas fluid levels within the intestine. In the small intestine, the presence of such fluid levels frequently indicates intestinal obstruction. Free intraperitoneal air is readily identifiable in this projection, because, unless trapped by intestinal adhesions, it will rise to reside beneath the domes of the hemidiaphragms. A rapid exposure technique is recommended to ensure the absence of diaphragmatic motion on the film. For the lateral decubitus film, the patient is recumbent lying on one side. A horizontal x-ray beam is directed at

(Continued)

Abdomen X-ray *(Continued)*

the abdomen from the anterior aspect. This film again will allow demonstration of fluid levels in patients who are unable to assume the upright position. If employed for identification of free intraperitoneal air, the patient's left side should be dependent. The patient should be placed in this position for at least 5 minutes prior to exposure of the film to ensure any free gas present within the peritoneal space will migrate to the highest point along the right lateral abdominal wall.

Causes for Rejection Barium in colon in cases to rule out kidney stone

Additional Information A PA view of the chest is sometimes included in this examination. This is because patients presenting with abdominal pain sometimes have pulmonary pathology such as lower lobe pneumonia. The upright PA chest film also facilitates recognition of free intraperitoneal air although a recent article suggests the upright lateral chest film is a more sensitive indicator of free intraperitoneal air. The presence of retroperitoneal air will not be appreciated as readily as free intraperitoneal air. This is because it will not migrate freely to a subphrenic location due to the configuration and confines of the retroperitoneal space. It will usually be recognized by its tendency to outline those organs which lie in the retroperitoneum such as the kidneys, ascending and descending colons, pancreas, and duodenum.

References

Baker SR, "The Abdominal Plain Film. What Will Be Its Role in the Future?" *Radiol Clin North Am*, 1993, 31(6):1335-44.

Baker SR, "Unenhanced Helical CT Versus Plain Abdominal Radiography: A Dissenting Opinion," *Radiology*, 1997, 205(1):45-7.

Kulshrestha MK, "Lead Poisoning Diagnosed by Abdominal X-rays," *J Toxicol Clin Toxicol*, 1996, 34(1):107-8.

Oliphant M, Berne AS, and Meyers MA, "The Subperitoneal Space of the Abdomen and Pelvis: Planes of Continuity," *AJR Am J Roentgenol*, 1996, 167(6):1433-9.

♦ **Air Contrast Study of Colon** *see* Colon Films *on page 352*

♦ **Barium Meal** *see* Gastrointestinal Series *on page 358*

♦ **Barium Swallow** *see* Esophagram *on page 355*

Bone Age

Procedure Commonly Includes Single AP view of the hand and wrist used to assess the physical development status of children

Indications Precocious puberty, marked hypogonadism, or eunuchoidism; evaluation of skeletal status and general body maturity

Equipment Standard radiography room

Technique Single AP view of the left hand

Additional Information There are a number of radiographic atlases of skeletal development of the hand and wrist. The patient's film is to be matched with a standard radiograph of the appropriate gender. The report should include information pertaining to skeletal age and chronological age. The standard deviation from the normal is included in the atlas. Comment can also be made on bone mineralization and any scars of interrupted growth that may provide a record of past illness or other misadventure.

References

Cole AJ, Webb L, and Cole TJ, "Bone Age Estimation: A Comparison of Methods," *Br J Radiol*, 1988, 61(728):683-6.

Oestreich AE, "Tanner-Whitehouse Versus Greulich-Pyle in Bone Age Determinations," *J Pediatr*, 1997, 131(1 Pt 1):5-6.

Tanner J, Oshman D, Bahhage F, et al, "Tanner-Whitehouse Bone Age Reference Values for North American Children," *J Pediatr*, 1997, 131(1 Pt 1):34-40.

Bone Biopsy

Applies to Percutaneous Biopsy of Musculoskeletal Lesions and Synovial Membranes

Procedure Commonly Includes This procedure involves the passage of a needle, either under fluoroscopic or computed tomographic guidance, into an area of bony abnormality to facilitate precise histologic and/or bacteriologic diagnosis. In many clinical situations, this procedure can establish definitive diagnosis without the disadvantages of surgery making it a useful alternative to open biopsy. In selected cases of arthritis, examination of the synovium may provide precise diagnostic clues or useful information about the nature of the arthritic process. A biopsy of the synovium can be performed through an open arthrotomy, percutaneous biopsy, or as part of an arthroscopic procedure during which the synovium can be visualized.

Indications The need for a tissue or bacteriologic diagnosis in situations where it is desirable to forego open biopsy

Patient Preparation Biopsies are performed in the Radiology Department. Skeletal biopsies are usually done under local anesthesia, with the exception of children and restless patients who are placed under general anesthesia or heavy sedation. Local anesthesia facilitates communication between the patient and the physician performing the procedure. Should the patient complain of radiating pain, the needle can be repositioned. Spinal biopsies necessitate a 24-hour hospitalization. Other anatomic areas may be biopsied on an outpatient basis. The patient should not eat the morning of the examination. An intravenous catheter is generally placed for I.V. access and the patient is usually administered both a sedative and a medication for pain.

Specimen There are a wide variety of commercially available needles for these procedures. A needle aspiration biopsy consists of aspiration of fluid for cytologic and/or bacteriologic analysis. A core biopsy, however, requires a larger needle and allows retrieval of a core of tissue for histopathologic interpretation.

References

Anderson MW, Temple HT, Dussault RG, et al, "Compartmental Anatomy: Relevance to Staging and Biopsy of Musculoskeletal Tumors," *AJR Am J Roentgenol*, 1999, 173(6):1663-71.

Fraser-Hill MA, Renfrew DL, Hilsenrath PE, "Percutaneous Needle Biopsy of Musculoskeletal Lesions. 1. Effective Accuracy and Diagnostic Utility," *AJR Am J Roentgenol*, 1992, 158(4):809-12.

Fraser-Hill MA, Renfrew DL, Hilsenrath PE, "Percutaneous Needle Biopsy of Musculoskeletal Lesions. 2. Cost-Effectiveness," *AJR Am J Roentgenol*, 1992, 158(4):813-8.

Jelinek JS, Krasndorf MJ, Gray R, et al, "Percutaneous Transpedicular Biopsy of Vertebral Body Lesions," *Spine*, 1996, 21(17):2035-40.

Leffler SG and Chew FS, "CT-Guided Percutaneous Biopsy of Sclerotic Bone Lesions: Diagnostic Yield and Accuracy," *AJR Am J Roentgenol*, 1999, 172(5):1389-92.

Yao L, Nelson SD, Seeger LL, et al, "Primary Musculoskeletal Neoplasms: Effectiveness of Core-Needle Biopsy," *Radiology*, 1999, 212(3):682-6.

♦ **Breast X-ray** *see* Mammogram *on page 361*

♦ **Cardiac Series** *see* Esophagram *on page 355*

Cervical Spine

Procedure Commonly Includes AP view of the cervical spine which is obtained with the patient in the supine position. Vertebral bodies below the level of C3 are well visualized in this view. An AP view of the upper cervical spine is obtained through the open mouth with the patient in the supine position. This allows good identification and evaluation of the odontoid process. Lateral view of the cervical spine may be performed in the upright or supine position. If the film is obtained to rule out fracture subsequent to trauma, the supine position should be maintained and the patient should not be moved until the films have been evaluated by the radiologist. The radiologist will decide if further views are necessary. In the nontraumatized patient, a lateral view of the cervical spine may be obtained with the patient in the upright position dropping the shoulders as much as possible to enhance visualization of C7. Traction on the arms by means of heavy weights held in the hands will aid in lowering the shoulders. Oblique views of the cervical spine are exposed in the supine position with the entire body rotated through 45° so that the head, neck, and torso are in straight alignment. Routine examination usually includes only the AP and lateral film. If oblique views are required, for example for evaluation of the neural foramina, then this should be written on the requisition.

Indications Evaluate cervical spine for presence of metastatic and primary neoplasm, trauma, infectious disease, degenerative and reactive processes

Patient Preparation If patients are being evaluated for fracture subluxation or dislocation, they may be wearing a cervical collar put in place either at the site of the trauma or in the emergency medicine department. In these circumstances, an AP and a lateral view are obtained in the supine position and then (Continued)

Cervical Spine *(Continued)*

shown to the radiologist who determines whether the collar can be removed for a complete examination.

Special Instructions Specify if patient can be removed from the stretcher in cases of injury.

Equipment Standard radiography equipment

References

Baker C, Kadish H, and Schunk JE, "Evaluation of Pediatric Cervical Spine Injuries," *Am J Emerg Med*, 1999, (1793):230-4.

Freemyer B, Knopp R, Piche J, et al, "Comparison of Five-View and Three-View Cervical Spine Series in the Evaluation of Patients With Cervical Trauma," *Ann Emerg Med*, 1989, 18(8):818-21.

Frohna WJ, "Emergency Department Evaluation and Treatment of the Neck and Cervical Spine Injuries," *Emerg Med Clin North Am*, 1999, 17(4):739-91.

Herman MJ and Pizzutillo PD, "Cervical Spine Disorders in Children," *Orthop Clin North Am*, 1999, 30(3):457-66.

Harris JH and Edeiken-Monroe B, *The Radiology of Acute Cervical Spine Trauma*, 2nd ed, St Louis, MO: CV Mosby, 1987.

Hughes SJ, "How Effective Is the Newport/Aspen Collar? A Prospective Radiographic Evaluation in Healthy Adult Volunteers," *J Trauma*, 1998, 45(2):374-8.

Kaiser JA and Holland BA, "Imaging of the Cervical Spine," *Spine*, 1998, 23(24):2701-12.

Klein GR, Vaccaro AR, Albert TJ, et al, "Efficacy of Magnetic Resonance Imaging in the Evaluation of Posterior Cervical Spine Fractures," *Spine* 1999, 24(8):771-4.

Mulcahey MJ, Betz RR, Smith BT, et al, "A Prospective Evaluation of Upper Extremity Tendon Transfers in Children With Cervical Spinal Cord Injury," *J Pediatr Orthop*, 1999, 19(3):319-28.

Vandemark RM, "Radiology of the Cervical Spine in Trauma Patients: Practice Pitfalls and Recommendations for Improving Efficiency and Communication," *AJR Am J Roentgenol*, 1990, 155(3):465-72.

Zabel DD, Tinkoff G, Wittenborn W, et al, "Adequacy and Efficacy of Lateral Cervical Spine Radiography in Alert, High-Risk Blunt Trauma Patient," *J Trauma*, 1997, 43(6):952-6.

Chest Films

Synonyms CXR; PA; PA and Lateral CXR

Procedure Commonly Includes PA and lateral exposures of the chest. Sagel and his colleagues published an article in 1974 questioning the efficacy of screening examinations of the chest and whether or not lateral views should be obtained. Both medical and economic factors were considered. The study was based on a review of PA and lateral views of the chest in 10,597 examinations and reached the following conclusions.

- Routine screening for hospital admission or for surgery was not warranted for patients younger than 20 years of age.
- Lateral projection could be eliminated in routine screening of patients 20-39 years of age.
- Lateral projection should be obtained at any age when disease of the chest is suspected.
- Lateral projection should be obtained in screening examinations of patients older than 40 years of age.

Indications Evaluate lungs and thoracic bones for presence of metastatic and primary neoplasm, infectious disease, degenerative and reactive processes, trauma, and surgical change. The chest film is also used to evaluate the heart and great vessels.

Patient Preparation Remove medals, lockets, and other jewelry from neck. Arrange hair, when long, high on head so that no locks hang over chest or shoulders.

Special Instructions The chest x-ray can be modified in various ways to answer specific questions. For example, while the standard PA view of the chest is obtained in full inspiration, a pneumothorax will be more readily appreciated when the film is exposed in expiration. Decubitus films are helpful in differentiating mobile fluid in the pleural space from fluid loculations or pleural thickening. A lordotic view of the chest may be helpful in evaluating the apices. Oblique views of the chest done with 45° angulation in the right anterior oblique projection and 60° angulation in the left anterior oblique projection with barium opacifying the esophagus at the time of exposure are helpful in evaluating the size of the various cardiac chambers. A standard radiographic examination of the chest in addition to the modifications mentioned may be scheduled by calling the Radiology Department.

References

Henschke CI, Yankelevitz DF, Wand A, et al, "Accuracy and Efficacy of Chest Radiography in the Intensive Care Unit," *Radiol Clin North Am*, 1996, 34(1):21-31.
Henschke CI, Yankelevitz DF, Wand A, et al, "Chest Radiography in the ICU," *Clin Imaging*, 1997, 21(2):90-103.
Sagel SS, Evens RG, Forrest JV, et al, "Efficacy of Routine Screening and Lateral Chest Radiographs in a Hospital-Based Population," *N Engl J Med*, 1974, 291(19):1001-4.
Woodard PK, Slone RM, Gierada DS, et al, "Chest Radiography: Depiction of Normal Anatomy and Pathologic Structures With Selenium-Based Digital Radiography Versus Conventional Screen-Film Radiography," *Radiology*, 1997, 203(1):197-201.

Cholangiogram, Operative

Synonyms Intraoperative Cholangiogram; Surgical Cholangiogram

Procedure Commonly Includes Visualization of the bile ducts by means of contrast agent injection through an indwelling T-tube at the time of surgery to assess for calculi within the biliary system. Radiographs are exposed in the operating room during the procedure in the AP and/or oblique projections.

Indications

- evaluate patency of biliary system
- evaluate filling defects in bile ducts
- demonstration of biliary anatomy

Contraindications History of allergic reaction to contrast media, barium in the bowel

Patient Preparation Procedure is performed in the operating room after cholecystectomy before closure of abdominal incision. Laparoscopic cholecystectomy is becoming increasingly popular as an alternative to open cholecystectomy. Operative cholangiography is feasible and useful in patients undergoing laparoscopic cholecystectomy.

Limitations Biliary duct system may not be optimally visualized due to respiratory motion or size of patient or barium in bowel

References

Heniford BT, Arca MJ, Gersin K, et al, "Intraoperative Dynamic Fluoroscopic Cholangiogram During Laparoscopic Cholecystectomy," *J Am Coll Surg*, 1999, 189(1):134-7.
Kondylis PD, Simmons DR, Agarwal SK, et al, "Abnormal Intraoperative Cholangiography. Treatment Options and Long-Term Follow-up," *Arch Surg*, 1997, 132(4):347-50.
Ladocsi LT, Benitez LD, Filippone DR, et al, "Intraoperative Cholangiography in Laparoscopic Cholecystectomy: A Review of 734 Consecutive Cases," *Am J Surg*, 1997, 63(2):150-6.
Sees DW and Martin RR, "Comparison of Preoperative Endoscopic Retrograde Cholangiopancreatography and Laparoscopic Cholecystectomy With Operative Management of Gallstone Pancreatitis," *Am J Surg*, 1997, 174(6):719-22.
Stuart SA, Simpson TI, Alvord LA, et al, "Routine Intraoperative Laparoscopic Cholangiography," *Am J Surg*, 1998, 176(6):632-7.
Van Campenhout I, Prosmanne O, Gagner M, et al, "Routine Operative Cholangiography During Laparoscopic Cholecystectomy: Feasibility and Value in 107 Patients," *AJR Am J Roentgenol*, 1993, 160:1209-11.
Weston AP, "Sincalide: A Cholecystokinin Agonist as an Aid in Endoscopic Retrograde Cholangiopancreatography - a Prospective Assessment," *J Clin Gastroenterol*, 1997, 24(4):227-30.
Weston SR, Jorgenson RA, Dickson ER, et al, "Is Routine Cholangiography Useful in Men With Suspected Primary Biliary Cirrhosis?" *J Clin Gastroenterol*, 1999, 29(1):68-70.

Cholangiography, Postoperative, T-Tube

Synonyms T-Tube

Applies to Postoperative Cholangiography

Procedure Commonly Includes Injection of contrast material through indwelling T-tube for visualization of bile ducts in the postoperative period in those patients who have had cholecystectomy and/or common bile duct exploration with placement of T-tube at the time of surgery.

Indications Evaluate the patency of the biliary system prior to removal of the T-tube. Evaluate for possible biliary leak in patients posthepatic transplantation.

Contraindications

- cholangitis
- sepsis without antibiotic cover

Aftercare Routine observation. Examination may be scheduled by calling the Radiology Department. Assuming the patient is not on dietary restriction, a light breakfast may be consumed the day of the procedure.

Special Instructions By appointment only. A completed and signed Radiology consult must be sent to Radiology before an appointment can be made.

(Continued)

Cholangiography, Postoperative, T-Tube *(Continued)*

Turnaround Time Written report available within 24 hours of completed exam. Verbal report will be supplied immediately postprocedure if requested.

Causes for Rejection Inadequate clinical information on the Radiology consult

Additional Information If sepsis is present the examination may be done in special circumstances following antibiotic care

References

Fallahzadeh H, "Common Duct Exploration During Laparoscopic Cholecystectomy," *Am J Surg*, 1997, 63(2):121-4.

Heniford BT, Arca MJ, Gersin K, et al, "Intraoperative Dynamic Fluoroscopic Cholangiogram During Laparoscopic Cholecystectomy," *J Am Coll Surg*, 1999, 189(1):134-7.

Ladocsi LT, Benitez LD, Filippone DR, et al, "Intraoperative Cholangiography in Laparoscopic Cholecystectomy: A Review of 734 Consecutive Cases," *Am Surg*, 1997, 63(2):150-6.

Rabkin JM, Orloff SL, Reed MH, et al, "Biliary Tract Complications of Side-to-Side Without T Tube Versus End-to-End With or Without T Tube Choledochocholedochostomy in Liver Transplant Recipients," *Transplantation*, 1998, 65(2):193-9.

♦ **Cholecystography** *see* Oral Cholecystogram, Gallbladder Series *on page 362*

Colon Films

Applies to Air Contrast Study of Colon

Indications Evaluate the colon for presence of embolism, aneurysm, neoplasms, hemorrhage, or atherosclerosis

Contraindications Known perforation of the colon

Patient Preparation Adequate bowel preparation is the key to the performance of a diagnostic barium enema. For appropriate preparation of the bowel we use a polyethylene glycol electrolyte gastrointestinal lavage solution. This product is contraindicated in patients with gastrointestinal obstruction, gastric retention, bowel perforation, toxic colitis, or megacolon. On the day prior to the examination, a clear liquid diet should start at lunchtime. Clear liquids include black tea or coffee, broth or bouillon, plain jello, strained fruit juice, popsicles, water, carbonated beverages or sherbet. The patient should not drink milk or cream. At 3 PM on the day before the examination, the patient should start drinking the product GoLYTELY® at a rate of 8 oz (240 mL) every 10 minutes until a total of 4 L has been consumed. Rapid drinking of each portion should be encouraged (as opposed to drinking sips continuously). It is important that each patient drink the entire volume of GoLYTELY® for an adequate GI examination. An alternative method of bowel cleansing may be required in patients with fluid restrictions, with renal failure, with congestive cardiac failure, or in patients younger than 18 years of age. The patient's primary physician should be consulted with regard to this. Orally administered GoLYTELY® induces a diarrhea which rapidly cleanses the bowel, usually within 4 hours. The material is available in a powdered form for oral administration as a solution following reconstitution. Other bowel cleansing preparations are available. See reference.

Aftercare Correct aftercare of the barium enema patient is essential if examination is to be followed by a GI series. If colon is not cleansed of residual barium following barium enema, patient will not be accepted for GI series on the following morning. The following is advised. All patients on return from barium enema examination should be given 10 oz of magnesium citrate at 4 PM. On the following morning, patient should have a Fleet® enema before being sent for GI series.

Special Instructions By appointment only. When a series of gastrointestinal examinations are desired, the procedures should be scheduled as follows.

- First day: Gallbladder series: If it is known that the patient is to have a barium enema following the gallbladder series, then preparation for the barium enema should begin on the same day as preparation for the gallbladder series. See Oral Cholecystogram, Gallbladder Series *on page 362.*
- Second day: Barium enema followed by adequate aftercare, consisting of 10 oz of magnesium citrate at 4 PM and a Fleet® enema on the following morning, if there is to be a GI series on the following morning. If this is not

done, residual barium may remain in the colon so that a GI series is not possible on the following morning.

- Third day: Gastrointestinal series and small bowel series. Barium enema will be supplemented by an air contrast study at the discretion of the radiologist. There is no need for the requisition to state "air contrast study". The decision whether to do an air contrast study will reside with the radiologist. An air contrast study may also be done after routine barium enema by consultation with the radiologist. Pyelograms should be scheduled before barium studies of the GI tract.

Causes for Rejection Barium in colon or inadequate preparation

Limitations If a rectal biopsy has been done, barium enema should not be ordered for 10 days. Exceptions to this will be permitted only after consultation with the surgeon involved. Hypotonic colon examination using glucagon will be ordered at the discretion of the radiologist or by consultation with the radiologist. If the patient is to have ultrasonography or computerized tomography, then barium enema should be delayed until these exams are completed. Barium in the abdomen will interfere with these exams. Air contrast examination is not optimally performed following sigmoidoscopy.

References

Gelfand DM and Ott DJ, "Double-Contrast Examination of the Colon Without Decubitus Films," *AJR Am J Roentgenol*, 1997, 169(6):1565-7.

Lai AK, Kwok PC, Man SW, "A Blinded Clinical Trial Comparing Conventional Cleansing Enema, Pico-Salax and GoLYTELY® for Barium Enema Bowel Preparation," *Clin Radiol*, 1996, 51(8):566-9.

Rex D, "Barium Enema and Colon Cancer Screening: Finally a Study," *Am J Gastroenterol*, 1997, 92(9):1570-2.

Tham RT, Korte JH, Bom EP, et al, "Preparation of the Colon for Single- and Double-Contrast Barium Enema Examination: A Simplified Method," *Radiology*, 1993, 188(2):578-80.

♦ **Contrast Study of the Esophagus and Pharynx** *see* Esophagram *on page 355*

♦ **CXR** *see* Chest Films *on page 350*

♦ **Cystogram** *see* Cystourethrogram *on page 353*

Cystourethrogram

Synonyms Cystogram; Voiding Cystourethrogram

Procedure Commonly Includes Catheterization of the urinary bladder which is then distended with contrast material until the patient feels the urge to micturate. Micturition is then recorded on videotape with appropriate views for confirmation or exclusion of ureteric reflux and appropriate evaluation of the urethra.

Indications Evaluation of the morphology of the urinary bladder, evaluation of the urethra for exclusion of obstructive processes such as posterior urethral valves or urethral strictures, evaluation for the presence and extent of ureteric reflux

Patient Preparation Obtain a signed procedure permit for cystourethrogram. Catheterization of the urinary bladder is performed.

Special Instructions Schedule this procedure before gastrointestinal barium studies.

Equipment The ability to videotape the fluoroscopic record of this procedure will be most beneficial in assuring documentation of the appropriate diagnostic information.

Causes for Rejection Barium in pelvic region

Limitations Previous barium studies within 24 hours

♦ **Decubitus Abdomen** *see* Abdomen X-ray *on page 347*

Dorsal Spine

Synonyms Thoracic Spine

Procedure Commonly Includes AP view of the thoracic spine obtained with the patient in the supine position. A lateral view of the thoracic spine obtained with the patient in the supine position. A lateral (slightly oblique) view of the upper two thoracic segments known as a Twining's or swimmer's view is obtained for evaluation of the lower cervical and upper thoracic spine.

Indications Evaluate thoracic spine for presence of metastasis and primary neoplasm, trauma, infectious disease, degenerative and reactive process

(Continued)

Dorsal Spine *(Continued)*

Patient Preparation No preparation required for the examination. To schedule a study, call X-ray Department.

References

Abraham DJ, Herkowitz HN, and Katz JN, "Indications for Thoracic and Lumbar Spine Fusion and Trends in Use," *Orthop Clin North Am*, 1998, 29(4):803.

Biyani A, Ebraheim NA, and Lu J, "Thoracic Spine Fractures in Patients Older Than 50 Years," *Clin Orthop*, 1996, (328):190-3.

Resnick DK and Benzel EC, "Lateral Extracavitary Approach for Thoracic and Thoracolumbar Spine Trauma: Operative Complications," *Neurosurgery*, 1998, 43(4):796-802.

Rosenthal D, Marquardt G, Lorenz R, et al, "Anterior Decompression and Stabilization Using a Microsurgical Endoscopic Technique for Metastatic Tumors of the Thoracic Spine," *J Neurosurg*, 1996, 84(4):565-72.

Sioutos P, Arbit E, Tsairis P, et al, "Spontaneous Thoracic Spinal Cord Herniation. A case report," *Spine*, 1996, 21(14):1710-3.

Tuli SK, Hurlbert RJ, Mikulis D, et al, "Ninety-Degree Rotation of the Thoracic Spinal Thecal Sac. Case Report," *J Neurosurg*, 1998, 89(1):133-8.

Enteroclysis

Synonyms Small Bowel Enema

Procedure Commonly Includes Intubation of the small bowel with a 12- or 14-gauge French catheter under fluoroscopic guidance. The catheter should be long enough to reach the first loop of jejunum. It should be the smallest possible diameter to minimize nasopharyngeal or oropharyngeal irritation. The catheter should possess an adaptation, such as a distensible balloon, to prevent reflux of contrast material thus preventing decompression of the small bowel during the examination. A barium mixture is then introduced into the small bowel. The examination may be performed in a single contrast or double contrast fashion. Where a double contrast examination is performed, methyl cellulose is introduced subsequent to infusion of high density contrast material.

Indications Enteroclysis is indicated after all radiologic and endoscopic tests have been unrevealing in the evaluation of gastrointestinal tract blood loss of unknown origin. Enteroclysis is the method of choice in the evaluation of malabsorptive states. While Crohn disease involving the distal ileum can be well demonstrated on a conventional small bowel study, enteroclysis excels in the demonstration of the proximal and distal extent of disease and the presence of skip lesions or fistulas in patients with Crohn disease. While contraindicated in patients with the clinical and radiographic findings of high grade obstruction, enteroclysis may be useful in determining the site, severity, and nature of the obstruction once the bowel has been satisfactorily decompressed. This method of examination may also be helpful in patients with periumbilical or right lower quadrant pain associated with abdominal distention, nausea, or vomiting, especially if the patient has had prior abdominal surgery.

Contraindications

- clinical and radiographic findings of high-grade obstruction
- extensive prior gastric surgery where the anatomy is ill-defined
- lack of patient compliance

Patient Preparation The patient should be fasting from midnight prior to the examination. A laxative or mild colon cleansing enema should be performed the day prior to the examination to ensure that not much fecal material is present in the ascending colon.

Special Instructions It is recommended that requests for enteroclysis be discussed with the attending radiologist prior to completion of the radiology consult. The importance of adequate bowel preparation is stressed. Metoclopramide administration prior to the study has been found useful as it eases transpyloric intubation and facilitates a faster infusion rate of contrast material. Intravenous diazepam in small doses (3-5 mg) may be helpful in particularly apprehensive patients.

Turnaround Time A written report available within 24 hours of the completed examination. Consultation with the radiologist prior to this upon request.

Additional Information This is a specialized examination of the small bowel. Routine enteroclysis in the absence of prior investigations or an attempt at small bowel examination is not usually performed.

References

Aliperti G, Zuckerman GR, Willis JR, et al, "Enteroscopy With Enteroclysis," *Gastrointest Endosc Clin N Am*, 1996, 6(4):803-10.

Barloon TJ, Lu CC, Honda H, et al, "Does a Normal Small-Bowel Enteroclysis Exclude Small-Bowel Disease? A Long-Term Follow-up of Consecutive Normal Studies," *Abdom Imaging*, 1994, 19(2):113-5.

Bender GN, "Radiographic Examination of the Small Bowel. An Application of Odds Ratio Analysis to Help Attain an Appropriate Mix of Small Bowel Follow Through and Enteroclysis in a Working-Clinical Environment," *Invest Radiol*, 1997, 32(6):357-62.

Bender GN, Maglinte DD, Kloppel VR, et al, "CT Enteroclysis: A Superfluous Diagnostic Procedure or Valuable When Investigating Small-Bowel Disease?" *AJR Am J Roentgenol*, 1999, 172(2):373-8.

Bender GN, Timmons JH, Williard WC, "Computed Tomographic Enteroclysis: One Methodology," *Invest Radiol*, 1996, 31(1):43-9.

Bernstein CN, Boult IF, Greenberg HM, et al, "A Prospective Randomized Comparison Between Small Enteroclysis and Small Bowel Follow-Through in Crohn's Disease," *Gastroenterology*, 1997, 113(2):390-8.

Hall F, "Enteroclysis," *AJR Am J Roentgenol*, 1996, 167(2):533-4.

Kelvin FM and Maglinte DD, "Enteroclysis or Small Bowel Follow-Through in Crohn's Disease?" *Gastroenterology*, 1998, 114(6):1349-51.

Lewis BS, "Radiology Versus Endoscopy of the Small Bowel," *Gastrointest Endosc Clin N Am*, 1999, 91(1):31-27.

Maglinte DD, Lappas JC, Kelvin FM, et al, "Small Bowel Radiography: How, When and Why?" *Radiology*, 1987, 163(2):297-305.

Ott DJ, "Celiac Disease: Biopsy or Enteroclysis Better for Evaluating Response to a Gluten-Free Diet?" *Am J Gastroenterol*, 1997, 92(4):715-6.

Willis JR, Chokshi HR, Zuckerman GR, "Enteroscopy-Enterolysis: Experience With a Combined Endoscopic-Radiographic Technique," *Gastrointest Endosc*, 1997, 45(2):163-7.

Esophagram

Synonyms Barium Swallow; Contrast Study of the Esophagus and Pharynx; Esophagus, X-ray

Applies to Cardiac Series; Heart Size; Positive Contrast Examinations of the Pharynx and Esophagus

Procedure Commonly Includes Fluoroscopy, spot films, and survey radiographs. Videotaping may be helpful in the further detailed analysis of the swallowing mechanism. Spot films are at the discretion of the radiologist and may be obtained in any projection to more clearly delineate pathology. Survey films obtained include an anteroposterior film of the barium distended esophagus extending from the neck to the diaphragm and right anterior oblique projection of the barium distended esophagus to include the neck and thorax. The left anterior oblique projection including the same anatomic area is occasionally included in the examination.

Indications

- establish the presence of intrinsic abnormalities of the pharynx and esophagus including neoplasms, webs, tracheoesophageal fistulas, gastroesophageal reflux, Barrett esophagus, and esophagitis
- demonstrate the type and location of foreign bodies within the pharynx and esophagus
- demonstrate narrowing or displacement of the barium-filled esophagus due to extrinsic pathology such as vascular rings, mediastinal masses, etc
- evaluate caliber and motility of the esophagus
- confirm the integrity of esophageal anastomoses in the postoperative patient

Contraindications While no definite contraindications to this examination are recognized, the study requires considerable modification under certain circumstances. Because of this, the type, location, and extent of suspected pathology should be clearly stated on the requisition.

Patient Preparation This examination is commonly performed in association with an upper GI series. Under these circumstances, the patient should have nothing to eat or drink after midnight before the examination. The morning of the examination, the patient may wash the mouth with water but should not swallow the water. If a foreign body is suspected, this should be clearly stated on the requisition, thus allowing the examination to be tailored accordingly.

Aftercare None or mild laxative

Special Instructions By appointment only. Where problem is complex, preliminary consultation with an attending radiologist is desirable. Such cases may require rapid serial spot filming or other modalities.

(Continued)

Esophagram *(Continued)*

Technique A comprehensive discussion of the methodology employed in the evaluation of the pharynx and esophagus is beyond the scope of this text. A reference for this information is supplied.

Additional Information The correct application of the full column technique, mucosal relief films, double contrast studies and motion recording is critical in obtaining maximum information from the examination. An article by Maglinte and his colleagues examines what constitutes a minimal esophageal survey in a patient referred for an upper GI series with nonspecific and/or vague upper abdominal complaints.[1] The author evaluated approximately 500 patients with nonspecific and/or vague upper GI complaints to examine what constituted a minimal esophageal survey and the extent of esophageal disease visible on radiography in these patients.

Footnotes

1. Maglinte DD, Schultheis TE, Krol KL, et al, "Survey of the Esophagus During the Upper Gastrointestinal Examination in 500 Patients," *Radiology*, 1983, 147(1):65-70.

References

de Oliveira JM, Birgisson S, Doinoff C, et al, "Timed Barium Swallow: A Simple Technique for Evaluating Esophageal Emptying in Patients With Achalasia," *AJR Am J Roentgenol*, 1997, 169(2):473-9.

Low VH and Rubesin SE, "Contrast Evaluation of the Pharynx and Esophagus," *Radiol Clin North Am*, 1993, 31(6):1265-91.

Ott DJ, Ledbetter MS, Chen MY, et al, "Correlation of Lower Esophageal Mucosal Ring and 24-h pH Monitoring of the Esophagus," *Am J Gastroenterol*, 1996, 91(1):61-4.

Richter JE, "Peptic Strictures of the Esophagus," *Gastroenterol Clin North Am*, 1999, 28(4):875-91.

Vaezi MF, Baker ME, and Richter JE, "Assessment of Esophageal Emptying Post-Pneumatic Dilation: Use of the Timed Barium Esophagram," *Am J Gastroenterol*, 1999, 94(7):1802-7.

♦ **Esophagus, X-ray** *see* Esophagram *on page 355*

Facet Joint Arthrography/Injection

Procedure Commonly Includes Arthrographic evaluation of facet joints or placement of needle within facet joints for injection of anti-inflammatory agents or a long-lasting anesthesia.

Indications

- facet syndrome
- nerve root compression by a facet joint synovial cyst
- narrowing of the lumbar canal caused primarily by degeneration of the facet joint
- prerhizolysis survey
- spondylolysis with nodule protruding from the bony defect which may be producing nerve root compression
- inflammatory spondyloarthropathy
- septic facet joint arthritis

Patient Preparation No alteration of the patient's diet is required for this procedure. Scheduling is accomplished by contacting the Radiology Department.

Special Instructions Examination will be performed by appointment following consultation with the neurosurgeon or neurologist.

References

Dreyer SJ and Dreyfuss PH, "Low Back Pain and the Zygapophyical (Facet) Joints," *Arch Phys Med Rehabil*, 1996, 77(3):290-300.

Lomasney LM and Cooper RA, "Distal Radioulnar Joint Arthrography: Simplified Technique," *Radiology*, 1996, 199(1):278-9.

Maldjian C, Mesgarzadeh M, and Tehranzadeh J, "Diagnostic and Therapeutic Features of Facet and Sacroiliac Joint Injection. Anatomy, Pathophysiology, and Technique," *Radiol Clin North Am*, 1998, 36(3):497-508.

Mann FA, "Performing a Satisfactory Arthrocentesis of the Distal Radioulnar Joint During Triple-Compartment Wrist Arthrography," *AJR Am J Roentgenol*, 1997, 168(3):840-1.

Mann FA, Wilson AJ, and Gilula LA, "Triple-Injection Wrist Arthrography: Unidirectional Communications Are Due to Technical Factors," *J Hand Surg*, 1998, 23(1):82-8.

McCormick CC, Taylor JR, and Twomey LT, "Facet Joint Arthrography in Lumbar Spondylolysis: Anatomic Basis for Spread of Contrast Medium," *Radiology*, 1989, 171(1):193-6.

Parlier-Cuau C, Champsaur P, Nizard R, et al, "Percutaneous Treatments of Painful Shoulder," *Radiol Clin North Am*, 1998, 36(3):589-96.

Revel M, Poiraudeau S, Auleley GR, et al, "Capacity of the Clinical Picture to Characterize low Back Pain Relieved by Facet Joint Anesthesia. Proposed Criteria to Identify Patients With Painful Facet Joints," *Spine*, 1998, 23(18):1972-6.

Shipley JA and Beukes CA, "The Nature of the Spondylolytic Defect. Demonstration of a Communicating Synovial Pseudarthrosis in the Pars Interarticularis," *J Bone Joint Surg Br*, 1998, 80(4):662-4.

Wybire M and Laredo JD, "Facet Joint Arthropathy and Steroid Injection," *Interventional Radiology in Bone and Joint*, Bard M and Laredo JD, eds, New York, NY: Springer-Verlag Wien, 1988.

Facial Bones

Related Information

Skull, X-ray *on page 367*

Applies to Zygomatic Arch, Left and Right

Procedure Commonly Includes Radiographic evaluation of the facial bones including three views of the bones of the face. The first is a posterior-anterior view obtained with the patient in the prone position. This projection provides a good view of the maxilla, the zygomatic arches, the orbits, and the nasal cavity. The second view is known as the submentovertical view of the skull. It is obtained with the patient in the supine position and the x-ray tube angled in a caudocephalad direction. This projection facilitates visualization of the foramina at the base of the skull, the petrous ridges, and the ethmoid and sphenoid bones. It also provides a tangential perspective on the zygomata, the zygomatic arches, and the maxillary bones. The third film in the facial bone series is a lateral view of the face. If a fracture of the zygomatic arch is suspected, a further view, entitled the verticosubmental projection, may be helpful.

Indications Facial trauma, specifically to exclude fracture of the facial bones

Patient Preparation No specific preparation required. The examination may be scheduled by contacting the Radiology Department.

References

Assael LA, "Clinical Aspects of Imaging in Maxillofacial Trauma," *Radiol Clin North Am*, 1993, 31(1):209-20.

Haug RH, "Retention of Asymptomatic Bone Plates Used for Orthognathic Surgery and Facial Fractures," *J Oral Maxillofac Surg*, 1996, 54(5):611-7.

Meaders RA and Sullivan SM, "The Development and Use of a Computerized Database for the Evaluation of Facial Fractures Incorporating Aspects of the AAOMS Parameters of Care," *J Oral Maxillofac Surg*, 1998, 56(8):924-9.

Schortinghuis J, Bos RR, and Vissink A, "Complications of Internal Fixation of Maxillofacial Fractures With Microplates," *J Oral Maxillofac Surg*, 1999, 57(2):130-4.

Tanaka N, Hayashi S, Amagasa T, et al, "Maxillofacial Fractures Sustained During Sports," *J Oral Maxillofac Surg*, 1996, 54(6):715-9.

Weil TS, Van Sickels JE, and Payne CJ, "Distraction Osteogenesis for Correction of Transverse Mandibular Deficiency: A Preliminary Report," *J Oral Maxillofac Surg*, 1997, 55(9):953-60.

♦ **Fistulogram** *see* Fistulous Tracts, X-ray *on page 357*

Fistulous Tracts, X-ray

Synonyms Fistulogram

Procedure Commonly Includes Opacification under fluoroscopic guidance of abnormal communications between two epithelial surfaces. Example: Between the skin and the bowel (enterocutaneous fistula), between the stomach and the colon (gastrocolic fistula), etc.

Indications Determine the extent and organs involved in the fistulous tract, to plan surgical therapeutic approach or to monitor healing

Contraindications Barium within the bowel may constitute a relative contraindication, depending upon whether it interferes with visualization of the opacified fistulous tract.

Special Instructions By appointment only

Additional Information In the case of enterocutaneous fistulas, opacification will require placement of an appropriate size catheter and injection of contrast material through the catheter to opacify the fistulous tract. This will generally be performed within the gastrointestinal radiology suite in the Radiology Department.

References

Chau WK and Chan SC, "Sonographic Diagnosis of a Small Fistulous Communication Between a Subphrenic Abscess and a Perforated Duodenal Ulcer," *J Clin Ultrasound*, 2000, 28(3):153-6.

Killen DA, Muehlebach GF, and Wathanacharoen S, "Aortopulmonary Fistula," *South Med J*, 2000, 93(2):195-8.

Older RA, Gizienski TA, Wilkowski MJ, et al, "Hemodialysis Access Stenosis: Early Detection With Color Doppler US," *Radiology*, 1998, 207(1):161-4.

(Continued)

Fistulous Tracts, X-ray *(Continued)*

Rocco MV, Bleyer AJ, and Burkart JM, "Utilization of Inpatient and Outpatient Resources for the Management of Hemodialysis Access Complications," *Am J Kidney Dis*, 1996, 28(2):250-6.

Sou S, Yao T, Matsui T, et al, "Preoperative Detection of Occult Enterovesical Fistulas in Patients With Crohn's Disease: Efficacy of Oral or Rectal Administration of Indocyanine Green Solution," *Dis Colon Rectum*, 1999, 42(2):266-70.

♦ **Gallbladder Series** *see* Oral Cholecystogram, Gallbladder Series *on page 362*

♦ **Gallbladder X-ray** *see* Oral Cholecystogram, Gallbladder Series *on page 362*

Gastrointestinal Series

Synonyms Barium Meal; GI Series; Upper GI Examination

Procedure Commonly Includes Radiographic and fluoroscopic evaluation of the esophagus, stomach, and duodenum while the patient is drinking a barium solution. Spot films will be obtained in various projections during the dynamic portion of the study. Subsequent to this, routine overhead films will also be obtained. The examination may be coupled with a study of the small bowel or may be done separately.

Indications Evaluation of the gastrointestinal tract for the presence of neoplasms, inflammatory diseases, ulcers, diverticula, obstruction, foreign body, hiatal hernia, and gastroesophageal reflux

Contraindications

- presence of barium within the colon
- presence of food within the stomach

Patient Preparation Adult patients should have a light, liquid supper the evening prior to the examination and should have nothing to eat or drink after midnight. Pediatric patients should refrain from eating or drinking for 4 hours prior to the examination. (The latter is at the discretion of the radiologist and depends on the age of the patient.) Some radiologists recommend a mild cathartic subsequent to the examination particularly in the case of older, chronically constipated patients.

Special Instructions Examination may be scheduled by calling the Radiology Department.

Limitations Pyelograms should be scheduled before barium studies of the GI tract. Hypotonic duodenography may be performed at the discretion of the radiologist. If the patient is scheduled to have sonographic examination of the abdomen or a CT examination, the gastrointestinal series should be delayed until these exams have been completed. High concentration of barium within the gastrointestinal tract will produce artifacts on CT scan. When the patient is scheduled for both an upper gastrointestinal series and a barium enema, the barium enema should be performed first and the patient given a cathartic such as magnesium citrate to facilitate evacuation prior to the gastrointestinal series.

Additional Information A number of different techniques are described for mucosal relief studies, double contrast examinations. There are also several different commercially available barium sulfate suspensions. In addition to this, pharmacological agents such as glucagon may be helpful in suppressing motility and facilitating hypotonic evaluation. A standard dose of 0.1 mg of glucagon diluted to 0.25 mL with sterile water is utilized routinely in some double contrast examinations.

References

Bender GN and Makuch RS, "Double-Contrast Barium Examination of the Upper Gastrointestinal Tract With Nonendoscopic Biopsy: Findings in 100 Patients," *Radiology*, 1997, 202(2):355-9.

Levine MS and Laufer I, "The Upper Gastrointestinal Series at a Crossroads," *AJR Am J Roentgenol*, 1993, 161(6):1131-7.

Levine MS, Rubesin SE, Herlinger H, et al, "Double-Contrast Upper Gastrointestinal Examination: Technique and Interpretation," *Radiology*, 1988, 168(3):593-602.

Lewis BS, "Radiology Versus Endoscopy of the Small Bowel," *Gastrointest Endosc Clin N Am*, 1999, 9(1):13-27.

♦ **GI Series** *see* Gastrointestinal Series *on page 358*

♦ **Heart Size** *see* Esophagram *on page 355*

High-Resolution CT

Synonyms HRCT

Procedure Commonly Includes Thin slices through the appropriate anatomic area for evaluation of suspected pathology

Indications High-resolution computed tomography is most frequently utilized in evaluation of pulmonary parenchymal pathology. Specifically in the evaluation of lung parenchyma for interstitial lung disease. The technique allows differentiation of entities such as lymphogenic spread of tumor and pulmonary edema. The technique is also utilized for evaluation of pulmonary nodules. Here it is helpful in the identification of fat within hamartomas and calcification within pulmonary nodules, the presence of which may aid in their characterization.

Contraindications Patient cooperation is of the utmost importance.

Patient Preparation The reader is referred to patient preparation for the area of anatomic interest.

Special Instructions While it does not replace other CT examinations it may be indicated in some clinical situations. The term high-resolution computed tomography refers to a modification of the computed transaxial tomography technique to maximize spacial resolution. This is accomplished by utilizing a thin slice thickness (1-2 mm), a high spacial frequency reconstruction algorithm, and retargeting the reconstruction to reduce pixel size.

Equipment Standard commercially available CT units are capable of this technique.

Technique The three major modifications of technique that constitute high-resolution computed tomography are thin slices to minimize partial lung imaging, reconstruction utilizing a high special frequency algorithm, and retargeting the area of interest to reduce pixel size.

References

Hansell DM, "High-Resolution Computed Tomography in the Evaluation of Fibrosing Alveolitis," *Clin Chest Med*, 1999, 20(4):739-60.

Heussel CP, Kauczor HU, Heussel GE, et al, "Pneumonia in Febrile Neutropenic Patients and in Bone Marrow and Blood Stem-Cell Transplant Recipients: Use of High-Resolution Computed Tomography," *J Clin Oncol*, 1999, 17(3):796-805.

Ikonen T, Kivisaari L, Taskinen E, et al, "High-Resolution CT in Long-Term Follow-up After Lung Transplantation," *Chest*, 1997, 111(2):370-6.

Kohlhaufl M, Brand P, Rock C, et al, "Noninvasive Diagnosis of Emphysema. Aerosol Morphometry and Aerosol Bolus Dispersion in Comparison to HRCT," *Am J Respir Crit Care Med*, 1999, 160(3):913-8.

Padley SP, Adler B, and Müller NL, "High-Resolution Computed Tomography of the Chest: Current Indications," *J Thorac Imaging*, 1993, 8(3):189-99.

Reuter M, Schnabel A, Wesner F, et al, "Pulmonary Wegener's Granulomatosis: Correlation Between High-Resolution CT Findings and Clinical Scoring of Disease Activity," *Chest*, 1998, 114(2):500-6.

Santamaria F, Grillo G, Guidi G, et al, "Cystic Fibrosis: When Should High-Resolution Computed Tomography of the Chest be Obtained?" *Pediatrics*, 1998, 101(5):908-13.

Syrjala H, Broas M, Suramo I, et al, "High-Resolution Computed Tomography for the Diagnosis of Community-Acquired Pneumonia," *Clin Infect Dis*, 1998, 27(2):358-63.

van Boxem TJ, Golding RP, Venmans BJ, et al, "High-Resolution CT in Patients With Intraluminal Typical Bronchial Carcinoid Tumors Treated With Bronchoscopic Therapy," *Chest*, 2000, 117(1):125-8.

Webb WR, Müller NL, and Naidich DP, "Standardized Terms for High-Resolution Computed Tomography of the Lung: A Proposed Glossary," *J Thorac Imaging*, 1993, 8(3):167-75.

Xaubet A, Agusti C, Luburich P, et al, "Pulmonary Function Tests and CT Scan in the Management of Idiopathic Pulmonary Fibrosis," *Am J Respir Crit Care Med*, 1998, 158(2):431-6.

Yassa NA and Wilcox AG, "High-Resolution CT Pulmonary Findings in Adults With Gaucher's Disease," *Clin Imaging*, 1998, 22(5):339-42.

♦ **HRCT** *see* High-Resolution CT *on page 359*

Hysterosalpingogram

Synonyms Uterogram

Procedure Commonly Includes Injection of a contrast agent into the uterus and fallopian tubes

Indications Examination allows demonstration and radiographic documentation of the outline of the uterine cavity. It also facilitates opacification of the fallopian tubes. Because of this, it is commonly part of the work-up in cases of infertility. Also used to evaluate the tubes subsequent to tubal ligation and to evaluate the results of reconstructive surgery.

(Continued)

Hysterosalpingogram *(Continued)*

Contraindications

- pregnancy
- active pelvic inflammatory disease (PID)

Complications While some procedural discomfort pain is frequently encountered, it is usually transient. Tubule granulomas are occasionally encountered and are thought to be more commonly related to the use of oil based contrast material.

Causes for Rejection Incorrect time in menstrual cycle. The exam is best performed following menstruation but before ovulation. This is usually between the 7th and 14th day of the menstrual cycle.

References

al-Badawi IA, Fluker MR, and Bebbington MW, "Diagnostic Laparoscopy in Infertile Women With Normal Hysterosalpingograms," *J Reprod Med*, 1999, 44(11):953-7.

Frye RE, Ascher SM, and Thomasson D, "MR Hysterosalpingography: Protocol Development and Refinement for Simulating Normal and Abnormal Fallopian Tube Patency - Feasibility Study With a Phantom," *Radiology*, 2000, 214(1):107-12.

Glatstein IZ, Sleeper LA, Lavy Y, et al, "Observer Variability in the Diagnosis and Management of the Hysterosalpingogram," *Fertil Steril*, 1997, 67(2):233-7.

Houmard BS and Seifer DB, "Infertility Treatment and Informed Consent: Current Practices of Reproductive Endocrinologists," *Obstet Gynecol*, 1999, 93(2):252-7.

Krysiewicz S, "Infertility in Women: Diagnostic Evaluation With Hysterosalpingography and Other Imaging Techniques," *AJR Am J Roentgenol*, 1992, 159(2):253-61.

McBean JH, Gibson M, and Brumsted JR, "The Association of Intrauterine Filling Defects on Hysterosalpingogram With Endometriosis," *Fertil Steril*, 1996, 66(4):522-6.

Mol BW, Swart P, Bossuyt PM, et al, "Is Hysterosalpingography an Important Tool in Predicting Fertility Outcome?" *Fertil Steril*, 1997, 67(4):663-9.

Soares SR, Barbosa dos Reis MM, and Camargos AF, "Diagnostic Accuracy of Sonohysterography, Transvaginal Sonography, and Hysterosalpingography in Patients With Uterine Cavity Disease," *Fertil Steril*, 2000, 73(2):406-11.

Stovall DW, "The Role of Hysterosalpingography in the Evaluation of Infertility," *Am Fam Physician*, 1997, 55(2):621-8.

Wolf DM and Spataro RF, "The Current State of Hysterosalpingography," *Radiographics*, 1988, 8(6):1041.

Yoder IC, "Diagnosis of Uterine Anomalies: Relative Accuracy of MR Imaging, Endovaginal Sonography, and Hysterosalpingography," *Radiology*, 1992, 185(2):343; discussion 344.

♦ **Infusion Pyelogram** *see* Urography *on page 367*

♦ **Intraoperative Cholangiogram** *see* Cholangiogram, Operative *on page 351*

♦ **Intravenous Pyelogram** *see* Urography *on page 367*

♦ **IVP** *see* Urography *on page 367*

♦ **KUB** *see* Abdomen X-ray *on page 347*

Laryngogram

Procedure Commonly Includes Fluoroscopic and radiographic evaluation of the larynx utilizing positive contrast material. CT scanning has replaced the use of tomography, xeroradiography, and laryngography for the radiologic evaluation of laryngeal tumors. This modality compliments direct laryngoscopy. Computed tomography demonstrates the status of the cartilage, tumor extension into the extralaryngeal and paralaryngeal spaces, and subglottic extensions.

References

Phelps PD, "Review: Carcinoma of the Larynx - The Role of Imaging in Staging and Pretreatment Assessments," *Clin Radiol*, 1992, 46(2):77-83.

Schuller DE and Bier-Laning CM, "Laryngeal Carcinoma Nodal Metastates and Their Management," *Otolaryngol Clin North Am*, 1997, 30(2):167-77.

Zbaren P, Becker M, and Lang H, "Pretherapeutic Staging of Laryngeal Carcinoma. Clinical Findings, Computed Tomography, and Magnetic Resonance Imaging Compared With Histopathology," *Cancer*, 1996, 77(7):1263-73.

Loop-O-Gram, X-ray

Procedure Commonly Includes Introduction of a catheter into the ileal conduit, injection of contrast material to reflux up the ureters and into the renal collecting systems.

Indications Evaluation of the collecting systems and ureters in patients who have previously undergone a urinary diversion

Patient Preparation Views on the necessity and the usefulness of cathartics in the preparation of patients for loop-o-grams vary. Some physicians advocate the routine use of 10 oz of magnesium citrate the evening before the examination. Alternatives would include a mild laxative such as $1^1/_4$ oz of a standard extract of senna fruit the evening before the examination. Others feel cathartics are not indicated.

Special Instructions Schedule this test before barium studies of the GI tract.

Turnaround Time Reports are mailed out within 24 hours after the examination is performed. If a preliminary reading is desired, please specify on the completed and signed requisition.

Causes for Rejection Residual barium

Lumbosacral Spine

Procedure Commonly Includes AP view of the lumbosacral spine obtained with the patient in the supine position and the knee flexed. Lateral view of the lumbosacral spine obtained with the patient recumbent. Oblique views of the lumbosacral spine are obtained, when requested, for demonstration of the pars interarticulares and the apophyseal joints to best advantage.

Indications Evaluate the bones for the presence of metastatic and primary neoplasms, trauma, infectious disease, degenerative, reactive, and post-surgical changes. Intervertebral disc spaces are also well evaluated by this method.

References

Carlson JR, Heller JG, Mansfield FL, et al, "Traumatic Open Anterior Lumbosacral Fracture Dislocation. A Report of Two Cases," *Spine*, 1999, 24(2):184-8.

Humke T, Grob D, Dvorak J, et al, "Translaminar Screw Fixation of the Lumbar and Lumbosacral Spine. A 5-Year Follow-up," *Spine*, 1998, 23(10):1180-4.

Miyake R, Ikata T, Katoh S, et al, "Morphologic Analysis of the Facet Joint in the Immature Lumbosacral Spine With Special Reference to Spondylolysis," *Spine*, 1996, 21(7):783-9.

Peh WC, Siu TH, and Chan JH, "Determining the Lumbar Vertebral Segments on Magnetic Resonance Imaging," *Spine*, 1999, 24(17):1852-5.

Reinus WR, Strome G, and Zwemer Fl Jr, "Use of Lumbosacral Spine Radiographs in a Level II Emergency Department," *AJR Am J Roentgenol*, 1998, 170(2):443-7.

van der Schaff DB, van Limbeek J, and Pavlov PW, "Temporary External Transpedicular Fixation of the Lumbosacral Spine," *Spine*, 1999, 24(5):481-4.

Viner A, Lee M, and Adams R, "Posteroanterior Stiffness in the Lumbosacral Spine. The Correlation Between Adjacent Vertebral Levels," *Spine*, 1997, 22(23):2724-9.

Weiner AL and MacKenzie RS, "Utilization of Lumbosacral Spine Radiographs for the Evaluation of Low Back Pain in the Emergency Department," *J Emerg Med*, 1999, 17(2):229-33.

Widmann RF, Hresko MT, and Hall JE, "Lumbosacral Fusion in Children and Adolescents Using the Modified Sacral Bar Technique," *Clin Orthop*, 1999, (364):85-91.

Mammogram

Synonyms Breast X-ray

Procedure Commonly Includes A minimum of two views of the breast

Indications A mammogram is indicated in the evaluation of any newly appearing breast lump considered suspicious for tumor. Because of the high incidence of breast cancer among the female population, the American Cancer Society recommends screening mammography for detection of cancer in the asymptomatic patient. The American Cancer Society sets down the following guidelines for screening. The society recommends a baseline mammogram be obtained in all females between the ages of 35 and 39. Between the ages of 40 and 49 they recommend a mammogram every 1-2 years. Patients 50 years of age or older are recommended to have a mammogram on an annual basis.

Patient Preparation Cleansing of the skin surface over both breasts and in the axilla is recommended prior to the examination. It should be noted that talcum powder and some deodorants may produce significant artifact on the film. Cleansing is therefore of the utmost importance to ensure no unnecessary repeat examinations.

Equipment The film screen mammogram is the best available method for radiographic examination of the breast.

Additional Information Nonpalpable breast lesions considered suspicious for malignancy should be excised. These abnormalities may be localized for the surgeon prior to surgery by the radiologist utilizing a localization needle. There are various localization markers commercially available. Subsequent to

(Continued)

Mammogram *(Continued)*

placement of the localization needle, its position within the abnormality is confirmed mammographically. The patient is then transported to the operating room. Once resected, the specimen is returned to Radiology where a further film is obtained to ensure that all the tissue believed to be suspicious in nature has been removed from the patient's breast.

References

Clark RA, "Economic Issues in Screening Mammography," *AJR Am J Roentgenol*, 1992, 158(3):527-34.

Hanchak NA, Kessler HB, MacPherson S, et al, "Screening Mammography: Experience in a Health Maintenance Organization," *Radiology*, 1997, 205(2):441-5.

Hindle WH, Davis L, and Wright D, "Clinical Value of Mammography for Symptomatic Women 35 Years of Age and Younger," *Am J Obstet Gynecol*, 1999, 180(6 Pt 1):1484-90.

Kalbhen CL, McGill JJ, Fendley PM, et al, "Mammographic Determination of Breast Volume: Comparing Different Methods," *AJR Am J Roentgenol*, 1999, 173(6):1643-9.

Lehman CD, White E, Peacock S, et al, "Effect of Age and Breast Density on Screening Mammograms With False-Positive Findings," *AJR Am J Roentgenol*, 1999, 173(6):1651-5.

Liberman L, Dershaw DD, Deutch BM, et al, "Screening Mammography: Value in Women 35-39 Years Old," *AJR Am J Roentgenol*, 1993, 161(1):53-6.

Parker JD, Sabogal F, and Gebretsadik T, "Relationship Between Earlier and Later Mammography Screening - California Medicare, 1992 Through 1994," *West J Med*, 1999, 170(1):25-7.

Wilson TE, Nijhawan VK, and Helvie MA, "Normal Mammograms and the Practice of Obtaining Previous Mammograms: Usefulness and Costs," *Radiology*, 1996, 198(3):661-3.

♦ **Mandible, Complete or Partial** *see* Skull, X-ray *on page 367*

♦ **Mastoids Complete** *see* Skull, X-ray *on page 367*

♦ **Maxilla** *see* Skull, X-ray *on page 367*

♦ **Metastatic Series Plus Long Bones** *see* Skeletal Survey *on page 366*

♦ **Nasal Bones** *see* Skull, X-ray *on page 367*

Oral Cholecystogram, Gallbladder Series

Related Information

Ultrasound, Gallbladder *on page 487*

Synonyms Cholecystography; Gallbladder Series; Gallbladder X-ray

Procedure Commonly Includes Radiographic examination of the gallbladder is performed subsequent to opacification of this organ by orally ingested contrast material. The patient ingests oral contrast material the evening prior to the radiographic examination. Radiographs of the right upper quadrant are obtained for evaluation of the opacified gallbladder.

Indications Cholelithiasis, cholecystitis, right upper quadrant pain. Ultrasound is the imaging method of choice for evaluation of the gallbladder. Oral cholecystography may be employed if the gallbladder is not visualized sonographically. It also may provide a measure of gallbladder function by allowing radiographic demonstration of contraction subsequent to ingestion of a fatty meal.

Contraindications

- prior cholecystectomy
- iodine allergy
- severe diarrhea

Patient Preparation Various oral contrast preparations are available. These are ingested the evening before the study and the dosage and timing of ingestion will be provided with the tablets. Some physicians advocate ingestion of a high fat lunch the day before the study. This stimulates evacuation of the gallbladder and refilling with opacified bile. The patient is to ingest nothing by mouth after midnight.

Special Instructions By appointment only

Complications The gallbladder may not be visualized for a number of reasons. This includes a lack of absorption of the contrast material from the patient's bowel. This may require an additional, repeat, or multiple day examination.

Equipment Standard radiography equipment

Additional Information This radiographic examination is rarely requested, having been almost totally supplanted by ultrasonography of the gallbladder. It is generally maintained among the radiology community that sonography warrants the pre-eminent position in the diagnosis of gallbladder disease.

References

Amberg JR and Leopold GR, "Is Oral Cholecystography Still Useful?" *Am J Roentgenol*, 1988, 151(1):73-4.

Chapman BA, Burt MJ, Chisholm RJ, et al, "Dissolution of Gallstones With Simvastatin, An HMG CoA Reductase Inhibitor," *Dig Dis Sci*, 1998, 43(2):349-53.

Chopra S, Chintapalli KN, Ramakrishna K, et al, "Helical CT Cholangiography With Oral Cholecystographic Contrast Material," *Radiology*, 2000, 214(2):596-601.

Gelfand DW, Wolfman NT, Ott DJ, et al, "Oral Cholecystography vs Gallbladder Sonography: A Prospective, Blinded Reappraisal," *AJR Am J Roentgenol*, 1988, 151(1):69-72.

Pereira SP, Veysey MJ, Kennedy C, et al, "Gallstone Dissolution With Oral Bile Acid Therapy. Importance of Pretreatment CT Scanning and Reasons for Nonresponse," *Dig Dis Sci*, 1997, 42(8):1775-82.

♦ **PA** *see* Chest Films *on page 350*

♦ **PA and Lateral CXR** *see* Chest Films *on page 350*

Paranasal Sinuses

Related Information

Computed Transaxial Tomography, Paranasal Sinuses *on page 337*

Synonyms Sinuses

Procedure Commonly Includes In the adult, the paranasal sinus radiographic evaluation usually includes four films. The first of these is obtained with the nose and forehead against the cassette and the x-ray beam passing in a posterior to anterior projection. The x-ray tube is tilted 15° caudally (Caldwell's projection). This projection demonstrates the frontal and ethmoid sinuses to best advantage. The maxillary sinuses are obscured by the petrous ridges in this projection. The maxillary antra are shown to best advantage with the Waters' projection. Here the beam again passes from a posterior to anterior direction and the patient's chin rests on the cassette. The nose is positioned 2-3 cm from the cassette. This view is generally obtained in both the recumbent and upright positions. The upright position allows demonstration of air fluid levels within the maxillary antra. The series is completed with a lateral projection of the paranasal sinuses. The sphenoid sinuses are seen to best advantage in this projection. The lateral projection also affords a good demonstration of the frontal sinuses.

Indications The examination is most commonly employed for the diagnosis of sinusitis. Films may demonstrate complete opacification of the sinuses, thickening of the mucoperiosteal lining of the sinuses, or air fluid levels. In addition to inflammatory conditions, this series of films may reveal congenital abnormalities, traumatic and neoplastic diseases. See Computed Transaxial Tomography, Paranasal Sinuses *on page 337.*

Patient Preparation No special preparation is required for this examination.

Special Instructions Relevant information pertinent to the examination should be indicated on the requisition which should accompany the patient to the Radiology Department.

Additional Information In the pediatric age group, the paranasal sinuses are difficult to evaluate due to variability in patterns of development. The maxillary and ethmoid sinuses are present and aerated at birth. The frontal sinuses usually do not develop until 7-10 years of age. The sphenoid sinuses develop shortly after the maxillary and ethmoid sinus cavities. The modified Waters' view and the lateral view suffice for evaluation of the paranasal sinuses in the pediatric population. In the pediatric population, the nose should be placed closer to the cassette for the Waters' projection. If the angulation is too steep, the sinuses may not be visualized or may appear falsely obliterated.

References

Phillips CD, "Current Status and New Developments in Techniques for Imaging the Nose and Sinuses," *Otolaryngol Clin North Am*, 1997, 30(3):371-87.

Rao VM and el-Noueam KL, "Sinonasal Imaging. Anatomy and Pathology," *Radiol Clin North Am*, 1998, 36(5):921-39, vi.

Witte RJ, Heurter JV, Orton DF, et al, "Limited Axial CT of the Paranasal Sinuses in Screening for Sinusitis," *AJR Am J Roentgenol*, 1996, 167(5):1313-5.

Yousem DM, "Imaging of Sinonasal Inflammatory Disease," *Radiology*, 1993, 188(2):303-14.

Pelvimetry

Procedure Commonly Includes Traditionally, pelvimetry has been performed utilizing the Colcher-Sussman pelvimeter with AP and lateral views

(Continued)

Pelvimetry *(Continued)*

of the pelvis. More recently, both computed tomography and magnetic resonance imaging have been used to diagnose cephalopelvic disproportion.

Indications Diagnosis of cephalopelvic disproportion

Patient Preparation Send patient with requisition to Radiology. The patient must wear x-ray gown to department.

References

Ferguson JE 2nd, De Angelis GA, Newberry YG, et al, "Fetal Radiation Exposure Is Minimal After Pelvimetry by Modified Digital Radiography," *Am J Obstet Gynecol*, 1996, 175(2):260-7; discussion: 267-9.

Freed KS, Kliewer MA, Hertzberg BS, et al, "Pelvic CT Morphometry in Down Syndrome: Implications for Prenatal US Evaluation - Preliminary Results," *Radiology*, 2000, 214(1):205-8.

Gherman RB, Tramont J, Muffley P, et al, "Analysis of McRoberts' Maneuver by X-ray Pelvimetry," *Obstet Gynecol*, 2000, 95(1):43-7.

Morris CW, Heggie JC, and Acton CM, "Computed Tomography Pelvimetry: Accuracy and Radiation Dose Compared With Conventional Pelvimetry," *Australas Radiol*, 1993, 37(2):186-91.

Sporri S, Hanggi W, Braghetti A, et al, "Pelvimetry by Magnetic Resonance Imaging as a Diagnostic Tool to Evaluate Dystocia," *Obstet Gynecol*, 1997, 89(6):902-8.

Sze EH, Kohli N, Miklos JR, et al, "Computed Tomography Comparison of Bony Pelvis Dimensions Between Women With and Without Genital Prolapse," *Obstet Gynecol*, 1999, 93(2):229-32.

Wade JP, "Accuracy of Pelvimetry Measurements on CT Scanners," *Br J Radiol*, 1992, 65(771):261-3.

Wright AR, English PT, Cameron HM, et al, "MR Pelvimetry - A Practical Alternative," *Acta Radiol*, 1992, 33(6):582-7.

♦ **Percutaneous Biopsy of Musculoskeletal Lesions and Synovial Membranes** *see* Bone Biopsy *on page 348*

♦ **Positive Contrast Examinations of the Pharynx and Esophagus** *see* Esophagram *on page 355*

♦ **Postoperative Cholangiography** *see* Cholangiography, Postoperative, T-Tube *on page 351*

Pyelogram, Retrograde

Related Information

Urography *on page 367*

Applies to Retrograde Pyelogram Generally Performed in the Operating Room

Procedure Commonly Includes AP view of the abdomen obtained prior to the introduction of any contrast material. Further films of the abdomen exposed subsequent to opacification of the ureters and renal collecting systems.

Indications Evaluation of renal collecting systems and ureters in cases where urography is unsatisfactory

Patient Preparation Obtain signed procedure permit for retrograde pyelogram. If the examination is to be done under general anesthesia, patient should have nothing by mouth after midnight. Bowel preparation recommendations are the same as those for urography.

Special Instructions Schedule this test before barium studies of the gastrointestinal tract.

Equipment When performed in the operating room, the room should be equipped with a standard overhead x-ray tube. If this is unavailable, portable radiographs may be obtained.

References

Babel SG and Winterkorn KG, "Retrograde Catheterization of the Ureter Without Cystoscopic Assistance: Preliminary Experience," *Radiology*, 1993, 187(2):547-9.

Chong PL and Thurston A, "Ureteric Calculus Diagnosed by Retrograde Ureterography During an Intravenous Urogram," *Urology*, 1999, 53(2):416.

Faerber GJ, Richardson TD, Farah N, et al, "Retrograde Treatment of Ureteropelvic Junction Obstruction Using the Ureteral Cutting Balloon Catheter," *J Urol*, 1997, 157(2):454-8.

Ghali AM, El Malik EM, Ibrahim, AL, et al, "Ureteric Injuries: Diagnosis, Management, and Outcome," *J Trauma*, 1999, 46(1):150-8.

Lugagne PM, Herve JM, Lebret T, et al, "Ureteroileal Implantation in Orthotopic Neobladder With the Le Duc-Camey Mucosal-Through Technique: Risk of Stenosis and Long-Term Follow-up," *J Urol*, 1997, 158(3 Pt 1):765-7.

Monga M, Smith R, Ferral H, et al, "Percutaneous Ablation of Caliceal Diverticulum: Long-Term Follow-up," *J Urol*, 2000, 163(1):28-32.

Nakada SY, "Acucise Endopyelotomy," *Urology*, 2000, 55(2):277-82.

Peuster M, Bertram H, Fink C, et al, "Percutaneous Transluminal Angioplasty for the Treatment of Complete Arterial Occlusion After Retrograde Cardiac Catheterization in Infancy," *Am J Cardiol*, 1999, 84(9):1124-6, A11.

Pienkos EJ, "Lumbar Ureteral Shunt: An Absolute Contraindication for Retrograde Pyelography," *J Urol*, 1996, 155(6):2026-7.

Platt JF, "Urinary Obstruction," *Radiol Clin North Am*, 1996, 34(6):1113-29.

Sadek S, Soloway MS, Hook S, et al, "The Value of Upper Tract Cytology After Transurethral Resection of Bladder Tumor in Patients With Bladder Transitional Cell Cancer," *J Urol*, 1999, 161(1):77-9; discussion: 79-80.

Ward AM, Kay R, and Ross JH, "Ureteropelvic Junction Obstruction in Children. Unique Considerations for Open Operative Intervention," *Urol Clin North Am*, 1998, 25(2):211-7.

♦ **Retrograde Pyelogram Generally Performed in the Operating Room** *see* Pyelogram, Retrograde *on page 364*

♦ **Scoliosis** *see* Scoliosis Series, X-ray *on page 365*

♦ **Scoliosis, Multiple Films** *see* Scoliosis Series, X-ray *on page 365*

Scoliosis Series, X-ray

Synonyms Scoliosis; Scoliosis, Multiple Films

Procedure Commonly Includes AP and lateral views of the spine are obtained at a standard 6 ft distance.

Indications Documentation of the type of curvature deformity and evaluation of the site and magnitude of deformity, assessment of the patient's skeletal maturity. Films of the spine are obtained for documentation of type and etiology of curvature deformity.

Technique Films are generally taken in the AP and lateral projections with the patient upright. Ideally, a 14" x 36" cassette is utilized so that the whole spine may be included. Film is exposed at standard 6 ft focal spot film distance to allow accurate measurement of growth. Ideally, an aluminum filter may be employed to achieve uniform radiographic density over the exposure.

Data Acquired The angular deformity may be measured by the Cobb-Lippman technique of measurement. These measurements are made by the orthopedist or orthopedic radiologist.

Turnaround Time Reports are mailed out within 24 hours after the examination is performed. If a preliminary reading is desired, please specify on the completed and signed requisition.

References

Bradford DS, Lonstein JE, Moe JH, et al, *Textbook of Scoliosis and Other Spinal Deformities*, 2nd ed, Philadelphia, PA: WB Saunders Co, 1987.

Burton DC, Asher MA, and Lai SM, "The Selection of Fusion Levels Using Torsional Correction Techniques in the Surgical Treatment of Idiopathic Scoliosis," *Spine*, 1999, 24(16):1728-39.

Comstock CP, Leach J, and Wenger DR, "Scoliosis in Total-Body-Involvement Cerebral Palsy. Analysis of Surgical Treatment and Patient and Caregiver Satisfaction," *Spine*, 1998, 23(12):1412-24; discussion: 1424-5.

Coonrad RW, Murrell GA, Motley G, et al, "A Logical Coronal Pattern Classification of 2,000 Consecutive Idiopathic Scoliosis Cases Based on the Scoliosis Research Society-Defined Apical Vertebra," *Spine*, 1998, 23(12):1380-91.

Grogan DP, Kalen V, Ross TI, et al, "Use of Allograft Bone for Posterior Spinal Fusion in Idiopathic Scoliosis," *Clin Orthop*, 1999, (369):273-8.

Luk KD, Cheung KM, Lu DS, et al, "Assessment of Scoliosis Correction in Relation to Flexibility Using the Fulcrum Bending Correction Index," *Spine*, 1998, 23(21):2303-7.

Matsui H, Ohmori K, Kanamori M, et al, "Significance of Sciatic Scoliotic List in Operated Patients With Lumbar Disc Herniation," *Spine*, 1998, 23(3):338-42.

Miladi LT, Ghanem IB, Draoui MM, et al, "Iliosacral Screw Fixation for Pelvic Obliquity in Neuromuscular Scoliosis. A Long-Term Follow-up Study," *Spine*, 1997, 22(15):1722-9.

Noordeen MH, Haddad FS, Edgar MA, et al, "Spinal Growth and a Histologic Evaluation of the Risser Grade in Idiopathic Scoliosis," *Spine*, 1999, 24(6):535-8.

Theologis TN, Fairbank JC, Turner-Smith AR, et al, "Early Detection of Progression in Adolescent Idiopathic Scoliosis by Measurement of Changes in Back Shape With the Integrated Shape Imaging System Scanner," *Spine*, 1997, 22(11):1223-7; discussion: 1228.

Tokunaga M, Minami S, Kitahara H, et al, "Vertebral Decancellation for Severe Scoliosis," *Spine*, 2000, 25(4):469-74.

♦ **Sella Turcica** *see* Skull, X-ray *on page 367*

Sialogram

Procedure Commonly Includes Placement of small catheter in the salivary duct and injection of contrast material with films obtained both preinjection and postinjection. Conventional radiography and sialography have proved very useful in the diagnosis of inflammatory disease of the salivary glands. The last

(Continued)

Sialogram *(Continued)*

decade has seen computed tomography emerge as the method of choice for evaluation of salivary gland neoplasms.

Indications These include recurrent sialoadenitis, pain, dryness of the mouth, postoperative or post-traumatic salivary fistula, or soft fluctuant swelling suggesting a sialocele. Sudden acute swelling of the gland especially during eating.

Contraindications

- acute infection
- sensitivity to iodine compounds

Patient Preparation The patient should be informed of the purpose of the study and its impact in determination of therapy. The patient should also be warned that the gland may enlarge as a result of this study but should return to normal size in the subsequent 24-48 hours.

Aftercare Evacuation of contrast material from the salivary glands may be facilitated by having the patient suck on a lemon or suck some citrate tablets. This will stimulate the flow of saliva and thus aid in the clearance of contrast material from the gland.

Limitations Cannot do bilateral sialogram; one side per day

References

Buckenham TM, George CD, MacVicar D, et al, "Digital Sialography: Imaging and Intervention," *Br J Radiol*, 1994, 67(798):524.

Drage NA, Brown JE, Wilson RF, et al, "Sialographic Changes in Sjögren and SOX Syndromes," *Oral Surg Oral Med Oral Pathol Oral Radiol Endod*, 1998, 86(1):104-9.

Nahlieli O and Baruchin AM, "Endoscopic Technique for the Diagnosis and Treatment of Obstructive Salivary Gland Diseases," *J Oral Maxillofac Surg*, 1999, 57(12):1394-401.

Shimizu M, Ussmuller J, Donath K, et al, "Sonographic Analysis of Recurrent Parotitis in Children: A Comparative Study With Sialographic Findings," *Oral Surg Oral Med Oral Pathol Oral Radiol Endod*, 1998, 86(5):606-15.

Stiller M, Golder W, Doring E, et al, "Diagnostic Value of Sialography With Both the Conventional and Digital Subtraction Techniques in Children With Primary and Secondary Sjögren Syndrome," *Oral Surg Oral Med Oral Pathol Oral Radiol Endod*, 1999, 88(5):620-7.

Varghese JC, Thornton F, Lucey BC, et al, "A Prospective Comparative Study of MR Sialography and Conventional Sialography of Salivary Duct Disease," *AJR Am J Roentgenol*, 1999, 173(6):1497-503.

Yoshiura K, Yuasa K, Tabata O, et al, "Reliability of Ultrasonography and Sialography in the Diagnosis of Sjögren Syndrome," *Oral Surg Oral Med Oral Pathol Oral Radiol Endod*, 1997, 83(3):400-7.

♦ **Sinuses** *see* Paranasal Sinuses *on page 363*

Skeletal Survey

Synonyms Metastatic Series Plus Long Bones

Procedure Commonly Includes Lateral skull, AP long bones, AP thorax with rib detail, AP lumbar with pelvis to include femoral heads, lateral cervical, dorsal, and lumbar spines

Indications Survey for metastatic disease, survey for battered child

Patient Preparation Any area to be radiographically examined should bare the lightest possible dressing and only if absolutely necessary.

Equipment Examination may be performed on commercially available radiography equipment.

Turnaround Time Report will be mailed out within 24 hours after the examination has been performed. If a preliminary reading is desired, please specify on the completed and signed requisition.

Limitations These examinations should be performed prior to barium studies of the gastrointestinal tract. Barium may obscure portions of the axial skeleton.

Additional Information A nuclear medicine bone scan is usually a more sensitive method of determining the presence of metastatic disease involving the skeleton. Whereas plain films of the bone may show no abnormality in the presence of considerable destruction. The bone scan reflects metabolic activity within the bone itself and is thus more sensitive in the detection of bone destruction. Rarely a tumor such as myeloma may be so aggressive as to produce a "cold spot" on the bone scan. In these cases a skeletal survey may be more effective in demonstrating the disseminated disease.

References

Kleinman PK, Nimkin K, Spevak MR, et al, "Follow-up Skeletal Surveys in Suspected Child Abuse," *AJR Am J Roentgenol*, 1996, 167(4):893-6.

- **Skull AP and Lateral** *see* Skull, X-ray *on page 367*
- **Skull Basilar View Only** *see* Skull, X-ray *on page 367*
- **Skull Series Complete** *see* Skull, X-ray *on page 367*

Skull, X-ray

Related Information

Facial Bones *on page 357*

Applies to Mandible, Complete or Partial; Mastoids Complete; Maxilla; Nasal Bones; Sella Turcica; Skull AP and Lateral; Skull Basilar View Only; Skull Series Complete; Temporomandibular Joints

Procedure Commonly Includes A series of radiographs, variable in number, obtained in projections designed to demonstrate the area of interest to maximum advantage.

Indications Establish the presence of fractures, infection, neoplastic destruction, degenerative and reactive processes of the skull, congenital anomalies

Patient Preparation Remove all jewelry, hairpins, glass eyes, braids, contact lenses, glasses, dentures, and dressings where possible.

Special Instructions Indicate if there is suspicion of neck injury since positioning requires considerable flexion and extension of neck.

Equipment Dedicated skull radiography unit desirable

References

Arana E and Marti-Bonmati L, "CT and MR Imaging of Focal Calvarial Lesions," *AJR Am J Roentgenol*, 1999, 172(6):1683-8.

Dahiya R, Keller JD, Litofsky NS, et al, "Temporal Bone Fractures: Otic Capsule Sparing Versus Otic Capsule Violating Clinical and Radiographic Considerations," *J Trauma*, 1999, 47(6):1079-83.

Damante JH, Filho LI, and Silva MA, "Radiographic Image of the Hard Palate and Nasal Fossa Floor in Panoramic Radiography," *Oral Surg oral Med Oral Pathol Oral Radiol Endod*, 1998, 85(4):479-84.

Frush DP, O'Hara SM, and Kliewer MA, "Pediatric Imaging Perspective: Acute Head Trauma - Is Skull Radiography Useful?" *J Pediatr*, 1998, 132(3 Pt 1):553-4.

Klufas RA, Hsu L, Patel MR, et al, "Unusual Manifestations of Head Trauma," *AJR Am J Roentgenol*, 1996, 166(3):675-81.

Masters SJ, "Evaluation of Head Trauma: Efficacy of Skull Films," *AJR Am J Roentgenol*, 1980, 135(3):539-47.

Miller EC, Derlet RW, and Kinser D, "Minor Head Trauma: Is Computed Tomography Always Necessary?" *Ann Emerg Med*, 1996, 27(3):290-4.

Tuli S, Tator Ch, Fehlings MG, et al, "Occipital Condyle Fractures," *Neurosurgery*, 1997, 41(2):368-76.

- **Small Bowel Enema** *see* Enteroclysis *on page 354*
- **Surgical Cholangiogram** *see* Cholangiogram, Operative *on page 351*
- **Temporomandibular Joints** *see* Skull, X-ray *on page 367*
- **Thoracic Spine** *see* Dorsal Spine *on page 353*
- **T-Tube** *see* Cholangiography, Postoperative, T-Tube *on page 351*
- **Upper GI Examination** *see* Gastrointestinal Series *on page 358*

Urography

Related Information

Pyelogram, Retrograde *on page 364*

Synonyms Infusion Pyelogram; Intravenous Pyelogram; IVP

Procedure Commonly Includes Intravenous administration of a contrast material. The contrast material is concentrated and excreted by the kidneys. Appropriate radiographs are exposed during the concentration and excretion of the contrast material for evaluation of the morphology and function of the urinary tract.

Indications This examination accurately demonstrates normal anatomy and a wide range of abnormalities involving the urinary tract.

Contraindications Allergy to iodine or a previous serious adverse reaction, advanced renal failure. A known diagnosis of multiple myeloma constitutes a relative contraindication. Every attempt should be made to hydrate patients

(Continued)

Urography *(Continued)*

with this diagnosis or with the diagnosis of diabetes mellitus prior to performance of a urogram as these patients run an increased risk of acute renal failure.

Patient Preparation Patients are encouraged to take nothing by mouth after midnight the night before the examination. This degree of fluid restriction will not produce significant dehydration but will improve the overall quality of the examination. If the urography examination is to be performed in the afternoon, a light liquid breakfast may be consumed. Views on the necessity and the usefulness of cathartics in the preparation of patients for urography vary. Some physicians advocate the routine use of 10 oz of magnesium citrate the evening before the examination. Alternatives would include a mild laxative such as 1¼ oz of a standard extract of senna fruit the evening before the examination.

Aftercare Encourage hydration by fluid ingestion.

Special Instructions All patients undergoing this examination should be questioned specifically with regard to drug allergies, particularly iodine. A recent serum creatinine is requested on patients 60 years of age or older, those with significant atherosclerotic disease, those with a known diagnosis of diabetes mellitus or with known pre-existing renal disease.

Complications Reactions to contrast material and specific treatment for such reactions are beyond the scope of this handbook. An appropriately equipped emergency cart should be immediately available should resuscitation be necessary.

Equipment Overhead radiography tube with float top table. Tomographic capabilities are desirable.

Limitations Urography should be performed prior to barium studies of the gastrointestinal tract. The presence of barium within the abdomen will compromise the urographic examination.

References

Clark RL, "IV Pyelography not for Diagnosis but in an Attempt to Flush Ureteral Calculi into the Urinary Bladder," *AJR Am J Roentgenol*, 1997, 169(6):1746.

Dorsam J, Knopp MV, Carl S, et al, "Ureteral Complications After Kidney Transplantation - Evaluation With Functional Magnetic Resonance Urography," *Transplant Proc*, 1997, 29(1-2):132-5.

Hattery RR, Williamson B Jr, Hartman GW, et al, "Intravenous Urographic Technique," *Radiology*, 1988, 167(3):593-9.

Holmang S, Hedelin H, Anderstrom C, et al, "Long-Term Follow-up of a Bladder Carcinoma Cohort: Routine Follow-up Urography Is not Necessary," *J Urol*, 1998, 160(1):45-8.

Katzberg RW, "Urography into the 21st Century: New Contrast Media, Renal Handling, Imaging Characteristics, and Nephrotoxicity," *Radiology*, 1997, 204(2):297-312.

Klein LT, Frager D, Subramanium A, et al, "Use of Magnetic Resonance Urography," *Urology*, 1998, 52(4):602-8.

Lautin EM, Schoenfeld A, and Choudhri A, "Subservience of Excretory Urography to Unenhanced CT in Evaluating Renal Colic: A Good Idea? - Benefits and Consequences," *Radiology*, 1998, 209(1):286-7.

Niall O, Russell J, MacGregor R, et al, "A Comparison of Noncontrast Computerized Tomography With Excretory Urography in the Assessment of Acute Flank Pain," *J Urol*, 1999, 161(2):534-7.

Nolte-Ernsting CC, Bucker A, Adam GB, et al, "Gadolinium-Enhanced Excretory MR Urography After Low-Dose Diuretic Injection: Comparison With Conventional Urography," *Radiology*, 1998, 209(1):147-57.

Sourtzis S, Thibeau JF, Damry N, et al, "Radiologic Investigation of Renal Colic: Unenhanced Helical CT Compared With Excretory Urography," *AJR Am J Roentgenol*, 1999, 172(6):1491-4.

♦ **Uterogram** *see* Hysterosalpingogram *on page 359*

♦ **Voiding Cystourethrogram** *see* Cystourethrogram *on page 353*

♦ **Zygomatic Arch, Left and Right** *see* Facial Bones *on page 357*

INVASIVE RADIOLOGY

- **Abdominal Aortogram** *see* Arteriogram, Transaxillary or Transbrachial Approach *on page 372*
- **Abdominal Aortogram** *see* Arteriogram, Transfemoral Approach *on page 373*

Abscess Drainage Under Fluoroscopic, Ultrasonic, or CT Guidance

Synonyms Catheter Drainage; External Decompression; Percutaneous Drainage

Applies to Drainage of Fluid Collection

Procedure Commonly Includes Placement of a catheter to drain or decompress an abscess or fluid collection. These examinations are typically performed under fluoroscopic, ultrasonic, or computed tomographic guidance. Aspirated material is usually sent for bacteriological, cytological, and/or chemical analysis.

Indications Determine the presence of an intra-abdominal, intrathoracic, or pelvic abscess; determine the presence of a symptomatic fluid collection (eg, hematoma, hygroma, lymphocele, urinoma, biloma, pseudocyst)

Contraindications An abscess or fluid collection which is inaccessible to percutaneous needle puncture, uncorrectable bleeding abnormalities, elevated laboratory coagulation parameters (INR, PTT, PTT), low platelet count

Patient Preparation Informed consent is obtained from the patient. The patient is placed on a clear liquid diet starting 4 hours before the procedure. Recent laboratory coagulation parameters (INR, PT, PTT, and platelet count) are recorded on the chart. In cases of abscesses and infected fluid collections, broad spectrum antibiotics are administered.

Aftercare The patient is placed on bedrest for approximately 4 hours after the procedure. Vital signs should be obtained every 30 minutes for 4 hours. During this time, the patient should be closely observed for any evidence of internal or external bleeding. The drainage catheters should be connected to a collection bag and output monitored. Appropriate precautions should be made that the catheter is not inadvertently pulled out. Catheter irrigation on a routine basis is essential to maintain catheter patency.

Special Instructions These examinations are usually arranged by the requesting physician in consultation with the physician performing the procedure. Any previous imaging studies of the area to be drained should be made available to the physician performing the procedure. Any bleeding abnormalities should be corrected beforehand.

Complications Most complications are related to either bleeding or sepsis from inadequate catheter placement. Delayed complications include fistula formation, plugging, pericatheter leakage or dislodgment of the drainage catheter.

Equipment Fluoroscopy, computed tomography, or ultrasonography; appropriate interventional needles, wires, and catheters

Technique The abscess or fluid collection is localized with ultrasound, CT, or occasionally fluoroscopy and the appropriate entry path is determined by the avoidance of critical organs. Local anesthesia is instilled at the appropriate site and a needle, with or without a sheath, is guided into the collection. Fluid

(Continued)

Abscess Drainage Under Fluoroscopic, Ultrasonic, or CT Guidance *(Continued)*

is aspirated and sent for appropriate bacteriological, cytological, and/or chemical analysis. If a sheathed needle system has been used, the sheath is advanced over the needle into the fluid collection. Otherwise, a wire is passed through the needle, the needle is removed, and a catheter is then inserted over the wire into the fluid collection. The catheter is then secured in place and connected to an external drainage bag. The catheter may need to be repositioned for optimal drainage.

Limitations Some fluid collections do not lend themselves to percutaneous drainage due to the presence of multiple septations within the collection and may require multiple catheter insertions. Some collections are inaccessible to percutaneous drainage secondary to overlying bony structures or close approximation to a vascular structure. If the material to be drained is very viscous, it may be necessary to place progressively larger drainage catheters.

References

Mueller PR, van Sonnenberg E, and Ferrucci JT Jr, "Percutaneous Drainage of 250 Abdominal Abscesses and Fluid Collections. Part II: Current Procedural Concepts," *Radiology*, 1984, 151(2):343-7.

Sones PJ, "Percutaneous Drainage of Abdominal Abscesses," *AJR Am J Roentgenol*, 1984, 142(1):35-9.

van Sonnenberg E, Mueller PR, and Ferrucci JT Jr, "Percutaneous Drainage of 250 Abdominal Abscesses and Fluid Collections. Part I: Results, Failures, and Complications," *Radiology*, 1984, 151(2):337-41.

- **Adrenal Arteriogram** *see* Arteriogram, Transfemoral Approach *on page 373*
- **Adrenal Venogram** *see* Venogram, Transfemoral or Transjugular Approach *on page 389*
- **Angiogram** *see* Arteriogram, Transfemoral Approach *on page 373*
- **Ankle Arthrogram** *see* Arthrogram *on page 374*

Antegrade Nephrostogram, Percutaneous

Synonyms Antegrade Pyelogram, Percutaneous

Procedure Commonly Includes Visualization of the upper urinary tract by the injection of contrast medium through a needle which has been percutaneously placed into a calix or the pelvis of the kidney.

Indications Determination of the cause and location of an obstruction of the upper urinary tract when an intravenous pyelogram or a retrograde pyelogram has not been helpful. Possible causes of obstruction include stone, neoplasm, compression from an extrinsic mass, retroperitoneal fibrosis, or an inflammatory, post-traumatic, or postsurgical stricture.

Patient Preparation Informed consent is obtained from the patient. The patient is placed on a clear liquid diet or NPO 4 hours before the procedure. Medications can be continued. An intravenous line is begun before the procedure to facilitate the administration of any medications or antibiotics required during the procedure. Most physicians will prescribe coverage with a broad spectrum antibiotic. Recent laboratory results (BUN, creatinine, platelet count, INR, PT, and PTT) should be recorded on the chart.

Aftercare The patient is placed on bedrest for approximately 4 hours. Vital signs should be obtained every 30 minutes for 2 hours, then every hour for 4 hours. The patient should be observed closely for any signs of sepsis or internal bleeding.

Special Instructions Any previous imaging study of the urinary tract should be made available to the interventional radiologist. Any bleeding abnormality should be corrected beforehand.

Complications Sepsis, shock, urinoma formation, hemorrhage

Equipment Fluoroscopy, ultrasound, needle, contrast medium, and method of x-ray film recording

Technique The patient is placed prone and a percutaneous entry site is chosen, usually with the assistance of ultrasound and/or fluoroscopy. If the kidney to be studied still functions adequately, contrast material can be injected intravenously to help localize the collecting system. Local anesthetic agent is instilled at the entry site which is usually located along the posterolateral aspect of the patient at approximately the level of the second lumbar vertebrae. A 21-gauge needle is then inserted into a calix or the pelvis of the kidney under fluoroscopic or ultrasonic guidance. Urine is aspirated and can be sent for Gram stain, culture, or cytology if desired. Contrast medium is then injected and x-ray films are obtained.

Data Acquired Opacification of an upper urinary tract

Normal Findings The pelvocalyceal system of the kidney and the ureter should be of normal caliber and configuration. There should be no evidence for any dilatation, filling defect, extrinsic compression, stricture formation, or extravasation. Contrast should flow freely down the ureter into the urinary bladder.

Limitations It can be difficult to successfully cannulate a urinary collection system which is both nondilated and not visualized from an intravenous injection of contrast medium.

References

Newhouse JH and Pfister RC, "Antegrade Pyelography," *Interventional Radiology*, Athanasoulis CA, Pfister RC, Green RE, et al, eds, Philadelphia, PA: WB Saunders Co, 1982, 437-54.

♦ **Antegrade Pyelogram, Percutaneous** *see* Antegrade Nephrostogram, Percutaneous *on page 370*

Aortogram, Translumbar Approach

Synonyms Translumbar Abdominal Aortogram; Translumbar Aortogram

Procedure Commonly Includes Visualization of the infrarenal abdominal aorta and iliac arteries by the injection of contrast medium through a needle which has been percutaneously placed through the lumbar region

Indications Evaluation of the abdominal aorta and iliac vessels for aneurysmal dilatation, atherosclerotic irregularity, stenosis, or occlusion

Contraindications

- acute renal failure
- known aneurysm at the projected site of puncture
- bleeding abnormalities
- elevated laboratory coagulation parameters (INR, PT, PTT)
- extremely high blood pressure
- shock

Patient Preparation Informed consent is obtained from the patient. If the procedure is to be performed under general anesthesia, the patient should be NPO; otherwise, the patient is placed on a clear liquid diet the morning of the procedure. An intravenous line is begun before the procedure in order to ensure that the patient is well hydrated and to facilitate the administration of any medications required during the procedure. Recent laboratory results (BUN, creatinine, platelet count, INR, PT, and PTT) should be recorded on the chart.

Aftercare Continued hydration is recommended. The patient is placed on bedrest for at least 6 hours after the procedure and often for the remainder of the day. Vital signs should be obtained at every 30 minutes for 2 hours then every hour for 4 hours. The patient should be observed for any signs of retroperitoneal hemorrhage, such as an unexplained decrease in blood pressure with an increase in pulse rate. Many physicians will obtain a follow-up hematocrit 12-24 hours after the procedure.

Special Instructions These examinations are often arranged by the requesting physician in consultation with the physician performing the procedure. Depending on the institution, the procedure may be performed in the operating room or in the angiography suite. Any previous imaging studies of the abdominal aorta or iliac arteries should be made available to the physician performing the procedure. Any patient problems (ie, renal insufficiency, bleeding abnormalities, diabetes, or history of severe contrast reaction) should be noted.

Complications Retroperitoneal or para-aortic hemorrhage, dissection of the abdominal aorta or one of its branches, hemothorax or pneumothorax, pseudoaneurysm, paraplegia, or osteomyelitis of the adjacent vertebral body or disc

(Continued)

Aortogram, Translumbar Approach *(Continued)*

Equipment 18-gauge needle, with or without a sheath; fluoroscopy; x-ray machine

Technique With the patient lying prone, local anesthesia is instilled in the lumbar region beneath the 12th rib and to the left of the midline. Under fluoroscopic guidance, the needle is inserted into the abdominal aorta at the level of the L2-3 lumbar vertebral bodies. Contrast is injected and films are obtained.

Data Acquired Visualization of the infrarenal abdominal aorta and of the iliac arteries

Normal Findings The abdominal aorta should be smooth and normal in caliber without evidence of irregularity, aneurysm, stenosis, or occlusion.

Limitations Anything which would obscure the blood vessels, such as overlying barium or patient motion.

References

Johnsrude IS, "Catheterization Techniques," *A Practical Approach to Angiography*, 2nd ed, Johnsrude IS, Jackson DC, and Dunnick NR, eds, Boston, MA: Little, Brown and Co, 1987, 44-70.

- ♦ **Arm Arteriogram** *see* Arteriogram, Transaxillary or Transbrachial Approach *on page 372*
- ♦ **Arm Arteriogram** *see* Arteriogram, Transfemoral Approach *on page 373*
- ♦ **Arm Venogram** *see* Venogram, Extremity *on page 389*
- ♦ **Arterial Study** *see* Arteriogram, Transfemoral Approach *on page 373*
- ♦ **Arterial Study via Upper Extremity Approach** *see* Arteriogram, Transaxillary or Transbrachial Approach *on page 372*

Arteriogram, Transaxillary or Transbrachial Approach

Synonyms Arterial Study via Upper Extremity Approach; Brachial Cut-Down; Transaxillary Angiogram; Transbrachial Angiogram

Applies to Abdominal Aortogram; Arm Arteriogram; Hepatic Arteriogram; Leg Arteriogram; Mesenteric Arteriogram; Pelvic Arteriogram; Renal Arteriogram; Splenic Arteriogram; Thoracic Aortogram; Vertebral Arteriogram

Procedure Commonly Includes Visualization of the arteries in the area of clinical concern by injection of contrast medium through a catheter which has been placed through the brachial or axillary artery. This upper extremity approach is an alternative to the femoral artery approach, especially when the femoral artery approach is not feasible secondary to femoral artery occlusion, aneurysm, or infection.

Indications Evaluation of the arteries in the area of clinical interest for abnormalities (eg, arterial aneurysm, atherosclerosis, embolism, fistula, hemorrhage, neoplasm, occlusion, arteriovenous shunting, stenosis, thrombosis, trauma, vasculitis).

Contraindications

- absence of axillary pulses
- acute renal failure
- bleeding abnormalities
- elevated laboratory coagulation parameters (INR, PT, PTT),
- extremely high blood pressure
- shock

Patient Preparation Informed consent is obtained from the patient. The patient is placed on a clear liquid diet on the morning of the procedure. All medications are continued. If the axillary approach is to be used, the appropriate axilla should be shaved. Similarly, if a brachial approach is anticipated, the antecubital fossa should be shaved if necessary. An intravenous line is begun in the opposite arm before the procedure in order to ensure that the patient is well hydrated (thus decreasing the risk of acute renal failure) and to facilitate the administration of any medications required during the procedure. Recent laboratory results (BUN, creatinine, platelet count, INR, PT, and PTT) should be recorded on the chart.

Aftercare The patient needs be on bedrest for only 3-4 hours after the procedure. The patient should keep the upper extremity used for the procedure at rest at his side for the remainder of the day. Eating and other activity should be performed with the opposite arm. Vital signs should be obtained every 30 minutes for the first 2 hours, then every hour for the next 4 hours. At these times, the axilla or brachial entry site should be examined for any evidence of bleeding or swelling and the arm should be evaluated for any change in pulses, color, or warmth. Also, the hand grasp should be evaluated at these times to evaluate for any potential nerve damage. No blood pressure should be obtained using that arm for the following 48 hours. If the procedure has been performed via a cut-down, skin sutures must be removed in 5-6 days.

Special Instructions These examinations are often arranged by the requesting physician in consultation with the cardiovascular radiologist. The requisition should state clearly the reason for the study as well as the specific vessels to be examined. Any previous imaging studies of the area to be examined should be made available to the cardiovascular radiologist. The performing physician should be alerted to any potential problem areas in the patient's condition (eg, renal insufficiency, bleeding abnormalities, or history of severe contrast reaction).

Complications Immediate complications include contrast reaction, acute renal failure, bleeding or hematoma formation at the puncture site or the site of the cut-down, vessel dissection or occlusion, and distal embolization of any clots which may have formed on the catheter. A complication unique to the axillary approach is the potential for brachial plexus neuropathy secondary to hematoma formation within the brachial plexus sheath.

Equipment Fluoroscopy, angiographic catheters and wires, a cut-down tray if a brachial artery cut-down approach is anticipated, and a method of film recording (either conventional cut-film or digital subtraction films).

Technique A local anesthetic agent is instilled over either the axillary artery or the brachial artery. For the axillary approach, the artery is percutaneously punctured. For the brachial approach, the artery can be either percutaneously punctured or a cut-down can be performed. After the catheter is inserted, it is fluoroscopically guided into the artery of interest. Contrast medium is injected and the films are obtained.

Data Acquired Visualization of the arteries in the area of clinical concern on either conventional x-ray film or on digitally subtracted images, sometimes referred to as intra-arterial DSA.

Normal Findings The opacified arteries should be smooth and gradually taper as they continue to branch. There should be no evidence of vessel wall irregularity, aneurysm, narrowing, occlusion, extravasation, or arteriovenous shunting.

Limitations Anything which would obscure the blood vessels, such as overlying barium or patient motion.

References

Johnsrude IS, "Catheterization Techniques," *A Practical Approach to Angiography*, 2nd ed, Johnsrude IS, Jackson DC, and Dunnick NR, eds, Boston, MA: Little, Brown and Co, 1987, 47-70.

Arteriogram, Transfemoral Approach

Synonyms Angiogram; Arterial Study; Percutaneous Transfemoral Angiogram

Applies to Abdominal Aortogram; Adrenal Arteriogram; Arm Arteriogram; Bronchial Arteriogram; Carotid Arteriogram; Cerebral Arteriogram; Coronary Arteriogram; Hepatic Arteriogram; Leg Arteriogram; Mesenteric Arteriogram; Pelvic Arteriogram; Renal Arteriogram; Splenic Arteriogram; Thoracic Aortogram; Vertebral Arteriogram

Procedure Commonly Includes Visualization of the arteries in the area of clinical concern by injection of contrast medium through a catheter which has been percutaneously placed through the femoral artery

Indications Evaluation of the arteries in the area of clinical interest for abnormalities such as arterial aneurysm, atherosclerosis, embolism, fistula, hemorrhage, neoplasm, occlusion, arteriovenous shunting, stenosis, thrombosis, trauma, vasculitis.

Contraindications

- inability of patient to lie supine
- absence of femoral pulses
- acute renal failure

(Continued)

Arteriogram, Transfemoral Approach *(Continued)*

- bleeding abnormalities
- elevated laboratory coagulation parameters (INR, PT, PTT)
- extremely high blood pressure
- shock

Patient Preparation Informed consent is obtained from the patient. The patient is placed on a clear liquid diet on the morning of the procedure. All medications are continued. An intravenous line is begun before the procedure in order to ensure that the patient is well hydrated (thus decreasing the risk of acute renal failure) and to facilitate the administration of any medications required during the procedure. Recent laboratory results (BUN, creatinine, platelet count, INR, PT, and PTT) should be recorded on the chart.

Aftercare The patient is placed on bedrest for at least 6 hours after the procedure and often for the remainder of the day. During this time, the patient should be flat in bed with the legs straight. Vital signs should be obtained every 30 minutes for the first 2 hours, then every hour for the next 4 hours. At these times, the femoral puncture site should be examined for any evidence of bleeding or swelling and the leg should be examined for any change in pulses, color, or warmth.

Special Instructions These examinations are often arranged by the requesting physician in consultation with the cardiovascular radiologist. The requisition should state clearly the reason for the study as well as the specific vessels to be examined. Any previous imaging studies of the area to be examined should be made available to the cardiovascular radiologist. The performing physician should be alerted to any potential problem areas in the patient's condition (eg, renal insufficiency, bleeding abnormalities, or history of severe contrast reaction).

Complications Immediate complications include contrast reaction, acute renal failure, bleeding or hematoma formation at the puncture site, vessel dissection or occlusion, and distal embolization of any clots which may have formed on the catheter. Delayed complications consist of formation of either a false aneurysm or arteriovenous fistula at the puncture site.

Equipment Fluoroscopy, angiographic catheter and wires, a cut-down tray if a brachial artery cut-down approach is anticipated and, a method of film recording (either conventional cut-film or digital subtraction films).

Technique A local anesthetic agent is instilled over the common femoral artery. The artery is percutaneously punctured and a catheter is inserted and fluoroscopically guided into the artery of interest. Contrast medium is injected and the films are obtained.

Data Acquired Visualization of the arteries in the area of clinical concern on either conventional x-ray film or on digitally subtracted images, sometimes referred to as intra-arterial DSA.

Normal Findings The opacified arteries should be smooth and gradually taper as they continue to branch. There should be no evidence of vessel wall irregularity, aneurysm, narrowing, occlusion, extravasation, or arteriovenous shunting.

Limitations Anything which would obscure the blood vessels, such as overlying barium or patient motion

References

Johnsrude IS, "Catheterization Techniques," *A Practical Approach to Angiography*, 2nd ed, Johnsrude IS, Jackson DC, and Dunnick NR, eds, Boston, MA: Little, Brown and Co, 1987, 33-44, 58-70.

♦ **Arteriovenous Fistulogram** *see* Dialysis Fistulogram *on page 378*

Arthrogram

Synonyms Joint Study

Applies to Ankle Arthrogram; Elbow Arthrogram; Hip Arthrogram; Knee Arthrogram; Shoulder Arthrogram; Temporomandibular Joint Arthrogram; Wrist Arthrogram

Indications Evaluation of any damage to the cartilage, ligaments, and bony structures composing the joint or soft tissue masses in the joint

Contraindications Bleeding abnormalities

Patient Preparation Informed consent is obtained from the patient.

Aftercare No strenuous activity involving the joint of interest for 24 hours.

Equipment 18- to 22-gauge needle (needle size will vary according to the joint being studied), contrast medium, fluoroscopic and x-ray equipment

Technique Local anesthesia is instilled at the appropriate site. A small gauge needle is inserted into the joint space. Any fluid within the joint space is aspirated and sent for appropriate chemical or bacteriologic analysis. Contrast medium, with or without air, is then inserted into the joint space under fluoroscopic guidance. Radiographs and occasionally tomograms are then obtained in multiple projections. In addition, CT imaging of the joint of study may also be performed.

Data Acquired Visualization of the components of the joint space including the cartilage, ligaments, menisci, and connecting bursa

Normal Findings The joint space should not contain fluid or masses. The cartilaginous surfaces and menisci should be smooth without evidence for erosions, tears, or disintegration.

Limitations Large joint effusions can be difficult to aspirate completely, thus resulting in dilution of the contrast material and poor visualization of the joint space structures.

References

Resnick D, "Arthrography, Tenography and Bursography," *Diagnosis of Bone and Joint Disorders*, 2nd ed, Philadelphia, PA: WB Saunders Co, 1996, 113-35.

♦ **Biliary Decompression** *see* Biliary Drainage, Percutaneous Transhepatic *on page 375*

Biliary Drainage, Percutaneous Transhepatic

Synonyms Biliary Decompression; External Biliary Drainage

Applies to Biliary Stent Placement, Percutaneous; Biliary Stricture Dilatation, Percutaneous; Cholecystostomy, Percutaneous; Gallbladder Drainage, Percutaneous

Procedure Commonly Includes Percutaneous placement of a drainage catheter in an obstructed biliary system

Indications Biliary obstruction resulting in jaundice, cholangitis, sepsis, or pain. The site of the obstruction should be in one of the larger ducts (ie, right hepatic, left hepatic, common hepatic, or common bile duct). The cause of obstruction can be secondary to malignancy, stone, pancreatitis, or stricture related to surgery, trauma, or infection. Drainage of the gallbladder can be performed in cases of cholecystitis and/or calculi when patients are at too high a risk for surgery.

Contraindications

- tense ascites
- bleeding abnormalities
- elevated laboratory coagulation parameters (INR, PT, PTT)
- low platelet count

Patient Preparation Informed consent is obtained from the patient. The patient is placed on a clear liquid diet or NPO 4 hours before the procedure. All medications are continued. An intravenous line is begun before the procedure in order to ensure that the patient is well hydrated and to facilitate the administration of any medications required during the procedure. If the patient is not already on antibiotics, a broad spectrum antibiotic should be administered intravenously 30 minutes before the procedure. Recent laboratory results (BUN, creatinine, platelet count, INR, PT, and PTT) should be recorded on the chart.

Aftercare The patient is placed on bedrest for approximately 4 hours. Vital signs should be obtained every 30 minutes for 2 hours, then every hour for 4 hours. The patient should be observed closely for any signs of internal bleeding or sepsis.

Special Instructions The volume of output from the biliary drain should be recorded. While the drainage may be blood tinged, any profuse bleeding from the catheter should be attended to promptly. If the drainage ceases completely, the catheter may be irrigated to remove blood clots or debris. (Continued)

Biliary Drainage, Percutaneous Transhepatic *(Continued)*

Drainage of bile around the catheter at the skin site is usually a sign that the catheter is at least partially obstructed.

Complications Bleeding and sepsis are the most common complications, occurring in as many as 5% to 10% of cases. Delayed complications include dislodgment or plugging of the drainage catheter, infection at the skin entry site, development of a biloma, or erosion of a hepatic blood vessel by the catheter resulting in hemobilia or pseudoaneurysm formation.

Equipment Fluoroscopy, steerable wires, and catheters

Technique The site of entry is determined using fluoroscopy and/or ultrasound. Local anesthetic agent is instilled at the entry site and a needle is inserted into the biliary system. After the ducts have been opacified with contrast, a steerable wire is maneuvered to the point of obstruction. A drainage catheter is then passed over this wire. The catheter is affixed to the skin to prevent dislodgment. This percutaneous access route can later be used for placement of a stent across the obstruction or for balloon dilatation of an obstructing stricture. Essentially, the same technique is used for drainage of the gallbladder.

Data Acquired A bile specimen can be sent for Gram stain and culture.

Limitations Obstructions cephalad to the level of the porta hepatis are usually not amenable to drainage.

References

Ferrucci JT Jr, Mueller PR, and Harbin WP, "Percutaneous Transhepatic Biliary Drainage: Technique, Results, and Applications," *Radiology*, 1980, 135(1):1-13.

McLean GK, Ring EJ, and Freiman DB, "Therapeutic Alternatives in the Treatment of Intrahepatic Biliary Obstruction," *Radiology*, 1982, 145(2):289-95.

♦ **Biliary Stent Placement, Percutaneous** *see* Biliary Drainage, Percutaneous Transhepatic *on page 375*

♦ **Biliary Stricture Dilatation, Percutaneous** *see* Biliary Drainage, Percutaneous Transhepatic *on page 375*

Biopsy, Percutaneous Needle, Under Fluoroscopic, CT, or Ultrasound Guidance

Synonyms Needle Aspiration Biopsy

Applies to Needle Biopsy Under CT Guidance; Needle Biopsy Under Ultrasound Guidance; Needle Localization; Transthoracic Needle Aspiration Biopsy

Procedure Commonly Includes Obtaining a sample of cells from a mass via a percutaneously placed needle. The needle placement can be performed using fluoroscopic, ultrasonic, or computed tomographic guidance. The specimen is then sent for cytologic, pathologic, or bacteriologic analysis.

Indications Determine the presence of a mass of unknown origin

Contraindications Masses of vascular origin (aneurysm, pseudoaneurysm, arteriovenous malformation, etc) are absolute contraindications for biopsy. Neoplasms that are highly vascular (hemangioma, meningioma, hypervascular malignant neoplasms, etc) are relative contraindications. Other contraindications are bleeding abnormalities, elevated laboratory coagulation parameters (INR, PT, PTT), low platelet count.

Patient Preparation Informed consent is obtained from the patient. The patient is placed on a clear liquid diet or NPO 4 hours before the procedure. An intravenous line is begun before the procedure to facilitate the administration of any medications required during the procedure. Recent laboratory results (BUN, creatinine, platelet count, INR, PT, and PTT) should be recorded on the chart.

Aftercare The patient is placed on bedrest for approximately 4 hours after the procedure. Vital signs should be obtained every 30 minutes for 2 hours, then every hour for 4 hours. During this time, the patient should be closely observed for any evidence of internal or external bleeding. If biopsy has involved the thoracic region, the patient should be observed for any signs of a pneumothorax or hemothorax.

Special Instructions These examinations are usually arranged by the requesting physician in consultation with the physician performing the procedure. Any previous imaging studies of the mass to be biopsied should be made available to the interventional radiologist. Any bleeding abnormalities should be corrected beforehand.

Complications Most complications are related to either bleeding, pneumothorax, or sepsis.

Equipment Fluoroscopy, computed tomography, or ultrasonography; aspiration or cutting biopsy needles; appropriate fixatives or culture media

Technique The mass or region to be biopsied is localized with ultrasound, CT, or fluoroscopy and the appropriate entry path is determined. Local anesthesia is instilled at the appropriate site and the aspiration or cutting biopsy needle is guided into the mass. The specimen is then sent to the laboratory for appropriate cytological, pathological, or bacteriological analysis. If a sufficient amount of cellular material is not obtained and the patient remains stable, the procedure can be repeated.

Data Acquired Cytologic, pathologic, or bacteriologic analysis of the cells within a mass

Limitations Some masses are inaccessible to percutaneous biopsy secondary to overlying bony structures or close approximation to vascular structures.

References

Bernardino ME, "Percutaneous Biopsy," *AJR Am J Roentgenol*, 1984, 142(1):41-5.

♦ **Bipedal Lymphangiography** *see* Lymphangiogram *on page 380*

♦ **Brachial Cut-Down** *see* Arteriogram, Transaxillary or Transbrachial Approach *on page 372*

♦ **Bronchial Arteriogram** *see* Arteriogram, Transfemoral Approach *on page 373*

♦ **Carotid Arteriogram** *see* Arteriogram, Transfemoral Approach *on page 373*

♦ **Catheter Drainage** *see* Abscess Drainage Under Fluoroscopic, Ultrasonic, or CT Guidance *on page 369*

♦ **Catheter Portography** *see* Portal Venogram, Percutaneous Transhepatic *on page 384*

♦ **Cerebral Arteriogram** *see* Arteriogram, Transfemoral Approach *on page 373*

♦ **Cervical Myelogram** *see* Myelogram *on page 381*

Cholangiogram, Percutaneous Transhepatic (PTC)

Applies to Cholecystogram, Percutaneous

Procedure Commonly Includes Visualization of the biliary system by the injection of contrast medium through a needle which has been percutaneously placed into the intrahepatic biliary system or, occasionally, the gallbladder

Indications Determination of the cause and location of an obstruction of the biliary system. Possible causes include stones, pancreatitis, sclerosing cholangitis, inflammatory or traumatic stricture, pancreatic carcinoma, cholangiocarcinoma, gallbladder carcinoma, and metastases.

Contraindications

- inability of patient to lie supine
- bleeding abnormalities
- elevated coagulation parameters (INR, PT, PTT)
- acute renal failure

Patient Preparation Informed consent is obtained from the patient. The patient is placed on a clear liquid diet or NPO 4 hours before the procedure. All medications are continued. An intravenous line is begun before the procedure in order to ensure that the patient is well hydrated (thus decreasing the risk of acute renal failure) and to facilitate the administration of any medications required during the procedure. Most physicians will prescribe coverage with broad spectrum antibiotics. Blood typing is often requested beforehand. Recent laboratory results (BUN, creatinine, platelet count, INR, PT, and PTT) should be recorded on the chart.

Aftercare The patient is placed on bedrest for approximately 4 hours. Vital signs should be obtained every 30 minutes for 2 hours, then every hour for 4

(Continued)

Cholangiogram, Percutaneous Transhepatic (PTC) *(Continued)*

hours. The patient should be observed closely for any signs of internal bleeding or sepsis.

Special Instructions Any previous imaging study of the hepatobiliary system should be made available to the interventional radiologist. Any potential problem areas should be noted (eg, renal insufficiency, bleeding abnormalities, history of severe contrast reaction).

Complications Most complications are secondary to either sepsis or hemorrhage.

Equipment Fluoroscopy, ultrasound, needle, contrast medium, and a method of x-ray film recording

Technique A percutaneous entry site is chosen, usually with the assistance of ultrasound and/or fluoroscopy. Local anesthetic agent is instilled at the entry site. A 20-gauge needle is inserted into the liver until a bile duct is encountered. This may require several passages with the needle until a duct is successfully cannulated. Contrast medium is then injected and x-ray films are obtained. A sample of bile is often sent for Gram stain and culture.

Data Acquired Opacification of the biliary system

Normal Findings The bile duct should be smooth and of normal caliber. There should be no evidence of any dilatation, filling defects, bile duct narrowing, or extravasation. Contrast should flow freely into the duodenum.

Limitations It can be difficult to successfully cannulate intrahepatic bile ducts which are not dilated, especially in cases of sclerosing cholangitis where the ducts are narrower than normal.

References

Mueller PR, Harbin WP, Ferrucci JT Jr, et al, "Fine-Needle Transhepatic Cholangiography: Reflections After 450 Cases," *AJR Am J Roentgenol*, 1981, 136(1):85-90.

Turner MA, Cho SR, and Messmer JM, "Pitfalls in Cholangiographic Interpretation," *Radiographics*, 1987, 7(6):1067-105.

♦ **Cholecystogram, Percutaneous** *see* Cholangiogram, Percutaneous Transhepatic (PTC) *on page 377*

♦ **Cholecystostomy, Percutaneous** *see* Biliary Drainage, Percutaneous Transhepatic *on page 375*

♦ **Coronary Arteriogram** *see* Arteriogram, Transfemoral Approach *on page 373*

Dialysis Fistulogram

Synonyms Arteriovenous Fistulogram; Dialysis Shuntogram

Procedure Commonly Includes Visualization of an arteriovenous fistula or graft which has been constructed as a vascular access for dialysis

Indications Evaluation of the cause of poor flow through or loss of pulse in a dialysis fistula or graft

Contraindications

- bleeding abnormalities
- elevated laboratory coagulation parameters (INR, PT, PTT)
- low platelet count

Patient Preparation Informed consent is obtained from the patient. The patient is placed on a clear liquid diet 2-4 hours before the procedure. An intravenous line is begun before the procedure in order to facilitate the administration of any medications required during the procedure. Recent laboratory results (platelet count, INR, PT, and PTT) should be recorded on the chart.

Aftercare The needle entry site should be observed for bleeding or hematoma formation.

Complications Bleeding or hematoma formation at the needle entry site, thrombosis of the graft or fistula, extravasation of contrast material into the surrounding soft tissues

Equipment Fluoroscopy, angiographic catheter or needle, and a method of film recording

Technique Local anesthetic agent is instilled over the fistula or graft. The fistula is palpated and punctured with a needle. Blood return will confirm that the needle tip is intraluminal. If desired, the needle can be exchanged for an angiographic catheter. Contrast material is injected and the films are obtained.

Data Acquired Visualization of the arteriovenous fistula, the surgical anastomoses, the artery supplying the fistula or graft and the veins draining it

Normal Findings The surgical anastomoses should be patent without evidence for stenosis. The artery supplying the fistula, as well as the veins draining it, should be normal in caliber without evidence of stricture or occlusion.

Limitations Inability to adequately and securely cannulate the fistula will preclude contrast injection

References

Gilula L, Staple TW, Anderson CB, et al, "Venous Angiography of Hemodialysis Fistulas, Experience With 52 Studies," *Radiology*, 1975, 115(3):555-62.

♦ **Dialysis Shuntogram** *see* Dialysis Fistulogram *on page 378*

Digital Subtraction Angiogram, Intravenous

Synonyms DSA; IV-DSA

Procedure Commonly Includes Visualization of the arteries in the area of clinical concern by injection of contrast medium into a catheter placed in an arm vein and recording the subsequent x-ray images using digital computer technology

Indications Screening evaluation of arteries for stenoses or occlusions, typically renal arteries for hypertension and carotid arteries for transient ischemic attacks (TIA). Also useful for follow-up evaluation of angioplasty sites and surgical grafts.

Contraindications

- inability of patient to lie flat and motionless
- acute renal failure

Patient Preparation Informed consent is obtained from the patient. The patient is placed on a clear liquid diet 2-4 hours before the procedure. Recent laboratory studies (BUN, creatinine) should be recorded on the chart.

Aftercare A small compression dressing is applied to the venous catheter entry site for the remainder of the day.

Complications Contrast reaction, acute renal failure, upper extremity vein thrombosis

Equipment An intracatheter or angiographic catheter, fluoroscopy, and a digital subtraction angiographic unit

Technique An intracatheter or an angiographic catheter is placed into a vein of the upper extremity, typically in the antecubital fossa. Most angiographers will advance the catheter under fluoroscopy into the superior vena cava or right atrium; others will merely place an angiocatheter through the vein up to the upper arm. Approximately 40-50 mL contrast material is then injected into the vein or right atrium and a series of x-rays are obtained over the area of clinical interest. The computer will then "subtract" an image of the area obtained after the arrival of contrast material from an image obtained before the arrival of contrast material, leaving only an image of the contrast material in the blood vessels.

Data Acquired Visualization of the arteries in the area of clinical concern in the form of digitally subtracted images

Normal Findings The opacified arteries should be smooth and gradually taper as they continue to branch. There should be no evidence of vessel wall irregularity, aneurysm, narrowing, occlusion, extravasation, neovascularity, or arteriovenous shunting.

Limitations Because the computer subtracts x-ray images after the arrival of contrast material from an image obtained before the arrival of contrast material, any patient motion which has occurred in the interval will create an artifact. This includes respiratory motion, bowel motion, or patient motion. These artifacts can considerably obscure the image. Also, there is global opacification of all arteries in the area, often resulting in overlapping of multiple arterial structures which can obscure an area of interest. Finally, image quality is considerably degraded in patients who have poor cardiac output.

(Continued)

Digital Subtraction Angiogram, Intravenous *(Continued)*

References

Meaney TF, Weinstein MA, Buonocore E, et al, "Digital Subtraction Angiography of the Human Cardiovascular System," *AJR Am J Roentgenol*, 1980, 135(6):1153-60.

- **Direct Portal Venography** *see* Portal Venogram, Percutaneous Transhepatic *on page 384*
- **Direct Portography** *see* Portal Venogram, Percutaneous Transhepatic *on page 384*
- **Direct Splenoportography** *see* Splenoportogram, Percutaneous *on page 386*
- **Drainage of Fluid Collection** *see* Abscess Drainage Under Fluoroscopic, Ultrasonic, or CT Guidance *on page 369*
- **DSA** *see* Digital Subtraction Angiogram, Intravenous *on page 379*
- **Elbow Arthrogram** *see* Arthrogram *on page 374*
- **Embolization of Gastroesophageal Varices** *see* Portal Venogram, Percutaneous Transhepatic *on page 384*
- **External Biliary Drainage** *see* Biliary Drainage, Percutaneous Transhepatic *on page 375*
- **External Decompression** *see* Abscess Drainage Under Fluoroscopic, Ultrasonic, or CT Guidance *on page 369*
- **Filter Insertion** *see* Vena Caval Filter Placement *on page 388*
- **Gallbladder Drainage, Percutaneous** *see* Biliary Drainage, Percutaneous Transhepatic *on page 375*
- **Greenfield Filter Placement** *see* Vena Caval Filter Placement *on page 388*
- **Hepatic Arteriogram** *see* Arteriogram, Transaxillary or Transbrachial Approach *on page 372*
- **Hepatic Arteriogram** *see* Arteriogram, Transfemoral Approach *on page 373*
- **Hepatic Venogram** *see* Venogram, Transfemoral or Transjugular Approach *on page 389*
- **Hip Arthrogram** *see* Arthrogram *on page 374*
- **Iliofemoral Venogram** *see* Venogram, Transfemoral or Transjugular Approach *on page 389*
- **Inferior Vena Cava Filter Placement** *see* Vena Caval Filter Placement *on page 388*
- **IV-DSA** *see* Digital Subtraction Angiogram, Intravenous *on page 379*
- **Joint Study** *see* Arthrogram *on page 374*
- **Knee Arthrogram** *see* Arthrogram *on page 374*
- **Leg Arteriogram** *see* Arteriogram, Transaxillary or Transbrachial Approach *on page 372*
- **Leg Arteriogram** *see* Arteriogram, Transfemoral Approach *on page 373*
- **Lower Extremity Venogram** *see* Venogram, Extremity *on page 389*
- **Lumbar Myelogram** *see* Myelogram *on page 381*

Lymphangiogram

Synonyms Bipedal Lymphangiography

Procedure Commonly Includes Visualization of the lymphatic vessels and associated lymph nodes in the extremities, the pelvis, and the retroperitoneum, as well as the thoracic duct in the thorax

Indications Evaluation of the lymph nodes for possible involvement with primary or metastatic cancer or for occlusion or interruption of the lymphatic vessels secondary to a traumatic, surgical, or congenital cause

Patient Preparation Informed consent is obtained from the patient. There are no dietary restrictions.

Aftercare Dressings are placed on the incision sites on the dorsum of the feet. The feet should not be emersed in water until the stitches are removed approximately 7-10 days after the procedure. The patient should be informed that his urine will have a blue-green color for several days. The patient should be kept on bedrest for the remainder of the day.

Special Instructions The patient should be informed that the procedure will require a second set of x-rays the day following the actual injection of contrast material.

Complications Infection at the incision site, contrast reaction, pulmonary oil emboli

Equipment A surgical cut down tray, small gauge needles (27- to 30-gauge), fluoroscopy, and an x-ray unit

Technique The dorsa of both feet are sterilely prepared and draped. A blue dye (Lymphazurin®) is injected intradermally into the webs between the toes. Within 30 minutes, this dye is picked up by the lymphatic system, and the lymphatic channels on the dorsum of the foot become evident. Local anesthetic is then instilled over one of these lymphatic channels and a small surgical cut-down is performed. The lymphatic channel is isolated and a small gauge needle is inserted into it under direct vision. Approximately 5-7 mL (bilateral lymphangiography) or 8-10 mL (unilateral lymphangiography) of oil-based contrast material (eg, Ethiodol®) is then injected at a rate of 0.1-0.15 mL/minute using an automated pump device. The needles are then removed and the incision sites are sutured. Radiographs are then obtained of the pelvis, abdomen, and thorax to display the major lymphatic channels. Repeat films are then performed 24 hours later after the contrast material has been picked up by the lymph nodes themselves.

Data Acquired The first day films demonstrate the lymphatic channels within the extremity, pelvis, and retroperitoneum, as well as the thoracic duct. The second day films demonstrate the lymph nodes in these regions.

Normal Findings The appropriate lymphatic channels should be visualized without evidence for occlusion, displacement, or leakage. The lymph nodes themselves should be of normal size and architecture without evidence for enlargement or partial or complete replacement by neoplasm.

Limitations Inability to isolate and cannulate a lymph vessel (a process which is more difficult in children and patients with swollen feet, lymphangiectasia or small, frail lymphatic vessels)

References

Fuchs WA, "Technique and Complications of Lymphangiography," *Abrams Angiography, Vascular and Interventional Radiology*, 4th ed, Baum S, ed, Boston, MA: Little, Brown and Co, 1997, 1864-70.

Jing B, Wallace S, and Zornoza J, "Metastases to Retroperitoneal and Pelvic Lymph Nodes, Computed Tomography and Lymphangiography," *Radiol Clin North Am*, 1982, 20(3):511-30.

♦ **Mesenteric Arteriogram** *see* Arteriogram, Transaxillary or Transbrachial Approach *on page 372*

♦ **Mesenteric Arteriogram** *see* Arteriogram, Transfemoral Approach *on page 373*

Myelogram

Related Information

Lumbar Puncture *on page 160*

Synonyms Cervical Myelogram; Lumbar Myelogram; Thoracic Myelogram

Applies to Spinal Tap Under Fluoroscopy

Procedure Commonly Includes Visualization of the cervical, thoracic, and/or lumbar spinal cord by the injection of contrast material into the thecal sac through a percutaneously placed spinal needle. Spinal fluid is usually aspirated before the contrast is instilled and sent for appropriate laboratory analysis.

Indications Visualization of spinal cord abnormalities; evaluation of signs and/or symptoms of compression of the spinal nerve roots or spinal cord by a herniated disc, degenerative spur, traumatic injury, neoplasm, or other mass; usually performed in patients unable to undergo MRI evaluation or those with equivocal MRI findings.

Contraindications

- evidence of raised intracranial pressure (eg, papilledema)
- bleeding abnormalities
- elevated laboratory coagulation parameters (INR, PT, PTT)
- low platelet count
- patients on anticoagulation

(Continued)

Myelogram *(Continued)*

Patient Preparation Informed consent is obtained from the patient. The patient is made NPO 2-4 hours before the procedure. Any bleeding abnormality is corrected beforehand.

Aftercare The patient is placed on bedrest with the head of the bed elevated at least 30° to 45° for 12 hours. Oral fluids are encouraged and the diet is as tolerated. Any nausea or vomiting which occurs should not be treated with phenothiazine antinauseants. The patient is advised to remain still in bed in a head up position for the remainder of the day. Restricted medications may be resumed after 24 hours.

Special Instructions Any previous spine x-rays or any prior CT or MR studies of the spine should be made available to the radiologist. Patients taking drugs that lower the seizure threshold (eg, phenothiazines, antipsychotics, etc) should stop these medications at least 24-48 hours before the study.

Complications Seizure, arachnoiditis, subarachnoid bleeding, spinal infection; nausea and vomiting are not infrequent side effects.

Equipment Spinal needle, nonionic contrast material, fluoroscopy, and x-ray equipment with a tilting table

Technique The patient is usually placed in a prone position. Under fluoroscopy, an appropriate entry site is selected over the lumbar spine or, occasionally, over the upper cervical spine. Local anesthetic is instilled and a 21-gauge spinal needle is fluoroscopically guided into the thecal sac. If desired, spinal fluid can be obtained and sent for appropriate laboratory analysis (eg, cell count, cytology, Gram stain, culture, protein, immunoglobulins). Approximately 10 mL nonionic contrast material is injected into the subarachnoid space of the spinal canal with the patient in a reverse Trendelenburg position. Films of the lumbar area are then obtained. Since the contrast material is heavier than spinal fluid, the patient is slowly tilted downward to obtain films of the thoracic and spinal regions. Care is made not to allow the contrast material to enter the intracranial region.

Data Acquired Visualization of the thecal sac of the lumbar, thoracic, and/or cervical spine

Normal Findings There should be no evidence for any filling defect within or extrinsic compression on the thecal sac. There should be no impingement upon or displacement of the nerve roots or the spinal cord.

Limitations Adhesions from arachnoiditis or areas of marked compression may impede the flow of contrast material. Severe kyphosis, scoliosis, or ankylosing spondylitis can make the examination technically difficult.

References

Benson JE and Han JS, "Examination of the Spine," *Radiology: Diagnosis, Imaging, Intervention*, Volume 3, Chapter 102, Taveras JM and Ferrucci JT, eds, Philadelphia, PA: JB Lippincott Co, 1992, 1-18.

Grossman RI and Yousem DM, "Techniques in Neuroimaging," *Neuroradiology, The Requisites*, Thrall JH, ed, St Louis, MO: CV Mosby Co, 1994, 1-23.

♦ **Needle Aspiration Biopsy** *see* Biopsy, Percutaneous Needle, Under Fluoroscopic, CT, or Ultrasound Guidance *on page 376*

♦ **Needle Biopsy Under CT Guidance** *see* Biopsy, Percutaneous Needle, Under Fluoroscopic, CT, or Ultrasound Guidance *on page 376*

♦ **Needle Biopsy Under Ultrasound Guidance** *see* Biopsy, Percutaneous Needle, Under Fluoroscopic, CT, or Ultrasound Guidance *on page 376*

♦ **Needle Localization** *see* Biopsy, Percutaneous Needle, Under Fluoroscopic, CT, or Ultrasound Guidance *on page 376*

Nephrostomy, Percutaneous

Synonyms Percutaneous Renal Drainage

Applies to Ureteral Stent Placement, Percutaneous; Ureteral Stricture Dilatation, Percutaneous; Whittaker Test

Procedure Commonly Includes Percutaneous placement of a drainage catheter in an obstructed kidney

Indications Partial or complete ureteral obstruction resulting in pain, infection, hydronephrosis, pyohydronephrosis, sepsis, or decreased renal function. The cause of obstruction may be secondary to stone, neoplasm, fibrosis, extrinsic compression, or a stricture related to surgery, trauma, infection, or radiation.

Contraindications

- bleeding abnormalities
- elevated laboratory coagulation parameters (INR, PT, PTT)
- low platelet count

Patient Preparation Informed consent is obtained from the patient. The patient is placed on a clear liquid diet or NPO 4 hours before the procedure. Medications may be continued. An intravenous line is begun before the procedure to facilitate the administration of any antibiotics or medications during the procedure. If the patient is not already on antibiotics and the kidney is obstructed, most physicians will prescribe a broad spectrum antibiotic to be administered intravenously before the procedure. Recent laboratory results (BUN, creatinine, platelet count, INR, PT, and PTT) should be recorded on the chart.

Aftercare The patient is placed on bedrest for approximately 4 hours. Vital signs should be obtained every 30 minutes for 2 hours, then every hour for the 4 hours. The patient should be observed closely for any signs of internal bleeding or sepsis.

Special Instructions The volume of output from the nephrostomy tube should be recorded. While the urine from the drainage tube may be blood tinged, any profuse bleeding from the catheter should be attended to promptly. If the drainage ceases completely, the catheter may be irrigated to remove blood clot or debris. Drainage of urine around the catheter at the skin site is usually a sign that the catheter is at least partially obstructed or that progressively larger catheters are needed. If the urine appears infected, the patient should be continued on antibiotics.

Complications Bleeding and sepsis are the most common complications occurring in the first several hours after the procedure. Pneumothorax and transcolonic catheter placement are also potential complications. Delayed complications include infection at the skin entry site and dislodgment or plugging of the drainage catheter.

Equipment Ultrasound, fluoroscopy, steerable wires, and catheter with an inner retention mechanism

Technique The patient is placed prone and a percutaneous entry site is chosen with the assistance of ultrasound, fluoroscopy, or even CT. If the kidney to be drained still functions adequately, contrast material can be injected intravenously to help localize the collecting system. Local anesthetic is instilled at the entry site which is usually located along the posterolateral aspect of the patient below the 11th or 12th rib at approximately the level of the second lumbar vertebrae. A needle is then percutaneously inserted into a posterolateral calyx of the renal collecting system. If no intravenous contrast was administered, contrast is injected through the needle into the renal pelvis to confirm insertion of the needle into a posterolateral calyx, A guidewire is placed through the needle and advanced into the renal pelvis. The needle is then removed and a drainage catheter is passed over the guidewire. The drainage catheter is fixed to the skin to prevent dislodgment. This percutaneous access route can later be used for placement of a ureteral stent across the point of obstruction or for balloon dilatation of an obstructing stricture. Also, a Whittaker test can be performed to determine if a narrowing is urodynamically significant by measuring pressures in the renal pelvis and the urinary bladder simultaneously as saline is instilled through the nephrostomy catheter.

Data Acquired A urine specimen from the obstructed urinary tract can be sent for culture, Gram stain, and cytology.

Limitations It can be technically difficult to place a drainage catheter into a renal collecting system which is completely occupied by a staghorn calculus. Multiple attempts may be necessary to achieve placement into a posterolateral calyx.

References

Castaneda-Zuniga WR, Brady TM, Thomas R, et al, "Interventional Uroradiology: Part 1. Percutaneous Uroradiologic Techniques," *Interventional Radiology*, 3rd ed, Castaneda-Zuniga WR, ed, Baltimore, MD: Williams & Wilkins, 1997, 1049-269.

Farrell TA and Hicks ME, "A Review of Radiologically Guided Percutaneous Nephrostomies in 303 Patients," *J Vasc Interv Radiol*, 1997, 8:769-74.

(Continued)

Nephrostomy, Percutaneous *(Continued)*

Lang EK and Price ET, "Redefinitions of Indications for Percutaneous Nephrostomy," *Radiology*, 1983, 147(2):419-26.

Pfister RC and Newhouse JH, "Interventional Percutaneous Pyeloureteral Techniques. II. Percutaneous Nephrostomy and Other Procedures," *Radiol Clin North Am*, 1979, 17(2):351-63.

♦ **Pelvic Arteriogram** *see* Arteriogram, Transaxillary or Transbrachial Approach *on page 372*

♦ **Pelvic Arteriogram** *see* Arteriogram, Transfemoral Approach *on page 373*

♦ **Percutaneous Drainage** *see* Abscess Drainage Under Fluoroscopic, Ultrasonic, or CT Guidance *on page 369*

♦ **Percutaneous Renal Drainage** *see* Nephrostomy, Percutaneous *on page 382*

♦ **Percutaneous Transfemoral Angiogram** *see* Arteriogram, Transfemoral Approach *on page 373*

♦ **Percutaneous Transfemoral Venogram** *see* Venogram, Transfemoral or Transjugular Approach *on page 389*

♦ **Percutaneous Transjugular Venogram** *see* Venogram, Transfemoral or Transjugular Approach *on page 389*

♦ **Portal or Mesenteric Venous Sampling** *see* Portal Venogram, Percutaneous Transhepatic *on page 384*

Portal Venogram, Percutaneous Transhepatic

Synonyms Catheter Portography; Direct Portal Venography; Direct Portography

Applies to Embolization of Gastroesophageal Varices; Portal or Mesenteric Venous Sampling

Procedure Commonly Includes Visualization of the portal vein and its connecting veins (eg, splenic, superior mesenteric, inferior mesenteric, gastroduodenal, or coronary veins) by the injection of contrast material through a catheter which has been placed through a percutaneous puncture of the liver. This catheter technique can also be used for obtaining venous samples from various regions to help localize an endocrine-secreting pancreatic tumor or for embolizing gastroesophageal varices in an attempt to control variceal bleeding.

Indications Elevation of the portal venous system, localization of endocrine pancreatic tumor, embolization of bleeding varices. Currently, percutaneous transhepatic portal venography is used infrequently due to the advent of endoscopic sclerotherapy of esophageal varices and percutaneous transhepatic portosystemic shunts.

Contraindications

- tense ascites
- bleeding abnormalities
- elevated laboratory coagulation parameters (INR, PT, PTT)
- low platelet count
- acute renal failure

Patient Preparation Informed consent is obtained from the patient. The patient is placed on a clear liquid diet or NPO 4 hours before the procedure. All medications are continued. An intravenous line is begun before the procedure in order to ensure that the patient is well hydrated and to facilitate the administration of any medications required during the procedure. Blood typing is often requested beforehand. Recent laboratory results (BUN, creatinine, platelet count, INR, PT, and PTT) should be recorded on the chart.

Aftercare The patient is placed on bedrest for approximately 4 hours. Vital signs should be obtained every 30 minutes for 2 hours, then every hour for 4 hours. The patient should be observed closely for any signs of internal bleeding or sepsis. Many physicians will routinely check a hematocrit 6-8 hours after the procedure.

Special Instructions Any previous imaging study of the upper abdomen should be made available to the interventional radiologist. Any bleeding abnormalities should be corrected beforehand. Any problem areas should be called attention to (eg, renal insufficiency or history of severe contrast reaction).

Complications Internal hemorrhage is the most feared and most common complication, but sepsis can also occur.

Equipment Fluoroscopy, x-ray equipment, and angiographic needles, wires, and catheters

Technique An appropriate entry site is determined with fluoroscopy or ultrasound. Typically, this is in a low intercostal space along the right midaxillary line below the costophrenic sulcus. Local anesthesia is instilled and a 10-15 cm 21-gauge needle or sheathed needle is advanced through the liver into a intrahepatic portal vein. A guidewire is then placed through the needle or sheath, the needle or sheath is removed leaving the wire in the portal vein. The angiographic catheter is then guided over wire under fluoroscopy into the vein of interest. Contrast material is injected and x-rays are obtained to demonstrate the portal venous system. When searching for an endocrine-secreting tumor (eg, insulinoma, gastrinoma, glucagonoma, APUDoma), venous samples are obtained at various sites as the catheter is manipulated. For embolization of bleeding varices, the catheter is advanced into the varices and embolic material is discharged through the catheter.

Data Acquired Visualization of the portal venous system

Normal Findings The portal veins and the veins draining into it should be of normal caliber without evidence for occlusion, filling defect, compression, displacement or variceal formation.

Limitations Anything which would obscure the portal veins (ie, overlying barium or patient motion). Also, a small, very firm, or cirrhotic liver can make the procedure technically difficult and increase the risk for complication.

References

L'Hermine CL, Chastanet P, Delemazure O, et al, "Percutaneous Transhepatic Embolization of Gastroesophageal Varices: Results in 400 Patients," *AJR Am J Roentgenol*, 1989, 152(4):755-60.

Lunderquist A, and Ivancev K, "Portal and Pancreatic Venography," *Abrams Angiography, Vascular and Interventional Radiology*, 4th ed, Baum S, ed, Boston, MA: Little, Brown and Co, 1997, 1422-32.

♦ **Pulmonary Angiogram** *see* Pulmonary Arteriogram, Transfemoral or Transjugular Approach *on page 385*

Pulmonary Arteriogram, Transfemoral or Transjugular Approach

Synonyms Pulmonary Angiogram

Procedure Commonly Includes Visualization of the pulmonary arteries and their branches by the injection of contrast material through a catheter which has been percutaneously placed through a common femoral or internal jugular vein

Indications Evaluation of the pulmonary arteries for the presence of pulmonary embolism, stenosis, arteriovenous malformation, fistula, stenosis, or aneurysm

Patient Preparation Informed consent is obtained from the patient. The patient is placed on a clear liquid diet the morning of the procedure if possible, although this procedure is often performed on an emergency basis. All medications are continued. An intravenous line is begun before the procedure in order to ensure that the patient is well hydrated and to facilitate the administration of any medications required during the procedure. The patient should also have electrocardiographic monitoring throughout the procedure. Recent laboratory results (BUN, creatinine, platelet count, INR, PT, and PTT) and an EKG should be recorded on the chart.

Aftercare If a femoral approach was used, the patient is placed on bedrest for 4 hours after the procedure. During this time, the patient should remain flat in bed with the legs straight. Vital signs should be observed every 30 minutes for the first 2 hours, then every hour for the next 2 hours. At these times, the femoral puncture site should be examined for any evidence of bleeding or swelling. The legs should be examined for any changes in color or warmth. If the jugular approach was used, the head of the bed should be elevated and the site should be observed for any signs of bleeding.

(Continued)

Pulmonary Arteriogram, Transfemoral or Transjugular Approach *(Continued)*

Special Instructions These examinations are often arranged by the requesting physician in consultation with the cardiovascular radiologist. Any prior chest x-rays, lung scans, or helical chest CTs should be made available. Any potential problem areas (eg, renal insufficiency, left bundle branch block, or history of severe contrast reaction) should be noted.

Complications Contrast reaction; acute renal failure; cardiopulmonary arrest; or venous thrombosis, bleeding, or hematoma formation at the puncture site

Equipment Fluoroscopy, angiographic catheters and wires, intravascular pressure transducers, and a method of film recording (either conventional cut films or digital subtraction films)

Technique Local anesthetic agent is instilled over the entry site, either the common femoral vein or the internal jugular vein. The vein is percutaneously punctured and a catheter is inserted and fluoroscopically maneuvered through the vena cava, right atrium, and right ventricle and then into the pulmonary arteries. Pulmonary artery pressures are then obtained. Contrast medium is injected through the catheter and the films are obtained.

Data Acquired Visualization of the pulmonary arterial tree. Also, pulmonary arterial pressures and pressures in the right atrium and ventricle can be obtained at this time.

Normal Findings The pulmonary arteries should taper gradually as they continue to branch. There should be no radiolucent filling defects (representing pulmonary emboli) and no evidence of arteriovenous malformation, fistula, vessel stenosis, or aneurysm.

Limitations Since these patients are often short of breath, breathing artifact may be present on the films and this can result in a considerable degradation of the image quality.

References

Alderson PO and Martin EC, "Pulmonary Embolism: Diagnosis With Multiple Imaging Modalities," *Radiology*, 1987, 164(2):297-312.

Barton RE, Lakin PC, and Rosch J, "Pulmonary Arteriography: Indications, Technique, Normal Findings, and Complications," *Abrams' Angiography, Vascular, and Interventional Radiology*, 4th ed, Baum S, ed, Boston, MA: Little, Brown and Co, 1997, 768-85.

♦ **Renal Arteriogram** *see* Arteriogram, Transaxillary or Transbrachial Approach *on page 372*

♦ **Renal Arteriogram** *see* Arteriogram, Transfemoral Approach *on page 373*

♦ **Renal Vein Renin Sampling** *see* Venogram, Transfemoral or Transjugular Approach *on page 389*

♦ **Renal Venogram** *see* Venogram, Transfemoral or Transjugular Approach *on page 389*

♦ **Shoulder Arthrogram** *see* Arthrogram *on page 374*

♦ **Spinal Tap Under Fluoroscopy** *see* Myelogram *on page 381*

♦ **Splenic Arteriogram** *see* Arteriogram, Transaxillary or Transbrachial Approach *on page 372*

♦ **Splenic Arteriogram** *see* Arteriogram, Transfemoral Approach *on page 373*

Splenoportogram, Percutaneous

Synonyms Direct Splenoportography

Procedure Commonly Includes Visualization of the splenic veins and portal venous system by the injection of contrast material through a needle which has been percutaneously placed into the pulp of the spleen

Indications Evaluation of the status of the splenic or portal veins when they are not adequately visualized on the venous phase of a celiac or splenic arteriogram. Most commonly used for cases of suspected splenic vein or portal vein thrombosis.

Contraindications

- bleeding abnormalities
- elevated laboratory coagulation parameters (INR, PT, PTT)
- low platelet count
- known splenic tumors

Patient Preparation Informed consent is obtained from the patient. The patient is placed on a clear liquid diet or NPO 4 hours before the procedure. All medications can be continued. An intravenous line is begun before the procedure in order to ensure adequate hydration and to facilitate the administration of any medications or blood products required during the procedure. Blood typing should be performed beforehand. Recent laboratory results (BUN, creatinine, platelet count, INR, PT, and PTT) should be recorded on the chart.

Aftercare The patient is placed on bedrest for approximately 8 hours. Vital signs should be obtained every 30 minutes for 2 hours, then every hour for 6 hours. The patient should be observed closely for any signs of internal bleeding or sepsis. Many physicians will routinely check a hematocrit 6-8 hours after the procedure.

Special Instructions Any previous imaging study of the upper abdomen should be made available to the interventional radiologist. Any bleeding abnormality should be corrected. Potential problem areas should be noted (eg, renal insufficiency or history of severe contrast reaction).

Complications Internal hemorrhage, shock, splenic rupture, puncture of adjacent organs, pneumothorax

Equipment Fluoroscopy, ultrasound, x-ray equipment, and a sheathed needle

Technique The appropriate entry site is localized with fluoroscopy and/or ultrasound. Typically, this is in a low intercostal space (8th to 10th) along the left mid to posterior axillary line. A sheathed needle is inserted into the splenic pulp and the needle is removed leaving only the sheath in place. Contrast material is injected at a rate of approximately 4-6 mL/second for 8-10 seconds and x-rays are obtained. Gelfoam embolization of the needle track may be performed as the needle is removed after the procedure.

Data Acquired Opacification of the splenic and portal veins as well as any collaterals or varices

Normal Findings The splenic and portal veins should be smooth and of normal caliber without evidence of occlusion, thrombosis, compression, filling defect, displacement, portosystemic shunting, or variceal formation.

Limitations Anything which would obscure the splenic or portal veins (ie, overlying barium or patient motion). Inflow of unopacified blood from vessels may cause nonvisualization of the splenic or portal veins.

References

Brazzini A, Hunter DW, Darcy MD, et al, "Safe Splenoportography," *Radiology*, 1987, 162(3):607-9.

Gardiner GA Jr and Bergstrand I, "Splenoportography and Portal Hypertension," *Abrams Angiography, Vascular and Interventional Radiology*, 4th ed, Baum S, ed, Boston, MA: Little, Brown and Co, 1997, 1497-1526.

♦ **Superior Vena Cavogram** *see* Venogram, Transfemoral or Transjugular Approach *on page 389*

♦ **Temporomandibular Joint Arthrogram** *see* Arthrogram *on page 374*

♦ **Thoracic Aortogram** *see* Arteriogram, Transaxillary or Transbrachial Approach *on page 372*

♦ **Thoracic Aortogram** *see* Arteriogram, Transfemoral Approach *on page 373*

♦ **Thoracic Myelogram** *see* Myelogram *on page 381*

♦ **Transaxillary Angiogram** *see* Arteriogram, Transaxillary or Transbrachial Approach *on page 372*

♦ **Transbrachial Angiogram** *see* Arteriogram, Transaxillary or Transbrachial Approach *on page 372*

♦ **Translumbar Abdominal Aortogram** *see* Aortogram, Translumbar Approach *on page 371*

♦ **Translumbar Aortogram** *see* Aortogram, Translumbar Approach *on page 371*

♦ **Transthoracic Needle Aspiration Biopsy** *see* Biopsy, Percutaneous Needle, Under Fluoroscopic, CT, or Ultrasound Guidance *on page 376*

♦ **Umbrella Insertion** *see* Vena Caval Filter Placement *on page 388*

♦ **Upper Extremity Venogram** *see* Venogram, Extremity *on page 389*

♦ **Ureteral Stent Placement, Percutaneous** *see* Nephrostomy, Percutaneous *on page 382*

♦ **Ureteral Stricture Dilatation, Percutaneous** *see* Nephrostomy, Percutaneous *on page 382*

Vena Caval Filter Placement

Synonyms Filter Insertion; Greenfield Filter Placement; Inferior Vena Cava Filter Placement; Umbrella Insertion

Procedure Commonly Includes Placement of a filtering device (sometimes referred to as an umbrella filter) into the inferior vena cava through a common femoral, internal jugular, or antecubital vein approach percutaneously

Indications Prevention of pulmonary emboli in patients with lower extremity deep venous thrombosis (DVT) or pelvic thrombosis, and for whom anticoagulation is contraindicated or ineffective

Contraindications There are no absolute contraindications to filter placement, however, complete thrombosis of the inferior vena cava would prevent placement.

Patient Preparation Informed consent is obtained from the patient. The patient is placed on a clear liquid diet the morning of the procedure if possible, although the procedure is often performed on an emergency basis. An intravenous line is begun before the procedure in order to ensure that the patient is well hydrated and to facilitate the administration of any medications required during the procedure. Recent laboratory results (BUN, creatinine, platelet count, INR, PT, and PTT) should be recorded on the chart.

Aftercare If the procedure was performed via a common femoral vein approach, the patient is placed on bedrest for approximately 4 hours. During this time, the patient should be flat in bed with the legs straight. Vital signs should be obtained every 30 minutes for 2 hours and then every hour for the next 2 hours. At these times, the femoral puncture site should be examined for any evidence of bleeding or swelling. If an internal jugular or antecubital vein approach was utilized, bedrest is not mandatory, but the patient's head should be elevated for 2 hours.

Special Instructions These examinations are usually arranged by the requesting physician in consultation with the physician performing the procedure. There should be a clear reason why the patient cannot be treated with anticoagulation rather than placement of a caval filter. The physician performing the procedure should be alerted to any potential problem areas (eg, history of severe contrast reaction, renal insufficiency, or bleeding abnormalities).

Complications Vein thrombosis at the insertion site, caval thrombosis at the filter site, filter migration or inadvertent placement of the filter in an inappropriate location, hematoma formation at the entry site, contrast reaction

Equipment Caval filter (several varieties are now available) and its delivery system, angiographic catheters and wires, fluoroscopy, and x-ray equipment

Technique Local anesthetic agent is instilled over either the common femoral vein, the internal jugular vein, or the antecubital vein. The vein is percutaneously punctured. A catheter is inserted and carefully advanced into the inferior vena cava. An inferior vena cavogram is performed in order to depict the anatomy, measure the cava, and assess for any thrombus within the cava. The catheter is then removed and an appropriately chosen filter delivery system is advanced into the cava. The filter is then extruded into the inferior vena cava, usually below the level of the renal veins and above the level of the confluence of the common iliac veins.

Normal Findings The caval filter should be expanded appropriately at the expected location without excessive tilting.

Limitations When thrombus is present within the inferior vena cava itself, there may not be sufficient room to place a filter if the thrombus extends into the intrahepatic segment of the inferior vena cava.

References

Dorfman GS, "Percutaneous Inferior Vena Caval Filters," *Radiology*, 1990, 174:987-992.

Greenfield LJ and Michna BA, "Twelve-Year Clinical Experience With the Greenfield Vena Caval Filter," *Surgery*, 1988, 104(4):706-12.

Hagspiel KD, et al, "Inferior Vena Cava Filters: An Update," *Applied Radiology*, 1998, 27(11)20-34.

Pais SO and Tobin KD, "Percutaneous Insertion of the Greenfield Filter," *AJR Am J Roentgenol*, 1989, 152(5):933-8.

Venogram, Extremity

Synonyms Arm Venogram; Lower Extremity Venogram; Upper Extremity Venogram

Procedure Commonly Includes Visualization of the veins of an extremity by injection of contrast material through a needle or angiocatheter which has been inserted into a vein on the dorsum of the foot or hand (of the extremity being examined)

Indications Suspicion of deep vein thrombosis, occlusion or compression, usually manifested by extremity swelling and/or pain; search for a source of pulmonary emboli

Contraindications Acute renal failure

Patient Preparation The patient is placed on a clear liquid diet for 4 hours prior to the procedure if possible, although the procedure is often performed on an emergency basis. Recent renal functions (BUN, creatinine) should be recorded on the chart.

Complications Contrast reaction, contrast-induced acute renal failure, contrast-induced venous thrombosis, extravasation of contrast at the needle puncture site

Equipment Various-sized angiocatheters or butterfly needles, contrast material, fluoroscopy, and x-ray equipment

Technique A butterfly needle or angiocatheter is inserted into a vein on the dorsum of the foot or distal calf for a lower extremity venogram, or on the dorsum of the hand or in the forearm for an upper extremity venogram. For lower extremity venograms, the patient is placed in a reverse Trendelenburg position (head up) as contrast is infused. Approximately 50-75 mL contrast is injected and films of the extremity are obtained. If necessary, the procedure is repeated in multiple projections and positions of the extremity. Tourniquets or inflated blood pressure cuffs may be used to help better visualize the deep veins.

Data Acquired Depiction of venous anatomy

Normal Findings There should be good opacification of the deep venous system. There should be no evidence of any radiolucent filling defects (representing clots) or venous occlusion or compression.

Limitations Inability to adequately cannulate a vein of the affected extremity. Also, prior venous thromboses may have resulted in chronic occlusions which can make visualization of any superimposed acute thrombi difficult.

References

Bettman MA, "Venography," *Abrams' Angiography, Vascular, and Interventional Radiology*, 4th ed, Baum S, ed, Boston, MA: Little, Brown, and Co, 1997, 1743-54.

Naidich JB, Feinberg AW, Karp-Harman H, et al, "Contrast Venography: Reassessment of Its Role," *Radiology*, 1988, 168(1):97-100.

Rabinov K and Paulin S, "Roentgen Diagnosis of Venous Thrombosis in the Leg," *Arch Surg*, 1972, 104(2):134-44.

Venogram, Transfemoral or Transjugular Approach

Synonyms Percutaneous Transfemoral Venogram; Percutaneous Transjugular Venogram

Applies to Adrenal Venogram; Hepatic Venogram; Iliofemoral Venogram; Renal Vein Renin Sampling; Renal Venogram; Superior Vena Cavogram; Venous Sampling

Procedure Commonly Includes Visualization of the veins of the pelvis, abdomen (excluding the portal venous system), thorax, or cervical region by the injection of contrast material through a catheter which has been percutaneously placed through the common femoral vein or, less frequently, the internal jugular vein. This catheter can also be used to obtain venous samples for endocrine assay (eg, renin levels from the renal veins, parathormone levels from the cervical veins or aldosterone, catechol, and cortisol levels from the adrenal veins).

Indications Evaluation of the pelvic, abdominal, or thoracic venous systems for thrombus formation, occlusion, compression, stenosis, trauma, or aneurysm

(Continued)

Venogram, Transfemoral or Transjugular Approach *(Continued)*

Contraindications

- inability of patient to lie supine
- acute renal failure
- bleeding abnormalities
- abnormal coagulation parameters (INR, PT, PTT)
- low platelet count

Patient Preparation Informed consent is obtained from the patient. The patient is placed on a clear liquid diet (not NPO) on the morning of the procedure. All medications are continued. An intravenous line is begun before the procedure in order to ensure that the patient is well hydrated (thus decreasing the risk of acute renal failure) and to facilitate the administration of any medications required during the procedure. Recent laboratory results (BUN, creatinine, platelet count, INR, PT, and PTT) should be recorded on the chart.

Aftercare If a femoral approach was used, the patient is placed on bedrest for 4 hours after the procedure. During this time, the patient should remain flat in bed with the legs straight. Vital signs should be observed every 30 minutes for the first 2 hours, then every hour for the next 2 hours. At these times, the femoral puncture site should be examined for any evidence of bleeding or swelling and the leg should be examined for any changes in color or warmth. If the jugular approach was used, the head of the bed should be elevated and the site should be observed for bleeding.

Special Instructions These examinations are often arranged by the requesting physician in consultation with the cardiovascular radiologist. The requisition should state clearly the reason for the study as well as the specific vessels to be examined or the specific veins which should be sampled for endocrine assays. The cardiovascular radiologist should be alerted to any potential problem areas (eg, renal insufficiency or history of severe contrast reaction).

Complications Contrast reaction; acute renal failure; venous thrombosis, bleeding, or hematoma formation at the puncture site

Equipment Fluoroscopy, angiographic catheters and wires, and a method of film recording (either conventional cut films or digital subtraction films)

Technique Local anesthetic agent is instilled over the common femoral vein or the internal jugular vein. The vein is percutaneously punctured and a catheter is inserted and fluoroscopically guided into the vein of interest. Contrast medium is injected and the films are obtained.

Data Acquired Visualization of the venous systems in the areas of clinical concern on either conventional x-ray film or on digitally subtracted images. If desired, venous samples can be assayed for the appropriate endocrine levels.

Normal Findings The veins should be smooth and of normal caliber. There should be no radiolucent filling defects (representing thrombi) and no evidence for vessel stenosis, occlusion, compression, extravasation, or aneurysm.

Limitations Anything which would obscure the blood vessels (ie, overlying barium or patient motion)

References

Johnsrude IS, "Catheterization Techniques," *A Practical Approach to Angiography*, 2nd ed, Johnsrude IS, Jackson DC, and Dunnick NR, eds, Boston, MA: Little, Brown and Co, 1987, 55-7.

♦ **Venous Sampling** *see* Venogram, Transfemoral or Transjugular Approach *on page 389*

♦ **Vertebral Arteriogram** *see* Arteriogram, Transaxillary or Transbrachial Approach *on page 372*

♦ **Vertebral Arteriogram** *see* Arteriogram, Transfemoral Approach *on page 373*

♦ **Whittaker Test** *see* Nephrostomy, Percutaneous *on page 382*

♦ **Wrist Arthrogram** *see* Arthrogram *on page 374*

MAGNETIC RESONANCE IMAGING

Magnetic Resonance Angiography, Brain

Related Information

Computed Transaxial Tomography, Head Studies *on page 332*

Applies to Magnetic Resonance Scan, Head

Indications Magnetic resonance angiography can be used in patients with a prior indication for parenchymal MRI, as well as in patients in whom the risk of conventional arteriography is considered too large. The major clinical indications are in extracranial and intracranial diseases such as atherosclerosis, fibromuscular dysplasia, occlusive disease, vasculitis, moyamoya, sickle cell vasculopathy, intracranial aneurysms, postoperative clipped aneurysm, pial arteriovenous malformations, cavernous malformation, capillary telangiectasia, venous malformation, dural arteriovenous fistulas, and venous occlusion.

Contraindications Patients weighing more than 300 lb and patients unable to squeeze into the magnet cannot undergo MRI. An absolute contraindication for MRI is a cardiac pacemaker. Relative contraindications to magnetic resonance imaging include intracranial aneurysm clips, cochlear implants, insulin infusion and chemotherapy pumps, neurocutaneous stimulators, prosthetic heart valves, ocular implants, penile implants, and artificial sphincters depending on date of manufacture and metallurgical composition. Please consult MRI physician if questions arise. Patients who have metallic foreign bodies within the eye or if the object is positioned near a vital neural, vascular, or soft tissue structure; or patients who have undergone recent surgery within

(Continued)

Magnetic Resonance Angiography, Brain *(Continued)*

the last 6 weeks requiring placement of a vascular surgical clip, should also not undergo MRI. The safety of MRI in pregnant patients has not been determined. In such cases, prior consultation with the MRI physician is required. Generally, patients who have undergone recent surgery not requiring vascular clips or who have had coronary artery bypass surgery in the past may undergo MRI. Patients who have shrapnel wounds or orthopedic prostheses can generally safely undergo MRI unless the metallic device is in the anatomic region to be scanned which results in degradation of the images. Patients with surgically implanted intravascular vena cava filters to prevent pulmonary embolism can usually be scanned if the device has been in place for at least 6 weeks. Patients requiring life support equipment, including ventilators, require special preparation. Please contact MRI physician ahead of time. Central venous lines, Swan-Ganz catheters, and nasogastric (NG) tubes usually present no problems. If the patient is positive when screened for metallic devices and you are uncertain of their significance, the MRI radiologist will provide additional information to assist you.

Patient Preparation Inpatient: The patient must be able to lie quietly while the scan is performed. The patient should be screened for metallic devices by nursing personnel. (See Contraindications.) This includes metal introduced into the patient either surgically or by trauma. All metallic objects must be removed from the patient, including jewelry or any other metal objects which may be in the patient's bedding. Dentures or other dental appliances must be removed. I.V.s which contain no metal are fine, but infusion pumps must be removed. Oxygen tanks and metallic backboards may come with the patient but will be removed prior to the patient entering the magnet room. Oxygen may be provided in the magnet room. Trauma, ICU, or CCU patients should be accompanied by a nurse. The patient needs to be NPO for abdominal MRI exams. If the patient is restless, combative, or claustrophobic, proper sedation may be administered on the floor prior to the MRI, or at the MRI Center. Consult the MRI radiologists with questions on proper sedation.

Outpatient: The patient should be screened for metallic devices. (See Contraindications.) If a question exists as to the patient's suitability for MRI, the MRI radiologist will assist you with your questions. If the patient is claustrophobic, oral or parenteral sedation may be necessary. If so, the patient should be accompanied by another adult to provide transportation home after the examination.

Aftercare If the patient received an MRI contrast agent (Magnevist®) and develops a delayed hypersensitivity reaction (ie, nausea, emesis, hives, or shortness of breath), the referring physician or MRI radiologist should be contacted immediately. If sedation is used, more time is required after the procedure for recovery period from the sedation.

Data Acquired Digital information with film reproduction

Limitations Generally, the greatest limitation of magnetic resonance imaging results from the patient's fear of the procedure. The patient must remain quiet and still for several scans, each lasting from several minutes to 10 minutes in length. Total examination time is usually 30-45 minutes and occasionally up to 1 hour. If the patient is restless during the examination, motion artifacts will be present on the images limiting their diagnostic value. If the patient is claustrophobic, mild oral sedation or occasionally parenteral sedation may be needed. Also, the patient can be accompanied by a family member or friend during the examination which may help to calm the patient's anxiety. Patients requiring life support equipment (ie, ventilators) require special preparation. Please refer to Contraindications for further causes for rejection.

Additional Information In some cases, an MRI contrast agent (Magnevist®) may be needed to increase the diagnostic accuracy of the MRI. This contrast agent can be administered to patients with a previous history of allergies to conventional iodinated x-ray agents, as it contains no iodine. Contraindications to its use include previous allergy to the contrast agent itself, renal failure, certain types of anemia, and Wilson disease. Nursing mothers should express their breasts and not breast-feed for 36-48 hours after the administration of an MRI contrast agent to ensure that the nursing child does not receive the drug in any notable quantity. The contrast agent is generally very safe and increases the diagnostic efficacy of the MRI.

References

Masaryk TJ, Perl J II, Dagirmanjian A, et al, "Magnetic Resonance Angiography: Neuroradiological Applications," *Magn Reson Imaging*, 3rd ed, Stark DD and Bradley WG Jr, St Louis, MO: CV Mosby Co, 1999, 1277-315.

Magnetic Resonance Scan, Abdomen

Related Information

Computed Transaxial Tomography, Abdomen Studies *on page 327*

Synonyms Abdomen MRI; MRI, Abdomen

Indications Evaluation of the liver, biliary system, spleen, pancreas, kidneys, adrenal glands, and the gastrointestinal tract as follows:

Liver and biliary system: MR is the diagnostic modality with the best accuracy for evaluation of liver iron deposition and fatty infiltration, and some focal lesions as hypervascular malignant lesions (hepatocellular carcinoma and metastases from hypervascular primary tumors). The MR cholangiopancreatography is a new technique which can depict bile ducts and pancreatic ducts, and can be used in patients who have undergone gastrectomy or pancreatoduodenectomy, and in whom endoscopic retrograde cholangiopancreatography cannot be performed.

Pancreas and spleen: Confirmation of a normal pancreas in patients in whom diffuse or focal pancreatic enlargement is detected incidentally by ultrasound or CT, staging of pancreatic carcinoma, localization of pancreatic islet cell tumors, evaluation of inflammatory recurrent pancreatic disease. Detection or evaluation of focal splenic lesions.

Kidneys: Mainly for the staging of renal neoplasms in patients in whom CT is contraindicated or the CT and US are indeterminate. Other use is in patients who cannot tolerate intravenous iodinated contrast agents and in patients with renal transplant dysfunction to evaluate post-transplant lymphoproliferative disorder.

Adrenal glands: Used as complement of CT. Other use is in patients who have had prior surgeries and the presence of metallic clips produce artifacts and in those patients unable to tolerate intravenous iodinated contrast agents. It is good to distinguish benign nonhyperfunctioning adenomas from other, potentially malignant lesions, especially metastases.

Gastrointestinal tract: Indicated in patients who cannot use iodinated contrast for CT and especially to evaluate intrinsic bowel diseases and for concurrent metastatic evaluation.

Contraindications Patients weighing more than 300 lb and patients unable to squeeze into the magnet cannot undergo MRI. An absolute contraindication for MRI is a cardiac pacemaker. Relative contraindications to magnetic resonance imaging include intracranial aneurysm clips, cochlear implants, insulin infusion and chemotherapy pumps, neurocutaneous stimulators, prosthetic heart valves, ocular implants, penile implants, and artificial sphincters depending on date of manufacture and metallurgical composition. Please consult MRI physician if questions arise. Patients who have metallic foreign bodies within the eye or if the object is positioned near a vital neural, vascular, or soft tissue structure; or patients who have undergone recent surgery within the last 6 weeks requiring placement of a vascular surgical clip, should also not undergo MRI. The safety of MRI in pregnant patients has not been determined. In such cases, prior consultation with the MRI physician is required. Generally, patients who have undergone recent surgery not requiring vascular clips or who have had coronary artery bypass surgery in the past may undergo MRI. Patients who have shrapnel wounds or orthopedic prostheses can generally safely undergo MRI unless the metallic device is in the anatomic region to be scanned which results in degradation of the images. Patients with surgically implanted intravascular vena cava filters to prevent pulmonary embolism can usually be scanned if the device has been in place for at least 6
(Continued)

Magnetic Resonance Scan, Abdomen *(Continued)*

weeks. Patients requiring life support equipment, including ventilators, require special preparation. Please contact MRI physician ahead of time. Central venous lines, Swan-Ganz catheters, and nasogastric (NG) tubes usually present no problems. If the patient is positive when screened for metallic devices and you are uncertain of their significance, the MRI radiologist will provide additional information to assist you.

Conflicting examination: Gastrointestinal tract barium studies

Patient Preparation Patients should remain NPO at least 4 hours prior to the exam.

Inpatient: The patient must be able to lie quietly while the scan is performed. The patient should be screened for metallic devices by nursing personnel. (See Contraindications.) This includes metal introduced into the patient either surgically or by trauma. All metallic objects must be removed from the patient, including jewelry or any other metal objects which may be in the patient's bedding. Dentures or other dental appliances must be removed. I.V.s which contain no metal are fine, but infusion pumps must be removed. Oxygen tanks and metallic backboards may come with the patient but will be removed prior to the patient entering the magnet room. Oxygen may be provided in the magnet room. Trauma, ICU, or CCU patients should be accompanied by a nurse. The patient needs to be NPO for abdominal MRI exams. If the patient is restless, combative, or claustrophobic, proper sedation may be administered on the floor prior to the MRI, or at the MRI Center. Consult the MRI radiologists with questions on proper sedation.

Outpatient: The patient should be screened for metallic devices. (See Contraindications.) If a question exists as to the patient's suitability for MRI, the MRI radiologist will assist you with your questions. If the patient is claustrophobic, oral or parenteral sedation may be necessary. If so, the patient should be accompanied by another adult to provide transportation home after the examination.

Aftercare If the patient received an MRI contrast agent (Magnevist®) and develops a delayed hypersensitivity reaction (ie, nausea, emesis, hives, or shortness of breath), the referring physician or MRI radiologist should be contacted immediately. If sedation is used, more time is required after the procedure for recovery period from the sedation.

Technique Unlike most conventional radiologic procedures, magnetic resonance imaging does not utilize ionizing radiation, but relies upon radio frequency or radio signals induced within the patient by the magnetic field to obtain images. There are no known biologic effects secondary to the magnetic fields currently used in clinical MRI. Prior to the scan, the patient will be asked to remove all metallic objects from their person, including loose change, hair pins, earrings, belts, etc. This is for safety reasons as the strong magnetic field could result in these and any other metal objects becoming projectiles resulting in injury to the patient or MRI personnel. Also the patient should not carry a purse or wallet into the magnetic room, as the magnetic field can permanently erase bank cards or credit cards. The magnet is open on both ends and music can be played for the patient if desired. Fresh air is constantly circulated through the magnet room and the patient is continually monitored by the MRI technologist. An intercom system is provided for communication between the patient and the technologist.

No surface coils are used in abdominal MRI and the patient is asked to remain as still as possible during the study.

Data Acquired Digital information with film reproduction

Limitations Generally, the greatest limitation of magnetic resonance imaging results from the patient's fear of the procedure. The patient must remain quiet and still for several scans, each lasting from several minutes to 10 minutes in length. Total examination time is usually 30-45 minutes and occasionally up to 1 hour. If the patient is restless during the examination, motion artifacts will be present on the images limiting their diagnostic value. If the patient is claustrophobic, mild oral sedation or occasionally parenteral sedation may be needed.

Also, the patient can be accompanied by a family member or friend during the examination which may help to calm the patient's anxiety. Patients requiring life support equipment (ie, ventilators) require special preparation. Please refer to Contraindications for further causes for rejection.

Additional Information In some cases, an MRI contrast agent (Magnevist®) may be needed to increase the diagnostic accuracy of the MRI. This contrast agent can be administered to patients with a previous history of allergies to conventional iodinated x-ray agents as it contains no iodine. Contraindications to its use include previous allergy to the contrast agent itself, renal failure, certain types of anemia, and Wilson disease. Nursing mothers should express their breasts and not breast-feed for 36-48 hours after the administration of an MRI contrast agent to ensure that the nursing child does not receive the drug in any notable quantity. The contrast agent is generally very safe and increases the diagnostic efficacy of the MRI. Intramuscular or subcutaneous injection of glucagon may be given to decrease motion artifacts from peristalsis.

References

Alagappan R and Hricak H, "The Kidneys," *Magn Reson Imaging of the Body*, Philadelphia, PA: Lippincott Williams & Wilkins, 1997, 725-60.

Ascher SM and Semelka RC, "The Gastrointestinal Tract," *Magn Reson Imaging of the Body*, New York, NY: Lippincott Williams & Wilkins, 1997, 677-700.

Breitenseher MJ, Metz VM, Gilula LA, et al, "Bioeffects and Safety," *Magn Reson Imaging of the Body*, Philadelphia, PA: Lippincott Williams & Wilkins, 1997, 175-204.

Debatin JF and Dunnick NR, "The Adrenal Glands," *Magn Reson Imaging of the Body*, New York, NY: Lippincott Williams & Wilkins, 1997, 701-24.

Irie H, Honda H, Tajima T, et al, "Optimal MR Cholangiopancreatographic Sequence and Its Clinical Application," *Radiology*, 1998, 206(2):379-87.

Mitchell DG and Semelka RC, "The Pancreas and Spleen," *Magn Reson Imaging of the Body*, Philadelphia, PA: Lippincott Williams & Wilkins, 1997, 639-76.

Semelka RC, Mitchell DG, Reinhold C, et al, "The Liver and Biliary System," *Magn Reson Imaging of the Body*, 3rd ed, Higgins CB, Hricak H, and Helms CA, eds, New York, NY: Lippincott Williams & Wilkins, 1997, 591-637.

Magnetic Resonance Scan, Ankle and Foot

Synonyms Ankle MRI; Foot MRI; MRI, Ankle and Foot

Indications The MRI is indicated to evaluated the tendons and ligaments of the ankle to depict tears, degeneration, subluxation, entrapment, and tenosynovitis. The MRI is useful to depict subtle bone edema in radiographically occult bone contusions and fractures and for detection of early marrow edema in avascular necrosis, and osteomyelitis, and stress fractures. Other pathologies where MRI has proved valuable include osteochondral lesions, arthritis, osteomyelitis, tarsal tunnel syndrome, tarsal coalition, plantar fibromatosis, and Morton's neuroma.

Contraindications Patients weighing more than 300 lb and patients unable to squeeze into the magnet cannot undergo MRI. An absolute contraindication for MRI is a cardiac pacemaker. Relative contraindications to magnetic resonance imaging include intracranial aneurysm clips, cochlear implants, insulin infusion and chemotherapy pumps, neurocutaneous stimulators, prosthetic heart valves, ocular implants, penile implants, and artificial sphincters depending on date of manufacture and metallurgical composition. Please consult MRI physician if questions arise. Patients who have metallic foreign bodies within the eye or if the object is positioned near a vital neural, vascular, or soft tissue structure; or patients who have undergone recent surgery within the last 6 weeks requiring placement of a vascular surgical clip, should also not undergo MRI. The safety of MRI in pregnant patients has not been determined. In such cases, prior consultation with the MRI physician is required. Generally, patients who have undergone recent surgery not requiring vascular clips or who have had coronary artery bypass surgery in the past may undergo MRI. Patients who have shrapnel wounds or orthopedic prostheses can generally safely undergo MRI unless the metallic device is in the anatomic region to be scanned which results in degradation of the images. Patients with surgically implanted intravascular vena cava filters to prevent pulmonary embolism can usually be scanned if the device has been in place for at least 6 weeks. Patients requiring life support equipment, including ventilators, require special preparation. Please contact MRI physician ahead of time. Central

(Continued)

Magnetic Resonance Scan, Ankle and Foot *(Continued)*

venous lines, Swan-Ganz catheters, and nasogastric (NG) tubes usually present no problems. If the patient is positive when screened for metallic devices and you are uncertain of their significance, the MRI radiologist will provide additional information to assist you.

Patient Preparation Inpatient: The patient must be able to lie quietly while the scan is performed. The patient should be screened for metallic devices by nursing personnel. (See Contraindications.) This includes metal introduced into the patient either surgically or by trauma. All metallic objects must be removed from the patient, including jewelry or any other metal objects which may be in the patient's bedding. Dentures or other dental appliances must be removed. I.V.s which contain no metal are fine, but infusion pumps must be removed. Oxygen tanks and metallic backboards may come with the patient but will be removed prior to the patient entering the magnet room. Oxygen may be provided in the magnet room. Trauma, ICU, or CCU patients should be accompanied by a nurse. The patient needs to be NPO for abdominal MRI exams. If the patient is restless, combative, or claustrophobic, proper sedation may be administered on the floor prior to the MRI, or at the MRI Center. Consult the MRI radiologists with questions on proper sedation.

Outpatient: The patient should be screened for metallic devices. (See Contraindications.) If a question exists as to the patient's suitability for MRI, the MRI radiologist will assist you with your questions. If the patient is claustrophobic, oral or parenteral sedation may be necessary. If so, the patient should be accompanied by another adult to provide transportation home after the examination.

Aftercare If the patient received an MRI contrast agent (Magnevist®) and develops a delayed hypersensitivity reaction (ie, nausea, emesis, hives, or shortness of breath), the referring physician or MRI radiologist should be contacted immediately. If sedation is used, more time is required after the procedure for recovery period from the sedation.

Data Acquired Digital information with film reproduction

Limitations Generally, the greatest limitation of magnetic resonance imaging results from the patient's fear of the procedure. The patient must remain quiet and still for several scans, each lasting from several minutes to 10 minutes in length. Total examination time is usually 30-45 minutes and occasionally up to 1 hour. If the patient is restless during the examination, motion artifacts will be present on the images limiting their diagnostic value. If the patient is claustrophobic, mild oral sedation or occasionally parenteral sedation may be needed. Also, the patient can be accompanied by a family member or friend during the examination which may help to calm the patient's anxiety. Patients requiring life support equipment (ie, ventilators) require special preparation. Please refer to Contraindications for further causes for rejection.

Additional Information In some cases, an MRI contrast agent (Magnevist®) may be needed to increase the diagnostic accuracy of the MRI. This contrast agent can be administered to patients with a previous history of allergies to conventional iodinated x-ray agents, as it contains no iodine. Contraindications to its use include previous allergy to the contrast agent itself, renal failure, certain types of anemia, and Wilson disease. Nursing mothers should express their breasts and not breast-feed for 36-48 hours after the administration of an MRI contrast agent to ensure that the nursing child does not receive the drug in any notable quantity. The contrast agent is generally very safe and increases the diagnostic efficacy of the MRI.

References

Erickson AS and Johnson JE, "MR Imaging of the Ankle and Foot," *Radiol Clin North Am*, 1997, 35(1):163-92.

Haygood TM, "Magnetic Resonance Imaging of the Musculoskeletal System. Part 7: The Ankle," *Clin Orthop*, 1997, 336:318-36.

Hochman MG, Min KK, and Zilberfarb JL, "The MR Imaging of the Symptomatic Ankle and Foot," *Orthop Clin North Am*, 1997, 28(4):659-83.

Magnetic Resonance Scan, Aorta

Synonyms Aorta MRI; MRI, Aorta

Indications Establish the diagnosis of aneurysm, dissection, occlusion, sinus of Valsalva aneurysm, and congenital abnormalities such as coarctation; follow-up of angioplasty, invasion or encasement of the aorta by lung, esophageal, and other tumors

Contraindications Patients weighing more than 300 lb and patients unable to squeeze into the magnet cannot undergo MRI. An absolute contraindication for MRI is a cardiac pacemaker. Relative contraindications to magnetic resonance imaging include intracranial aneurysm clips, cochlear implants, insulin infusion and chemotherapy pumps, neurocutaneous stimulators, prosthetic heart valves, ocular implants, penile implants, and artificial sphincters, depending on date of manufacture and metallurgical composition. Please consult MRI physician if questions arise. Patients who have metallic foreign bodies within the eye or if the object is positioned near a vital neural, vascular, or soft tissue structure; or patients who have undergone recent surgery within the last 6 weeks requiring placement of a vascular surgical clip, should also not undergo MRI. The safety of MRI in pregnant patients has not been determined. In such cases, prior consultation with the MRI physician is required. Generally, patients who have undergone recent surgery not requiring vascular clips or who have had coronary artery bypass surgery in the past may undergo MRI. Patients who have shrapnel wounds or orthopedic prostheses can generally safely undergo MRI unless the metallic device is in the anatomic region to be scanned which results in degradation of the images. Patients with surgically implanted intravascular vena cava filters to prevent pulmonary embolism can usually be scanned if the device has been in place for at least 6 weeks. Patients requiring life support equipment, including ventilators, require special preparation. Please contact MRI physician ahead of time. Central venous lines, Swan-Ganz catheters, and nasogastric (NG) tubes usually present no problems. If the patient is positive when screened for metallic devices and you are uncertain of their significance, the MRI radiologist will provide additional information to assist you.

Patient Preparation Inpatient: The patient must be able to lie quietly while the scan is performed. The patient should be screened for metallic devices by nursing personnel. (See Contraindications.) This includes metal introduced into the patient either surgically or by trauma. All metallic objects must be removed from the patient, including jewelry or any other metal objects which may be in the patient's bedding. Dentures or other dental appliances must be removed. I.V.s which contain no metal are fine, but infusion pumps must be removed. Oxygen tanks and metallic backboards may come with the patient but will be removed prior to the patient entering the magnet room. Oxygen may be provided in the magnet room. Trauma, ICU, or CCU patients should be accompanied by a nurse. If the patient is restless, combative, or claustrophobic, proper sedation may be administered on the floor prior to the MRI, or at the MRI Center. Consult the MRI radiologists with questions on proper sedation.

Outpatient: The patient should be screened for metallic devices. (See Contraindications.) If a question exists as to the patient's suitability for MRI, the MRI radiologist will assist you with your questions. If the patient is claustrophobic, oral or parenteral sedation may be necessary. If so, the patient should be accompanied by another adult to provide transportation home after the examination.

Aftercare If the patient received an MRI contrast agent (Magnevist®) and develops a delayed hypersensitivity reaction (ie, nausea, emesis, hives, or shortness of breath), the referring physician or MRI radiologist should be contacted immediately. If sedation is used, more time is required after the procedure for recovery period from the sedation.

Data Acquired Digital information with film reproduction

Limitations Generally, the greatest limitation of magnetic resonance imaging results from the patient's fear of the procedure. The patient must remain quiet and still for several scans, each lasting from several minutes to 10 minutes in length. Total examination time is usually 30-45 minutes and occasionally up to

(Continued)

Magnetic Resonance Scan, Aorta *(Continued)*

1 hour. If the patient is restless during the examination, motion artifacts will be present on the images limiting their diagnostic value. If the patient is claustrophobic, mild oral sedation or occasionally parenteral sedation may be needed. Also, the patient can be accompanied by a family member or friend during the examination which may help to calm the patient's anxiety. Patients requiring life support equipment (ie, ventilators) require special preparation. Please refer to Contraindications for further causes for rejection.

Additional Information In some cases, an MRI contrast agent (Magnevist®) may be needed to increase the diagnostic accuracy of the MRI. This contrast agent can be administered to patients with a previous history of allergies to conventional iodinated x-ray agents, as it contains no iodine. Contraindications to its use include previous allergy to the contrast agent itself, renal failure, certain types of anemia, and Wilson disease. Nursing mothers should express their breasts and not breast-feed for 36-48 hours after the administration of an MRI contrast agent to ensure that the nursing child does not receive the drug in any notable quantity. The contrast agent is generally very safe and increases the diagnostic efficacy of the MRI.

References

Dinsmore R, "Examination of the Adult Heart and Great Vessels," *Clinical Magnetic Resonance Imaging*, Edelman RR and Hesselink JR, eds, Philadelphia, PA: WB Saunders Co, 1990, 773-829.

Higgins CB, "The Thoracic Aorta," *Magn Reson Imaging of the Body*, Philadelphia, PA: Lippincott Williams & Wilkins, 1997, 519-53.

Smyth RH and Grist TM, "MR Angiography of the Abdominal Aorta," *Magn Reson Imaging Clin N Am*, 1998, 6(2):321-9.

Soler R, Rodriguez E, Requejo I, et al, "Magn Reson Imaging of Congenital Abnormalities of the Thoracic Aorta," *Eur J Radiol*, 1998, 8(4):540-6.

Magnetic Resonance Scan, Bone Marrow

Synonyms Bone Marrow MRI; MRI, Bone Marrow

Indications Define marrow anatomy and assess its morphologic appearance. MRI can determine the normal chronologic changes in fatty marrow conversion, and evaluate many pathologies with bone marrow involvement, such as multiple myeloma, metastases, lymphoma, primary bone tumors, leukemia, reconversion (anemia or incidental), myelofibrosis, polycythemia vera, hemosiderosis, Gaucher disease, osteomyelitis, aplastic anemia, hyperemia, and ischemia.

Contraindications Patients weighing more than 300 lb and patients unable to squeeze into the magnet cannot undergo MRI. An absolute contraindication for MRI is a cardiac pacemaker. Relative contraindications to magnetic resonance imaging include intracranial aneurysm clips, cochlear implants, insulin infusion and chemotherapy pumps, neurocutaneous stimulators, prosthetic heart valves, ocular implants, penile implants, and artificial sphincters depending on date of manufacture and metallurgical composition. Please consult MRI physician if questions arise. Patients who have metallic foreign bodies within the eye or if the object is positioned near a vital neural, vascular, or soft tissue structure; or patients who have undergone recent surgery within the last 6 weeks requiring placement of a vascular surgical clip, should also not undergo MRI. The safety of MRI in pregnant patients has not been determined. In such cases, prior consultation with the MRI physician is required. Generally, patients who have undergone recent surgery not requiring vascular clips or who have had coronary artery bypass surgery in the past may undergo MRI. Patients who have shrapnel wounds or orthopedic prostheses can generally safely undergo MRI unless the metallic device is in the anatomic region to be scanned which results in degradation of the images. Patients with surgically implanted intravascular vena cava filters to prevent pulmonary embolism can usually be scanned if the device has been in place for at least 6 weeks. Patients requiring life support equipment, including ventilators, require special preparation. Please contact MRI physician ahead of time. Central venous lines, Swan-Ganz catheters, and nasogastric (NG) tubes usually present no problems. If the patient is positive when screened for metallic devices and you are uncertain of their significance, the MRI radiologist will provide additional information to assist you.

Patient Preparation Inpatient: The patient must be able to lie quietly while the scan is performed. The patient should be screened for metallic devices by nursing personnel. (See Contraindications.) This includes metal introduced into the patient either surgically or by trauma. All metallic objects must be removed from the patient, including jewelry or any other metal objects which may be in the patient's bedding. Dentures or other dental appliances must be removed. I.V.s which contain no metal are fine, but infusion pumps must be removed. Oxygen tanks and metallic backboards may come with the patient but will be removed prior to the patient entering the magnet room. Oxygen may be provided in the magnet room. Trauma, ICU, or CCU patients should be accompanied by a nurse. The patient needs to be NPO for abdominal MRI exams. If the patient is restless, combative, or claustrophobic, proper sedation may be administered on the floor prior to the MRI, or at the MRI Center. Consult the MRI radiologists with questions on proper sedation.

Outpatient: The patient should be screened for metallic devices. (See Contraindications.) If a question exists as to the patient's suitability for MRI, the MRI radiologist will assist you with your questions. If the patient is claustrophobic, oral or parenteral sedation may be necessary. If so, the patient should be accompanied by another adult to provide transportation home after the examination.

Aftercare If the patient received an MRI contrast agent (Magnevist®) and develops a delayed hypersensitivity reaction (ie, nausea, emesis, hives, or shortness of breath), the referring physician or MRI radiologist should be contacted immediately. If sedation is used, more time is required after the procedure for recovery period from the sedation.

Technique Unlike most conventional radiologic procedures, magnetic resonance imaging does not utilize ionizing radiation, but relies upon radio frequency or radio signals induced within the patient by the magnetic field to obtain images. There are no known biologic effects secondary to the magnetic fields currently used in clinical MRI. Prior to the scan, the patient will be asked to remove all metallic objects from their person, including loose change, hair pins, earrings, belts, etc. This is for safety reasons as the strong magnetic field could result in these and any other metal objects becoming projectiles resulting in injury to the patient or MRI personnel. Also the patient should not carry a purse or wallet into the magnetic room, as the magnetic field can permanently erase bank cards or credit cards. The magnet is open on both ends and music can be played for the patient if desired. Fresh air is constantly circulated through the magnet room and the patient is continually monitored by the MRI technologist. An intercom system is provided for communication between the patient and the technologist. A surface coil will be utilized in areas of the body where applicable.

Data Acquired Digital information with film reproduction

Limitations Generally, the greatest limitation of magnetic resonance imaging results from the patient's fear of the procedure. The patient must remain quiet and still for several scans, each lasting from several minutes to 10 minutes in length. Total examination time is usually 30-45 minutes and occasionally up to 1 hour. If the patient is restless during the examination, motion artifacts will be present on the images limiting their diagnostic value. If the patient is claustrophobic, mild oral sedation or occasionally parenteral sedation may be needed. Also, the patient can be accompanied by a family member or friend during the examination which may help to calm the patient's anxiety. Patients requiring life support equipment (ie, ventilators) require special preparation. Please refer to Contraindications for further causes for rejection. Implanted orthopedic appliances may limit the usefulness of the scan in the area being imaged.

Additional Information In some cases, an MRI contrast agent (Magnevist®) may be needed to increase the diagnostic accuracy of the MRI. This contrast agent can be administered to patients with a previous history of allergies to conventional iodinated x-ray agents, as it contains no iodine. Contraindications to its use include previous allergy to the contrast agent itself, renal

(Continued)

Magnetic Resonance Scan, Bone Marrow *(Continued)*

failure, certain types of anemia, and Wilson disease. Nursing mothers should express their breasts and not breast-feed for 36-48 hours after the administration of an MRI contrast agent to ensure that the nursing child does not receive the drug in any notable quantity. The contrast agent is generally very safe and increases the diagnostic efficacy of the MRI.

References

Deely DM and Schweitzer ME, "MR Imaging of Bone Marrow Disorders," *Radiol Clin North Am*, 1997, 35(1):193-212.

Kaplan PA and Dussault RG, "Bone Marrow," *Magn Reson Imaging of the Body*, Philadelphia, PA: Lippincott Williams & Wilkins, 1997, 1295-320.

Koo KH, Dussault R, Kaplan P, et al, "Age-Related Marrow Conversion in the Proximal Metaphysis of the Femur: Evaluation With T1-Weighted MR Imaging," *Radiology*, 1998, 206(3):745-8.

Magnetic Resonance Scan, Brachial Plexus

Synonyms Brachial Plexus MRI; MRI, Brachial Plexus

Indications Diagnostic questions regarding the brachial plexus arise from the occurrence of symptoms consistent with a brachial plexopathy, or the presence of a pathological lesion located in proximity to the course of the brachial plexus, including primary or secondary tumors. Two of the most common malignant tumors, bronchogenic carcinoma and breast carcinoma, may affect the brachial plexus. Other indications include trauma of the neck, shoulder, or upper extremity which may involve the brachial plexus causing avulsion injuries, radiation therapy of the lung or breast, or intrinsic diseases of the brachial plexus (ie, neuritis and the so-called idiopathic brachial plexopathy).

Contraindications Patients weighing more than 300 lb and patients unable to squeeze into the magnet cannot undergo MRI. An absolute contraindication for MRI is a cardiac pacemaker. Relative contraindications to magnetic resonance imaging include intracranial aneurysm clips, cochlear implants, insulin infusion and chemotherapy pumps, neurocutaneous stimulators, prosthetic heart valves, ocular implants, penile implants, and artificial sphincters depending on date of manufacture and metallurgical composition. Please consult MRI physician if questions arise. Patients who have metallic foreign bodies within the eye or if the object is positioned near a vital neural, vascular, or soft tissue structure; or patients who have undergone recent surgery within the last 6 weeks requiring placement of a vascular surgical clip, should also not undergo MRI. The safety of MRI in pregnant patients has not been determined. In such cases, prior consultation with the MRI physician is required. Generally, patients who have undergone recent surgery not requiring vascular clips or who have had coronary artery bypass surgery in the past may undergo MRI. Patients who have shrapnel wounds or orthopedic prostheses can generally safely undergo MRI unless the metallic device is in the anatomic region to be scanned which results in degradation of the images. Patients with surgically implanted intravascular vena cava filters to prevent pulmonary embolism can usually be scanned if the device has been in place for at least 6 weeks. Patients requiring life support equipment, including ventilators, require special preparation. Please contact MRI physician ahead of time. Central venous lines, Swan-Ganz catheters, and nasogastric (NG) tubes usually present no problems. If the patient is positive when screened for metallic devices and you are uncertain of their significance, the MRI radiologist will provide additional information to assist you.

Patient Preparation Inpatient: The patient must be able to lie quietly while the scan is performed. The patient should be screened for metallic devices by nursing personnel. (See Contraindications.) This includes metal introduced into the patient either surgically or by trauma. All metallic objects must be removed from the patient, including jewelry or any other metal objects which may be in the patient's bedding. Dentures or other dental appliances must be removed. I.V.s which contain no metal are fine, but infusion pumps must be removed. Oxygen tanks and metallic backboards may come with the patient but will be removed prior to the patient entering the magnet room. Oxygen may be provided in the magnet room. Trauma, ICU, or CCU patients should be accompanied by a nurse. The patient needs to be NPO for abdominal MRI exams. If the patient is restless, combative, or claustrophobic, proper sedation may be administered on the floor prior to the MRI, or at the MRI Center. Consult the MRI radiologists with questions on proper sedation.

Outpatient: The patient should be screened for metallic devices. (See Contraindications.) If a question exists as to the patient's suitability for MRI, the MRI radiologist will assist you with your questions. If the patient is claustrophobic, oral or parenteral sedation may be necessary. If so, the patient should be accompanied by another adult to provide transportation home after the examination.

Aftercare If the patient received an MRI contrast agent (Magnevist®) and develops a delayed hypersensitivity reaction (ie, nausea, emesis, hives, or shortness of breath), the referring physician or MRI radiologist should be contacted immediately. If sedation is used, more time is required after the procedure for recovery period from the sedation.

Data Acquired Digital information with film reproduction

Limitations Generally, the greatest limitation of magnetic resonance imaging results from the patient's fear of the procedure. The patient must remain quiet and still for several scans, each lasting from several minutes to 10 minutes in length. Total examination time is usually 30-45 minutes and occasionally up to 1 hour. If the patient is restless during the examination, motion artifacts will be present on the images limiting their diagnostic value. If the patient is claustrophobic, mild oral sedation or occasionally parenteral sedation may be needed. Also, the patient can be accompanied by a family member or friend during the examination which may help to calm the patient's anxiety. Patients requiring life support equipment (ie, ventilators) require special preparation. Please refer to Contraindications for further causes for rejection.

Additional Information In some cases, an MRI contrast agent (Magnevist®) may be needed to increase the diagnostic accuracy of the MRI. This contrast agent can be administered to patients with a previous history of allergies to conventional iodinated x-ray agents, as it contains no iodine. Contraindications to its use include previous allergy to the contrast agent itself, renal failure, certain types of anemia, and Wilson disease. Nursing mothers should express their breasts and not breast-feed for 36-48 hours after the administration of an MRI contrast agent to ensure that the nursing child does not receive the drug in any notable quantity. The contrast agent is generally very safe and increases the diagnostic efficacy of the MRI.

References

Hayashi N, Yamamoto S, Okubo T, et al, "Avulsion Injury of Cervical Nerve Roots: Enhanced Intradural Nerve Roots at MR Imaging," *Radiology*, 1998, 206(3):817-22.

Higgins CB, "The Brachial Plexus," *Clinical Magnetic Resonance Imaging*, Philadelphia, PA: WB Saunders Co, 1997, 291-315.

Magnetic Resonance Scan, Brain

Related Information

Computed Transaxial Tomography, Head Studies *on page 332*

Synonyms Brain MRI; MRI, Brain

Applies to Magnetic Resonance Scan, Head

Indications Diagnose intracranial abnormalities including intra- and extra-axial tumors, vascular malformations and aneurysm, ischemia and infarction, head trauma, infection, white matter diseases, phakomatosis, inherited syndromes, or any abnormalities relating to the brain or calvarium. MRI is an excellent modality for assessment of congenital brain abnormalities or relating to the status of brain maturation in the pediatric population. In addition, the MRI can investigate cerebral physiology, using diffusion and perfusion techniques, which can characterize the time of stroke. The neurospectroscopy is other new technique that can be useful in cases of dementia, hepatic encephalopathy, hypoxic encephalopathy, neonatal hypoxia, closed head trauma, and also to differentiate tumor recurrence from radiation necrosis.

Contraindications Patients weighing more than 300 lb and patients unable to squeeze into the magnet cannot undergo MRI. An absolute contraindication for MRI is a cardiac pacemaker. Relative contraindications to magnetic resonance imaging include intracranial aneurysm clips, cochlear implants, insulin infusion and chemotherapy pumps, neurocutaneous stimulators, prosthetic heart valves, ocular implants, penile implants, and artificial sphincters

(Continued)

Magnetic Resonance Scan, Brain *(Continued)*

depending on date of manufacture and metallurgical composition. Please consult MRI physician if questions arise. Patients who have metallic foreign bodies within the eye or if the object is positioned near a vital neural, vascular, or soft tissue structure; or patients who have undergone recent surgery within the last 6 weeks requiring placement of a vascular surgical clip, should also not undergo MRI. The safety of MRI in pregnant patients has not been determined. In such cases, prior consultation with the MRI physician is required. Generally, patients who have undergone recent surgery not requiring vascular clips or who have had coronary artery bypass surgery in the past may undergo MRI. Patients who have shrapnel wounds or orthopedic prostheses can generally safely undergo MRI unless the metallic device is in the anatomic region to be scanned which results in degradation of the images. Patients with surgically implanted intravascular vena cava filters to prevent pulmonary embolism can usually be scanned if the device has been in place for at least 6 weeks. Patients requiring life support equipment, including ventilators, require special preparation. Please contact MRI physician ahead of time. Central venous lines, Swan-Ganz catheters, and nasogastric (NG) tubes usually present no problems. If the patient is positive when screened for metallic devices and you are uncertain of their significance, the MRI radiologist will provide additional information to assist you.

Patient Preparation Inpatient: The patient must be able to lie quietly while the scan is performed. The patient should be screened for metallic devices by nursing personnel. (See Contraindications.) This includes metal introduced into the patient either surgically or by trauma. All metallic objects must be removed from the patient, including jewelry or any other metal objects which may be in the patient's bedding. Dentures or other dental appliances must be removed. I.V.s which contain no metal are fine, but infusion pumps must be removed. Oxygen tanks and metallic backboards may come with the patient but will be removed prior to the patient entering the magnet room. Oxygen may be provided in the magnet room. Trauma, ICU, or CCU patients should be accompanied by a nurse. The patient needs to be NPO for abdominal MRI exams. If the patient is restless, combative, or claustrophobic, proper sedation may be administered on the floor prior to the MRI, or at the MRI Center. Consult the MRI radiologists with questions on proper sedation.

Outpatient: The patient should be screened for metallic devices. (See Contraindications.) If a question exists as to the patient's suitability for MRI, the MRI radiologist will assist you with your questions. If the patient is claustrophobic, oral or parenteral sedation may be necessary. If so, the patient should be accompanied by another adult to provide transportation home after the examination.

Aftercare If the patient received an MRI contrast agent (Magnevist®) and develops a delayed hypersensitivity reaction (ie, nausea, emesis, hives, or shortness of breath), the referring physician or MRI radiologist should be contacted immediately. If sedation is used, more time is required after the procedure for recovery period from the sedation.

Technique Unlike most conventional radiologic procedures, magnetic resonance imaging does not utilize ionizing radiation, but relies upon radio frequency or radio signals induced within the patient by the magnetic field to obtain images. There are no known biologic effects secondary to the magnetic fields currently used in clinical MRI. Prior to the scan, the patient will be asked to remove all metallic objects from their person, including loose change, hair pins, earrings, belts, etc. This is for safety reasons as the strong magnetic field could result in these and any other metal objects becoming projectiles resulting in injury to the patient or MRI personnel. Also the patient should not carry a purse or wallet into the magnetic room, as the magnetic field can permanently erase bank cards or credit cards. The magnet is open on both ends and music can be played for the patient if desired. Fresh air is constantly circulated through the magnet room and the patient is continually monitored by the MRI technologist. An intercom system is provided for communication between the patient and the technologist. For MRI of the brain, a special coil surrounds, but does not touch the patient's head. The patient will be asked to remain very still while scans are being obtained. In certain cases, an MRI contrast agent, Gadopentetate Dimeglumine (Magnevist®) may be necessary to increase the diagnostic accuracy of the MRI examination. This is administered intravenously, via an antecubital vein in a small volume (less than 20 mL). This contrast agent may be used in patients who are allergic to conventional iodinated contrast agents such as is used in IVPs or CT examination without difficulty. There are very few contraindications to its use. (See Contraindications.)

Data Acquired Digital information with film reproduction

Limitations Generally, the greatest limitation of magnetic resonance imaging results from the patient's fear of the procedure. The patient must remain quiet and still for several scans, each lasting from several minutes to 10 minutes in length. Total examination time is usually 30-45 minutes and occasionally up to 1 hour. If the patient is restless during the examination, motion artifacts will be present on the images limiting their diagnostic value. If the patient is claustrophobic, mild oral sedation or occasionally parenteral sedation may be needed. Also, the patient can be accompanied by a family member or friend during the examination which may help to calm the patient's anxiety. Patients requiring life support equipment (ie, ventilators) require special preparation. Please refer to Contraindications for further causes for rejection.

Additional Information In some cases, an MRI contrast agent (Magnevist®) may be needed to increase the diagnostic accuracy of the MRI. This contrast agent can be administered to patients with a previous history of allergies to conventional iodinated x-ray agents, as it contains no iodine. Contraindications to its use include previous allergy to the contrast agent itself, renal failure, certain types of anemia, and Wilson disease. Nursing mothers should express their breasts and not breast-feed for 36-48 hours after the administration of an MRI contrast agent to ensure that the nursing child does not receive the drug in any notable quantity. The contrast agent is generally very safe and increases the diagnostic efficacy of the MRI.

References

Danielsen ER and Ross BD, "Neurospectroscopy," *Magn Reson Imaging*, 3rd ed, Stark DD and Bradley WG Jr, eds, St Louis, MO: CV Mosby Co, 1999, 1595-635.

Moseley ME and Butts K, "Diffusion and Perfusion," *Magn Reson Imaging*, 3rd ed, Stark DD and Bradley WG Jr, eds, St Louis, MO: CV Mosby Co, 1999, 1515-38.

Sorensen AG and Rosen BR, "Functional MRI of the Brain," *Magnetic Resonance Imaging of the Brain and Spine*, Philadelphia, PA: Lippincott Williams & Wilkins, 1996, 1501-45.

Magnetic Resonance Scan, Breast

Synonyms Breast MRI; MRI, Breast

Indications Evaluation of the breast in cases where other techniques (ie, mammography and ultrasound) are limited. These include patients with silicone implants after mastectomy or augmentation mammoplasty (detection of recurrence/prosthesis rupture/silicon leakage); patients whose breasts are difficult to evaluate by combined mammography and ultrasound, who have had breast conservation therapy, or who have proven carcinoma in one or proven axillary lymph node metastases from an unknown primary tumor, especially when these are hormone receptor-positive; and finally, patients with extensive postoperative scarring.

Contraindications Patients weighing more than 300 lb and patients unable to squeeze into the magnet cannot undergo MRI. An absolute contraindication for MRI is a cardiac pacemaker. Relative contraindications to magnetic resonance imaging include intracranial aneurysm clips, cochlear implants, insulin infusion and chemotherapy pumps, neurocutaneous stimulators, prosthetic heart valves, ocular implants, penile implants, and artificial sphincters depending on date of manufacture and metallurgical composition. Please consult MRI physician if questions arise. Patients who have metallic foreign bodies within the eye or if the object is positioned near a vital neural, vascular, or soft tissue structure; or patients who have undergone recent surgery within the last 6 weeks requiring placement of a vascular surgical clip, should also not undergo MRI. The safety of MRI in pregnant patients has not been determined. In such cases, prior consultation with the MRI physician is required. Generally, patients who have undergone recent surgery not requiring vascular

(Continued)

Magnetic Resonance Scan, Breast *(Continued)*

clips or who have had coronary artery bypass surgery in the past may undergo MRI. Patients who have shrapnel wounds or orthopedic prostheses can generally safely undergo MRI unless the metallic device is in the anatomic region to be scanned which results in degradation of the images. Patients with surgically implanted intravascular vena cava filters to prevent pulmonary embolism can usually be scanned if the device has been in place for at least 6 weeks. Patients requiring life support equipment, including ventilators, require special preparation. Please contact MRI physician ahead of time. Central venous lines, Swan-Ganz catheters, and nasogastric (NG) tubes usually present no problems. If the patient is positive when screened for metallic devices and you are uncertain of their significance, the MRI radiologist will provide additional information to assist you.

Patient Preparation Inpatient: The patient must be able to lie quietly while the scan is performed. The patient should be screened for metallic devices by nursing personnel. (See Contraindications.) This includes metal introduced into the patient either surgically or by trauma. All metallic objects must be removed from the patient, including jewelry or any other metal objects which may be in the patient's bedding. Dentures or other dental appliances must be removed. I.V.s which contain no metal are fine, but infusion pumps must be removed. Oxygen tanks and metallic backboards may come with the patient but will be removed prior to the patient entering the magnet room. Oxygen may be provided in the magnet room. Trauma, ICU, or CCU patients should be accompanied by a nurse. If the patient is restless, combative, or claustrophobic, proper sedation may be administered on the floor prior to the MRI, or at the MRI Center. Consult the MRI radiologists with questions on proper sedation.

Outpatient: The patient should be screened for metallic devices. (See Contraindications.) If a question exists as to the patient's suitability for MRI, the MRI radiologist will assist you with your questions. If the patient is claustrophobic, oral or parenteral sedation may be necessary. If so, the patient should be accompanied by another adult to provide transportation home after the examination.

Aftercare If the patient received an MRI contrast agent (Magnevist®) and develops a delayed hypersensitivity reaction (ie, nausea, emesis, hives, or shortness of breath), the referring physician or MRI radiologist should be contacted immediately. If sedation is used, more time is required after the procedure for recovery period from the sedation.

Data Acquired Digital information with film reproduction

Limitations Generally, the greatest limitation of magnetic resonance imaging results from the patient's fear of the procedure. The patient must remain quiet and still for several scans, each lasting from several minutes to 10 minutes in length. Total examination time is usually 30-45 minutes and occasionally up to 1 hour. If the patient is restless during the examination, motion artifacts will be present on the images limiting their diagnostic value. If the patient is claustrophobic, mild oral sedation or occasionally parenteral sedation may be needed. Also, the patient can be accompanied by a family member or friend during the examination which may help to calm the patient's anxiety. Patients requiring life support equipment (ie, ventilators) require special preparation. Please refer to Contraindications for further causes for rejection.

Additional Information In some cases, an MRI contrast agent (Magnevist®) may be needed to increase the diagnostic accuracy of the MRI. This contrast agent can be administered to patients with a previous history of allergies to conventional iodinated x-ray agents, as it contains no iodine. Contraindications to its use include previous allergy to the contrast agent itself, renal failure, certain types of anemia, and Wilson disease. Nursing mothers should express their breasts and not breast-feed for 36-48 hours after the administration of an MRI contrast agent to ensure that the nursing child does not receive the drug in any notable quantity. The contrast agent is generally very safe and increases the diagnostic efficacy of the MRI.

References

Friedrich M, "MRI of the Breast: State of the Art," *Eur J Radiol*, 1998, 8(5):707-25.

Heywang-Kobrunner S and Hilbertz T, "The Breast," *Magn Reson Imaging of the Body*, Philadelphia, PA: Lippincott Williams & Wilkins, 1997, 379-95.

Magnetic Resonance Scan, Cardiac

Synonyms Cardiac MRI; MRI, Cardiac

Indications The use of MRI in congenital and acquired diseases is for the most part supplemental to echocardiography and its applications are related to the capability for morphologic diagnoses. The major clinical indications for acquired disease include determination of the presence and location of previous myocardial infarctions, constrictive pericardial disease, hypertrophic cardiomyopathy, right ventricular dysplasia, valvular disease, and paracardiac and intracardiac disease. For the congenital diseases the major indications are pulmonary atresia, tetralogy of Fallot, transposition of great arteries, double outlet right ventricle, truncus arteriosus, all types of ventricular septal defect, abnormalities of atrioventricular connections, and atrial abnormalities. MRI imaging can be also helpful to characterize ischemic syndromes such as ischemia, myocardial infarction, stunned myocardium, and hibernating myocardium.

Contraindications Patients weighing more than 300 lb and patients unable to squeeze into the magnet cannot undergo MRI. An absolute contraindication for MRI is a cardiac pacemaker. Relative contraindications to magnetic resonance imaging include intracranial aneurysm clips, cochlear implants, insulin infusion and chemotherapy pumps, neurocutaneous stimulators, prosthetic heart valves, ocular implants, penile implants, and artificial sphincters depending on date of manufacture and metallurgical composition. Please consult MRI physician if questions arise. Patients who have metallic foreign bodies within the eye or if the object is positioned near a vital neural, vascular, or soft tissue structure; or patients who have undergone recent surgery within the last 6 weeks requiring placement of a vascular surgical clip, should also not undergo MRI. The safety of MRI in pregnant patients has not been determined. In such cases, prior consultation with the MRI physician is required. Generally, patients who have undergone recent surgery not requiring vascular clips or who have had coronary artery bypass surgery in the past may undergo MRI. Patients who have shrapnel wounds or orthopedic prostheses can generally safely undergo MRI unless the metallic device is in the anatomic region to be scanned which results in degradation of the images. Patients with surgically implanted intravascular vena cava filters to prevent pulmonary embolism can usually be scanned if the device has been in place for at least 6 weeks. Patients requiring life support equipment, including ventilators, require special preparation. Please contact MRI physician ahead of time. Central venous lines, Swan-Ganz catheters, and nasogastric (NG) tubes usually present no problems. If the patient is positive when screened for metallic devices and you are uncertain of their significance, the MRI radiologist will provide additional information to assist you.

Patient Preparation Inpatient: The patient must be able to lie quietly while the scan is performed. The patient should be screened for metallic devices by nursing personnel. (See Contraindications.) This includes metal introduced into the patient either surgically or by trauma. All metallic objects must be removed from the patient, including jewelry or any other metal objects which may be in the patient's bedding. Dentures or other dental appliances must be removed. I.V.s which contain no metal are fine, but infusion pumps must be removed. Oxygen tanks and metallic backboards may come with the patient but will be removed prior to the patient entering the magnet room. Oxygen may be provided in the magnet room. Trauma, ICU, or CCU patients should be accompanied by a nurse. If the patient is restless, combative, or claustrophobic, proper sedation may be administered on the floor prior to the MRI, or at the MRI Center. Consult the MRI radiologists with questions on proper sedation.

Outpatient: The patient should be screened for metallic devices. (See Contraindications.) If a question exists as to the patient's suitability for MRI, the MRI radiologist will assist you with your questions. If the patient is claustrophobic, oral or parenteral sedation may be necessary. If so, the patient should be

(Continued)

Magnetic Resonance Scan, Cardiac *(Continued)*

accompanied by another adult to provide transportation home after the examination.

Aftercare If the patient received an MRI contrast agent (Magnevist®) and develops a delayed hypersensitivity reaction (ie, nausea, emesis, hives, or shortness of breath), the referring physician or MRI radiologist should be contacted immediately. If sedation is used, more time is required after the procedure for recovery period from the sedation.

Data Acquired Digital information displayed as static film based images and cine loop. Data is EKG gated.

Limitations The patient's motion and cardiac rhythm abnormalities will degrade the study, limiting interpretation. Generally, the greatest limitation of magnetic resonance imaging results from the patient's fear of the procedure. The patient must remain quiet and still for several scans, each lasting from several minutes to 10 minutes in length. Total examination time is usually up to 1 hour. If the patient is restless during the examination, motion artifacts will be present on the images limiting their diagnostic value. If the patient is claustrophobic, oral or parenteral sedation may be needed. Patients requiring life support equipment (ie, ventilators) require special preparation. Please refer to Contraindications for further causes for rejection.

Additional Information In some cases, an MRI contrast agent (Magnevist®) may be needed to increase the diagnostic accuracy of the MRI. This contrast agent can be administered to patients with a previous history of allergies to conventional iodinated x-ray agents as it contains no iodine. Contraindications to its use include previous allergy to the contrast agent itself, renal failure, certain types of anemia, and Wilson disease. Nursing mothers should express their breasts and not breast-feed for 36-48 hours after the administration of an MRI contrast agent to ensure that the nursing child does not receive the drug in any notable quantity. The contrast agent is generally very safe and increases the diagnostic efficacy of the MRI.

References

Geskin G, Kramer CM, Rogers WJ, et al, "Quantitative Assessment of Myocardial Viability After Infarction by Dobutamine Magnetic Resonance Tagging," *Circulation*, 1998, 98(3):217-23.

Higgins CB, "Acquired Heart Disease," *Magn Reson Imaging of the Body*, Philadelphia, PA: Lippincott Williams & Wilkins, 1997, 409-60, 461-518.

Higgins CB, "Ischemic Heart Disease," *Magn Reson Imaging of the Body*, Philadelphia, PA: Lippincott Williams & Wilkins, 1997, 567-87.

Magnetic Resonance Scan, Cervical and Thoracic Spine

Related Information

Computed Transaxial Tomography, Spine *on page 340*

Synonyms Cervical Spine MRI; MRI, Cervical and Thoracic Spine; Spinal MRI; Thoracic Spine MRI

Replaces Discogram

Indications Assessment of intramedullary spinal cord disease (eg, tumors, infection, ischemia, vascular malformation, hemorrhage, inflammatory conditions, and demyelination); extramedullary-intradural disease (eg, tumors, infection, disc degeneration, herniation); evaluate the skull base (cervicomedullary junction); evaluate congenital abnormalities (eg, Chiari malformation, myelocele, myelomeningocele, lipomyelomeningocele, diastematomyelia)

Contraindications Patients weighing more than 300 lb and patients unable to squeeze into the magnet cannot undergo MRI. An absolute contraindication for MRI is a cardiac pacemaker. Relative contraindications to magnetic resonance imaging include intracranial aneurysm clips, cochlear implants, insulin infusion and chemotherapy pumps, neurocutaneous stimulators, prosthetic heart valves, ocular implants, penile implants, and artificial sphincters depending on date of manufacture and metallurgical composition. Please consult MRI physician if questions arise. Patients who have metallic foreign bodies within the eye or if the object is positioned near a vital neural, vascular, or soft tissue structure; or patients who have undergone recent surgery within the last 6 weeks requiring placement of a vascular surgical clip, should also not undergo MRI. The safety of MRI in pregnant patients has not been determined. In such cases, prior consultation with the MRI physician is required. Generally, patients who have undergone recent surgery not requiring vascular clips or who have had coronary artery bypass surgery in the past may undergo MRI. Patients who have shrapnel wounds or orthopedic prostheses can generally safely undergo MRI unless the metallic device is in the anatomic region to be scanned which results in degradation of the images. Patients with surgically implanted intravascular vena cava filters to prevent pulmonary embolism can usually be scanned if the device has been in place for at least 6 weeks. Patients requiring life support equipment, including ventilators, require special preparation. Please contact MRI physician ahead of time. Central venous lines, Swan-Ganz catheters, and nasogastric (NG) tubes usually present no problems. If the patient is positive when screened for metallic devices and you are uncertain of their significance, the MRI radiologist will provide additional information to assist you.

Patient Preparation **Inpatient**: The patient must be able to lie quietly while the scan is performed. The patient should be screened for metallic devices by nursing personnel. (See Contraindications.) This includes metal introduced into the patient either surgically or by trauma. All metallic objects must be removed from the patient, including jewelry or any other metal objects which may be in the patient's bedding. Dentures or other dental appliances must be removed. I.V.s which contain no metal are fine, but infusion pumps must be removed. Oxygen tanks and metallic backboards may come with the patient but will be removed prior to the patient entering the magnet room. Oxygen may be provided in the magnet room. Trauma, ICU, or CCU patients should be accompanied by a nurse. The patient needs to be NPO for abdominal MRI exams. If the patient is restless, combative, or claustrophobic, proper sedation may be administered on the floor prior to the MRI, or at the MRI Center. Consult the MRI radiologists with questions on proper sedation.

Outpatient: The patient should be screened for metallic devices. (See Contraindications.) If a question exists as to the patient's suitability for MRI, the MRI radiologist will assist you with your questions. If the patient is claustrophobic, oral or parenteral sedation may be necessary. If so, the patient should be accompanied by another adult to provide transportation home after the examination.

Aftercare If the patient received an MRI contrast agent (Magnevist®) and develops a delayed hypersensitivity reaction (ie, nausea, emesis, hives, or shortness of breath), the referring physician or MRI radiologist should be contacted immediately. If sedation is used, more time is required after the procedure for recovery period from the sedation.

Technique Unlike most conventional radiologic procedures, magnetic resonance imaging does not utilize ionizing radiation, but relies upon radio frequency or radio signals induced within the patient by the magnetic field to obtain images. There are no known biologic effects secondary to the magnetic fields currently used in clinical MRI. Prior to the scan, the patient will be asked to remove all metallic objects from their person, including loose change, hair pins, earrings, belts, etc. This is for safety reasons as the strong magnetic field could result in these and any other metal objects becoming projectiles resulting in injury to the patient or MRI personnel. Also the patient should not carry a purse or wallet into the magnetic room, as the magnetic field can permanently erase bank cards or credit cards. The magnet is open on both ends and music can be played for the patient if desired. Fresh air is constantly circulated through the magnet room and the patient is continually monitored by the MRI technologist. An intercom system is provided for communication between the patient and the technologist. For MRI of the cervical spine, the patient will be asked to lie on a surface coil on the posterior neck and asked to remain still during scanning. In certain cases, an MRI contrast agent, Gadopentetate Dimeglumine (Magnevist®) may be necessary to increase the diagnostic accuracy of the MRI examination. This is administered intravenously, via an antecubital vein in a small volume (less than 20 mL). This contrast agent may be used in patients who are allergic to conventional iodinated

(Continued)

Magnetic Resonance Scan, Cervical and Thoracic Spine *(Continued)*

contrast agents such as is used in IVPs or CT examination without difficulty. There are very few contraindications to its use. (See Contraindications.)

Data Acquired Digital information with film reproduction

Limitations Generally, the greatest limitation of magnetic resonance imaging results from the patient's fear of the procedure. The patient must remain quiet and still for several scans, each lasting from several minutes to 10 minutes in length. Total examination time is usually 30-45 minutes and occasionally up to 1 hour. If the patient is restless during the examination, motion artifacts will be present on the images limiting their diagnostic value. If the patient is claustrophobic, mild oral sedation or occasionally parenteral sedation may be needed. Also, the patient can be accompanied by a family member or friend during the examination which may help to calm the patient's anxiety. Patients requiring life support equipment (ie, ventilators) require special preparation. Please refer to Contraindications for further causes for rejection.

Additional Information In some cases, an MRI contrast agent (Magnevist®) may be needed to increase the diagnostic accuracy of the MRI. This contrast agent can be administered to patients with a previous history of allergies to conventional iodinated x-ray agents, as it contains no iodine. Contraindications to its use include previous allergy to the contrast agent itself, renal failure, certain types of anemia, and Wilson disease. Nursing mothers should express their breasts and not breast-feed for 36-48 hours after the administration of an MRI contrast agent to ensure that the nursing child does not receive the drug in any notable quantity. The contrast agent is generally very safe and increases the diagnostic efficacy of the MRI.

References

Schenk M and Masaryk TJ, "The Cervical-Thoracic Spine," *Magn Reson Imaging of the Body*, 3rd ed, Higgins CB, Hricak H, and Helms CA, eds, Philadelphia, PA: Lippincott Williams & Wilkins, 1997, 987-1043.

Simon JE and Lukin RR, "Diskogenic Disease of the Cervical Spine," *Semin Roentgenol*, 1988, 23(2):118-24.

Magnetic Resonance Scan, Chest

Synonyms Chest MRI; MRI, Chest

Applies to Magnetic Resonance Scan, Thorax

Indications Evaluation of the chest for pathology including the heart, major vessels, mediastinum, hilar lesions, lungs, pleura, and chest wall. From a clinical viewpoint, the most important task for thoracic magnetic resonance is the pretherapeutic evaluation of intrathoracic masses, the differential diagnosis of benign versus malignant lesions, and the accurate documentation of tumor extent in malignancies, including three dimensional display, to improve surgical or radiation planning.

Contraindications Patients weighing more than 300 lb and patients unable to squeeze into the magnet cannot undergo MRI. An absolute contraindication for MRI is a cardiac pacemaker. Relative contraindications to magnetic resonance imaging include intracranial aneurysm clips, cochlear implants, insulin infusion and chemotherapy pumps, neurocutaneous stimulators, prosthetic heart valves, ocular implants, penile implants, and artificial sphincters depending on date of manufacture and metallurgical composition. Please consult MRI physician if questions arise. Patients who have metallic foreign bodies within the eye or if the object is positioned near a vital neural, vascular, or soft tissue structure; or patients who have undergone recent surgery within the last 6 weeks requiring placement of a vascular surgical clip, should also not undergo MRI. The safety of MRI in pregnant patients has not been determined. In such cases, prior consultation with the MRI physician is required. Generally, patients who have undergone recent surgery not requiring vascular clips or who have had coronary artery bypass surgery in the past may undergo MRI. Patients who have shrapnel wounds or orthopedic prostheses can generally safely undergo MRI unless the metallic device is in the anatomic region to be scanned which results in degradation of the images. Patients with surgically implanted intravascular vena cava filters to prevent pulmonary embolism can usually be scanned if the device has been in place for at least 6 weeks. Patients requiring life support equipment, including ventilators, require special preparation. Please contact MRI physician ahead of time. Central venous lines, Swan-Ganz catheters, and nasogastric (NG) tubes usually present no problems. If the patient is positive when screened for metallic devices and you are uncertain of their significance, the MRI radiologist will provide additional information to assist you.

Conflicting examination: Gastrointestinal tract barium studies

Patient Preparation Inpatient: The patient must be able to lie quietly while the scan is performed. The patient should be screened for metallic devices by nursing personnel. (See Contraindications.) This includes metal introduced into the patient either surgically or by trauma. All metallic objects must be removed from the patient, including jewelry or any other metal objects which may be in the patient's bedding. Dentures or other dental appliances must be removed. I.V.s which contain no metal are fine, but infusion pumps must be removed. Oxygen tanks and metallic backboards may come with the patient but will be removed prior to the patient entering the magnet room. Oxygen may be provided in the magnet room. Trauma, ICU, or CCU patients should be accompanied by a nurse. The patient needs to be NPO for abdominal MRI exams. If the patient is restless, combative, or claustrophobic, proper sedation may be administered on the floor prior to the MRI, or at the MRI Center. Consult the MRI radiologists with questions on proper sedation.

Outpatient: The patient should be screened for metallic devices. (See Contraindications.) If a question exists as to the patient's suitability for MRI, the MRI radiologist will assist you with your questions. If the patient is claustrophobic, oral or parenteral sedation may be necessary. If so, the patient should be accompanied by another adult to provide transportation home after the examination.

Aftercare If the patient received an MRI contrast agent (Magnevist®) and develops a delayed hypersensitivity reaction (ie, nausea, emesis, hives, or shortness of breath), the referring physician or MRI radiologist should be contacted immediately. If sedation is used, more time is required after the procedure for recovery period from the sedation.

Technique Unlike most conventional radiologic procedures, magnetic resonance imaging does not utilize ionizing radiation, but relies upon radio frequency or radio signals induced within the patient by the magnetic field to obtain images. There are no known biologic effects secondary to the magnetic fields currently used in clinical MRI. Prior to the scan, the patient will be asked to remove all metallic objects from their person, including loose change, hair pins, earrings, belts, etc. This is for safety reasons as the strong magnetic field could result in these and any other metal objects becoming projectiles resulting in injury to the patient or MRI personnel. Also the patient should not carry a purse or wallet into the magnetic room, as the magnetic field can permanently erase bank cards or credit cards. The magnet is open on both ends and music can be played for the patient if desired. Fresh air is constantly circulated through the magnet room and the patient is continually monitored by the MRI technologist. An intercom system is provided for communication between the patient and the technologist. Surface coils are generally not used in chest MRI.

Data Acquired Digital information with film reproduction

Limitations Generally, the greatest limitation of magnetic resonance imaging results from the patient's fear of the procedure. The patient must remain quiet and still for several scans, each lasting from several minutes to 10 minutes in length. Total examination time is usually 30-45 minutes and occasionally up to 1 hour. If the patient is restless during the examination, motion artifacts will be present on the images limiting their diagnostic value. If the patient is claustrophobic, mild oral sedation or occasionally parenteral sedation may be needed. Also, the patient can be accompanied by a family member or friend during the examination which may help to calm the patient's anxiety. Patients requiring life support equipment (ie, ventilators) require special preparation. Please refer to Contraindications for further causes for rejection.

Additional Information In some cases, an MRI contrast agent (Magnevist®) may be needed to increase the diagnostic accuracy of the MRI. This contrast

(Continued)

Magnetic Resonance Scan, Chest *(Continued)*

agent can be administered to patients with a previous history of allergies to conventional iodinated x-ray agents, as it contains no iodine. Contraindications to its use include previous allergy to the contrast agent itself, renal failure, certain types of anemia, and Wilson disease. Nursing mothers should express their breasts and not breast-feed for 36-48 hours after the administration of an MRI contrast agent to ensure that the nursing child does not receive the drug in any notable quantity. The contrast agent is generally very safe and increases the diagnostic efficacy of the MRI.

References

Bittner RC and Felix R, "Magnetic Resonance (MR) Imaging of the Chest: State-of-the-Art," *Eur Respir J*, 1998, 11(6):1392-404.

Gefter WB, "Chest Applications of Magnetic Resonance Imaging: An Update," *Radiol Clin North Am*, 1988, 26(3):573-88

Swensen SJ, Ehman RL, and Brown LR, "Magnetic Resonance Imaging of the Thorax," *J Thorac Imaging*, 1989, 4(2):19-33.

Magnetic Resonance Scan, Elbow

Synonyms Elbow MRI; MRI, Elbow

Indications The MRI study can depict accurately the presence and extent of many abnormal conditions such as degeneration and tearing of the medial and lateral collateral ligaments, medial epicondylitis (pitchers' elbow or golfers' elbow), lateral epicondylitis (tennis elbow), posterior dislocation injury, fracture of the coronoid process, supracondylar fracture in children not visualized on plain x-ray, fracture of the lateral humeral condyle in children (longitudinal Salter-Harris type IV), osteochondritis dissecans, loose bodies, biceps and triceps tendon injury, and ulnar nerve entrapment.

Contraindications Patients weighing more than 300 lb and patients unable to squeeze into the magnet cannot undergo MRI. An absolute contraindication for MRI is a cardiac pacemaker. Relative contraindications to magnetic resonance imaging include intracranial aneurysm clips, cochlear implants, insulin infusion and chemotherapy pumps, neurocutaneous stimulators, prosthetic heart valves, ocular implants, penile implants, and artificial sphincters depending on date of manufacture and metallurgical composition. Please consult MRI physician if questions arise. Patients who have metallic foreign bodies within the eye or if the object is positioned near a vital neural, vascular, or soft tissue structure; or patients who have undergone recent surgery within the last 6 weeks requiring placement of a vascular surgical clip, should also not undergo MRI. The safety of MRI in pregnant patients has not been determined. In such cases, prior consultation with the MRI physician is required. Generally, patients who have undergone recent surgery not requiring vascular clips or who have had coronary artery bypass surgery in the past may undergo MRI. Patients who have shrapnel wounds or orthopedic prostheses can generally safely undergo MRI unless the metallic device is in the anatomic region to be scanned which results in degradation of the images. Patients with surgically implanted intravascular vena cava filters to prevent pulmonary embolism can usually be scanned if the device has been in place for at least 6 weeks. Patients requiring life support equipment, including ventilators, require special preparation. Please contact MRI physician ahead of time. Central venous lines, Swan-Ganz catheters, and nasogastric (NG) tubes usually present no problems. If the patient is positive when screened for metallic devices and you are uncertain of their significance, the MRI radiologist will provide additional information to assist you.

Patient Preparation Inpatient: The patient must be able to lie quietly while the scan is performed. The patient should be screened for metallic devices by nursing personnel. (See Contraindications.) This includes metal introduced into the patient either surgically or by trauma. All metallic objects must be removed from the patient, including jewelry or any other metal objects which may be in the patient's bedding. Dentures or other dental appliances must be removed. I.V.s which contain no metal are fine, but infusion pumps must be removed. Oxygen tanks and metallic backboards may come with the patient but will be removed prior to the patient entering the magnet room. Oxygen may be provided in the magnet room. Trauma, ICU, or CCU patients should be accompanied by a nurse. If the patient is restless, combative, or claustrophobic, proper sedation may be administered on the floor prior to the MRI, or at the MRI Center. Consult the MRI radiologists with questions on proper sedation.

Outpatient: The patient should be screened for metallic devices. (See Contraindications.) If a question exists as to the patient's suitability for MRI, the MRI radiologist will assist you with your questions. If the patient is claustrophobic, oral or parenteral sedation may be necessary. If so, the patient should be accompanied by another adult to provide transportation home after the examination.

Aftercare If the patient received an MRI contrast agent (Magnevist®) and develops a delayed hypersensitivity reaction (ie, nausea, emesis, hives, or shortness of breath), the referring physician or MRI radiologist should be contacted immediately. If sedation is used, more time is required after the procedure for recovery period from the sedation.

Data Acquired Digital information with film reproduction

Limitations Implanted orthopedic devices in the anatomical area being imaged may limit the usefulness of the test. Generally, the greatest limitation of magnetic resonance imaging results from the patient's fear of the procedure. The patient must remain quiet and still for several scans, each lasting from several minutes to 10 minutes in length. Total examination time is usually 30-45 minutes and occasionally up to 1 hour. If the patient is restless during the examination, motion artifacts will be present on the images limiting their diagnostic value. If the patient is claustrophobic, mild oral sedation or occasionally parenteral sedation may be needed. Also, the patient can be accompanied by a family member or friend during the examination which may help to calm the patient's anxiety. Patients requiring life support equipment (ie, ventilators) require special preparation. Please refer to Contraindications for further causes for rejection.

Additional Information In some cases, an MRI contrast agent (Magnevist®) may be needed to increase the diagnostic accuracy of the MRI. This contrast agent can be administered to patients with a previous history of allergies to conventional iodinated x-ray agents as it contains no iodine. Contraindications to its use include previous allergy to the contrast agent itself, renal failure, certain types of anemia, and Wilson disease. Nursing mothers should express their breasts and not breast-feed for 36-48 hours after the administration of an MRI contrast agent to ensure that the nursing child does not receive the drug in any notable quantity. The contrast agent is generally very safe and increases the diagnostic efficacy of the MRI. As the positioning for elbow MR imaging is often uncomfortable for the patient, an effort should be made to streamline the examination as much as possible.

References

Fritz RC, Steinbach LS, Tirman PF, et al, "MR Imaging of the Elbow. An Update," *Radiol Clin North Am*, 1997, 35(1):117-44.

Sonin AH and Fitzgerald SW, "MR Imaging of Sports Injuries in the Adult Elbow: A Tailored Approach," *AJR Am J Roentgenol*, 1996, 167(2):325-31.

Magnetic Resonance Scan, Female Pelvis

Synonyms MRI, Pelvis, Female; Pelvis MRI, Female

Indications Define and characterize pathology of the pelvis including lymphadenopathy and urinary bladder diseases (eg, tumors, diverticula, ureterocele, hernia, fistula); uterine abnormalities (eg, congenital diseases, leiomyomas, adenomyosis, endometrial carcinoma, endometrial polyps gestational trophoblastic neoplasia, cervical carcinoma); ovarian diseases (eg, cysts, torsion, tumors, endometriosis); and fallopian tube diseases (eg, hydrosalpinx, tuboovarian abscess, and tumors)

Contraindications Patients weighing more than 300 lb and patients unable to squeeze into the magnet cannot undergo MRI. An absolute contraindication for MRI is a cardiac pacemaker. Relative contraindications to magnetic resonance imaging include intracranial aneurysm clips, cochlear implants, insulin infusion and chemotherapy pumps, neurocutaneous stimulators, prosthetic heart valves, ocular implants, penile implants, and artificial sphincters depending on date of manufacture and metallurgical composition. Please

(Continued)

Magnetic Resonance Scan, Female Pelvis *(Continued)*

consult MRI physician if questions arise. Patients who have metallic foreign bodies within the eye or if the object is positioned near a vital neural, vascular, or soft tissue structure; or patients who have undergone recent surgery within the last 6 weeks requiring placement of a vascular surgical clip, should also not undergo MRI. The safety of MRI in pregnant patients has not been determined. In such cases, prior consultation with the MRI physician is required. Generally, patients who have undergone recent surgery not requiring vascular clips or who have had coronary artery bypass surgery in the past may undergo MRI. Patients who have shrapnel wounds or orthopedic prostheses can generally safely undergo MRI unless the metallic device is in the anatomic region to be scanned which results in degradation of the images. Patients with surgically implanted intravascular vena cava filters to prevent pulmonary embolism can usually be scanned if the device has been in place for at least 6 weeks. Patients requiring life support equipment, including ventilators, require special preparation. Please contact MRI physician ahead of time. Central venous lines, Swan-Ganz catheters, and nasogastric (NG) tubes usually present no problems. If the patient is positive when screened for metallic devices and you are uncertain of their significance, the MRI radiologist will provide additional information to assist you.

Conflicting examination: Gastrointestinal tract barium studies

Patient Preparation Inpatient: The patient must be able to lie quietly while the scan is performed. The patient should be screened for metallic devices by nursing personnel. (See Contraindications.) This includes metal introduced into the patient either surgically or by trauma. All metallic objects must be removed from the patient, including jewelry or any other metal objects which may be in the patient's bedding. Dentures or other dental appliances must be removed. I.V.s which contain no metal are fine, but infusion pumps must be removed. Oxygen tanks and metallic backboards may come with the patient but will be removed prior to the patient entering the magnet room. Oxygen may be provided in the magnet room. Trauma, ICU, or CCU patients should be accompanied by a nurse. The patient needs to be NPO for abdominal MRI exams. If the patient is restless, combative, or claustrophobic, proper sedation may be administered on the floor prior to the MRI, or at the MRI Center. Consult the MRI radiologists with questions on proper sedation.

Outpatient: The patient should be screened for metallic devices. (See Contraindications.) If a question exists as to the patient's suitability for MRI, the MRI radiologist will assist you with your questions. If the patient is claustrophobic, oral or parenteral sedation may be necessary. If so, the patient should be accompanied by another adult to provide transportation home after the examination.

Aftercare If the patient received an MRI contrast agent (Magnevist®) and develops a delayed hypersensitivity reaction (ie, nausea, emesis, hives, or shortness of breath), the referring physician or MRI radiologist should be contacted immediately. If sedation is used, more time is required after the procedure for recovery period from the sedation.

Data Acquired Digital information with film reproduction

Limitations Generally, the greatest limitation of magnetic resonance imaging results from the patient's fear of the procedure. The patient must remain quiet and still for several scans, each lasting from several minutes to 10 minutes in length. Total examination time is usually 30-45 minutes and occasionally up to 1 hour. If the patient is restless during the examination, motion artifacts will be present on the images limiting their diagnostic value. If the patient is claustrophobic, mild oral sedation or occasionally parenteral sedation may be needed. Also, the patient can be accompanied by a family member or friend during the examination which may help to calm the patient's anxiety. Patients requiring life support equipment (ie, ventilators) require special preparation. Please refer to Contraindications for further causes for rejection.

Additional Information In some cases, an MRI contrast agent (Magnevist®) may be needed to increase the diagnostic accuracy of the MRI. This contrast agent can be administered to patients with a previous history of allergies to conventional iodinated x-ray agents, as it contains no iodine. Contraindications to its use include previous allergy to the contrast agent itself, renal failure, certain types of anemia, and Wilson disease. Nursing mothers should express their breasts and not breast-feed for 36-48 hours after the administration of an MRI contrast agent to ensure that the nursing child does not receive the drug in any notable quantity. The contrast agent is generally very safe and increases the diagnostic efficacy of the MRI. Intramuscular or subcutaneous injection of glucagon may be given to decrease motion artifacts from peristalsis. Use of a vaginal tampon in female patients may be required.

References

Cohen EK and Kressel HY, "MR Imaging of the Pelvis," *Clinical Magnetic Resonance Imaging*, Edelman RR and Hesselink JR, eds, Philadelphia, PA: WB Saunders Co, 1990, 915-37.

Scoutt LM and McCarthy SM, "Female Pelvis," *Magnetic Resonance Imaging*, 3rd ed, Stark DD and Bradley WG Jr, eds, St Louis, MO: CV Mosby Co, 1999, 557-90.

Siegelman ES and Scnall MD, "Urinary Bladder," *Magnetic Resonance Imaging*, 3rd ed, Stark DD and Bradley WG Jr, eds, St Louis, MO: CV Mosby Co, 1999, 545-55.

♦ **Magnetic Resonance Scan, Head** *see* Magnetic Resonance Angiography, Brain *on page 391*

♦ **Magnetic Resonance Scan, Head** *see* Magnetic Resonance Scan, Brain *on page 401*

Magnetic Resonance Scan, Hip

Synonyms Hip MRI Scan; MRI, Hip

Indications Evaluation of the intra- and extra-articular soft tissues. One of the conditions where the use of MRI of the hip is well established, and is considered the most sensitive noninvasive technique, is for the diagnosis and monitoring of avascular necrosis. Other conditions such as abnormalities of articular cartilage, labral tears, loose bodies, synovial pathology, and joint effusion are less well defined.

Contraindications Patients weighing more than 300 lb and patients unable to squeeze into the magnet cannot undergo MRI. An absolute contraindication for MRI is a cardiac pacemaker. Relative contraindications to magnetic resonance imaging include intracranial aneurysm clips, cochlear implants, insulin infusion and chemotherapy pumps, neurocutaneous stimulators, prosthetic heart valves, ocular implants, penile implants, and artificial sphincters depending on date of manufacture and metallurgical composition. Please consult MRI physician if questions arise. Patients who have metallic foreign bodies within the eye or if the object is positioned near a vital neural, vascular, or soft tissue structure; or patients who have undergone recent surgery within the last 6 weeks requiring placement of a vascular surgical clip, should also not undergo MRI. The safety of MRI in pregnant patients has not been determined. In such cases, prior consultation with the MRI physician is required. Generally, patients who have undergone recent surgery not requiring vascular clips or who have had coronary artery bypass surgery in the past may undergo MRI. Patients who have shrapnel wounds or orthopedic prostheses can generally safely undergo MRI unless the metallic device is in the anatomic region to be scanned which results in degradation of the images. Patients with surgically implanted intravascular vena cava filters to prevent pulmonary embolism can usually be scanned if the device has been in place for at least 6 weeks. Patients requiring life support equipment, including ventilators, require special preparation. Please contact MRI physician ahead of time. Central venous lines, Swan-Ganz catheters, and nasogastric (NG) tubes usually present no problems. If the patient is positive when screened for metallic devices and you are uncertain of their significance, the MRI radiologist will provide additional information to assist you.

Patient Preparation Inpatient: The patient must be able to lie quietly while the scan is performed. The patient should be screened for metallic devices by nursing personnel. (See Contraindications.) This includes metal introduced into the patient either surgically or by trauma. All metallic objects must be removed from the patient, including jewelry or any other metal objects which may be in the patient's bedding. Dentures or other dental appliances must be removed. I.V.s which contain no metal are fine, but infusion pumps must be removed. Oxygen tanks and metallic backboards may come with the patient but will be removed prior to the patient entering the magnet room. Oxygen

(Continued)

Magnetic Resonance Scan, Hip *(Continued)*

may be provided in the magnet room. Trauma, ICU, or CCU patients should be accompanied by a nurse. If the patient is restless, combative, or claustrophobic, proper sedation may be administered on the floor prior to the MRI, or at the MRI Center. Consult the MRI radiologists with questions on proper sedation.

Outpatient: The patient should be screened for metallic devices. (See Contraindications.) If a question exists as to the patient's suitability for MRI, the MRI radiologist will assist you with your questions. If the patient is claustrophobic, oral or parenteral sedation may be necessary. If so, the patient should be accompanied by another adult to provide transportation home after the examination.

Aftercare If the patient received an MRI contrast agent (Magnevist®) and develops a delayed hypersensitivity reaction (ie, nausea, emesis, hives, or shortness of breath), the referring physician or MRI radiologist should be contacted immediately. If sedation is used, more time is required after the procedure for recovery period from the sedation.

Data Acquired Digital information with film reproduction

Limitations Implanted orthopedic devices in the anatomical area being imaged may limit the usefulness of the test. Generally, the greatest limitation of magnetic resonance imaging results from the patient's fear of the procedure. The patient must remain quiet and still for several scans, each lasting from several minutes to 10 minutes in length. Total examination time is usually 30-45 minutes and occasionally up to 1 hour. If the patient is restless during the examination, motion artifacts will be present on the images limiting their diagnostic value. If the patient is claustrophobic, mild oral sedation or occasionally parenteral sedation may be needed. Also, the patient can be accompanied by a family member or friend during the examination which may help to calm the patient's anxiety. Patients requiring life support equipment (ie, ventilators) require special preparation. Please refer to Contraindications for further causes for rejection.

Additional Information In some cases, an MRI contrast agent (Magnevist®) may be needed to increase the diagnostic accuracy of the MRI. This contrast agent can be administered to patients with a previous history of allergies to conventional iodinated x-ray agents as it contains no iodine. Contraindications to its use include previous allergy to the contrast agent itself, renal failure, certain types of anemia, and Wilson disease. Nursing mothers should express their breasts and not breast-feed for 36-48 hours after the administration of an MRI contrast agent to ensure that the nursing child does not receive the drug in any notable quantity. The contrast agent is generally very safe and increases the diagnostic efficacy of the MRI.

References

Bluemke DA, Petri M, and Zerhouni EA, "Femoral Head Perfusion and Composition: MR Imaging and Spectroscopic Evaluation of Patients With Systemic Lupus Erythematosus and at Risk for Avascular Necrosis," *Radiology*, 1995, 197(2):433-8.

Edwards DJ, Lomas D, and Villar RN, "Diagnosis of the Painful Hip by Magnetic Resonance Imaging and Arthroscopy," *J Bone Joint Surg [Br]*, 1995, 77(3):374-6.

Moss SG, Schweitzer ME, Jacobson JA, et al, "Hip Joint Fluid: Detection and Distribution at MR Imaging and US With Cadaveric Correlation" *Radiology*, 1998, 208(1):43-8.

Magnetic Resonance Scan, Knee

Synonyms Knee MRI; MRI, Knee

Indications Diagnose internal derangements of the knee, including meniscal tears and degeneration, anterior and posterior cruciate ligament tears, avulsion fractures, fractures with articular surface extension, lesions of the bones, and bone marrow of the knee joint as well as surrounding tissue

Contraindications Patients weighing more than 300 lb and patients unable to squeeze into the magnet cannot undergo MRI. An absolute contraindication for MRI is a cardiac pacemaker. Relative contraindications to magnetic resonance imaging include intracranial aneurysm clips, cochlear implants, insulin infusion and chemotherapy pumps, neurocutaneous stimulators, prosthetic heart valves, ocular implants, penile implants, and artificial sphincters depending on date of manufacture and metallurgical composition. Please consult MRI physician if questions arise. Patients who have metallic foreign bodies within the eye or if the object is positioned near a vital neural, vascular, or soft tissue structure; or patients who have undergone recent surgery within the last 6 weeks requiring placement of a vascular surgical clip, should also not undergo MRI. The safety of MRI in pregnant patients has not been determined. In such cases, prior consultation with the MRI physician is required. Generally, patients who have undergone recent surgery not requiring vascular clips or who have had coronary artery bypass surgery in the past may undergo MRI. Patients who have shrapnel wounds or orthopedic prostheses can generally safely undergo MRI unless the metallic device is in the anatomic region to be scanned which results in degradation of the images. Patients with surgically implanted intravascular vena cava filters to prevent pulmonary embolism can usually be scanned if the device has been in place for at least 6 weeks. Patients requiring life support equipment, including ventilators, require special preparation. Please contact MRI physician ahead of time. Central venous lines, Swan-Ganz catheters, and nasogastric (NG) tubes usually present no problems. If the patient is positive when screened for metallic devices and you are uncertain of their significance, the MRI radiologist will provide additional information to assist you.

Patient Preparation Inpatient: The patient must be able to lie quietly while the scan is performed. The patient should be screened for metallic devices by nursing personnel. (See Contraindications.) This includes metal introduced into the patient either surgically or by trauma. All metallic objects must be removed from the patient, including jewelry or any other metal objects which may be in the patient's bedding. Dentures or other dental appliances must be removed. I.V.s which contain no metal are fine, but infusion pumps must be removed. Oxygen tanks and metallic backboards may come with the patient but will be removed prior to the patient entering the magnet room. Oxygen may be provided in the magnet room. Trauma, ICU, or CCU patients should be accompanied by a nurse. The patient needs to be NPO for abdominal MRI exams. If the patient is restless, combative, or claustrophobic, proper sedation may be administered on the floor prior to the MRI, or at the MRI Center. Consult the MRI radiologists with questions on proper sedation.

Outpatient: The patient should be screened for metallic devices. (See Contraindications.) If a question exists as to the patient's suitability for MRI, the MRI radiologist will assist you with your questions. If the patient is claustrophobic, oral or parenteral sedation may be necessary. If so, the patient should be accompanied by another adult to provide transportation home after the examination.

Aftercare If the patient received an MRI contrast agent (Magnevist®) and develops a delayed hypersensitivity reaction (ie, nausea, emesis, hives, or shortness of breath), the referring physician or MRI radiologist should be contacted immediately. If sedation is used, more time is required after the procedure for recovery period from the sedation.

Technique Unlike most conventional radiologic procedures, magnetic resonance imaging does not utilize ionizing radiation, but relies upon radio frequency or radio signals induced within the patient by the magnetic field to obtain images. There are no known biologic effects secondary to the magnetic fields currently used in clinical MRI. Prior to the scan, the patient will be asked to remove all metallic objects from their person, including loose change, hair pins, earrings, belts, etc. This is for safety reasons as the strong magnetic field could result in these and any other metal objects becoming projectiles resulting in injury to the patient or MRI personnel. Also the patient should not carry a purse or wallet into the magnetic room, as the magnetic field can permanently erase bank cards or credit cards. The magnet is open on both ends and music can be played for the patient if desired. Fresh air is constantly circulated through the magnet room and the patient is continually monitored by the MRI technologist. An intercom system is provided for communication between the patient and the technologist. The patient must be supine on the scan table for 20-30 minutes with the knee supported in a surface coil.

Data Acquired Digital information with film reproduction

(Continued)

Magnetic Resonance Scan, Knee *(Continued)*

Limitations Generally, the greatest limitation of magnetic resonance imaging results from the patient's fear of the procedure. The patient must remain quiet and still for several scans, each lasting from several minutes to 10 minutes in length. Total examination time is usually 30-45 minutes and occasionally up to 1 hour. If the patient is restless during the examination, motion artifacts will be present on the images limiting their diagnostic value. If the patient is claustrophobic, mild oral sedation or occasionally parenteral sedation may be needed. Also, the patient can be accompanied by a family member or friend during the examination which may help to calm the patient's anxiety. Patients requiring life support equipment (ie, ventilators) require special preparation. Please refer to Contraindications for further causes for rejection.

Additional Information In some cases, an MRI contrast agent (Magnevist) may be needed to increase the diagnostic accuracy of the MRI. This contrast agent can be administered to patients with a previous history of allergies to conventional iodinated x-ray agents, as it contains no iodine. Contraindications to its use include previous allergy to the contrast agent itself, renal failure, certain types of anemia, and Wilson disease. Nursing mothers should express their breasts and not breast-feed for 36-48 hours after the administration of an MRI contrast agent to ensure that the nursing child does not receive the drug in any notable quantity. The contrast agent is generally very safe and increases the diagnostic efficacy of the MRI.

References

Burk DL Jr, Mitchell DG, Rifkin MD, et al, "Recent Advances in Magnetic Resonance Imaging of the Knee," *Radiol Clin North Am*, 1990, 28(2):379-93.

Walker CW and Moore TE, "Imaging of Skeletal and Soft Tissue Injuries in and Around the Knee," *Radiol Clin North Am*, 1997, 35(3):631-53.

Magnetic Resonance Scan, Larynx

Related Information

Computed Transaxial Tomography, Larynx *on page 333*
Computed Transaxial Tomography, Neck *on page 335*

Synonyms Larynx MRI; MRI, Larynx

Indications Evaluate deep structures inaccessible to endoscopy, mainly in cases of tumors and evaluation after radiation therapy

Contraindications Patients weighing more than 300 lb and patients unable to squeeze into the magnet cannot undergo MRI. An absolute contraindication for MRI is a cardiac pacemaker. Relative contraindications to magnetic resonance imaging include intracranial aneurysm clips, cochlear implants, insulin infusion and chemotherapy pumps, neurocutaneous stimulators, prosthetic heart valves, ocular implants, penile implants, and artificial sphincters depending on date of manufacture and metallurgical composition. Please consult MRI physician if questions arise. Patients who have metallic foreign bodies within the eye or if the object is positioned near a vital neural, vascular, or soft tissue structure; or patients who have undergone recent surgery within the last 6 weeks requiring placement of a vascular surgical clip, should also not undergo MRI. The safety of MRI in pregnant patients has not been determined. In such cases, prior consultation with the MRI physician is required. Generally, patients who have undergone recent surgery not requiring vascular clips or who have had coronary artery bypass surgery in the past may undergo MRI. Patients who have shrapnel wounds or orthopedic prostheses can generally safely undergo MRI unless the metallic device is in the anatomic region to be scanned which results in degradation of the images. Patients with surgically implanted intravascular vena cava filters to prevent pulmonary embolism can usually be scanned if the device has been in place for at least 6 weeks. Patients requiring life support equipment, including ventilators, require special preparation. Please contact MRI physician ahead of time. Central venous lines, Swan-Ganz catheters, and nasogastric (NG) tubes usually present no problems. If the patient is positive when screened for metallic devices and you are uncertain of their significance, the MRI radiologist will provide additional information to assist you.

Patient Preparation Inpatient: The patient must be able to lie quietly while the scan is performed. The patient should be screened for metallic devices by

supine position on a special surface coil during the study and remain still. In certain cases, an MRI contrast agent, Gadopentetate Dimeglumine (Magnevist®) may be necessary to increase the diagnostic accuracy of the MRI examination. This is administered intravenously, via an antecubital vein in a small volume (less than 20 mL). This contrast agent may be used in patients who are allergic to conventional iodinated contrast agents such as is used in IVPs or CT examination without difficulty. There are very few contraindications to its use. (See Contraindications.)

Data Acquired Digital information with film reproduction

Limitations Generally, the greatest limitation of magnetic resonance imaging results from the patient's fear of the procedure. The patient must remain quiet and still for several scans, each lasting from several minutes to 10 minutes in length. Total examination time is usually 30-45 minutes and occasionally up to 1 hour. If the patient is restless during the examination, motion artifacts will be present on the images limiting their diagnostic value. If the patient is claustrophobic, mild oral sedation or occasionally parenteral sedation may be needed. Also, the patient can be accompanied by a family member or friend during the examination which may help to calm the patient's anxiety. Patients requiring life support equipment (ie, ventilators) require special preparation. Please refer to Contraindications for further causes for rejection. Patients with intraspinal metallic rods may be scanned; however, images may not be optimal due to metallic distortion artifacts.

Additional Information In some cases, an MRI contrast agent (Magnevist®) may be needed to increase the diagnostic accuracy of the MRI. This contrast agent can be administered to patients with a previous history of allergies to conventional iodinated x-ray agents, as it contains no iodine. Contraindications to its use include previous allergy to the contrast agent itself, renal failure, certain types of anemia, and Wilson disease. Nursing mothers should express their breasts and not breast-feed for 36-48 hours after the administration of an MRI contrast agent to ensure that the nursing child does not receive the drug in any notable quantity. The contrast agent is generally very safe and increases the diagnostic efficacy of the MRI.

References

Ross JS, Masaryk TJ, and Modic MT, *Magn Reson Imaging*, 3rd ed, Stark DD and Bradley WG Jr, eds, St Louis, MO: CV Mosby Co, 1999, 1883-906.

Magnetic Resonance Scan, Male Pelvis and Scrotum

Synonyms MRI, Pelvis (Male) and Scrotum; Pelvis (Male) MRI; Scrotum MRI

Indications Define and characterize pathology of the pelvis including lymphadenopathy, urinary bladder diseases (eg, tumors, diverticula, ureterocele, hernia, fistula); prostate diseases (eg, benign hyperplasia, prostatitis, calculi, cystic lesions, cancer and staging of known cancer); and seminal vesicles. The evaluation of the scrotum and testes has been improved and is now considered the best technique for localizing and assessing undescended testes and complications of cryptorchidism, as well as the most specific imaging modality for the differential diagnosis of ischemia, inflammation, and tumor.

Contraindications Patients weighing more than 300 lb and patients unable to squeeze into the magnet cannot undergo MRI. An absolute contraindication for MRI is a cardiac pacemaker. Relative contraindications to magnetic resonance imaging include intracranial aneurysm clips, cochlear implants, insulin infusion and chemotherapy pumps, neurocutaneous stimulators, prosthetic heart valves, ocular implants, penile implants, and artificial sphincters depending on date of manufacture and metallurgical composition. Please consult MRI physician if questions arise. Patients who have metallic foreign bodies within the eye or if the object is positioned near a vital neural, vascular, or soft tissue structure; or patients who have undergone recent surgery within the last 6 weeks requiring placement of a vascular surgical clip, should also not undergo MRI. The safety of MRI in pregnant patients has not been determined. In such cases, prior consultation with the MRI physician is required. Generally, patients who have undergone recent surgery not requiring vascular clips or who have had coronary artery bypass surgery in the past may undergo MRI. Patients who have shrapnel wounds or orthopedic prostheses

(Continued)

Magnetic Resonance Scan, Male Pelvis and Scrotum *(Continued)*

can generally safely undergo MRI unless the metallic device is in the anatomic region to be scanned which results in degradation of the images. Patients with surgically implanted intravascular vena cava filters to prevent pulmonary embolism can usually be scanned if the device has been in place for at least 6 weeks. Patients requiring life support equipment, including ventilators, require special preparation. Please contact MRI physician ahead of time. Central venous lines, Swan-Ganz catheters, and nasogastric (NG) tubes usually present no problems. If the patient is positive when screened for metallic devices and you are uncertain of their significance, the MRI radiologist will provide additional information to assist you.

Conflicting examination: Gastrointestinal tract barium studies

Patient Preparation Inpatient: The patient must be able to lie quietly while the scan is performed. The patient should be screened for metallic devices by nursing personnel. (See Contraindications.) This includes metal introduced into the patient either surgically or by trauma. All metallic objects must be removed from the patient, including jewelry or any other metal objects which may be in the patient's bedding. Dentures or other dental appliances must be removed. I.V.s which contain no metal are fine, but infusion pumps must be removed. Oxygen tanks and metallic backboards may come with the patient but will be removed prior to the patient entering the magnet room. Oxygen may be provided in the magnet room. Trauma, ICU, or CCU patients should be accompanied by a nurse. The patient needs to be NPO for abdominal MRI exams. If the patient is restless, combative, or claustrophobic, proper sedation may be administered on the floor prior to the MRI, or at the MRI Center. Consult the MRI radiologists with questions on proper sedation.

Outpatient: The patient should be screened for metallic devices. (See Contraindications.) If a question exists as to the patient's suitability for MRI, the MRI radiologist will assist you with your questions. If the patient is claustrophobic, oral or parenteral sedation may be necessary. If so, the patient should be accompanied by another adult to provide transportation home after the examination.

Aftercare If the patient received an MRI contrast agent (Magnevist®) and develops a delayed hypersensitivity reaction (ie, nausea, emesis, hives, or shortness of breath), the referring physician or MRI radiologist should be contacted immediately. If sedation is used, more time is required after the procedure for recovery period from the sedation.

Technique Unlike most conventional radiologic procedures, magnetic resonance imaging does not utilize ionizing radiation, but relies upon radio frequency or radio signals induced within the patient by the magnetic field to obtain images. There are no known biologic effects secondary to the magnetic fields currently used in clinical MRI. Prior to the scan, the patient will be asked to remove all metallic objects from their person, including loose change, hair pins, earrings, belts, etc. This is for safety reasons as the strong magnetic field could result in these and any other metal objects becoming projectiles resulting in injury to the patient or MRI personnel. Also the patient should not carry a purse or wallet into the magnetic room, as the magnetic field can permanently erase bank cards or credit cards. The magnet is open on both ends and music can be played for the patient if desired. Fresh air is constantly circulated through the magnet room and the patient is continually monitored by the MRI technologist. An intercom system is provided for communication between the patient and the technologist. No surface coils are used for MRI of the pelvis. The patient is asked to remain as still as possible during the study.

Data Acquired Digital information with film reproduction

Limitations Generally, the greatest limitation of magnetic resonance imaging results from the patient's fear of the procedure. The patient must remain quiet and still for several scans, each lasting from several minutes to 10 minutes in length. Total examination time is usually 30-45 minutes and occasionally up to 1 hour. If the patient is restless during the examination, motion artifacts will be present on the images limiting their diagnostic value. If the patient is claustrophobic, mild oral sedation or occasionally parenteral sedation may be needed. Also, the patient can be accompanied by a family member or friend during the examination which may help to calm the patient's anxiety. Patients requiring life support equipment (ie, ventilators) require special preparation. Please refer to Contraindications for further causes for rejection.

Additional Information In some cases, an MRI contrast agent (Magnevist®) may be needed to increase the diagnostic accuracy of the MRI. This contrast agent can be administered to patients with a previous history of allergies to conventional iodinated x-ray agents, as it contains no iodine. Contraindications to its use include previous allergy to the contrast agent itself, renal failure, certain types of anemia, and Wilson disease. Nursing mothers should express their breasts and not breast-feed for 36-48 hours after the administration of an MRI contrast agent to ensure that the nursing child does not receive the drug in any notable quantity. The contrast agent is generally very safe and increases the diagnostic efficacy of the MRI. Intramuscular or subcutaneous injection of glucagon may be given to decrease motion artifacts from peristalsis. In prostate examinations, a special type of endorectal coil can be used to increase the accuracy of the exam.

References

Cohen EK and Kressel HY, "MR Imaging of the Pelvis," *Clinical Magnetic Resonance Imaging*, Edelman RR and Hesselink JR, eds, Philadelphia, PA: WB Saunders Co, 1990, 915-37.

Mattrey RF, "Scrotum and Testes," *Magn Reson Imaging*, 3rd ed, Stark DD, Bradley WG Jr, eds, St Louis, MO: CV Mosby Co, 1999, 635-52.

Schwartz CP, MaCauley TR, and Rifkin MD, "Prostate and Seminal Vesicles," *Magn Reson Imaging*, 3rd ed, Stark DD and Bradley WG Jr, eds, St Louis, MO: CV Mosby Co, 1999, 617-34.

Siegelman ES and Scnall MD, "Urinary Bladder," *Magn Reson Imaging*, 3rd ed, Stark DD and Bradley WG Jr, eds, St Louis, MO: CV Mosby Co, 1999, 545-55.

Magnetic Resonance Scan, Muscles

Synonyms MRI, Muscles; Muscle MRI

Indications Assess the morphologic appearance as well as physiology (spectroscopy). MRI can determine a normal transient alteration of specific muscles after acute exercise, and evaluate abnormalities of the muscles such as acute strain, muscle tears, delayed-onset muscle soreness, direct trauma with edema, compartment syndrome, acute rhabdomyolysis, muscle infarct, denervation injuries, dystrophies, myopathies, infectious diseases, inflammatory diseases, and neoplasms.

Contraindications Patients weighing more than 300 lb and patients unable to squeeze into the magnet cannot undergo MRI. An absolute contraindication for MRI is a cardiac pacemaker. Relative contraindications to magnetic resonance imaging include intracranial aneurysm clips, cochlear implants, insulin infusion and chemotherapy pumps, neurocutaneous stimulators, prosthetic heart valves, ocular implants, penile implants, and artificial sphincters depending on date of manufacture and metallurgical composition. Please consult MRI physician if questions arise. Patients who have metallic foreign bodies within the eye or if the object is positioned near a vital neural, vascular, or soft tissue structure; or patients who have undergone recent surgery within the last 6 weeks requiring placement of a vascular surgical clip, should also not undergo MRI. The safety of MRI in pregnant patients has not been determined. In such cases, prior consultation with the MRI physician is required. Generally, patients who have undergone recent surgery not requiring vascular clips or who have had coronary artery bypass surgery in the past may undergo MRI. Patients who have shrapnel wounds or orthopedic prostheses can generally safely undergo MRI unless the metallic device is in the anatomic region to be scanned which results in degradation of the images. Patients with surgically implanted intravascular vena cava filters to prevent pulmonary embolism can usually be scanned if the device has been in place for at least 6 weeks. Patients requiring life support equipment, including ventilators, require special preparation. Please contact MRI physician ahead of time. Central venous lines, Swan-Ganz catheters, and nasogastric (NG) tubes usually present no problems. If the patient is positive when screened for metallic devices and you are uncertain of their significance, the MRI radiologist will provide additional information to assist you.

(Continued)

Magnetic Resonance Scan, Muscles *(Continued)*

Patient Preparation Inpatient: The patient must be able to lie quietly while the scan is performed. The patient should be screened for metallic devices by nursing personnel. (See Contraindications.) This includes metal introduced into the patient either surgically or by trauma. All metallic objects must be removed from the patient, including jewelry or any other metal objects which may be in the patient's bedding. Dentures or other dental appliances must be removed. I.V.s which contain no metal are fine, but infusion pumps must be removed. Oxygen tanks and metallic backboards may come with the patient but will be removed prior to the patient entering the magnet room. Oxygen may be provided in the magnet room. Trauma, ICU, or CCU patients should be accompanied by a nurse. The patient needs to be NPO for abdominal MRI exams. If the patient is restless, combative, or claustrophobic, proper sedation may be administered on the floor prior to the MRI, or at the MRI Center. Consult the MRI radiologists with questions on proper sedation.

Outpatient: The patient should be screened for metallic devices. (See Contraindications.) If a question exists as to the patient's suitability for MRI, the MRI radiologist will assist you with your questions. If the patient is claustrophobic, oral or parenteral sedation may be necessary. If so, the patient should be accompanied by another adult to provide transportation home after the examination.

Aftercare If the patient received an MRI contrast agent (Magnevist®) and develops a delayed hypersensitivity reaction (ie, nausea, emesis, hives, or shortness of breath), the referring physician or MRI radiologist should be contacted immediately. If sedation is used, more time is required after the procedure for recovery period from the sedation.

Data Acquired Digital information with film reproduction

Limitations Generally, the greatest limitation of magnetic resonance imaging results from the patient's fear of the procedure. The patient must remain quiet and still for several scans, each lasting from several minutes to 10 minutes in length. Total examination time is usually 30-45 minutes and occasionally up to 1 hour. If the patient is restless during the examination, motion artifacts will be present on the images limiting their diagnostic value. If the patient is claustrophobic, mild oral sedation or occasionally parenteral sedation may be needed. Also, the patient can be accompanied by a family member or friend during the examination which may help to calm the patient's anxiety. Patients requiring life support equipment (ie, ventilators) require special preparation. Please refer to Contraindications for further causes for rejection. Implanted orthopedic appliances may limit the usefulness of the scan in the area being imaged.

Additional Information In some cases, an MRI contrast agent (Magnevist®) may be needed to increase the diagnostic accuracy of the MRI. This contrast agent can be administered to patients with a previous history of allergies to conventional iodinated x-ray agents, as it contains no iodine. Contraindications to its use include previous allergy to the contrast agent itself, renal failure, certain types of anemia, and Wilson disease. Nursing mothers should express their breasts and not breast-feed for 36-48 hours after the administration of an MRI contrast agent to ensure that the nursing child does not receive the drug in any notable quantity. The contrast agent is generally very safe and increases the diagnostic efficacy of the MRI.

References

Anderson MW, "Muscles," *Magn Reson Imaging of the Body*, Philadelphia, PA: Lippincott Williams & Wilkins, 1997, 1321-41.

Magnetic Resonance Scan, Nasopharynx, Oropharynx, and Hypopharynx

Related Information

Computed Transaxial Tomography, Larynx *on page 333*

Computed Transaxial Tomography, Neck *on page 335*

Synonyms Hypopharynx MRI; MRI, Nasopharynx, Oropharynx, and Hypopharynx; Nasopharynx MRI; Oropharynx MRI

Indications Evaluate the nasopharynx, oropharynx, and hypopharynx to detect inflammatory disease, benign and malignant tumors. MRI can help to differentiate inflammatory from neoplastic disease, as well as indicate the extension of the tumor into the deep.

Contraindications Patients weighing more than 300 lb and patients unable to squeeze into the magnet cannot undergo MRI. An absolute contraindication for MRI is a cardiac pacemaker. Relative contraindications to magnetic resonance imaging include intracranial aneurysm clips, cochlear implants, insulin infusion and chemotherapy pumps, neurocutaneous stimulators, prosthetic heart valves, ocular implants, penile implants, and artificial sphincters depending on date of manufacture and metallurgical composition. Please consult MRI physician if questions arise. Patients who have metallic foreign bodies within the eye or if the object is positioned near a vital neural, vascular, or soft tissue structure; or patients who have undergone recent surgery within the last 6 weeks requiring placement of a vascular surgical clip, should also not undergo MRI. The safety of MRI in pregnant patients has not been determined. In such cases, prior consultation with the MRI physician is required. Generally, patients who have undergone recent surgery not requiring vascular clips or who have had coronary artery bypass surgery in the past may undergo MRI. Patients who have shrapnel wounds or orthopedic prostheses can generally safely undergo MRI unless the metallic device is in the anatomic region to be scanned which results in degradation of the images. Patients with surgically implanted intravascular vena cava filters to prevent pulmonary embolism can usually be scanned if the device has been in place for at least 6 weeks. Patients requiring life support equipment, including ventilators, require special preparation. Please contact MRI physician ahead of time. Central venous lines, Swan-Ganz catheters, and nasogastric (NG) tubes usually present no problems. If the patient is positive when screened for metallic devices and you are uncertain of their significance, the MRI radiologist will provide additional information to assist you.

Patient Preparation Inpatient: The patient must be able to lie quietly while the scan is performed. The patient should be screened for metallic devices by nursing personnel. (See Contraindications.) This includes metal introduced into the patient either surgically or by trauma. All metallic objects must be removed from the patient, including jewelry or any other metal objects which may be in the patient's bedding. Dentures or other dental appliances must be removed. I.V.s which contain no metal are fine, but infusion pumps must be removed. Oxygen tanks and metallic backboards may come with the patient but will be removed prior to the patient entering the magnet room. Oxygen may be provided in the magnet room. Trauma, ICU, or CCU patients should be accompanied by a nurse. The patient needs to be NPO for abdominal MRI exams. If the patient is restless, combative, or claustrophobic, proper sedation may be administered on the floor prior to the MRI, or at the MRI Center. Consult the MRI radiologists with questions on proper sedation.

Outpatient: The patient should be screened for metallic devices. (See Contraindications.) If a question exists as to the patient's suitability for MRI, the MRI radiologist will assist you with your questions. If the patient is claustrophobic, oral or parenteral sedation may be necessary. If so, the patient should be accompanied by another adult to provide transportation home after the examination.

Aftercare If the patient received an MRI contrast agent (Magnevist®) and develops a delayed hypersensitivity reaction (ie, nausea, emesis, hives, or shortness of breath), the referring physician or MRI radiologist should be contacted immediately. If sedation is used, more time is required after the procedure for recovery period from the sedation.

Technique Unlike most conventional radiologic procedures, magnetic resonance imaging does not utilize ionizing radiation, but relies upon radio frequency or radio signals induced within the patient by the magnetic field to obtain images. There are no known biologic effects secondary to the magnetic fields currently used in clinical MRI. Prior to the scan, the patient will be asked to remove all metallic objects from their person, including loose change, hair pins, earrings, belts, etc. This is for safety reasons as the strong magnetic

(Continued)

Magnetic Resonance Scan, Nasopharynx, Oropharynx, and Hypopharynx *(Continued)*

field could result in these and any other metal objects becoming projectiles resulting in injury to the patient or MRI personnel. Also the patient should not carry a purse or wallet into the magnetic room, as the magnetic field can permanently erase bank cards or credit cards. The magnet is open on both ends and music can be played for the patient if desired. Fresh air is constantly circulated through the magnet room and the patient is continually monitored by the MRI technologist. An intercom system is provided for communication between the patient and the technologist. A special surface coil will be placed over the area to be studied and the patient will be asked to remain still during the study. In certain cases, an MRI contrast agent, Gadopentetate Dimeglumine (Magnevist®) may be necessary to increase the diagnostic accuracy of the MRI examination. This is administered intravenously, via an antecubital vein in a small volume (less than 20 mL). This contrast agent may be used in patients who are allergic to conventional iodinated contrast agents such as is used in IVPs or CT examination without difficulty. There are very few contraindications to its use. (See Contraindications.)

Data Acquired Digital information with film reproduction

Limitations Generally, the greatest limitation of magnetic resonance imaging results from the patient's fear of the procedure. The patient must remain quiet and still for several scans, each lasting from several minutes to 10 minutes in length. Total examination time is usually 30-45 minutes and occasionally up to 1 hour. If the patient is restless during the examination, motion artifacts will be present on the images limiting their diagnostic value. If the patient is claustrophobic, mild oral sedation or occasionally parenteral sedation may be needed. Also, the patient can be accompanied by a family member or friend during the examination which may help to calm the patient's anxiety. Patients requiring life support equipment (ie, ventilators) require special preparation. Please refer to Contraindications for further causes for rejection.

Additional Information In some cases, an MRI contrast agent (Magnevist®) may be needed to increase the diagnostic accuracy of the MRI. This contrast agent can be administered to patients with a previous history of allergies to conventional iodinated x-ray agents, as it contains no iodine. Contraindications to its use include previous allergy to the contrast agent itself, renal failure, certain types of anemia, and Wilson disease. Nursing mothers should express their breasts and not breast-feed for 36-48 hours after the administration of an MRI contrast agent to ensure that the nursing child does not receive the drug in any notable quantity. The contrast agent is generally very safe and increases the diagnostic efficacy of the MRI.

References

Vogl TJ and Steger W, "The Head and Neck: Nasopharynx, Oropharynx, and Hypopharynx," *Magn Reson Imaging of the Body*, 3rd ed, Higgins CB, Hricak H, and Helms CA, eds, Philadelphia, PA: Lippincott Williams & Wilkins, 1997, 223-41.

Magnetic Resonance Scan, Obstetrics

Synonyms MRI, Obstetrics; Obstetrics MRI

Indications Magnetic resonance examination during pregnancy should be performed in only those patients for whom the diagnostic benefits are believed to outweigh the theoretical risks, since at the present there is no conclusive evidence of safety to the developing fetus. In those cases where ultrasound examination is equivocal (ie, presence of oligohydramnios, suspicion of placenta accreta with a scar in the posterior uterus - limiting factors to ultrasound), the MR scan can help.

Contraindications Patients weighing more than 300 lb and patients unable to squeeze into the magnet cannot undergo MRI. An absolute contraindication for MRI is a cardiac pacemaker. Relative contraindications to magnetic resonance imaging include intracranial aneurysm clips, cochlear implants, insulin infusion and chemotherapy pumps, neurocutaneous stimulators, prosthetic heart valves, ocular implants, penile implants, and artificial sphincters depending on date of manufacture and metallurgical composition. Please consult MRI physician if questions arise. Patients who have metallic foreign bodies within the eye or if the object is positioned near a vital neural, vascular, or soft tissue structure; or patients who have undergone recent surgery within the last 6 weeks requiring placement of a vascular surgical clip, should also not undergo MRI. The safety of MRI in pregnant patients has not been determined. In such cases, prior consultation with the MRI physician is required. Generally, patients who have undergone recent surgery not requiring vascular clips or who have had coronary artery bypass surgery in the past may undergo MRI. Patients who have shrapnel wounds or orthopedic prostheses can generally safely undergo MRI unless the metallic device is in the anatomic region to be scanned which results in degradation of the images. Patients with surgically implanted intravascular vena cava filters to prevent pulmonary embolism can usually be scanned if the device has been in place for at least 6 weeks. Patients requiring life support equipment, including ventilators, require special preparation. Please contact MRI physician ahead of time. Central venous lines, Swan-Ganz catheters, and nasogastric (NG) tubes usually present no problems. If the patient is positive when screened for metallic devices and you are uncertain of their significance, the MRI radiologist will provide additional information to assist you.

Patient Preparation Inpatient: The patient must be able to lie quietly while the scan is performed. The patient should be screened for metallic devices by nursing personnel. (See Contraindications.) This includes metal introduced into the patient either surgically or by trauma. All metallic objects must be removed from the patient, including jewelry or any other metal objects which may be in the patient's bedding. Dentures or other dental appliances must be removed. I.V.s which contain no metal are fine, but infusion pumps must be removed. Oxygen tanks and metallic backboards may come with the patient but will be removed prior to the patient entering the magnet room. Oxygen may be provided in the magnet room. Trauma, ICU, or CCU patients should be accompanied by a nurse. The patient needs to be NPO for abdominal MRI exams. If the patient is restless, combative, or claustrophobic, proper sedation may be administered on the floor prior to the MRI, or at the MRI Center. Consult the MRI radiologists with questions on proper sedation.

Outpatient: The patient should be screened for metallic devices. (See Contraindications.) If a question exists as to the patient's suitability for MRI, the MRI radiologist will assist you with your questions. If the patient is claustrophobic, oral or parenteral sedation may be necessary. If so, the patient should be accompanied by another adult to provide transportation home after the examination.

Aftercare If the patient received an MRI contrast agent (Magnevist®) and develops a delayed hypersensitivity reaction (ie, nausea, emesis, hives, or shortness of breath), the referring physician or MRI radiologist should be contacted immediately. If sedation is used, more time is required after the procedure for recovery period from the sedation.

Data Acquired Digital information with film reproduction

Limitations Generally, the greatest limitation of magnetic resonance imaging results from the patient's fear of the procedure. The patient must remain quiet and still for several scans, each lasting from several minutes to 10 minutes in length. Total examination time is usually 30-45 minutes and occasionally up to 1 hour. If the patient is restless during the examination, motion artifacts will be present on the images limiting their diagnostic value. If the patient is claustrophobic, mild oral sedation or occasionally parenteral sedation may be needed. Also, the patient can be accompanied by a family member or friend during the examination which may help to calm the patient's anxiety. Patients requiring life support equipment (ie, ventilators) require special preparation. Please refer to Contraindications for further causes for rejection.

Additional Information In some cases, an MRI contrast agent (Magnevist®) may be needed to increase the diagnostic accuracy of the MRI. This contrast agent can be administered to patients with a previous history of allergies to conventional iodinated x-ray agents, as it contains no iodine. Contraindications to its use include previous allergy to the contrast agent itself, renal failure, certain types of anemia, and Wilson disease. Nursing mothers should

(Continued)

Magnetic Resonance Scan, Obstetrics *(Continued)*

express their breasts and not breast-feed for 36-48 hours after the administration of an MRI contrast agent to ensure that the nursing child does not receive the drug in any notable quantity. The contrast agent is generally very safe and increases the diagnostic efficacy of the MRI.

References

Levine D, Barnes PD, Sher S, et al, "Fetal Fast MR Imaging: Reproducibility, Technical Quality, and Conspicuity of Anatomy," *Radiology*, 1998, 206(2):549-54.

Levine D, Hulka CA, Ludmir J, et al, "Placenta Accreta: Evaluation With Color Doppler US, Power Doppler US, and MR Imaging," *Radiology*, 1997, 205(3):773-6.

Magnetic Resonance Scan, Orbit

Related Information

Computed Transaxial Tomography, Orbits *on page 336*

Synonyms MRI, Orbit; Orbit MRI

Indications Diagnose pathology of the orbit including tumors of the orbit such as meningioma, optic nerve glioma, metastases, lacrimal gland tumors, and ocular melanoma; lymphoproliferative disease; inflammatory diseases such as pseudotumor, cellulitis, abscess, and thyroid orbitopathy; vascular abnormalities; nonmetallic foreign bodies; trauma; mucocele; hyperostosis; retinal detachment, etc

Contraindications Patients weighing more than 300 lb and patients unable to squeeze into the magnet cannot undergo MRI. An absolute contraindication for MRI is a cardiac pacemaker. Relative contraindications to magnetic resonance imaging include intracranial aneurysm clips, cochlear implants, insulin infusion and chemotherapy pumps, neurocutaneous stimulators, prosthetic heart valves, ocular implants, penile implants, and artificial sphincters depending on date of manufacture and metallurgical composition. Please consult MRI physician if questions arise. Patients who have metallic foreign bodies within the eye or if the object is positioned near a vital neural, vascular, or soft tissue structure; or patients who have undergone recent surgery within the last 6 weeks requiring placement of a vascular surgical clip, should also not undergo MRI. The safety of MRI in pregnant patients has not been determined. In such cases, prior consultation with the MRI physician is required. Generally, patients who have undergone recent surgery not requiring vascular clips or who have had coronary artery bypass surgery in the past may undergo MRI. Patients who have shrapnel wounds or orthopedic prostheses can generally safely undergo MRI unless the metallic device is in the anatomic region to be scanned which results in degradation of the images. Patients with surgically implanted intravascular vena cava filters to prevent pulmonary embolism can usually be scanned if the device has been in place for at least 6 weeks. Patients requiring life support equipment, including ventilators, require special preparation. Please contact MRI physician ahead of time. Central venous lines, Swan-Ganz catheters, and nasogastric (NG) tubes usually present no problems. If the patient is positive when screened for metallic devices and you are uncertain of their significance, the MRI radiologist will provide additional information to assist you.

Patient Preparation All cosmetic make-up must be removed prior to the scan in addition to contact lenses.

Inpatient: The patient must be able to lie quietly while the scan is performed. The patient should be screened for metallic devices by nursing personnel. (See Contraindications.) This includes metal introduced into the patient either surgically or by trauma. All metallic objects must be removed from the patient, including jewelry or any other metal objects which may be in the patient's bedding. Dentures or other dental appliances must be removed. I.V.s which contain no metal are fine, but infusion pumps must be removed. Oxygen tanks and metallic backboards may come with the patient but will be removed prior to the patient entering the magnet room. Oxygen may be provided in the magnet room. Trauma, ICU, or CCU patients should be accompanied by a nurse. The patient needs to be NPO for abdominal MRI exams. If the patient is restless, combative, or claustrophobic, proper sedation may be administered on the floor prior to the MRI, or at the MRI Center. Consult the MRI radiologists with questions on proper sedation.

Outpatient: The patient should be screened for metallic devices. (See Contraindications.) If a question exists as to the patient's suitability for MRI, the MRI radiologist will assist you with your questions. If the patient is claustrophobic, oral or parenteral sedation may be necessary. If so, the patient should be accompanied by another adult to provide transportation home after the examination.

Aftercare If the patient received an MRI contrast agent (Magnevist®) and develops a delayed hypersensitivity reaction (ie, nausea, emesis, hives, or shortness of breath), the referring physician or MRI radiologist should be contacted immediately. If sedation is used, more time is required after the procedure for recovery period from the sedation.

Technique Unlike most conventional radiologic procedures, magnetic resonance imaging does not utilize ionizing radiation, but relies upon radio frequency or radio signals induced within the patient by the magnetic field to obtain images. There are no known biologic effects secondary to the magnetic fields currently used in clinical MRI. Prior to the scan, the patient will be asked to remove all metallic objects from their person, including loose change, hair pins, earrings, belts, etc. This is for safety reasons as the strong magnetic field could result in these and any other metal objects becoming projectiles resulting in injury to the patient or MRI personnel. Also the patient should not carry a purse or wallet into the magnetic room, as the magnetic field can permanently erase bank cards or credit cards. The magnet is open on both ends and music can be played for the patient if desired. Fresh air is constantly circulated through the magnet room and the patient is continually monitored by the MRI technologist. An intercom system is provided for communication between the patient and the technologist. For MRI of the orbit or face, a special surface coil will be placed over the orbit or face and the patient will be asked to remain still while the scans are obtained. In certain cases, an MRI contrast agent, Gadopentetate Dimeglumine (Magnevist®) may be necessary to increase the diagnostic accuracy of the MRI examination. This is administered intravenously, via an antecubital vein in a small volume (less than 20 mL). This contrast agent may be used in patients who are allergic to conventional iodinated contrast agents such as is used in IVPs or CT examination without difficulty. There are very few contraindications to its use. (See Contraindications.)

Data Acquired Digital information with film reproduction

Limitations Generally, the greatest limitation of magnetic resonance imaging results from the patient's fear of the procedure. The patient must remain quiet and still for several scans, each lasting from several minutes to 10 minutes in length. Total examination time is usually 30-45 minutes and occasionally up to 1 hour. If the patient is restless during the examination, motion artifacts will be present on the images limiting their diagnostic value. If the patient is claustrophobic, mild oral sedation or occasionally parenteral sedation may be needed. Also, the patient can be accompanied by a family member or friend during the examination which may help to calm the patient's anxiety. Patients requiring life support equipment (ie, ventilators) require special preparation. Please refer to Contraindications for further causes for rejection.

Additional Information In some cases, an MRI contrast agent (Magnevist®) may be needed to increase the diagnostic accuracy of the MRI. This contrast agent can be administered to patients with a previous history of allergies to conventional iodinated x-ray agents, as it contains no iodine. Contraindications to its use include previous allergy to the contrast agent itself, renal failure, certain types of anemia, and Wilson disease. Nursing mothers should express their breasts and not breast-feed for 36-48 hours after the administration of an MRI contrast agent to ensure that the nursing child does not receive the drug in any notable quantity. The contrast agent is generally very safe and increases the diagnostic efficacy of the MRI.

References

Atlas SW, "MR Imaging of the Orbit: Current Status," *Magn Reson Q*, 1989, 5(1):39-96.

Atlas SW, "Orbit," *Magn Reson Imaging*, 3rd ed, Stark DD, Bradley WG Jr, eds, St Louis, MO: CV Mosby Co, 1999, 1637-66.

Weber AL, Jakobiec FA, and Sabates NR, "Lymphoproliferative Disease of the Orbit," *Neuroimaging Clin N Am*, 1996, 6(1):93-111.

(Continued)

Magnetic Resonance Scan, Orbit *(Continued)*

Weber AL, Jakobiec FA, and Sabates NR, "Pseudotumor of the Orbit," *Neuroimaging Clin N Am*, 1996, 6(1):73-92.

Wheatcroft S and Benjamin L, "Magnetic Resonance Imaging and the Dangers of Orbital Foreign Bodies," *Br J Ophthalmol*, 1996, 80(12):1116.

Magnetic Resonance Scan, Peripheral Vascular

Synonyms Magnetic Resonance Angiography; MRI, Peripheral Vascular; MRI, Venography; Peripheral Vascular MRI

Indications Diagnose and characterize peripheral vascular abnormalities (eg, atherosclerosis thrombosis, occlusions, vascular malformations)

Contraindications Patients weighing more than 300 lb and patients unable to squeeze into the magnet cannot undergo MRI. An absolute contraindication for MRI is a cardiac pacemaker. Relative contraindications to magnetic resonance imaging include intracranial aneurysm clips, cochlear implants, insulin infusion and chemotherapy pumps, neurocutaneous stimulators, prosthetic heart valves, ocular implants, penile implants, and artificial sphincters depending on date of manufacture and metallurgical composition. Please consult MRI physician if questions arise. Patients who have metallic foreign bodies within the eye or if the object is positioned near a vital neural, vascular, or soft tissue structure; or patients who have undergone recent surgery within the last 6 weeks requiring placement of a vascular surgical clip, should also not undergo MRI. The safety of MRI in pregnant patients has not been determined. In such cases, prior consultation with the MRI physician is required. Generally, patients who have undergone recent surgery not requiring vascular clips or who have had coronary artery bypass surgery in the past may undergo MRI. Patients who have shrapnel wounds or orthopedic prostheses can generally safely undergo MRI unless the metallic device is in the anatomic region to be scanned which results in degradation of the images. Patients with surgically implanted intravascular vena cava filters to prevent pulmonary embolism can usually be scanned if the device has been in place for at least 6 weeks. Patients requiring life support equipment, including ventilators, require special preparation. Please contact MRI physician ahead of time. Central venous lines, Swan-Ganz catheters, and nasogastric (NG) tubes usually present no problems. If the patient is positive when screened for metallic devices and you are uncertain of their significance, the MRI radiologist will provide additional information to assist you.

Patient Preparation **Inpatient:** The patient must be able to lie quietly while the scan is performed. The patient should be screened for metallic devices by nursing personnel. (See Contraindications.) This includes metal introduced into the patient either surgically or by trauma. All metallic objects must be removed from the patient, including jewelry or any other metal objects which may be in the patient's bedding. Dentures or other dental appliances must be removed. I.V.s which contain no metal are fine, but infusion pumps must be removed. Oxygen tanks and metallic backboards may come with the patient but will be removed prior to the patient entering the magnet room. Oxygen may be provided in the magnet room. Trauma, ICU, or CCU patients should be accompanied by a nurse. The patient needs to be NPO for abdominal MRI exams. If the patient is restless, combative, or claustrophobic, proper sedation may be administered on the floor prior to the MRI, or at the MRI Center. Consult the MRI radiologists with questions on proper sedation.

Outpatient: The patient should be screened for metallic devices. (See Contraindications.) If a question exists as to the patient's suitability for MRI, the MRI radiologist will assist you with your questions. If the patient is claustrophobic, oral or parenteral sedation may be necessary. If so, the patient should be accompanied by another adult to provide transportation home after the examination.

Aftercare If the patient received an MRI contrast agent (Magnevist®) and develops a delayed hypersensitivity reaction (ie, nausea, emesis, hives, or shortness of breath), the referring physician or MRI radiologist should be contacted immediately. If sedation is used, more time is required after the procedure for recovery period from the sedation.

Data Acquired Digital information with film reproduction

Limitations Generally, the greatest limitation of magnetic resonance imaging results from the patient's fear of the procedure. The patient must remain quiet and still for several scans, each lasting from several minutes to 10 minutes in length. Total examination time is usually 30-45 minutes and occasionally up to 1 hour. If the patient is restless during the examination, motion artifacts will be present on the images limiting their diagnostic value. If the patient is claustrophobic, mild oral sedation or occasionally parenteral sedation may be needed. Also, the patient can be accompanied by a family member or friend during the examination which may help to calm the patient's anxiety. Patients requiring life support equipment (ie, ventilators) require special preparation. Please refer to Contraindications for further causes for rejection.

Additional Information In some cases, an MRI contrast agent (Magnevist®) may be needed to increase the diagnostic accuracy of the MRI. This contrast agent can be administered to patients with a previous history of allergies to conventional iodinated x-ray agents, as it contains no iodine. Contraindications to its use include previous allergy to the contrast agent itself, renal failure, certain types of anemia, and Wilson disease. Nursing mothers should express their breasts and not breast-feed for 36-48 hours after the administration of an MRI contrast agent to ensure that the nursing child does not receive the drug in any notable quantity. The contrast agent is generally very safe and increases the diagnostic efficacy of the MRI.

References

Baum RA and Carpenter JP, "Magnetic Resonance Angiography: Peripheral Vasculature," *Magn Reson Imaging*, 3rd ed, Stark DD and Bradley WG Jr, eds, St Louis, MO: CV Mosby Co, 1999, 1097-108.

Bongartz GM, Boos M, Winter K, et al, "Clinical Utility of Contrast-Enhanced MR Angiography," *Eur J Radiol*, 1997, 7(Suppl 5):178-86.

Disa JJ, Chung KC, Gellad FE, et al, "Efficacy of Magnetic Resonance Angiography in the Evaluation of Vascular Malformations of the Hand," *Plast Reconstr Surg*, 1997, 99(1):136-44.

Masaryk TJ and Ross JS, "MR Angiography: Clinical Applications," *Magnetic Resonance Imaging of the Brain and Spine*, Atlas SW, ed, New York, NY: Raven Press, 1991, 1079-97.

Magnetic Resonance Scan, Shoulder

Synonyms MRI, Shoulder; Shoulder MRI

Indications The MRI and MR arthrography are used to diagnose derangements of the shoulder joint including impingement syndrome (extrinsic and intrinsic), rotator cuff tendinopathy and tears, glenohumeral joint instability, and anterior labra abnormalities. The MRI is also indicated to evaluate osteonecrosis of the humeral head and shoulder masses such as ganglion, distended bursa, hemangioma, hematoma, and lipoma.

Contraindications Patients weighing more than 300 lb and patients unable to squeeze into the magnet cannot undergo MRI. An absolute contraindication for MRI is a cardiac pacemaker. Relative contraindications to magnetic resonance imaging include intracranial aneurysm clips, cochlear implants, insulin infusion and chemotherapy pumps, neurocutaneous stimulators, prosthetic heart valves, ocular implants, penile implants, and artificial sphincters depending on date of manufacture and metallurgical composition. Please consult MRI physician if questions arise. Patients who have metallic foreign bodies within the eye or if the object is positioned near a vital neural, vascular, or soft tissue structure; or patients who have undergone recent surgery within the last 6 weeks requiring placement of a vascular surgical clip, should also not undergo MRI. The safety of MRI in pregnant patients has not been determined. In such cases, prior consultation with the MRI physician is required. Generally, patients who have undergone recent surgery not requiring vascular clips or who have had coronary artery bypass surgery in the past may undergo MRI. Patients who have shrapnel wounds or orthopedic prostheses can generally safely undergo MRI unless the metallic device is in the anatomic region to be scanned which results in degradation of the images. Patients with surgically implanted intravascular vena cava filters to prevent pulmonary embolism can usually be scanned if the device has been in place for at least 6 weeks. Patients requiring life support equipment, including ventilators, require special preparation. Please contact MRI physician ahead of time. Central venous lines, Swan-Ganz catheters, and nasogastric (NG) tubes usually

(Continued)

Magnetic Resonance Scan, Shoulder *(Continued)*

present no problems. If the patient is positive when screened for metallic devices and you are uncertain of their significance, the MRI radiologist will provide additional information to assist you.

Patient Preparation Inpatient: The patient must be able to lie quietly while the scan is performed. The patient should be screened for metallic devices by nursing personnel. (See Contraindications.) This includes metal introduced into the patient either surgically or by trauma. All metallic objects must be removed from the patient, including jewelry or any other metal objects which may be in the patient's bedding. Dentures or other dental appliances must be removed. I.V.s which contain no metal are fine, but infusion pumps must be removed. Oxygen tanks and metallic backboards may come with the patient but will be removed prior to the patient entering the magnet room. Oxygen may be provided in the magnet room. Trauma, ICU, or CCU patients should be accompanied by a nurse. If the patient is restless, combative, or claustrophobic, proper sedation may be administered on the floor prior to the MRI, or at the MRI Center. Consult the MRI radiologists with questions on proper sedation.

Outpatient: The patient should be screened for metallic devices. (See Contraindications.) If a question exists as to the patient's suitability for MRI, the MRI radiologist will assist you with your questions. If the patient is claustrophobic, oral or parenteral sedation may be necessary. If so, the patient should be accompanied by another adult to provide transportation home after the examination.

Aftercare If the patient received an MRI contrast agent (Magnevist®) and develops a delayed hypersensitivity reaction (ie, nausea, emesis, hives, or shortness of breath), the referring physician or MRI radiologist should be contacted immediately. If sedation is used, more time is required after the procedure for recovery period from the sedation.

Technique Unlike most conventional radiologic procedures, magnetic resonance imaging does not utilize ionizing radiation, but relies upon radio frequency or radio signals induced within the patient by the magnetic field to obtain images. There are no known biologic effects secondary to the magnetic fields currently used in clinical MRI. Prior to the scan, the patient will be asked to remove all metallic objects from their person, including loose change, hair pins, earrings, belts, etc. This is for safety reasons as the strong magnetic field could result in these and any other metal objects becoming projectiles resulting in injury to the patient or MRI personnel. Also the patient should not carry a purse or wallet into the magnetic room, as the magnetic field can permanently erase bank cards or credit cards. The magnet is open on both ends and music can be played for the patient if desired. Fresh air is constantly circulated through the magnet room and the patient is continually monitored by the MRI technologist. An intercom system is provided for communication between the patient and the technologist. A special surface coil will be placed over the affected shoulder and images obtained. The patient will need to remain motionless during the exam.

Data Acquired Digital information with film reproduction

Limitations Generally, the greatest limitation of magnetic resonance imaging results from the patient's fear of the procedure. The patient must remain quiet and still for several scans, each lasting from several minutes to 10 minutes in length. Total examination time is usually 30-45 minutes and occasionally up to 1 hour. If the patient is restless during the examination, motion artifacts will be present on the images limiting their diagnostic value. If the patient is claustrophobic, mild oral sedation or occasionally parenteral sedation may be needed. Also, the patient can be accompanied by a family member or friend during the examination which may help to calm the patient's anxiety. Patients requiring life support equipment (ie, ventilators) cannot undergo MRI. Please refer to Contraindications for further causes for rejection. The exam may be somewhat limited if orthopedic appliances have been placed previously on the affected shoulder.

Additional Information In some cases, an MRI contrast agent (Magnevist®) may be needed to increase the diagnostic accuracy of the MRI. This contrast agent can be administered to patients with a previous history of allergies to conventional iodinated x-ray agents as it contains no iodine. Contraindications to its use include previous allergy to the contrast agent itself, renal failure, certain types of anemia, and Wilson disease. Nursing mothers should express their breasts and not breast-feed for 36-48 hours after the administration of an MRI contrast agent to ensure that the nursing child does not receive the drug in any notable quantity. The contrast agent is generally very safe and increases the diagnostic efficacy of the MRI.

References

Oxner KG, "Magnetic Resonance Imaging of the Musculoskeletal System. Part 6. The Shoulder," *Clin Orthop*, 1997, 334:354-73.

Stoller DW, "MR Arthrography of the Glenohumeral Joint," *Radiol Clin North Am*, 1997, 35(1):97-116.

Tirman PF, Steinbach LS, Belzer JP, et al, "A Practical Approach to Imaging of the Shoulder With Emphasis on MR Imaging," *Orthop Clin North Am*, 1997, 28(4):483-515.

Uri DS, "MR Imaging of Shoulder Impingement and Rotator Cuff Disease," *Radiol Clin North Am*, 1997, 35(1):77-96.

Magnetic Resonance Scan, Sinuses

Related Information

Computed Transaxial Tomography, Paranasal Sinuses *on page 337*

Synonyms MRI Sinuses; Sinuses, MRI

Indications Evaluate infection, cysts, polyps, granulomatous diseases, mucocele, tumors of sinus cavities, vascular tumors, fibroosseous lesions, Paget disease, odontogenic cysts, and fracture

Contraindications Patients weighing more than 300 lb and patients unable to squeeze into the magnet cannot undergo MRI. An absolute contraindication for MRI is a cardiac pacemaker. Relative contraindications to magnetic resonance imaging include intracranial aneurysm clips, cochlear implants, insulin infusion and chemotherapy pumps, neurocutaneous stimulators, prosthetic heart valves, ocular implants, penile implants, and artificial sphincters depending on date of manufacture and metallurgical composition. Please consult MRI physician if questions arise. Patients who have metallic foreign bodies within the eye or if the object is positioned near a vital neural, vascular, or soft tissue structure; or patients who have undergone recent surgery within the last 6 weeks requiring placement of a vascular surgical clip, should also not undergo MRI. The safety of MRI in pregnant patients has not been determined. In such cases, prior consultation with the MRI physician is required. Generally, patients who have undergone recent surgery not requiring vascular clips or who have had coronary artery bypass surgery in the past may undergo MRI. Patients who have shrapnel wounds or orthopedic prostheses can generally safely undergo MRI unless the metallic device is in the anatomic region to be scanned which results in degradation of the images. Patients with surgically implanted intravascular vena cava filters to prevent pulmonary embolism can usually be scanned if the device has been in place for at least 6 weeks. Patients requiring life support equipment, including ventilators, require special preparation. Please contact MRI physician ahead of time. Central venous lines, Swan-Ganz catheters, and nasogastric (NG) tubes usually present no problems. If the patient is positive when screened for metallic devices and you are uncertain of their significance, the MRI radiologist will provide additional information to assist you.

Patient Preparation All cosmetic make-up must be removed prior to the scan in addition to contact lenses.

Inpatient: The patient must be able to lie quietly while the scan is performed. The patient should be screened for metallic devices by nursing personnel. (See Contraindications.) This includes metal introduced into the patient either surgically or by trauma. All metallic objects must be removed from the patient, including jewelry or any other metal objects which may be in the patient's bedding. Dentures or other dental appliances must be removed. I.V.s which contain no metal are fine, but infusion pumps must be removed. Oxygen tanks and metallic backboards may come with the patient but will be removed prior to the patient entering the magnet room. Oxygen may be provided in the

(Continued)

Magnetic Resonance Scan, Sinuses *(Continued)*

magnet room. Trauma, ICU, or CCU patients should be accompanied by a nurse. If the patient is restless, combative, or claustrophobic, proper sedation may be administered on the floor prior to the MRI, or at the MRI Center. Consult the MRI radiologists with questions on proper sedation.

Outpatient: The patient should be screened for metallic devices. (See Contraindications.) If a question exists as to the patient's suitability for MRI, the MRI radiologist will assist you with your questions. If the patient is claustrophobic, oral or parenteral sedation may be necessary. If so, the patient should be accompanied by another adult to provide transportation home after the examination.

Aftercare If the patient received an MRI contrast agent (Magnevist®) and develops a delayed hypersensitivity reaction (ie, nausea, emesis, hives, or shortness of breath), the referring physician or MRI radiologist should be contacted immediately. If sedation is used, more time is required after the procedure for recovery period from the sedation.

Data Acquired Digital information with film reproduction

Limitations Generally, the greatest limitation of magnetic resonance imaging results from the patient's fear of the procedure. The patient must remain quiet and still for several scans, each lasting from several minutes to 10 minutes in length. Total examination time is usually 30-45 minutes and occasionally up to 1 hour. If the patient is restless during the examination, motion artifacts will be present on the images limiting their diagnostic value. If the patient is claustrophobic, mild oral sedation or occasionally parenteral sedation may be needed. Also, the patient can be accompanied by a family member or friend during the examination which may help to calm the patient's anxiety. Patients requiring life support equipment (ie, ventilators) require special preparation. Please refer to Contraindications for further causes for rejection.

Additional Information In some cases, an MRI contrast agent (Magnevist®) may be needed to increase the diagnostic accuracy of the MRI. This contrast agent can be administered to patients with a previous history of allergies to conventional iodinated x-ray agents, as it contains no iodine. Contraindications to its use include previous allergy to the contrast agent itself, renal failure, certain types of anemia, and Wilson disease. Nursing mothers should express their breasts and not breast-feed for 36-48 hours after the administration of an MRI contrast agent to ensure that the nursing child does not receive the drug in any notable quantity. The contrast agent is generally very safe and increases the diagnostic efficacy of the MRI. Common sinonasal inflammatory disease is best imaged by CT.

References

Hudgins PA, "Sinonasal Imaging," *Neuroimaging Clin N Am*, 1996, 6(2):319-31.

Som PM and Curtin HD, "Sinuses," *Magnetic Resonance Imaging*, 3rd ed, Stark DD and Bradley WG Jr, eds, St Louis, MO: CV Mosby Co, 1999, 1675-94.

Magnetic Resonance Scan, Temporomandibular Joint

Synonyms MRI, Temporomandibular Joint; Temporomandibular Joint MRI

Indications Evaluate temporomandibular joint disorders such as internal derangements (abnormal disk position), articular disease (inflammatory arthritis, rheumatoid arthritis, ankylosing spondylitis, systemic lupus erythematosus, juvenile chronic arthritis, crystalline arthropathies), trauma, adhesions, congenital variations; evaluate implanted prostheses

Contraindications Patients weighing more than 300 lb and patients unable to squeeze into the magnet cannot undergo MRI. An absolute contraindication for MRI is a cardiac pacemaker. Relative contraindications to magnetic resonance imaging include intracranial aneurysm clips, cochlear implants, insulin infusion and chemotherapy pumps, neurocutaneous stimulators, prosthetic heart valves, ocular implants, penile implants, and artificial sphincters depending on date of manufacture and metallurgical composition. Please consult MRI physician if questions arise. Patients who have metallic foreign bodies within the eye or if the object is positioned near a vital neural, vascular, or soft tissue structure; or patients who have undergone recent surgery within the last 6 weeks requiring placement of a vascular surgical clip, should also not undergo MRI. The safety of MRI in pregnant patients has not been determined. In such cases, prior consultation with the MRI physician is required. Generally, patients who have undergone recent surgery not requiring vascular clips or who have had coronary artery bypass surgery in the past may undergo MRI. Patients who have shrapnel wounds or orthopedic prostheses can generally safely undergo MRI unless the metallic device is in the anatomic region to be scanned which results in degradation of the images. Patients with surgically implanted intravascular vena cava filters to prevent pulmonary embolism can usually be scanned if the device has been in place for at least 6 weeks. Patients requiring life support equipment, including ventilators, require special preparation. Please contact MRI physician ahead of time. Central venous lines, Swan-Ganz catheters, and nasogastric (NG) tubes usually present no problems. If the patient is positive when screened for metallic devices and you are uncertain of their significance, the MRI radiologist will provide additional information to assist you.

Patient Preparation Inpatient: The patient must be able to lie quietly while the scan is performed. The patient should be screened for metallic devices by nursing personnel. (See Contraindications.) This includes metal introduced into the patient either surgically or by trauma. All metallic objects must be removed from the patient, including jewelry or any other metal objects which may be in the patient's bedding. Dentures or other dental appliances must be removed. I.V.s which contain no metal are fine, but infusion pumps must be removed. Oxygen tanks and metallic backboards may come with the patient but will be removed prior to the patient entering the magnet room. Oxygen may be provided in the magnet room. Trauma, ICU, or CCU patients should be accompanied by a nurse. The patient needs to be NPO for abdominal MRI exams. If the patient is restless, combative, or claustrophobic, proper sedation may be administered on the floor prior to the MRI, or at the MRI Center. Consult the MRI radiologists with questions on proper sedation.

Outpatient: The patient should be screened for metallic devices. (See Contraindications.) If a question exists as to the patient's suitability for MRI, the MRI radiologist will assist you with your questions. If the patient is claustrophobic, oral or parenteral sedation may be necessary. If so, the patient should be accompanied by another adult to provide transportation home after the examination.

Aftercare If the patient received an MRI contrast agent (Magnevist®) and develops a delayed hypersensitivity reaction (ie, nausea, emesis, hives, or shortness of breath), the referring physician or MRI radiologist should be contacted immediately. If sedation is used, more time is required after the procedure for recovery period from the sedation.

Technique Unlike most conventional radiologic procedures, magnetic resonance imaging does not utilize ionizing radiation, but relies upon radio frequency or radio signals induced within the patient by the magnetic field to obtain images. There are no known biologic effects secondary to the magnetic fields currently used in clinical MRI. Prior to the scan, the patient will be asked to remove all metallic objects from their person, including loose change, hair pins, earrings, belts, etc. This is for safety reasons as the strong magnetic field could result in these and any other metal objects becoming projectiles resulting in injury to the patient or MRI personnel. Also the patient should not carry a purse or wallet into the magnetic room, as the magnetic field can permanently erase bank cards or credit cards. The magnet is open on both ends and music can be played for the patient if desired. Fresh air is constantly circulated through the magnet room and the patient is continually monitored by the MRI technologist. An intercom system is provided for communication between the patient and the technologist. A special surface coil will be placed over the affected TMJ and images obtained in both open and closed positions.

Data Acquired Digital information with film reproduction

Limitations Generally, the greatest limitation of magnetic resonance imaging results from the patient's fear of the procedure. The patient must remain quiet and still for several scans, each lasting from several minutes to 10 minutes in

(Continued)

Magnetic Resonance Scan, Temporomandibular Joint *(Continued)*

length. Total examination time is usually 30-45 minutes and occasionally up to 1 hour. If the patient is restless during the examination, motion artifacts will be present on the images limiting their diagnostic value. If the patient is claustrophobic, mild oral sedation or occasionally parenteral sedation may be needed. Also, the patient can be accompanied by a family member or friend during the examination which may help to calm the patient's anxiety. Patients requiring life support equipment (ie, ventilators) require special preparation. Please refer to Contraindications for further causes for rejection.

Additional Information In some cases, an MRI contrast agent (Magnevist®) may be needed to increase the diagnostic accuracy of the MRI. This contrast agent can be administered to patients with a previous history of allergies to conventional iodinated x-ray agents, as it contains no iodine. Contraindications to its use include previous allergy to the contrast agent itself, renal failure, certain types of anemia, and Wilson disease. Nursing mothers should express their breasts and not breast-feed for 36-48 hours after the administration of an MRI contrast agent to ensure that the nursing child does not receive the drug in any notable quantity. The contrast agent is generally very safe and increases the diagnostic efficacy of the MRI. Positioning apparatus (Burnett opening device) is used to guide kinematic, open-mouth, and closed-mouth views and it is controlled by the patient.

References

Harms SE and Wilk RM, "Magnetic Resonance Imaging of the Temporomandibular Joint," *Radiographics*, 1987, 7(3):521-42.

Harms EH, "Temporomandibular Joint," *Magn Reson Imaging*, 3rd ed, Stark DD, Bradley WG Jr, eds, St Louis, MO: CV Mosby Co, 1999, 673-90.

Küseler A, Pedersen TK, Herlin T, et al, "Contrast Enhanced Magnetic Resonance Imaging as a Method to Diagnose Early Inflammatory Changes in the Temporomandibular Joint in Children With Juvenile Chronic Arthritis," *J Rheumatol*, 1998, 25(7):1406-12.

Rao VM, Farole A, and Karasick D, "Temporomandibular Joint Dysfunction: Correlation of MR Imaging, Arthrography, and Arthroscopy," *Radiology*, 1990, 174(3 Pt 1):663-7.

♦ **Magnetic Resonance Scan, Thorax** *see* Magnetic Resonance Scan, Chest *on page 408*

Magnetic Resonance Scan, Wrist

Synonyms MRI, Wrist; Wrist MRI

Indications Evaluate abnormalities of the wrist including tears of the intrinsic ligaments and of the triangular fibrocartilage complex, tendinopathy, tenosynovitis, tendon rupture, carpal tunnel syndrome, osteonecrosis, tumors, and ganglia; detect fractures of the scaphoid bone not evident on plain radiography

Contraindications Patients weighing more than 300 lb and patients unable to squeeze into the magnet cannot undergo MRI. An absolute contraindication for MRI is a cardiac pacemaker. Relative contraindications to magnetic resonance imaging include intracranial aneurysm clips, cochlear implants, insulin infusion and chemotherapy pumps, neurocutaneous stimulators, prosthetic heart valves, ocular implants, penile implants, and artificial sphincters depending on date of manufacture and metallurgical composition. Please consult MRI physician if questions arise. Patients who have metallic foreign bodies within the eye or if the object is positioned near a vital neural, vascular, or soft tissue structure; or patients who have undergone recent surgery within the last 6 weeks requiring placement of a vascular surgical clip, should also not undergo MRI. The safety of MRI in pregnant patients has not been determined. In such cases, prior consultation with the MRI physician is required. Generally, patients who have undergone recent surgery not requiring vascular clips or who have had coronary artery bypass surgery in the past may undergo MRI. Patients who have shrapnel wounds or orthopedic prostheses can generally safely undergo MRI unless the metallic device is in the anatomic region to be scanned which results in degradation of the images. Patients with surgically implanted intravascular vena cava filters to prevent pulmonary embolism can usually be scanned if the device has been in place for at least 6 weeks. Patients requiring life support equipment, including ventilators, require special preparation. Please contact MRI physician ahead of time. Central venous lines, Swan-Ganz catheters, and nasogastric (NG) tubes usually present no problems. If the patient is positive when screened for metallic devices and you are uncertain of their significance, the MRI radiologist will provide additional information to assist you.

Patient Preparation Inpatient: The patient must be able to lie quietly while the scan is performed. The patient should be screened for metallic devices by nursing personnel. (See Contraindications.) This includes metal introduced into the patient either surgically or by trauma. All metallic objects must be removed from the patient, including jewelry or any other metal objects which may be in the patient's bedding. Dentures or other dental appliances must be removed. I.V.s which contain no metal are fine, but infusion pumps must be removed. Oxygen tanks and metallic backboards may come with the patient but will be removed prior to the patient entering the magnet room. Oxygen may be provided in the magnet room. Trauma, ICU, or CCU patients should be accompanied by a nurse. If the patient is restless, combative, or claustrophobic, proper sedation may be administered on the floor prior to the MRI, or at the MRI Center. Consult the MRI radiologists with questions on proper sedation.

Outpatient: The patient should be screened for metallic devices. (See Contraindications.) If a question exists as to the patient's suitability for MRI, the MRI radiologist will assist you with your questions. If the patient is claustrophobic, oral or parenteral sedation may be necessary. If so, the patient should be accompanied by another adult to provide transportation home after the examination.

Aftercare If the patient received an MRI contrast agent (Magnevist®) and develops a delayed hypersensitivity reaction (ie, nausea, emesis, hives, or shortness of breath), the referring physician or MRI radiologist should be contacted immediately. If sedation is used, more time is required after the procedure for recovery period from the sedation.

Data Acquired Digital information with film reproduction

Limitations Implanted orthopedic devices in the anatomical area being imaged may limit the usefulness of the test. Generally, the greatest limitation of magnetic resonance imaging results from the patient's fear of the procedure. The patient must remain quiet and still for several scans, each lasting from several minutes to 10 minutes in length. Total examination time is usually 30-45 minutes and occasionally up to 1 hour. If the patient is restless during the examination, motion artifacts will be present on the images limiting their diagnostic value. If the patient is claustrophobic, mild oral sedation or occasionally parenteral sedation may be needed. Also, the patient can be accompanied by a family member or friend during the examination which may help to calm the patient's anxiety. Patients requiring life support equipment (ie, ventilators) require special preparation. Please refer to Contraindications for further causes for rejection.

Additional Information In some cases, an MRI contrast agent (Magnevist®) may be needed to increase the diagnostic accuracy of the MRI. This contrast agent can be administered to patients with a previous history of allergies to conventional iodinated x-ray agents as it contains no iodine. Contraindications to its use include previous allergy to the contrast agent itself, renal failure, certain types of anemia, and Wilson disease. Nursing mothers should express their breasts and not breast-feed for 36-48 hours after the administration of an MRI contrast agent to ensure that the nursing child does not receive the drug in any notable quantity. The contrast agent is generally very safe and increases the diagnostic efficacy of the MRI.

References

Breitenseher MJ, Metz VM, Gilula LA, et al, "Radiographically Occult Scaphoid Fractures: Value of MR Imaging in Detection," *Radiology*, 1997, 203(1):245-50.

Potter HG, Asnis-Ernberg L, Weiland AJ, et al, "The Utility of High-Resolution Magnetic Resonance Imaging in the Evaluation of the Triangular Fibrocartilage Complex of the Wrist," *J Bone Joint Surg [Am]*, 1997, 79(11):1675-84.

Pretorius ES, Epstein RE, and Dalinka MK, "MR Imaging of the Wrist," *Radiol Clin North Am*, 1997, 35(1):145-61.

♦ **MRI, Abdomen** *see* Magnetic Resonance Scan, Abdomen *on page 393*

NUCLEAR MEDICINE

- **Acute Myocardial Infarction Scan** *see* Myocardial Infarction Scan *on page 456*
- **Aerosol Lung Scan** *see* Lung Scan, Ventilation *on page 454*

Angiogram, Radionuclide

Related Information

Cardiac Blood Pool Scan, First Pass *on page 443*
Renal Scan *on page 463*

Synonyms Arterial Flow Study; Vascular Dynamic Study; Vascular Flow Study

Applies to Brain Flow Only; Superior Venacavagram

Procedure Commonly Includes The patient receives an intravenous injection of a technetium-99m (^{99m}Tc) compound. During and immediately following injection, rapid sequence images of the vascular structures and/or organs of interest are acquired. With computer assistance, a cine display of initial perfusion through major vascular structures can be made. Additional computer analysis can generate organ perfusion curves and other quantitative information.

Indications Radionuclide angiograms are helpful in noninvasively evaluating perfusion to many organ systems. They are often used to assess the functional significance of known or suspected anatomic abnormalities such as vascular stenoses or obstructions. They are a routine part of many dynamic organ imaging procedures (see Cardiac Blood Pool Scan, First Pass *on page 443* and Renal Scan *on page 463*). Additional applications include the detection of superior vena cava obstruction or documentation of absent cerebral perfusion (brain death).

Patient Preparation The patient does not need to be fasting or NPO for this procedure. The patient should have all RIA blood work performed, or at least drawn, prior to the injection of any radioactive material.

Special Instructions Requisition must state the current patient diagnosis in order to select the most appropriate radiopharmaceutical and/or imaging technique.

Duration of Procedure: 30 minutes

Radiopharmaceutical: ^{99m}Tc DTPA or other ^{99m}Tc compound

Turnaround Time A written report will be sent to the patient's chart and/or to the referring physician.

Causes for Rejection Other recent Nuclear Medicine procedure may interfere.

Normal Findings Prompt transit of the radionuclide bolus through arterial vascular structures and homogeneous perfusion of the organs supplied by these vessels

Limitations Radionuclide angiograms provide accurate screening for functional aspects of vascular flow and organ perfusion. However, image resolution is not good enough to accurately assess the exact anatomy (eg, the precise location and the extent of an obstruction). Radionuclide angiography is often used as a screening test to better select patients who may need a more invasive contrast angiographic procedure.

References

Coltart RS and Wraight EP, "The Value of Radionuclide Venography in Superior Vena Caval Obstruction," *Clin Radiol*, 1985, 36(4):415-8.

(Continued)

Angiogram, Radionuclide *(Continued)*

Muramatsu T, Miyamae T, and Dohi Y, "Collateral Pathways Observed by Radionuclide Superior Cavography in 70 Patients With Superior Vena Caval Obstruction," *Clin Nucl Med*, 1991, 16(5):332-6.

Rudavsky AZ, "Radionuclide Angiography in the Evaluation of Arterial and Venous Grafts," *Semin Nucl Med*, 1988, 18(3):261-8.

Turoglu Ht, Elmquist T, and Abdel-Dayem HM, "Incidence of Subclavian Vein Thrombosis Detected During First-Pass Phase of Radionuclide Angiocardiogram," *J Nucl Med*, 1997, 38(1):101-3.

♦ **Arterial Flow Study** *see* Angiogram, Radionuclide *on page 437*

♦ **Biliary Patency Scan** *see* Biliary Scan *on page 438*

♦ **Biliary Reflux Scan** *see* Biliary Scan *on page 438*

Biliary Scan

Synonyms Biliary Patency Scan; Choletec® Scan; DISIDA® Scan; Disofenin Scan; Gallbladder Ejection Fraction Scan; Gallbladder Scan; Hepatobiliary Scan; Hepatobiliary Scintigraphy; HIDA® Liver Scan; Mebrofenin® Scan

Applies to Biliary Reflux Scan

Replaces Rose Bengal Liver Scan

Procedure Commonly Includes The patient receives an intravenous injection of a technetium-99m (^{99m}Tc) IDA radiopharmaceutical which is excreted through the biliary system. Multiple images are acquired serially until appearance of the radiopharmaceutical in the gallbladder and small bowel or a sufficient period of time has passed.

Indications Biliary imaging has become the procedure of choice in evaluating patients with suspected acute cholecystitis because in virtually all cases of acute cholecystitis there is obstruction of the cystic duct with no passage of radionuclide into the gallbladder. The test can also be used to detect enterogastric reflux of bile and neonatal biliary atresia as well as to assess biliary kinetics (gallbladder ejection fraction) in suspected chronic cholecystitis.

Patient Preparation The patient should have all RIA blood work performed, or at least drawn, prior to injection of any radioactive material. The patient must be fasting (NPO) 4 hours before scan. If a patient has been NPO for longer than 24 hours, pretreatment with CCK (0.02 µg/kg I.V.) is sometimes used to avoid a false-positive scan. Infants being scanned to detect biliary atresia should receive oral phenobarbital 2.5 mg/kg twice daily for 5 days prior to the scan procedure.

Special Instructions Requisition must state the current patient diagnosis in order to select the most appropriate radiopharmaceutical and/or imaging technique. A serum bilirubin level is needed and should be noted on request form in order to administer the proper dose of radiopharmaceutical.

Duration of Procedure: 1-4 hours although additional delayed images for up to 24 hours may be required

Radiopharmaceutical: ^{99m}Tc IDA or related compound

Technique The application of single-photon emission tomography (SPECT) techniques may contribute significantly to the diagnostic accuracy of this imaging study.

Turnaround Time A written report will be sent to the patient's chart and/or to the referring physician.

Causes for Rejection Nonfasting patient, other recent Nuclear Medicine procedure may interfere. If uncertain, call the Nuclear Medicine Department.

Normal Findings Early tracer accumulation within the liver with rapid excretion into the extrahepatic biliary ductal system and subsequent visualization of the gallbladder and small bowel within 1 hour after injection

Limitations Sensitivity/specificity for acute cholecystitis decrease as bilirubin levels rise >5 mg/dL.

Additional Information Intravenous CCK is employed in selected patients to assess biliary kinetics quantitatively (gallbladder ejection fraction).

References

Cooperberg PL and Gibney RG, "Imaging of the Gallbladder, 1997," *Radiology*, 1987, 163(3):605-13.

Fidler J, Paulson EK, and Layfield L, "CT Evaluation of Acute Cholecystitis: Findings and Usefulness in Diagnosis," *AJR Am J Roentgenol*, 1996, 166(5):1085-8.

Freitas JE, Coleman RE, Nagle CE, et al, "Influence of Scan and Pathologic Criteria on the Specificity of Cholescintigraphy: Concise Communication," *J Nucl Med*, 1983, 24:876-9.

Kloiber R, AuCoin R, Hershfield NB, et al, "Biliary Obstruction After Cholecystectomy: Diagnosis With Quantitative Cholescintigraphy," *Radiology*, 1988, 169(3):643-7.

♦ **Bladder Reflux Study** *see* Voiding Cystourethrogram, Radionuclide *on page 473*

♦ **Blood Loss Localization Study** *see* Gastrointestinal Bleed Localization Study *on page 449*

Blood Volume

Related Information
Red Cell Volume *on page 462*

Synonyms Plasma/Blood Volume; Total Blood Volume

Applies to Plasma Volume Measurement; Red Cell Mass; Red Cell Mass Measurement

Procedure Commonly Includes Determinations of red blood cell and plasma volumes are nonimaging procedures in which the patient receives intravenous injections of radiolabeled autologous red cells, sometimes followed later by radiolabeled albumin (RISA). The respective volumes in the circulation are measured in subsequent timed blood samples.

Indications Red cell volume measurement is helpful in the differential diagnosis of polycythemia. Plasma volumes assist in therapeutic management of patients with fluid losses such as from burns, severe diarrhea, or surgery.

Contraindications
- active bleeding
- edema

Patient Preparation The patient should have all RIA blood work performed, or at least drawn, prior to injection of any radioactive material. The patient does not need to be fasting or NPO for this procedure. Other blood samples should not be taken during this procedure nor should transfusions of blood products be given.

Special Instructions Requisition must state the current patient diagnosis in order to select the most appropriate radiopharmaceutical and/or imaging technique. Before the test is ordered it should be verified that the patient has **not** recently received an isotope *in vivo* (eg, bone scans, liver scans, brain scans). Include patient's height and weight on requisition because it is needed for calculations.

Duration of Procedure: 2-4 hours

Radiopharmaceutical: Chromium-51 chromate for RBC label and iodine-131 or iodine-125 human serum albumin

Turnaround Time A written report will be sent to the patient's chart and/or to the referring physician.

Causes for Rejection Active bleeding or recent blood transfusions, other recent Nuclear Medicine procedure may interfere. If uncertain, call the Nuclear Medicine Department.

Normal Findings Normal blood volumes are a function of the size and sex of the patient. Expected blood volumes are estimated based on body surface area. Measured volumes are compared to the expected results and normally can vary ±20%. Obese patients may have volumes somewhat less than expected.

Limitations Any *in vivo* isotope test will affect blood volume (eg, bone scans, liver scans, brain scans). The procedure is technically difficult with multiple laboratory steps which tend to introduce errors.

References

Jones JG and Wardrop CA, "Measurement of Blood Volume in Surgical and Intensive Care Practice," *Br J Anaesth*, 2000, 84(2):226-35.

Pollycove M and Tono M, "Blood Volume," *Diagnostic Nuclear Medicine*, 2nd ed, Gottschalk A, Hoffer PB, and Potchen EJ, eds, Baltimore, MD: Williams & Wilkins, 1988, 690-8.

Srivastava SC and Chervu LR, "Radionuclide-Labeled Red Blood Cells: Current Status and Future Prospects," *Semin Nucl Med*, 1984, 14(2):68-82.

♦ **Bone Marrow Function Scan** *see* Bone Marrow Scan *on page 440*

Bone Marrow Scan

Synonyms Bone Marrow Function Scan; Marrow Scan

Procedure Commonly Includes The patient receives an intravenous injection of a technetium-99m (^{99m}Tc) colloid compound which localizes in the reticuloendothelial cells of the bone marrow. Whole body or appropriate regional images of active marrow sites in the skeleton are acquired.

Indications Bone marrow imaging is helpful in detecting the presence and distribution of active functioning marrow versus alterations due to a variety of hematologic disorders such as myelofibrosis, leukemia, lymphoma, and anemia including sickle cell anemia with marrow infarction. Additional applications include estimation of bone marrow function in oncology before or after radiation or chemotherapy, determining the best site for bone marrow biopsy, and assessment of blood supply to the femoral head in possible avascular necrosis.

Patient Preparation The patient should have all RIA blood work performed, or at least drawn, prior to injection of any radioactive material. The patient does not need to be fasting or NPO for this procedure.

Special Instructions Requisition must state the current patient diagnosis in order to select the most appropriate radiopharmaceutical and/or imaging technique.

Duration of Procedure: 1-2 hours **Radiopharmaceutical:** ^{99m}Tc sulfur colloid

Turnaround Time A written report will be sent to the patient's chart and/or to the referring physician.

Causes for Rejection Other recent Nuclear Medicine procedure may interfere. If uncertain, call the Nuclear Medicine Department.

Normal Findings Homogenous and symmetric distribution of activity in sites of functioning marrow reticuloendothelial cells. In adults this includes the skull, axial skeleton, and proximal third of the humeral and femoral shafts. Active marrow extends more distally in children.

Limitations Reticuloendothelial cell distribution varies somewhat from that of functioning hematopoietic cells. Asymmetric activity patterns are nonspecific and should be correlated with other radiographic and clinical findings.

References

Alavi A and Heyman S, "Bone Marrow Imaging," *Diagnostic Nuclear Medicine*, 2nd ed, Gottschalk A, Hoffer PB, and Potchen EJ, eds, Baltimore, MD: Williams & Wilkins, 1988, 707-24.

Freedman GM, Negendank WG, Hudes GR, et al, "Preliminary Results of a Bone Marrow Magnetic Resonance Imaging Protocol for Patients With High-Risk Prostate Cancer," *Urology*, 1999, 54(1):118-23.

Gruning T and Franke WG, "Bone Marrow Scqan Using Tc-99m Labeled Antigranulocyte Antibody to Evaluate Hematopoiesis in Osteomyelofibrosis," *Clin Nucl Med*, 2000, 25(3):222-3.

Huic D, Ivancevic V, Richter WS, et al, "Immunoscintigraphy of the Bone Marrow: Normal Uptake Values of Technetium-99m Labeled Monoclonal Antigranulocyte Antibodies," *J Nucl Med*, 1997, 38(11):1755-8.

Vogler JB and Murphy WA, "Bone Marrow Imaging," *Radiology*, 1988, 168(3):679-93.

Bone Scan

Synonyms Bone Scintigraphy; Radionuclide Bone Scan; Whole Body Bone Scan

Applies to Bone Scan With Flow; Three-Phase Bone Scan

Procedure Commonly Includes The patient receives an intravenous injection of a technetium-99m (^{99m}Tc) phosphonate radiopharmaceutical which localizes in bone with intensity proportional to the degree of metabolic activity present. Three hours after the injection, whole body and appropriate regional skeletal images are acquired. An initial dynamic flow study and/or early blood pool images (phase 1 and 2) may also be acquired if osteomyelitis, osteonecrosis, Legg-Calvé-Perthes disease, septic arthritis, or other inflammatory disease is suspected (three-phase technique).

Indications Bone imaging is extremely sensitive for the detection of infection or malignancy involving any part of the skeleton. It is the most appropriate screening test for these conditions, since scan abnormalities are present long before structural defects develop radiographically. Bone scans are also accurate for localizing lesions for biopsy, excision, or debridement. Stress fractures can be diagnosed by bone scan when radiographs are completely normal.

Patient Preparation The patient should have all RIA blood work performed, or at least drawn, prior to injection of any radioactive material. The patient does not need to be fasting or NPO for this procedure. The patient should be encouraged to drink fluids during the waiting period before scanning and will be asked to void just before scanning begins.

Special Instructions Requisition must state the current patient diagnosis in order to select the most appropriate radiopharmaceutical and/or imaging technique. When ordering liver and bone scans for the same patient, schedule liver scan at least 1 day before the bone scan.

Duration of Procedure: 3-4.5 hours; this includes a 3-hour delay after tracer injection to allow adequate localization in bone.

Radiopharmaceutical: ^{99m}Tc phosphonate compound (MDP or HDP)

Technique The application of single-photon emission tomography (SPECT) techniques may contribute significantly to the diagnostic accuracy of this imaging study.

Turnaround Time A written report will be sent to the patient's chart and/or to the referring physician.

Causes for Rejection Other recent Nuclear Medicine procedure may interfere. If uncertain, call the Nuclear Medicine Department.

Normal Findings Homogeneous and symmetric distribution of activity throughout all skeletal structures

Limitations In postoperative orthopedic patients and diabetics, additional imaging with gallium-67 or radiolabeled white blood cells may help to confirm the presence of active infection and serve as a baseline for later comparison

References

Bernard EJ, Nicholls WD, Howman-Giles RB, et al, "Patterns of Abnormality on Bone Scans in Acute Childhood Leukemia," *J Nucl Med*, 1998, 39(11):1983-6.

Datz FL, "Radionuclide Imaging of Joint Inflammation in the '90s," *J Nucl Med*, 1990, 31(5):684-7.

Duncan I, Dorai-Raj A, Khoo K, et al, "The Utility of Bone Scans in Rheumatology," *Clin Nucl Med*, 1999, 24(1):9-14.

Even-Sapir E, Martin RH, Barnes DC, et al, "Role of SPECT in Differentiating Malignant From Benign Lesions in the Lower Thoracic and Lumbar Vertebrae," *Radiology*, 1993, 187(1):193-8.

Holder LE, "Clinical Radionuclide Bone Imaging," *Radiology*, 1990, 176(3):607-14.

Jacobson AF, Cronin EB, Stomper PC, et al, "Bone Scans With One or Two Abnormalities in Cancer Patients With No Known Metastases: Frequency and Serial Scintigraphic Behavior of Benign and Malignant Lesions," *Radiology*, 1990, 175(1):229-32.

Kloos RT, Rufini V, Gross MD, et al, "Bone Scans in Neurofibromatosis: Neurofibroma, Plexiform Neuroma and Neurofibrosarcoma," *J Nucl Med*, 1996, 37(11):1778-83.

Lusins JO, Danielski EF, and Goldsmith SJ, "Bone SPECT in Patients With Persistent Back Pain After Lumbar Spine Surgery," *J Nucl Med*, 1989, 30(4):490-6.

Matin P, "Basic Principles of Nuclear Medicine Techniques for Detection and Evaluation of Trauma and Sports Medicine Injuries," *Semin Nucl Med*, 1988, 18(2):90-112.

McNeil BJ, "Value of Bone Scanning in Neoplastic Disease," *Semin Nucl Med*, 1985, 14(4):277-86.

Mohamed A, Ryan P, Lewis M, et al, "Registration Bone Scan in the Evaluation of Wrist Pain," *J Hand Surg*, 1997, 22(2):161-6.

Samuelson DR and Cram RL, "The Three-Phase Bone Scan and Exercise Induced Lower-leg Pain. The Tibial Stress Test," *Clin Nucl Med*, 1996, 21(2):89-93.

Schauwecker DS, "The Scintigraphic Diagnosis of Osteomyelitis," *AJR Am J Roentgenol*, 1992, 158(1):9-18.

Sutter CW and Shelton DK, "Three-Phase Bone Scan in Osteomyelitis and Other Musculoskeletal Disorders," *Am Fam Physician*, 1996, 54(5):1639-47.

♦ **Bone Scan With Flow** *see* Bone Scan *on page 440*

♦ **Bone Scintigraphy** *see* Bone Scan *on page 440*

♦ **Brain Flow Only** *see* Angiogram, Radionuclide *on page 437*

♦ **Brain Perfusion Scan** *see* Brain Scan *on page 441*

Brain Scan

Synonyms Brain Scintigraphy; Ceretec® Brain Scan; Neurolite® Brain Scan

Applies to Brain Perfusion Scan; Brain Scan With Flow

Procedure Commonly Includes The patient receives an intravenous injection of a radiopharmaceutical which crosses the blood-brain barrier and localizes in the brain proportionate to regional brain perfusion. Images are then obtained which demonstrate the presence and symmetry of regional perfusion and metabolism within the brain.

Indications Brain imaging is useful for the early diagnosis of cerebrovascular disease. Thrombotic stroke and/or transient ischemic episodes can be

(Continued)

Brain Scan *(Continued)*

detected before anatomic abnormalities develop on CT or MR scans. Anatomic imaging with CT or MRI is indicated initially if acute stroke is suspected due to its ability to differentiate hemorrhagic from thrombotic causes. Other indications for perfusion brain scans include localization of seizure foci, detection of tumors, and the assessment of neuropsychiatric disorders such as schizophrenia, depression, organic brain syndromes, and dementias (especially Alzheimer's vs multi-infarct).

Patient Preparation The patient should have all RIA blood work performed, or at least drawn, prior to injection of any radioactive material. The patient should be in a quiet area with low lighting for several minutes before tracer injection. Motion during image acquisition will degrade the quality and accuracy of the procedure. If sedation is necessary, it is preferable to administer it after tracer injection.

Special Instructions Requisition must state the current patient diagnosis in order to select the most appropriate radiopharmaceutical and/or imaging technique.

Duration of Procedure: 1 hour; additional delayed images may be required.
Radiopharmaceutical: Technetium-99m (^{99m}Tc) HMPAO (Ceretec®) or Tc-99m ECD (Neurolite®)

Technique The application of single-photon emission tomography (SPECT) techniques contributes significantly to the diagnostic accuracy of this imaging study and should be performed.

Turnaround Time A written report will be sent to the patient's chart and/or to the referring physician.

Causes for Rejection Other recent Nuclear Medicine procedure may interfere. If uncertain, call the Nuclear Medicine Department.

Normal Findings Homogeneous and symmetric distribution of activity throughout the brain. Cerebellar activity is usually somewhat greater than in other structures.

References

Biersack NJ, Grünwald F, Reichmann K, et al, "Functional Brain Imaging With Single-Photon Emission Computed Tomography Using ^{99m}Tc-Labeled HM-PAO," *Nucl Med Ann*, 1990, 59-94.

Holman BL and Devous MD Sr, "Functional Brain SPECT: The Emergence of a Powerful Clinical Method," *J Nucl Med*, 1992, 33(10):1888-904.

Kao CH, Hung DZ, Chang Lai SP, et al, "HMPAO Brain SPECT in Acute Carbon Monoxide Poisoning," *J Nucl Med*, 1998, 39(5):769-72.

Licho R, Glick SJ, Xia W, et al, "Attenuation Compensation in 99m Tc SPECT Brain Imaging: A Comparison of the Use of Attenuation Maps Derived From Transmission Versus Emission Data in Normal Scans," *J Nucl Med*, 1999, 40(3):456-63.

Mountz JM, Modell JG, Foster NL, et al, "Prognostication of Recovery Following Stroke Using the Comparison of CT and Technetium-99m HM-PAO SPECT," *J Nucl Med*, 1990, 31(1):61-6.

Reid RH, Gulenchyn KY, Ballinger JR, et al, "Cerebral Perfusion Imaging With Technetium-99m HMPAO Following Cerebral Trauma. Initial Experience," *Clin Nucl Med*, 1990, 15(6):383-8.

Rupright J, Woods EA, and Singh A, "Hypoxic Brain Injury: Evaluation by Single Photon Emission Computed Tomography," *Arch Phys Med Rehabil*, 1996, 77(11):1205-8.

San Pedro EC, Mountz JM, Liu HG, et al, "Postinfectious Cerebellitis: Clinical Significance of Tc-99m HMPAO Brain SPECT Compared With MRI," *Clin Nucl Med*, 1998, 23(4):212-6.

Sataloff RT, Mandel S, Muscal E, et al, "Single-Photon-Emission Computed Tomography (SPECT) in Neurotologic Assessment: A Preliminary Report," *Am J Otol*, 1996, 17(6):909-16.

Vera P, Rohrlich P, Stievenart JL, et al, "Contribution of Single-Photon Emission Computed Tomography in the Diagnosis and Follow-up of CNS Toxicity of a Cytarabine-Containing Regimen in Pediatric Leukemia," *J Clin Oncol*, 1999, 17(9):2804-10.

♦ **Brain Scan With Flow** *see* Brain Scan *on page 441*

♦ **Brain Scintigraphy** *see* Brain Scan *on page 441*

Cardiac Blood Pool Scan, EKG-Gated

Related Information

Cardiac Blood Pool Scan, First Pass *on page 443*
Venogram, Radionuclide *on page 472*

Synonyms Ejection Fraction Study; Gated Cardiac Scan, Rest and/or Exercise; Gated Study; MUGA; Radionuclide Angiography; Radionuclide Ventriculogram; Wall Motion Study

Applies to Exercise Radionuclide Angiography; Radionuclide Angiography, Stress; Stress Gated Study

Procedure Commonly Includes The patient receives an intravenous injection of either technetium-99m (^{99m}Tc) pertechnetate in a technique to radiolabel circulating erythrocytes (^{99m}Tc RBC) or ^{99m}Tc albumin (HSA). Multiple images of the heart synchronized to the electrocardiographic R-R interval (EKG-gated) are then acquired several minutes later at equilibrium. These images are acquired into a Nuclear Medicine computer to achieve a cine display of cardiac chamber size and wall motion, calculation of ventricular ejection fractions (global and regional), and functional images based on mathematical manipulation of the initially acquired data. Repetitive data acquisition is possible during graded levels of exercise, usually either bicycle ergometer or handgrip, to assess ventricular functional response to exercise.

Indications Cardiac blood pool imaging is used to assess the functional status of the heart at rest and/or in response to physiologic stress. Quantification of ventricular ejection fractions calculated by this technique are quite accurate and are independent of chamber geometry, relying on the proportionality of blood volume with the amount of radioactivity in the cardiac chambers. Routine uses include evaluation of effects of coronary artery disease, heart failure, cardiomyopathies, and cardiotoxic drugs. Repetitive studies to assess response to therapeutic interventions can give accurate follow-up information.

Contraindications Cardiac arrhythmia, especially atrial fibrillation, will degrade image resolution.

Patient Preparation The patient does not need to be fasting or NPO for this procedure. The patient should have all RIA blood work performed, or at least drawn, prior to the injection of any radioactive material.

Special Instructions Requisition must state the current patient diagnosis in order to select the most appropriate radiopharmaceutical and/or imaging technique.

Duration of Procedure: 1 hour
Radiopharmaceutical: ^{99m}Tc labeled RBC or ^{99m}Tc HSA (albumin)

Technique The application of single-photon emission tomography (SPECT) techniques may contribute significantly to the diagnostic accuracy of this imaging study.

Turnaround Time A written report will be sent to the patient's chart and/or to the referring physician.

Causes for Rejection Other recent Nuclear Medicine procedure may interfere. If uncertain, call the Nuclear Medicine Department.

Normal Findings Normal biventricular size and regional wall motion with ejection fractions >50% (left) and/or >45% (right).

Limitations The technique of gating involves synchronization of image acquisition with the patient's electrocardiographic rhythm. Patients who have arrhythmias will have degraded image resolution and calculations of ejection fraction and other parameters will only be approximate. Rapid atrial fibrillation will give particularly poor results. When arrhythmias are severe, a first-pass technique may provide more accurate information. Right ventricular ejection fractions by a gated technique are limited by underlying right atrial isotope activity and sometimes by poor separation from left ventricular activity. A more accurate right ventricular ejection fraction may be gained from a first pass study. This can often be performed dynamically during isotope injection for the equilibrium EKG-gated study.

References

Chin BB, Bloomgarden DC, Xia W, et al, "Right and Left Ventricular Volume and Ejection Fraction by Tomographic Gated Blood-Pool Scintigraphy," *J Nucl Med*, 1997, 38(6):942-8.

Dilsizian V, Rocco TP, Bonow RO, et al, "Cardiac Blood-Pool Imaging II: Applications in Noncoronary Heart Disease," *J Nucl Med*, 1990, 31(1):10-22.

Mochizuki T, Murase K, Tanaka H, et al, "Assessment of Left Ventricular Volume Using ECG-Gated SPECT With Technetium-99m-MIBI and Technetium-99m-Tetrofosmin," *J Nucl Med*, 1997, 38(1):53-7.

Nichols K, Dorbala S, De Puey EG, et al, "Influence of Arrhythmias on Gated SPECT Myocardial Perfusion and Function Quantification," *J Nucl Med*, 1999, 40(6):924-34.

Cardiac Blood Pool Scan, First Pass

Related Information

Angiogram, Radionuclide *on page 437*
Cardiac Blood Pool Scan, EKG-Gated *on page 442*

(Continued)

Cardiac Blood Pool Scan, First Pass *(Continued)*

Synonyms Cardiac Scan, First Pass; First Pass Ejection Fraction; Radionuclide Cineangiography; Radionuclide Ventriculogram, First Pass

Applies to Exercise Radionuclide Angiography, First Pass

Procedure Commonly Includes The patient receives an intravenous injection of a technetium-99m (^{99m}Tc) radiopharmaceutical with acquisition of image data on computer in a rapid sequence as the isotope first passes through the cardiac chambers. Similar information to EKG-gated procedures (see Cardiac Blood Pool Scan, EKG-Gated *on page 442*) can be obtained without the need for synchronization with the patient's EKG.

Indications First pass cardiac blood pool imaging can provide information about the functional status of the heart at rest and/or in response to physiologic stress. Quantification of both right and left ventricular ejection fractions is possible. A first pass right ventricular ejection fraction is usually more accurate than by EKG-gated technique (see Cardiac Blood Pool Scan, EKG-Gated *on page 442*).

Patient Preparation The patient should have all RIA blood work performed, or at least drawn, prior to injection of any radioactive material. The patient does not need to be fasting or NPO for this procedure.

Special Instructions Requisition must state the current patient diagnosis in order to select the most appropriate radiopharmaceutical and/or imaging technique.

Duration of Procedure: 30 minutes

Radiopharmaceutical: ^{99m}Tc DTPA, pertechnetate, or other compound

Turnaround Time A written report will be sent to the patient's chart and/or to the referring physician at the completion of the procedure.

Causes for Rejection Other recent Nuclear Medicine procedure may interfere. If uncertain, call the Nuclear Medicine Department.

Normal Findings Normal biventricular size and regional wall motion with ejection fractions >50% (left) and/or >45% (right).

References

Benedetto AR and Nusynowitz ML, "Correlation of Right and Left Ventricular Ejection Fraction and Volume Measurements," *J Nucl Med*, 1988, 29(6):1114-7.

Faber TL, Cooke CD, Folks RD, et al, "Left Ventricular Function and Perfusion From Gated SPECT Perfusion Images: An Integrated Method," *J Nucl Med*, 1999, 40(4):650-9.

Rumberger JA, Behrenbeck T, Bell MR, et al, "Determination of Ventricular Ejection Fraction: A Comparison of Available Imaging Methods. The Cardiovascular Imaging Working Group," *Mayo Clin Proc*, 1997, 72(9):860-70.

Yoshioka J, Hasegawa S, Yamaguchi H, et al, "Left Ventricular Volumes and Ejection Fraction Calculated From Quantitative Electrocardiographic-Gated 99m Tc-Tetrofosmin Myocardial SPECT," *J Nucl Med*, 1999, 40(10):1693-8.

◆ **Cardiac Scan, First Pass** *see* Cardiac Blood Pool Scan, First Pass *on page 443*

◆ **Cardiolite® Scan** *see* Myocardial Perfusion Scan *on page 457*

◆ **Cerebrospinal Fluid Scan** *see* Cisternogram *on page 445*

◆ **Ceretec® Brain Scan** *see* Brain Scan *on page 441*

◆ **Choletec® Scan** *see* Biliary Scan *on page 438*

Chromium-51 Red Cell Survival

Synonyms Erythrocyte Survival; RBC Survival Test; Red Blood Cell Sequestration; Red Cell Survival; Survival of Red Blood Cells

Applies to Splenic Sequestration Study

Procedure Commonly Includes Determinations of red blood cell survival and splenic sequestration are nonimaging procedures in which the patient receives an intravenous injection of radiolabeled autologous red cells. Blood samples are then drawn after 24 hours and periodically for approximately 3 weeks. The half-life of the circulating radiolabeled red cells is then calculated. Additionally, periodic external measurements of radioactivity from the heart (blood pool), liver, and spleen help to assess the role of the spleen in a possible hemolytic condition.

Indications This procedure is helpful in the differential diagnosis and management of hemolytic anemia including conditions such as spherocytosis, red cell enzyme deficiency, and various hemoglobinopathies. Occult blood loss can also be evaluated. Evaluation of red cell sequestration within the spleen demonstrates the possible role of the spleen in the hemolytic process and may predict the therapeutic value of splenectomy.

Patient Preparation The patient should have all RIA blood work performed, or at least drawn, prior to injection of any radioactive material. The patient does not need to be fasting or NPO for this procedure. Transfusions of blood products should be avoided during this procedure. The Nuclear Medicine Department will provide a schedule for drawing of serial blood samples.

Special Instructions Requisition must state the current patient diagnosis in order to select the most appropriate radiopharmaceutical technique. At least 21 days should be allowed for this study. When selective splenic sequestration as cause of hemolysis is suspected, liver and spleen readings are performed in conjunction with chromium-51 RBC survival test. Please notify the Nuclear Medicine Department if the patient is to be discharged.

Duration of Procedure: 3-4 weeks

Radiopharmaceutical: Chromium-51 chromate for RBC label

Turnaround Time A written report will be sent to the patient's chart and/or to the referring physician.

Causes for Rejection Active or known intermittent bleeding, recent blood transfusions, other recent Nuclear Medicine procedure may interfere.

Normal Findings The normal red cell survival half-time (50% survival) range is 25-30 days. Shorter half-times indicate excessive red cell destruction and/or blood loss. The normal spleen to liver (or spleen to precordium) ratio is 1:1. Splenomegaly alone may show a ratio of 1 to 2:1. Ratios >2.5:1 indicate significant splenic sequestration of red cells.

Limitations This procedure cannot discriminate between red cell loss due to intravascular hemolysis and red cell loss due to bleeding. The procedure is also technically difficult and requires a prolonged period of time to obtain results.

References

Baker WJ and Datz FL, "Preparation and Clinical Utility of Labeled Blood Products," *Essentials of Nuclear Medicine Science*, Hladik WB, Saha GB, and Study KT, eds, Baltimore, MD: Williams & Wilkins, 1987, 91-2.

Bax BE, Bain MD, Talbot PJ, et al, "Survival of Human Carrier Erythrocytes *In Vivo*," *Clin Sci*, 1999, 96(2):127-8

Kumpel BM, Austin EB, Lee D, et al, "Comparison of Flow Cytometric Assays With Isotopic Assays of (51)Chromium-Labeled Cells for Estimation of Red Cell Clearance or Survival *In Vivo*," *Transfusion*, 2000, 40(2):228-39.

Mock DM, Lankford GL, Widness JA, et al, "Measurement of Red Cell Survival Using Biotin-Labeled Red Cells: Validation Against 51Cr-Labeled Red Cells," *Transfusion*, 1999, 39(2):156-62.

♦ **Chromium-Labeled Red Cell Volume** *see* Red Cell Volume *on page 462*

Cisternogram

Synonyms Cerebrospinal Fluid Scan; CSF Scan; CSF Scintigraphy; Radionuclide Cisternography

Procedure Commonly Includes The patient undergoes a lumbar puncture under sterile conditions with subarachnoid injection of a water-soluble radiopharmaceutical which distributes into the cerebrospinal fluid (CSF). For patients with ventricular shunts or implanted CSF reservoirs, the radiopharmaceutical may be injected into these directly by appropriate personnel. Images of the spinal canal and CSF spaces of the brain are acquired intermittently for up to 72 hours to assess CSF pathways and/or shunt patency.

Indications Cisternography is helpful in the differential diagnosis of hydrocephalus. In normal pressure hydrocephalus (NPH) there is a typical pattern of abnormal CSF movement. Additional indications are the detection of traumatic or postoperative CSF leaks as well as determination of CSF shunt patency.

Patient Preparation The patient should have all RIA blood work performed, at least drawn, prior to injection of any radioactive material. The patient does not need to be fasting or NPO for this procedure.

Special Instructions Requisition must state the current patient diagnosis in order to select the most appropriate radiopharmaceutical and/or imaging technique.

(Continued)

Cisternogram *(Continued)*

Duration of Procedure: 4-72 hours

Radiopharmaceutical: Pyrogen-free indium-111 DTPA or ^{169}Y6 DTPA

Technique CSF samples should not be taken during the lumbar puncture for this procedure. This would lower CSF volume and alter the physiologic flow pattern.

Turnaround Time A written report will be sent to the patient's chart and/or to the referring physician.

Causes for Rejection Other recent Nuclear Medicine procedure may interfere. If uncertain, call the Nuclear Medicine Department.

Normal Findings The normal CSF pattern of flow is from the lumbar region to the basal cisterns within 2-4 hours. There is progressive passage symmetrically over the cerebral convexities during the first 24 hours with no reflux into the lateral ventricles. From 24-72 hours there should be gradual clearance from the CSF via the choroid plexus.

Limitations Inadequate images may result from other than a true subarachnoid injection of tracer. Early images of the injection site confirm the technique success or failure.

Additional Information For detection of CSF rhinorrhea or otorrhea, cotton pledgets may be placed in the nasal turbinates or external ear canals. These are removed within 4-6 hours for weighing and counting the radioactivity present. Notify the Nuclear Medicine Department when scheduling the procedure if a CSF leak is suspected.

References

Ali SA, Cesani F, Zuckermann JA, et al, "Spinal-Cerebrospinal Fluid Leak Demonstrated by Radiopharmaceutical Cisternography," *Clin Nucl Med,* 1998, 23(3):152-5.

Ashley DM, Coleman RE, Fuchs H, et al, "Chronic CSF Leak Into the Peritoneal Cavity Shown by Radionuclide Cisternography. Successful Treatment With an Epidural Blood Patch," *Clin Nucl Med,* 1997, 22(6):390-2.

Benamor M, Tainturier C, Graveleau P, et al, "Radionuclide Cisternography in Spontaneous Intracranial Hypotension," *Clin Nucl Med,* 1998, 23(3):150-1.

Brigham M, Korzec KR, and Yobbagy J, "Resolution of Primary Spontaneous Cerebrospinal Fluid Rhinorrhea After Computed Tomographic Cisternography," *Otolaryngol Head Neck Surg,* 1997, 116(4):533-5.

Krasnow AZ, Collier BD, Isitman AT, et al, "The Use of Radionuclide Cisternography in the Diagnosis of Pleural Cerebrospinal Fluid Fistulae," *J Nucl Med,* 1989, 30(1):120-3.

Sandler MP, Price AC, Runge VM, et al, "Cerebrospinal Fluid Cisternography," *Diagnostic Nuclear Medicine,* Gottschalk A, Hoffer PB, and Potchen EJ, eds, Baltimore, MD: Williams & Wilkins, 1988, 888-98.

Wax MK, Ramadan HH, Ortiz O, et al, "Contemporary Management of Cerebrospinal Fluid Rhinorrhea," *Otolaryngol Head Neck Surg,* 1997, 116(4):442-9.

♦ **CSF Scan** *see* Cisternogram *on page 445*

♦ **CSF Scintigraphy** *see* Cisternogram *on page 445*

♦ **DISIDA® Scan** *see* Biliary Scan *on page 438*

♦ **Disofenin Scan** *see* Biliary Scan *on page 438*

♦ **Diuretic Renal Scan** *see* Renal Scan *on page 463*

♦ **Ectopic Gastric Mucosa Scan** *see* Meckel's Diverticulum Scan *on page 455*

♦ **Ejection Fraction Study** *see* Cardiac Blood Pool Scan, EKG-Gated *on page 442*

♦ **Erythrocyte Survival** *see* Chromium-51 Red Cell Survival *on page 444*

♦ **Exercise Radionuclide Angiography** *see* Cardiac Blood Pool Scan, EKG-Gated *on page 442*

♦ **Exercise Radionuclide Angiography, First Pass** *see* Cardiac Blood Pool Scan, First Pass *on page 443*

♦ **First Pass Ejection Fraction** *see* Cardiac Blood Pool Scan, First Pass *on page 443*

♦ **Gallbladder Ejection Fraction Scan** *see* Biliary Scan *on page 438*

♦ **Gallbladder Scan** *see* Biliary Scan *on page 438*

♦ **Gallium Abscess Scan** *see* Gallium Scan, Abscess and/or Tumor *on page 447*

Gallium Scan, Abscess and/or Tumor

Applies to Gallium Abscess Scan; Gallium Tumor Scan; Soft Tissue Scan

Procedure Commonly Includes The patient receives an intravenous injection of gallium-67 citrate. Images are then acquired for some combination of 24, 48, and 72 hours after injection.

Indications Gallium localizes at sites of active inflammation or infection as well as in some neoplasms. Gallium imaging is very sensitive in detection of abscesses, pneumonia, pyelonephritis, active sarcoidosis, and active tuberculosis. Even in immunocompromised patients (eg, those with AIDS, gallium imaging can detect early complications such as *Pneumocystis carinii* pneumonitis). The nonspecificity of gallium activity, however, requires that correlation with other radiographic studies and clinical findings be given close attention. Gallium imaging is very useful in the differential diagnosis and staging of some neoplasms, notably Hodgkin disease, lymphoma, hepatocellular carcinoma, bronchogenic carcinoma, melanoma, and leukemia. Recent evidence has shown a correlation of gallium localization in the lungs with the activity of disease in pulmonary fibrosis and asbestosis. Gallium is also used in addition to bone scintigraphy for detecting osteomyelitis, especially in its chronic stages. A common indication for gallium imaging is as a screening procedure for infection in fever of unknown origin (FUO).

Patient Preparation The patient should have all RIA blood work performed, or at least drawn, prior to injection of any radioactive material. The patient does not need to be fasting or NPO for this procedure.

Special Instructions Requisition must state the current patient diagnosis in order to select the most appropriate radiopharmaceutical and/or imaging technique. Other Nuclear Medicine procedures (bone, liver, lung) should be completed prior to gallium injection. If abdominal abscess/infection is suspected, laxatives, and/or enemas may be ordered for the patient prior to delayed imaging at 48 or 72 hours. This will help clear normal intestinal gallium activity from the colon.

Duration of Procedure: 24-72 hours

Radiopharmaceutical: Gallium-67 citrate

Technique The application of single-photon emission tomography (SPECT) techniques may contribute significantly to the diagnostic accuracy of this imaging study.

Turnaround Time A written report will be sent to the patient's chart and/or to the referring physician.

Normal Findings Gallium will localize to some degree in liver and spleen, bone, nasopharynx, lacrimal glands, and breast tissue. There is normally some secretion of gallium into the bowel. This may require laxatives and/or enemas for the patient to evacuate this normal activity before additional imaging of possible abdominal infection or abscess. Abnormal accumulation of gallium will usually be asymmetric, increase in later images, and remain in the same location (normal bowel luminal gallium activity will transit).

Limitations There is variable normal excretion of gallium via the intestinal tract. This contributes to the nonspecificity of gallium imaging in suspected abdominal or pelvic infections. Previous treatment with antibiotics or high doses of steroids may decrease the inflammatory response and result in false-negative gallium imaging.

Additional Information Other isotope studies may need to be postponed up to 7 days after a gallium scan has been done due to its slow elimination from soft tissue.

References

Bisson G, Lamoureux G, and Bégin R, "Quantitative Gallium-67 Lung Scan to Assess the Inflammatory Activity in the Pneumoconioses," *Semin Nucl Med*, 1987, 17(1):72-80.

Chan WL, Fernandes VB, and Carolan MG, "Retropharyngeal Abscess on a Ga-67 Scan: A Case Report," *Clin Nucl Med*, 1999, 24(12):942-4.

Gasparini M, Bombardieri E, Castellani M, et al, "Gallium-67 Scintigraphy Evaluation of Therapy in non-Hodgkin's Lymphoma," *J Nucl Med*, 1998, 39(9):1586-90.

Hussain R, Christie DR, Gebski V, et al, "The Role of the Gallium Scan in Primary Extranodal Lymphoma," *J Nucl Med*, 1998, 39(1):95-8.

Israel O, Front D, Epelbaum R, et al, "Residual Mass and Negative Gallium Scintigraphy in Treated Lymphoma," *J Nucl Med*, 1990, 31(3):365-8.

(Continued)

Gallium Scan, Abscess and/or Tumor *(Continued)*

Kumar M, Naddaf S, Abujudeh HH, et al, "Ga-67 Imaging of Perisplenic Abscess After Splenic Embolization," *Clin Nucl Med*, 1998, 23(6):394-5.

Lee KS, Kim JS, Ha CS, et al, "Correlation of Gallium-67 SPECT and CT Findings in Primary Gynecologic Lymphoma," *Clin Imaging*, 1999, 23(2):119-24.

Lee VW, Antonacci V, Tilak S, et al, "Intracranial Mass Lesions: Sequential Thallium and Gallium Scintigraphy in Patients With AIDS," *Radiology*, 1999, 211(2):507-12.

Turoglu HT, Akisik MF, Naddaf SY, et al, "Tumor and Infection Localization in AIDS Patients: Ga-67 and Tl-201 Findings," *Clin Nucl Med*, 1998, 23(7):446-59.

Yen TC, Tsai MF, and Tzen KY, "Biliary and Liver Abscesses Demonstrated With Tc-99m DISIDA and Ga-67 Imaging," *Clin Nucl Med*, 1998, 23(12):853-4.

Zinzani PL, Martelli M, Magagnoli M, et al, "Treatment and Clinical Management of Primary Mediastinal Large B-Cell Lymphoma With Sclerosis: MACOP-B Regimen and Mediastinal Radiotherapy Monitored by (67)Gallium Scan in 50 Patients," *Blood*, 1999, 94(10):3289-93.

♦ **Gallium Tumor Scan** *see* Gallium Scan, Abscess and/or Tumor *on page 447*

♦ **Gastric Emptying Quantitation** *see* Gastric Emptying Scan *on page 448*

Gastric Emptying Scan

Synonyms Gastric Emptying Quantitation; Gastric Emptying Scintigraphy

Procedure Commonly Includes The patient receives an oral radiolabeled solid-phase meal. Sequential computer assisted images of the gastric region are acquired over the next 2 hours. Gastric emptying lines are calculated based on the decrease in radioactivity with time after ingestion of the meal. If emptying of solids is abnormally prolonged, a repeat procedure assessing the emptying of a liquid radiolabeled bolus can be performed 1-2 days later. Some departments employ a dual isotope technique (eg, technetium-99m (^{99m}Tc) solid and indium-111 liquid) to quantify solid and liquid emptying simultaneously.

Indications Quantification of gastric emptying physiology is helpful in evaluating patients with suspected gastric motility disorders. These include diagnoses of diabetic gastroparesis, anorexia nervosa, gastric outlet obstruction syndromes, postvagotomy, and postgastrectomy syndromes, and other systemic diseases known to affect motility. Treatment responses can also be assessed.

Patient Preparation The patient should be NPO from midnight the night before this procedure. The procedure itself should be scheduled for the early AM time period. The patient should also abstain from alcohol and smoking for the previous 24 hours. Other medications should be noted. The patient should have all RIA blood work performed, or at least drawn, prior to administration of any radioactive material.

Special Instructions Requisition must state the current patient diagnosis in order to select the most appropriate radiopharmaceutical and/or imaging technique.

Duration of Procedure: 2 hours

Radiopharmaceutical: ^{99m}Tc sulfur colloid (solid), ^{99m}Tc DTPA (liquid), indium-111 DTPA (liquid if simultaneous with solid)

Technique Routinely, ^{99m}Tc sulfur colloid is mixed with two eggs and then cooked as scrambled eggs in a microwave oven. This is then served as a sandwich. Multiple alternative "recipes" exist but many do not sufficiently bind the isotope to a true solid phase to assess emptying accurately. If a simultaneous dual isotope technique is utilized, the usual liquid phase is indium-111 DTPA mixed in 6 oz orange juice.

Turnaround Time A written report will be sent to the patient's chart and/or to the referring physician.

Causes for Rejection Other recent Nuclear Medicine procedure may interfere. If uncertain, call the Nuclear Medicine Department.

Normal Findings Normal half-emptying (T½) times for gastric contents are 45-90 minutes for solids and 5-30 minutes for a liquid phase.

Limitations These are approximations for the meals described above in a sitting patient. Results will vary markedly as a function of alternative meals, time of day, patient positioning, and the medication status of the patient.

References

Alexander F, Whllie R, Jirousek K, et al, "Delayed Gastric Emptying Affects Outcome of Nissen Fundoplication in Neurologically Impaired Children," *Surgery*, 1997, 122(4):690-7.

Borovicka J, Lehmann R, Kunz P, et al, "Evaluation of Gastric Emptying and Motility in Diabetic Gastroparesis With Magnetic Resonance Imaging: Effects of Cisapride," *Am J Gastroenterol*, 1999, 94(10):2866-73.

Choi MG, Camilleri M, Burton DD, et al, "Octanoic Acid Breath Test for Gastric Emptying of Solids: Accuracy, Reproducibility, and Comparison With Scintigraphy," *Gastroenterology*, 1997, 112(4):1155-62.

Datz FL, Christian PE, and Moore J, "Gender-Related Differences in Gastric Emptying," *J Nucl Med*, 1987, 28(7):1204-7.

Ehrenpreis ED and Zaitman D, "Improved Computer Analysis of Solid Phase Gastric Emptying Scans," *Am J Gastroenterol*, 1996, 91(4):674-9.

Ross EA and Koo LC, "Improved Nutrition After the Detection and Treatment of Occult Gastroparesis in Nondiabetic Dialysis Patients," *Am J Kidney Dis*, 1998, 31(1):62-6.

Schwizer W, Fraser R, Borovicka J, et al, "Measurement of Proximal and Distal Gastric Motility With Magnetic Resonance Imaging," *Am J Physiol*, 1996, 271(1 Pt 1):G217-22.

Tougas G, Chen Y, Coates G, et al, "Standardization of a Simplified Scintigraphic Methodology for the Assessment of Gastric Emptying in a Multicenter Setting," *Am J Gastroenterol*, 2000, 95(1):78-86.

Velchik MG, Reynolds JC, and Alavi A, "The Effect of Meal Energy Content on Gastric Emptying," *J Nucl Med*, 1989, 30(6):1106-10.

♦ **Gastric Emptying Scintigraphy** *see* Gastric Emptying Scan *on page 448*

Gastrointestinal Bleed Localization Study

Synonyms Blood Loss Localization Study; Gastrointestinal Blood Loss Scan; GI Bleed Scintigraphy; Lower GI Blood Loss Scan

Procedure Commonly Includes The patient receives an intravenous injection of a technetium-99m (^{99m}Tc) radiopharmaceutical which remains in the circulation for sufficient time to extravasate and accumulate within the bowel lumen at the site of active bleeding. Depending on the radiopharmaceutical used, delayed images or repetitive injections may demonstrate intermittent bleeding.

Indications Gastrointestinal bleeding, even severe hemorrhage, is intermittent. Scintigraphy is a noninvasive method of detecting and localizing active lower (and sometimes upper) GI tract bleeding in order to better direct endoscopic or angiographic studies. Two scan techniques are available. ^{99m}Tc labeled red blood cells are accurate in detecting intermittent bleeding if serial images are acquired for up to 24 hours. ^{99m}Tc sulfur colloid, which rapidly localizes in the liver and spleen, is very sensitive for detecting active bleeding at the time of injection. Very small amounts of extravasated activity in the bowel lumen can be detected. Repetitive injections can detect intermittent bleeding.

Patient Preparation The patient should have all RIA blood work performed, or at least drawn, prior to the injection of any radioactive material. The patient does not need to be fasting or NPO for this procedure.

Special Instructions Requisition must state the current patient diagnosis in order to select the most appropriate radiopharmaceutical and/or imaging technique.

Duration of Procedure: 1-2 hours; additional delayed images may be required.

Radiopharmaceutical: ^{99m}Tc sulfur colloid or ^{99m}Tc labeled RBC

Turnaround Time A written report will be sent to the patient's chart and/or to the referring physician.

Causes for Rejection Recent radiographic barium studies within 24-48 hours, other recent Nuclear Medicine procedure may interfere. If uncertain, call the Nuclear Medicine Department.

Normal Findings Uptake by the liver and spleen (^{99m}Tc colloid) or circulating activity in the large vessels (^{99m}Tc RBC) with no ectopic extravascular activity

Limitations The scan only detects intermittent active bleeding. It is of little use in the patient with chronic anemia or slowly decreasing hematocrit. The scan is less accurate for bleeding in the upper gastrointestinal tract (ie, stomach or small bowel).

References

Bagga S, Gupta SM, and Johns W, "Scintigraphic Localization of Recurrent Anastomotic Site Bleeding in the Gastrointestinal Tract," *Clin Nucl Med*, 1996, 21(4):296-8.

(Continued)

Gastrointestinal Bleed Localization Study *(Continued)*

Bennett JS, Cynamon J, and Zuckier LS, "Use of a Water Enema to Facilitate Localization of Gastrointestinal Hemorrhage During Tc-99m Labeled RBC Scintigraphy," *Clin Nucl Med*, 1996, 21(6):463-4.

Emslie JT, Zarnegar K, Siegel ME, et al, "Technetium-99m-Labeled Red Blood Cell Scans in the Investigation of Gastrointestinal Bleeding," *Dis Colon Rectum*, 1996, 39(7):750-4.

Garofalo TE and Abdu RA, "Accuracy and Efficacy of Nuclear Scintigraphy for the Detection of Gastrointestinal Bleeding," *Arch Surg*, 1997, 132(9):196-9.

Gutierrez C, Mariano M, Vander Lann T, et al, "The Use of Technetium-Labeled Erythrocyte Scintigraphy in the Evaluation and Treatment of Lower Gastrointestinal Hemorrhage," *Am Surg*, 1998, 64(10):989-92.

Han DC and Feliciano DV, "The Clinical Complexity of Splenic Vein Thrombosis," *Am Surg*, 1998, 64(6):558-61, 561-2.

Hilfiker PR, Zimmermann-Paul GG, Schmidt M, et al, "Intestinal and Peritoneal Bleeding: Detection With an Intravascular Contrast Agent and Fast Three-Dimensional MR Imaging - Preliminary Experience From an Experimental Study," *Radiology*, 1998, 209(3):769-74.

Krestan CR, Pokieser P, Wenzl E, et al, "Localization of Gastrointestinal Bleeding With Contrast-Enhanced Helical CT," *AJR Am J Roentgenol*, 2000, 174(1):265-6.

Maurer AH, Rodman MS, Vitti RA, et al, "Gastrointestinal Bleeding: Improved Localization With Cine Scintigraphy," *Radiology*, 1992, 185(1):187-92.

Oliveras A, Aubia J, Cao H, et al, "99m Tc-Labeled Red Blood Cell Scintigraphy for Localization of Gastrointestinal Bleeding in Chronic Renal Failure," *Nephron*, 1998, 80(1):76-8.

Suzman MS, Talmor M, Jennis R, et al, "Accurate Localization and Surgical Management of Active Lower Gastrointestinal Hemorrhage With Technetium-Labeled Erythrocyte Scintigraphy," *Ann Surg*, 1996, 224(1):29-36.

Vernava AM III, Moore BA, Longo WE, et al, "Lower Gastrointestinal Bleeding," *Dis Colon Rectum*, 1997, 40(7):846-58.

Winzelberg GG, McKusick KA, Froelich JW, et al, "Detection of Gastrointestinal Bleeding With ^{99m}Tc-Labeled Red Blood Cells," *Semin Nucl Med*, 1982, 12(2):139-46.

Wyatt RA, "Detection and Localization of Gastrointestinal Bleeding," *West J Med*, 1996, 165(5):306.

♦ **Gastrointestinal Blood Loss Scan** *see* Gastrointestinal Bleed Localization Study *on page 449*

♦ **Gated Cardiac Scan, Rest and/or Exercise** *see* Cardiac Blood Pool Scan, EKG-Gated *on page 442*

♦ **Gated Study** *see* Cardiac Blood Pool Scan, EKG-Gated *on page 442*

♦ **GI Bleed Scintigraphy** *see* Gastrointestinal Bleed Localization Study *on page 449*

♦ **Hepatobiliary Scan** *see* Biliary Scan *on page 438*

♦ **Hepatobiliary Scintigraphy** *see* Biliary Scan *on page 438*

♦ **HIDA® Liver Scan** *see* Biliary Scan *on page 438*

♦ **Hippuran Scan** *see* Renal Scan *on page 463*

♦ **^{131}I Body Scan** *see* Thyroid Metastatic Survey, Iodine-131 *on page 468*

♦ **^{131}I Metastatic Survey** *see* Thyroid Metastatic Survey, Iodine-131 *on page 468*

♦ **Indium-111 Labeled Leukocyte Scan** *see* Indium Leukocyte Scan *on page 450*

Indium Leukocyte Scan

Synonyms Indium-111 Labeled Leukocyte Scan; Infection Scan; Infection Scintigraphy; Leukocyte Scintigraphy; WBC Scan; White Blood Cell Scan

Procedure Commonly Includes The patient receives an intravenous reinjection of radiolabeled leukocytes. The patient initially has a 60-80 mL sample of blood drawn for an *in vitro* process of labeling and separating the leukocyte component. Images are acquired at intervals between 2-24 hours after subsequent reinjection of radiolabeled cells.

Indications Radiolabeled leukocyte imaging is useful either in determining the site of an occult infection or in confirming the presence or absence of infection at a suspected site. This technique has largely replaced gallium-67 imaging for acute infections because of the better image resolution and greater specificity. Some chronic infections (eg, chronic osteomyelitis) may be better imaged with gallium-67. Radiolabeled leukocyte imaging is especially helpful in detecting postoperative infection sites and in documenting lack of residual infection after a course of therapy.

Patient Preparation The patient does not need to be fasting or NPO for this procedure. The patient should have all RIA blood work performed, or at least drawn, prior to injection of any radioactive material.

Special Instructions Requisition must state the current patient diagnosis in order to select the most appropriate radiopharmaceutical and/or imaging technique.

Duration of Procedure: 2 hours from blood draw to reinjection of labeled cells; 2-24 hours for imaging at intervals
Radiopharmaceutical: Indium-111 labeled leukocytes

Turnaround Time A written report will be sent to the patient's chart and/or to the referring physician.

Causes for Rejection Other recent Nuclear Medicine procedure may interfere. If uncertain, call the Nuclear Medicine Department.

Normal Findings Radiolabeled leukocytes will localize to some degree in the liver, spleen, and bone marrow. Focal accumulations in soft tissue or asymmetric uptake in bone will be seen in infected or inflamed sites. For osteomyelitis, a bone scan is usually performed first for comparison with the radiolabeled leukocyte scan findings.

Limitations Leukocyte radiolabeling is a complex process and is usually performed on-site only where there are dedicated Radiopharmacy Laboratories. Most commercial radiopharmacies will also provide this service locally.

Additional Information An alternative method of leukocyte radiolabeling with technetium-99m (^{99m}Tc) HMPAO is possible. Advantages of this method include earlier imaging times and better sensitivity for infections in extremities with utilization of higher doses of ^{99m}Tc versus indium-111.

References

Abreu SH, "Skeletal Uptake of Indium-111 Labeled White Blood Cells," *Semin Nucl Med*, 1989, 19(2):152-5.

Burris GW and Gordon BM, "Cold Defect on Indium Leukocyte Scanning of a Hepatic Abscess," *Clin Nucl Med*, 1998, 23(1):26-8.

Campeau RJ and Ingram C, "Perivalvular Abscess Complicating Infective Endocarditis: Complementary Role of Echocardiography and Indium-111-Labeled Leukocytes," *Clin Nucl Med*, 1998, 23(9):582-4.

Datz FL and Thorne DA, "Effect of Antibiotic Therapy on the Sensitivity of Indium-111 Labeled Leukocyte Scans," *J Nucl Med*, 1986, 27(12):1849-53.

Elgazzar AH, Yeung HW, and Webner PJ, "Indium-111-Leukocyte and Technetium-99m-Sulfur Colloid Uptake in Paget's Disease," *J Nucl Med*, 1996, 37(5):858-61.

Froelich JW and Field SA, "The Role of Indium-111 White Blood Cells in Inflammatory Bowel Disease," *Semin Nucl Med*, 1988, 18(4):300-7.

Gobar LS, Graham R, and Harrison KA, "Indium-111-Leukocyte Imaging: A Case of Peritonitis Mimicking Inflammatory Bowel Disease," *J Nucl Med*, 1997, 38(7):1138-40.

Ho Y and Hennessy O, "Indium-111 WBC Scan to Diagnose Mycotic Aneurysm," *Clin Nucl Med*, 1999, 24(11):903-4.

Kolindou A, Liu Y, Ozker K, et al, "In-111 WBC Imaging of Osteomyelitis in Patients With Underlying Bone Scan Abnormalities," *Clin Nucl Med*, 1996, 21(3):183-91.

Lahiri SA, Halff GA, Speeg KV, et al, "In-111 WBC Scan Localized Infected Hepatic Cysts and Confirms Their Complete Resection in Adult Polycystic Kidney Disease," *Clin Nucl Med*, 1998, 23(1):33-4.

Laitinen R, Tähtinen J, Lantto T, et al, "^{99m}Tc Labeled Leukocytes in Imaging of Patients With Suspected Acute Abdominal Inflammation," *Clin Nucl Med*, 1990, 15(9):597-602.

Larcos G, Brown ML, and Sutton RT, "Diagnosis of Osteomyelitis of the Foot in Diabetic Patients: Value of 111In-Leukocyte Scintigraphy," *AJR Am J Roentgenol*, 1991, 157(3):527-31.

Moser AS and Siegel A, "Metastatic Disease to the Thoracic Spine. Simultaneous In-111 WBC and Bone Scan Findings After Radiation Therapy," *Clin Nucl Med*, 1997, 22(5):333-4.

Palestro CJ, Mehta HH, Patel M, et al, "Marrow Versus Infection in the Charcot Joint: Indium-111 Leukocyte and Technetium-99m Sulfur Colloid Scintigraphy," *J Nucl Med*, 1998, 39(2):346-50.

Posillico LF and Shah AN, "A Wandering Spleen. Detection by In-111 Leukocyte Imaging," *Clin Nucl Med*, 1996, 21(4):287-9.

Roddie ME, Peters AM, Danpure HJ, et al, "Inflammation: Imaging With ^{99m}Tc HMPAO-Labeled Leukocytes," *Radiology*, 1988, 166(3):767-72.

♦ **^{131}I Neck and Chest Survey** *see* Thyroid Metastatic Survey, Iodine-131 *on page 468*

♦ **Infarct-Avid Scan** *see* Myocardial Infarction Scan *on page 456*

♦ **Infection Scan** *see* Indium Leukocyte Scan *on page 450*

♦ **Infection Scintigraphy** *see* Indium Leukocyte Scan *on page 450*

♦ **Iodine Thyroid Scan** *see* Thyroid Scan *on page 469*

♦ **Isotope Venogram** *see* Venogram, Radionuclide *on page 472*

♦ **^{131}I Whole Body Survey** *see* Thyroid Metastatic Survey, Iodine-131 *on page 468*

♦ **Kidney Scan** *see* Renal Scan *on page 463*

♦ **Leukocyte Scintigraphy** *see* Indium Leukocyte Scan *on page 450*

Liver and Spleen Scan

Synonyms Liver Scintigraphy; Liver-Spleen Scan; Radioisotope Hepatic Scan; Radionuclide Liver Scan; Spleen Scan

Procedure Commonly Includes The patient receives an intravenous injection of a technetium-99m (^{99m}Tc) colloidal radiopharmaceutical which is rapidly accumulated in reticuloendothelial cells of the liver and spleen. Multiple images of the liver and spleen are then acquired after 20-30 minutes. An initial dynamic flow study may also be acquired to assess hepatic and/or splenic perfusion, especially in cases of trauma.

Indications Liver and spleen imaging is an accurate noninvasive method to delineate overall organ size, the presence of focal lesions, and/or the degree of hepatocellular dysfunction in diffuse liver disease. It has been used to detect and document later resolution of traumatic splenic hematomas or infarcts.

Patient Preparation The patient should have all RIA blood work performed, or at least drawn, prior to injection of any radioactive material. The patient does not need to be fasting or NPO for this procedure.

Special Instructions Requisition must state the current patient diagnosis in order to select the most appropriate radiopharmaceutical and/or imaging technique. Schedule a liver scan at least 1 day before a bone scan if both are ordered for the same patient.

Duration of Procedure: 30 minutes to 1 hour

Radiopharmaceutical: ^{99m}Tc sulfur colloid or other microcolloid compound

Technique The application of single-photon emission tomography (SPECT) techniques contributes significantly to the diagnostic accuracy of this imaging study.

Turnaround Time A written report will be sent to the patient's chart and/or to the referring physician.

Causes for Rejection Residual barium in GI tract from recent x-rays, other recent Nuclear Medicine procedure may interfere. If uncertain, call the Nuclear Medicine Department.

Normal Findings Homogeneous distribution of activity throughout both liver and spleen with no organomegaly or focal defects. The ratio of spleen:liver activity should be about equal. Increased relative splenic uptake, especially if accompanied by visualization of bone marrow reticuloendothelial uptake, indicates at least some degree of hepatocellular dysfunction.

References

Derbekyan VA, Pham C, Emond C, et al, "Scintigraphic Diagnosis of Polysplenia in the Adult," *Clin Nucl Med*, 1999, 24(3):161-3.

Hoefs JC, Wang FW, Lilien DL, et al, "A Novel, Simple Method of Functional Spleen Volume Calculation by Liver-Spleen Scan," *J Nucl Med*, 1999, 40(10):1745-55.

Kao CH, "Incidental Detection of Bilateral Kidney Calyces in Tc-99m Phytate Liver and Spleen Scan," *Clin Nucl Med*, 1999, 24(9):720-1.

Kempf JS, Hudak R, Abdel-Dayem HM, et al, "Tl-201 Chloride SPECT Imaging of Hepatocellular Carcinoma," *Clin Nucl Med*, 1996, 21(12):953-7.

Krishnamurthy S and Krishnamurthy GT, "Nuclear Hepatology: Where Is it Heading Now?" *J Nucl Med*, 1988, 29(6):1144-9.

Morio S, Oh H, Endo N, et al, "Magnetic Resonance Imaging of Reticulo-Endothelial System in Patients With Idiopathic Thrombocytopenic Purpura," *Am J Hematol*, 1997, 56(1):52-8.

Oppenheim BE, Wellman HN, and Hoffer PB, "Liver Imaging," *Diagnostic Nuclear Medicine*, Gottschalk A, Hoffer PB, and Potchen EJ, eds, Baltimore, MD: Williams & Wilkins, 1988, 538-65.

Powsner RA, Simms RW, Chudnovsky A, et al, "Scintigraphic Functional Hyposplenism in Amyloidosis," *J Nucl Med*, 1998, 39(2):221-3.

Toro JR, Stoll HL Jr, Stomper PC, et al, "Prognostic Factors and Evaluation of Mycosis Fungoides and Sezary Syndrome," *J Am Acad Dermatol*, 1997, 37(1):58-67.

Van Heertum RL, Brunetti JC, and Yudd AP, "Abdominal SPECT Imaging," *Semin Nucl Med*, 1987, 17(3):230-46.

♦ **Liver Scintigraphy** *see* Liver and Spleen Scan *on page 452*

♦ **Liver-Spleen Scan** *see* Liver and Spleen Scan *on page 452*

♦ **Lower Extremity Venogram, Radionuclide** *see* Venogram, Radionuclide *on page 472*

♦ **Lower GI Blood Loss Scan** *see* Gastrointestinal Bleed Localization Study *on page 449*

♦ **Lung-Liver Scan for Subdiaphragmatic Abscesses** *see* Radioisotope Liver-Lung Scan for Subdiaphragmatic Abscesses *on page 461*

♦ **Lung Perfusion Scintigraphy** *see* Lung Scan, Perfusion *on page 453*

Lung Scan, Perfusion

Related Information

Lung Scan, Ventilation *on page 454*

Synonyms Lung Perfusion Scintigraphy; Perfusion Lung Scan; Perfusion-Ventilation Scan; Pulmonary Scan; Radionuclide Perfusion Lung Scan; V/Q Scan

Applies to Quantitative Perfusion Lung Scan; Ventilation-Perfusion Lung Scan

Procedure Commonly Includes The patient receives an intravenous injection of a technetium-99m (^{99m}Tc) macroaggregated albumin radiopharmaceutical which is trapped by the small arterioles of the pulmonary circulation. Multiple images of the lungs are then acquired to assess lung perfusion. **Special note:** This procedure is almost always combined with a lung ventilation scan to detect a characteristic pattern of segmental perfusion deficits with normal corresponding regional ventilation that is the hallmark of pulmonary emboli. (See Lung Scan, Ventilation *on page 454*.) A perfusion scan performed alone or in conjunction with a ventilation scan, but with computer image acquisition and quantification of regional perfusion and ventilation, is sometimes used to predict the prognosis in patients under consideration for pneumonectomy or lobectomy surgery.

Indications The primary indication for lung perfusion and ventilation imaging is the detection of acute pulmonary emboli. These procedures together provide an accurate noninvasive screening test both for the detection of emboli and for documentation of resolution during and after therapy. Perfusion lung scans are also used to assess regional pulmonary perfusion preoperatively in patients undergoing lung resection surgery.

Contraindications Caution should be exercised in performing this procedure for patients with known primary or secondary pulmonary hypertension. The microembolization with the ^{99m}Tc macroaggregated albumin may worsen the underlying condition temporarily. The procedure can usually still be performed with a freshly prepared lower dose.

Patient Preparation The patient should have all RIA blood work performed, or at least drawn, prior to injection of any radioactive material. The patient does not need to be fasting or NPO for this procedure. The patient should have a routine chest radiograph performed within 12 hours prior to imaging or receive one immediately after.

Special Instructions Requisition must state the current patient diagnosis in order to select the most appropriate radiopharmaceutical and/or imaging technique.

Duration of Procedure: 30 minutes to 1 hour

Radiopharmaceutical: ^{99m}Tc macroaggregated albumin (MAA) or albumin microspheres (HAM)

Technique The application of single-photon emission tomography (SPECT) techniques may contribute significantly to the diagnostic accuracy of this imaging study.

Turnaround Time A written report will be sent to the patient's chart and/or to the referring physician.

Causes for Rejection Other recent Nuclear Medicine procedure may interfere. If uncertain, call the Nuclear Medicine Department.

Normal Findings Homogeneous distribution of activity throughout the lungs

Limitations The procedure is somewhat nonspecific in the presence of underlying lung conditions such as pneumonia or chronic obstructive disease. A same day chest radiograph is necessary for review and comparison with scan findings.

References

Davey NC, Smith TP, Hanson MW, et al, "Ventilation-Perfusion Lung Scintigraphy as a Guide for Pulmonary Angiography in the Localization of Pulmonary Emboli," *Radiology*, 1999, 213(1):51-7.

Hauck RW, Romer W, Schulz C, et al, "Ventilation Perfusion Scintigraphy and Lung Function Testing to Assess Metal Stent Efficacy," *J Nucl Med*, 1997, 38(10):1584-9.

(Continued)

Lung Scan, Perfusion *(Continued)*

Kahn D, Bushnell DL, Dean R, et al, "Clinical Outcome of Patients With a "Low Probability" of Pulmonary Embolism on Ventilation-Perfusion Lung Scan," *Arch Intern Med*, 1989, 149(2):377-9.

Kim JH, Lee DS, Chung JK, et al, "Quantitative Lung Perfusion Scintigraphy in Postoperative Evaluation of Congenital Right Ventricular Outflow Tract Obstructive Lesions," *Clin Nucl Med*, 1996, 21(6):471-6.

Mele FM and Caride VJ, "Pleural Effusions: Patterns on Ventilation-Perfusion Lung Scans," *Clin Nucl Med*, 1998, 23(9):571-5.

Miniati M, Pistolesi M, Marini C, et al, "Value of Perfusion Lung Scan in the Diagnosis of Pulmonary Embolism: Results of the Prospective Investigative Study of Acute Pulmonary Embolism Diagnosis (PISA-PED)," *Am J Respir Crit Care Med*, 1996, 154(5):1387-93.

Mitomo O, Aoki S, Tsunoda T, et al, "Quantitative Analysis of Nonuniform Distributions in Lung Perfusion Scintigraphy," *J Nucl Med*, 1998, 39(9):1630-5.

Pace WM and Goris ML, "Pulmonary SPECT Imaging and the Stripe Sign," *J Nucl Med*, 1998, 39(4):721-3.

Thurnheer R, Engel H, Weder W, et al, "Role of Lung Perfusion Scintigraphy in Relation to Chest Computed Tomography and Pulmonary Function in the Evaluation of Candidates for Lung Volume Reduction Surgery," *Am J Respir Crit Care Med*, 1999, 159(1):301-10.

Trujillo NP, Pratt JP, Talusani S, et al, "DTPA Aerosol in Ventilation/Perfusion Scintigraphy for Diagnosing Pulmonary Embolism," *J Nucl Med*, 1997, 38(11):1781-3.

"Value of the Ventilation/Perfusion Scan in Acute Pulmonary Embolism. Results of the Prospective Investigation of Pulmonary Embolism Diagnosis (PIOPED). The PIOPED Investigators," *JAMA*, 1990, 263(20):2753-9.

Lung Scan, Ventilation

Related Information

Lung Scan, Perfusion *on page 453*

Synonyms Aerosol Lung Scan; Radionuclide Ventilation Lung Scan; Ventilation Lung Scan; Xenon Lung Scan

Applies to Quantitative Ventilation Lung Scan; Ventilation-Perfusion Lung Scan

Procedure Commonly Includes The patient inhales a radioactive gas or nebulized aerosol and multiple images of the lungs are then acquired to assess lung ventilation. **Special note:** This procedure is almost always combined with a lung perfusion scan to detect a characteristic pattern of segmental perfusion deficits with normal corresponding regional ventilation that is the hallmark of pulmonary emboli. (See Lung Scan, Perfusion *on page 453.*)

Indications The primary indication for lung ventilation and perfusion imaging is the detection of acute pulmonary emboli. These procedures together provide an accurate noninvasive screening test both for the detection of emboli and for documentation of resolution during and after therapy. Lung ventilation imaging is also helpful in quantifying regional pulmonary ventilation in patients with severe obstructive lung disease or who are being considered for lung resection surgery.

Radiopharmaceuticals for Lung Ventilation Imaging

Agent	Isotope Half-Life	Timing vs Perfusion Scan	Advantages	Disadvantages
^{99m}Tc DTPA aerosol	6 h	Before	Multiple views of ventilation	Turbulent air flow can cause patchy distribution; no washout phase
^{133}Xe gas	5 d	Before	Single view with equilibrium and washout phases	Requires good single-breath effort; single view (usually posterior)
^{127}Xe gas	36 d	After	Single view with equilibrium and washout phases; may be performed after perfusion scan	
^{81m}Kr gas	13 sec	During	Multiple views of ventilation; no gas trap required	Nonavailability on 24-hour basis; expense

Patient Preparation The patient should have all RIA blood work performed, or at least drawn, prior to injection of any radioactive material. The patient does not need to be fasting or NPO for this procedure. The patient should have a routine chest radiograph performed within 12 hours prior to imaging or receive one immediately after. Notify the Nuclear Medicine Department if patients require high flow oxygen or respirator assistance.

Special Instructions Requisition must state the current patient diagnosis in order to select the most appropriate radiopharmaceutical and/or imaging technique.

Duration of Procedure: 30 minutes to 1 hour

Radiopharmaceutical: See table.

Turnaround Time A written report will be sent to the patient's chart and/or to the referring physician.

Causes for Rejection Other recent Nuclear Medicine procedure may interfere. If uncertain, call the Nuclear Medicine Department.

Normal Findings Homogeneous distribution of activity throughout the lungs

Limitations Patients must be able to cooperate in performing this test. They will be required to breathe through a mouthpiece or mask, remain still for approximately 15 minutes, (usually in the supine position) and if xenon gas is used, hold their breath for 10 seconds or longer. The procedure is somewhat nonspecific in the presence of underlying lung conditions such as pneumonia or chronic obstructive disease. A same day chest radiograph is necessary for review and comparison with scan findings.

Additional Information Patients on high flow oxygen or respirator assistance can undergo ventilation scans with radioactive aerosols using special nebulizer adaptors.

References

Davey NC, Smith TP, Hanson MW, et al, "Ventilation-Perfusion Lung Scintigraphy as a Guide for Pulmonary Angiography in the Localization of Pulmonary Emboli," *Radiology*, 1999, 213(1):51-7.

Hauck RW, Romer W, Schulz C, et al, "Ventilation Perfusion Scintigraphy and Lung Function Testing to Assess Metal Stent Efficacy," *J Nucl Med*, 1997, 38(10):1584-9.

Kahn D, Bushnell DL, Dean R, et al, "Clinical Outcome of Patients With a "Low Probability" of Pulmonary Embolism on Ventilation-Perfusion Lung Scan," *Arch Intern Med*, 1989, 149(2):377-9.

Kim JH, Lee DS, Chung JK, et al, "Quantitative Lung Perfusion Scintigraphy in Postoperative Evaluation of Congenital Right Ventricular Outflow Tract Obstructive Lesions," *Clin Nucl Med*, 1996, 21(6):471-6.

Mele FM and Caride VJ, "Pleural Effusions: Patterns on Ventilation-Perfusion Lung Scans," *Clin Nucl Med*, 1998, 23(9):571-5.

Miniati M, Pistolesi M, Marini C, et al, "Value of Perfusion Lung Scan in the Diagnosis of Pulmonary Embolism: Results of the Prospective Investigative Study of Acute Pulmonary Embolism Diagnosis (PISA-PED)," *Am J Respir Crit Care Med*, 1996, 154(5):1387-93.

Mitomo O, Aoki S, Tsunoda T, et al, "Quantitative Analysis of Nonuniform Distributions in Lung Perfusion Scintigraphy," *J Nucl Med*, 1998, 39(9):1630-5.

Pace WM and Goris ML, "Pulmonary SPECT Imaging and the Stripe Sign," *J Nucl Med*, 1998, 39(4):721-3.

Thurnheer R, Engel H, Weder W, et al, "Role of Lung Perfusion Scintigraphy in Relation to Chest Computed Tomography and Pulmonary Function in the Evaluation of Candidates for Lung Volume Reduction Surgery," *Am J Respir Crit Care Med*, 1999, 159(1):301-10.

Trujillo NP, Pratt JP, Talusani S, et al, "DTPA Aerosol in Ventilation/Perfusion Scintigraphy for Diagnosing Pulmonary Embolism," *J Nucl Med*, 1997, 38(11):1781-3.

"Value of the Ventilation/Perfusion Scan in Acute Pulmonary Embolism. Results of the Prospective Investigation of Pulmonary Embolism Diagnosis (PIOPED). The PIOPED Investigators," *JAMA*, 1990, 263(20):2753-9.

♦ **Marrow Scan** *see* Bone Marrow Scan *on page 440*

♦ **Mebrofenin® Scan** *see* Biliary Scan *on page 438*

Meckel's Diverticulum Scan

Synonyms Ectopic Gastric Mucosa Scan; Meckel's Scan; Meckel's Scintigraphy

Procedure Commonly Includes The patient receives an intravenous injection of technetium-99m (^{99m}Tc) pertechnetate which is quickly secreted by

(Continued)

Meckel's Diverticulum Scan *(Continued)*

gastric mucosa cells including sites of ectopic tissue, the Meckel's diverticulum. Sequential images of the abdomen are then acquired. The abnormality usually visualizes early, but delayed images are sometimes necessary.

Indications The procedure is useful in detecting the presence and location of a Meckel's diverticulum, a collection of functioning ectopic gastric mucosa usually located in the ileum and in the right lower quadrant of the abdomen. The abnormality usually occurs in young children and 50% of cases that bleed symptomatically will present before the age of 2 years.

Patient Preparation The patient should have all RIA blood work performed, or at least drawn, prior to injection of any radioactive material. The patient must be fasting at least 4 hours before scan.

Special Instructions Requisition must state the current patient diagnosis in order to select the most appropriate radiopharmaceutical and/or imaging technique.

Duration of Procedure: 30 minutes to 1 hour although additional delayed images may be required.

Radiopharmaceutical: ^{99m}Tc pertechnetate

Turnaround Time A written report will be sent to the patient's chart and/or to the referring physician.

Causes for Rejection Residual barium in GI tract from recent x-rays, other recent Nuclear Medicine procedure may interfere. If uncertain, call the Nuclear Medicine Department.

Normal Findings Lack of any focal secreted activity in the abdomen. Patients are often placed in a slightly left oblique decubitus position to slow transit of normal secreted activity from the stomach into the small bowel.

Limitations A Meckel's diverticulum without functioning gastric mucosa will not visualize. However, those lacking mucosa are also unlikely to bleed. Some false-positives may result from nondiverticular bleeding, intussusception, duplication cysts, or inflammatory bowel disease.

References

Connolly LP, Treves ST, Bozorgi F, et al, "Meckel's Diverticulum: Demonstration of Heterotopic Gastric Mucosa With Technetium 99m Pertechnetate SPECT," *J Nucl Med*, 1998, 39(8):1458-60.

Ford PV, Bartold SP, Fink-Bennett DM, et al, "Procedure Guideline for Gastrointestinal Bleeding and Meckel's Diverticulum Scintigraphy. Society of Nuclear Medicine," *J Nucl Med*, 1999, 40(7):1226-32.

Molmenti EP and Thompson RW, "Images in Clinical Medicine. Meckel's Diverticulum," *N Engl J Med*, 1999, 340(1):31.

Omar AM, Al-Saee'd TA, Elgazzar A, "Scintigraphic Pattern of Intestinal Duplication on a Meckel's Diverticulum Scan," *Clin Nucl Med*, 1998, 23(10):708-9.

Pantongrag-Brown L, Levine MS, Elsayed AM, et al, "Inverted Meckel's Diverticulum: Clinical, Radiologic, and Pathologic Findings," *Radiology*, 1996, 199(3):693-6.

♦ **Meckel's Scan** *see* Meckel's Diverticulum Scan *on page 455*

♦ **Meckel's Scintigraphy** *see* Meckel's Diverticulum Scan *on page 455*

♦ **MUGA** *see* Cardiac Blood Pool Scan, EKG-Gated *on page 442*

Myocardial Infarction Scan

Synonyms Acute Myocardial Infarction Scan; Infarct-Avid Scan; PYP Cardiac Scan; Pyrophosphate Cardiac Scan

Procedure Commonly Includes The patient receives an intravenous injection of a ^{99m}Tc pyrophosphate radiopharmaceutical which localizes in recently infarcted myocardial tissue. Multiple images of the heart are acquired at 1-3 hours after isotope injection.

Indications The primary indication for pyrophosphate cardiac imaging is the detection of recent myocardial infarction. Pyrophosphate will localize in damaged myocardium as a result of necrosis and disruption of myocardial cell membranes. This procedure is not useful in the first 24 hours after acute infarction. Maximum localization will occur from 24-72 hours after an acute event and then gradually diminish over the next 10-14 days. Vary rarely, especially in elderly patients, pyrophosphate will continue to localize indefinitely. Positive scans in patients with unstable angina indicate a higher risk of subsequent infarction. Pyrophosphate imaging has also been used to detect non-necrotic damage in cardiac contusions as well as some cardiomyopathies, amyloidosis, and sarcoidosis.

Patient Preparation The patient does not need to be fasting or NPO for this procedure. The patient should have all RIA blood work performed, or at least drawn, prior to injection of any radioactive material. If not contraindicated by the cardiac status, patients should be encouraged to ingest fluids and to void frequently in order to enhance renal excretion of isotope and decrease background activity.

Special Instructions Requisition must state the current patient diagnosis in order to select the most appropriate radiopharmaceutical and/or imaging technique.

Duration of Procedure: 2-4 hours
Radiopharmaceutical: ^{99m}Tc pyrophosphate

Technique The application of single-photon emission tomography (SPECT) techniques contributes significantly to the diagnostic accuracy of this imaging study.

Turnaround Time A written report will be sent to the patient's chart and/or to the referring physician.

Causes for Rejection Other recent Nuclear Medicine procedure may interfere. If uncertain, call the Nuclear Medicine Department.

Normal Findings The radiopharmaceutical normally localizes in bone. There should be no uptake above background activity in the myocardium. When there is localization in the myocardium it is usually graded (1+ to 4+) relative to rib uptake.

Limitations The timing of this procedure is important and should be from 1-3 days after an acute onset of symptoms. Earlier or later timing may give false-negative results. Cardioversion causing localized chest wall burns or cracked ribs may complicate interpretation. Use in other conditions such as cardiomyopathy or amyloidosis is less specific. False-positive scans may result from pericarditis or myocarditis, cardiac neoplasms, aneurysms, or calcifications in valves and coronary arteries.

References

Ando H, Fukuyama T, Mitsuoka W, et al, "Influence of Downscatter in Simultaneously Acquired Thallium 201/Technetium 99m PYP SPECT," *J Nucl Med*, 1996, 37(5):781-5.

Antunes ML, Seldin DW, Wall RM, et al, "Measurement of Acute Q-Wave Myocardial Infarct Size With Single Photon Emission Computed Tomography Imaging of Indium-111 Antimyosin," *Am J Cardiol*, 1989, 63(12):777-83.

Badner NH, Knill RL, Brown JE, et al, "Myocardial Infarction After Noncardiac Surgery," *Anesthesiology*, 1998, 88(3):572-8.

Botvinick EH, ""Hot Spot" Imaging Agents for Acute Myocardial Infarction," *J Nucl Med*, 1990, 31(2):143-6.

Emmett LM, Patel NC, Thanakrishnan K, et al, "Extensive Rhabdomyolysis After Streptokinase Therapy for Acute Myocardial Infarction Demonstrated by Tc-99m PYP Scintigraphy," *Clin Nucl Med*, 1999, 24(12):991-2.

Isoda H, Itagaki Y, Nomura N, et al, "Usefulness of Dual-SPECT With Tc-99m Pyrophosphate and Ti-201 to Predict Further Events After Acute Myocardial Infarction With Single-Vessel Coronary Artery Disease," *Clin Nucl Med*, 1999, 24(4):227-31.

Lewis SE, Parkey RW, Bonte FJ, et al, "Infarct-Avid Imaging in Acute Myocardial Infarction," *Diagnostic Nuclear Medicine*, Gottschalk A, Hoffer PB, and Potchen EJ, eds, Baltimore, MD: Williams & Wilkins, 1988, 399-413.

Mariani G, Villa G, Rossettin PF, et al, "Detection of Acute Myocardial Infarction by 99m Tc-Labeled D-Glucaric Acid Imaging in Patients With Acute Chest Pain," *J Nucl Med*, 1999, 40(11):1832-9.

Masuda T, Akiyama H, Kurosawa T, et al, "Long-Term Follow-up of Coronary Artery Dissection Due to Blunt Chest Trauma With Spontaneous Healing in a Young Woman," *Intensive Care Med*, 1996, 22(5):450-2.

Romero B, Candell-Riera J, Gracia RM, et al, "Myocardial Necrosis by Electrocution: Evaluation of Noninvasive Methods," *J Nucl Med*, 1997, 38(2):251-1.

Schmermund A, Gerber T, Behrenbeck T, et al, "Measurement of Myocardial Infarct Size by Electron Beam Computed Tomography: A Comparison With 99m Tc Sestamibi," *Invest Radiol*, 1998, 33(6):313-21.

Myocardial Perfusion Scan

Synonyms Cardiolite® Scan; Myoview® Scan; Sestamibi Scan; Stress Thallium Scan; Tetrofosmin Scan; Thallium-201 Scan; Thallium Stress Test

Applies to Rest Thallium Scan; Thallium Scan, Rest Only

Procedure Commonly Includes The patient undergoes either treadmill exercise stress or pharmacologic stress with an intravenous infusion of a

(Continued)

Myocardial Perfusion Scan *(Continued)*

vasodilator (eg, dipyridamole, adenosine, or dobutamine). At maximum stress, the patient receives an intravenous injection of radiopharmaceutical. Images of the heart are then acquired to assess regional myocardial perfusion. These images are compared to similar images which are acquired at rest (either before or late after the stress portion of the procedure). A transient stress defect which is normal in the rest phase implies ischemia. A persistent or fixed defect indicates scarring. Protocols in various Nuclear Medicine Departments may vary, depending on the radiopharmaceutical used. The use of ^{99}Tc compounds allows for acquisition of EKG gated data for wall motion analysis (CPT 78478) and calculation of ventricular ejection fraction (CPT).

Indications Myocardial perfusion imaging is employed to evaluate patients with known or suspected coronary artery stenoses. Regional areas of stress-induced myocardial ischemia or residual scarring (infarction) can be identified. Routine applications are in the differential diagnosis of chest pain and in the follow-up of patients who have had myocardial infarctions and/or who have undergone interventions such as coronary bypass surgery or balloon angioplasty. The prognostic information gained by this procedure can be extremely important in the management of patients with known coronary artery disease.

Patient Preparation Must be fasting from midnight the night before the test. The patient should have all RIA blood work performed, or at least drawn, prior to the injection of any radioactive material. If possible, patients having pharmacologic stress with dipyridamole (Persantine®) or adenosine (Adenocard®) should discontinue xanthine medications (eg, aminophylline) for 48 hours before testing. They should also refrain from any caffeine beverages (coffee, tea, cola) for at least 24 hours before testing.

Special Instructions Requisition must state the current patient diagnosis in order to select the most appropriate radiopharmaceutical and/or imaging technique.

Duration of Procedure: 4 hours

Radiopharmaceutical: Thallium-201 thallous chloride, ^{99m}TC sestamibi (Cardiolite®), or ^{99m}TC tetrofosmin (Myoview®)

Technique The application of single-photon emission tomography (SPECT) techniques contributes significantly to the diagnostic accuracy of this imaging study. A variety of protocols are employed for this procedure based on the sequence of stress and rest, the duration (1 vs 2 days), the choice of radiopharmaceutical, and the use of treadmill stress vs pharmacologic stress. The most common is a same-day rest followed by treadmill stress, Tc-99m tracer (8-10 mCi rest and 25-30 mCi stress) protocol. Acquisition of stress images in an EKG-gated format allows for evaluation of left ventricular function parameters of ED/ES volumes, regional wall motion, and LV ejection fraction.

Turnaround Time A written report will be sent to the patient's chart and/or to the referring physician.

Causes for Rejection Other recent Nuclear Medicine procedure may interfere. If uncertain, call the Nuclear Medicine Department.

Normal Findings Homogeneous distribution of isotope throughout all segments of the left ventricle with no transient (ischemia) or fixed (scar/infarct) regional perfusion defects. If EKG-gating is employed: good regional wall motion with an LV ejection fraction >50%.

Limitations Some false-positive results occur in females, patients with valvular disease, and patients with hypertrophic cardiomyopathies. Inadequate submaximal treadmill stress may result in false-negative results. Quantitative computer processing techniques may help refine the diagnostic accuracy of myocardial perfusion imaging. These techniques should be validated with a normal population at each clinical site for optimum application. Myocardial perfusion imaging is unable to distinguish the age of a persistent defect - scarring or infarction (ie, between old or new infarction). Arrhythmias will degrade the quality of EKG-gated image information.

Additional Information This procedure is normally performed in conjunction with standard stress electrocardiography and treadmill exercise.

References

Agati L, Autore C, Iaoboni C, et al, "The Complex Relation Between Myocardial Viability and Functional Recovery in Chronic Left Ventricular Dysfunction," *Am J Cardiol*, 1998, 81(12A):33G-5G.

Dilsizian V and Bonow RO, "Current Diagnostic Techniques of Assessing Myocardial Viability in Patients With Hibernating and Stunned Myocardium," *Circulation*, 1993, 87(1):1-20.

Hör G, Kober G, Maul F-D, et al, "Assessing Coronary Angioplasty With Myocardial Perfusion Imaging," *Nucl Med Ann*, 1990, 95-112.

Kang X, Berman DS, Van Train KF, et al, "Clinical Validation of Automatic Quantitative Defect Size in Rest Technetium 99m Sestamibi Myocardial Perfusion SPECT," 1997, 38(9):1441-6.

Mannting F and Morgan-Mannting MG, "Gated SPECT With Technetium-99m-Sestamibi for Assessment of Myocardial Perfusion Abnormalities," *J Nucl Med*, 1993, 34(4):601-8.

Medrano R, Lowry RW, Young JB, "Assessment of Myocardial Viability With 99m Tc Sestamibi in Patients Undergoing Cardiac Transplantation. A Scintigraphic/Pathological Study," *Circulation*, 1996, 94(5):1010-7.

Nigam A and Humen DP, "Prognostic Value of Myocardial Perfusion Imaging With Exercise and/or Dipyridamole Hyperemia in Patients With Preexisting Left Bundle Branch Block," *J Nucl Med*, 1998, 39(4):579-81.

Nunn AD, "Radiopharmaceuticals for Imaging Myocardial Perfusion," *Semin Nucl Med*, 1990, 20(2):111-8.

Passariello R and DeSantis M, "Magnetic Resonance Imaging Evaluation of Myocardial Perfusion," *Am J Cardiol*, 1998, 81(12A):68G-73G.

Ranhosky A and Kempthorne-Rawson J, "The Safety of Intravenous Dipyridamole Thallium Myocardial Perfusion Imaging. Intravenous Dipyridamole Thallium Imaging Study Group," *Circulation*, 1990, 81(4):1205-9.

Vernon S, Kaul S, Powers ER, et al, "Myocardial Viability in Patients With Chronic Coronary Artery Disease and Previous Myocardial Infarction: Comparison of Myocardial Contrast Echocardiography and Myocardial Perfusion Scintigraphy," *Am Heart J*, 1997, 134(5pt1):835-40.

Villanueva-Meyer J, Mena I, and Narahara KA, "Simultaneous Assessment of Left Ventricular Wall Motion and Myocardial Perfusion With Technetium-99m-Methoxy Isobutyl Isonitrile at Stress and Rest in Patients With Angina: Comparison With Thallium-201 SPECT," *J Nucl Med*, 1990, 31(4):457-63.

vom Dahl J, Altehoefer C, Sheehan FH, et al, "Recovery of Regional Left Ventricular Dysfunction After Coronary Revascularization. Impact of Myocardial Viability Assessed by Nuclear Imaging and Vessel Patency at Follow-up Angiography," *J Am Coll Cardiol*, 1996, 28(4):948-58.

♦ **Myoview® Scan** *see* Myocardial Perfusion Scan *on page 457*

♦ **Neurolite® Brain Scan** *see* Brain Scan *on page 441*

♦ **Parathyroid Localization Scan** *see* Parathyroid Scan *on page 459*

Parathyroid Scan

Synonyms Parathyroid Localization Scan; Parathyroid Scintigraphy

Replaces Selenium-75 Parathyroid Scan

Procedure Commonly Includes The patient receives an intravenous injection of Tc-99m sestamibi (Cardiolite®) followed by high resolution images of the anterior neck and upper chest at 30 minutes and again at 2 hours.

Indications Parathyroid imaging is useful in the preoperative localization of overactive parathyroid glands, especially in differentiating a solitary adenoma from a generalized parathyroid hyperplasia. The sensitivity of the technique is approximately 85%.

Patient Preparation The patient should have all RIA blood work performed, or at least drawn, prior to injection of any radioactive material. The patient does not need to be fasting or NPO for this procedure.

Special Instructions Requisition must state the current patient diagnosis in order to select the most appropriate radiopharmaceutical and/or imaging technique.

Duration of Procedure: 30 minutes to 1 hour

Radiopharmaceutical: Tc-99m sestamibi (Cardiolite®). An alternative method employs a combination of thallium-201 thallous chloride and ^{99m}Tc pertechnetate in a dual-isotope technique with computer-assisted subtraction of thyroid activity.

Turnaround Time A written report will be sent to the patient's chart and/or to the referring physician.

Causes for Rejection Other recent Nuclear Medicine procedure may interfere. Recent radiographic procedure involving iodinated contrast administration may preclude thyroid localization of ^{99m}Tc pertechnetate. If uncertain, call the Nuclear Medicine Department.

Normal Findings No tracer activity above background in the thyroid/parathyroid region of the neck or upper mediastinum

(Continued)

Parathyroid Scan *(Continued)*

Limitations Poor localization of ^{99m}Tc pertechnetate (if used) in the thyroid gland due to exogenous iodine or hypothyroidism may give erroneous results. Nodular disease (eg, multinodular goiter, neoplasm, and cysts) will also frequently give false-positive results.

References

Bergenfelz A, Tennvall J, Valdermarsson S, et al, "Sestamibi Versus Thallium Subtraction Scintigraphy in Parathyroid Localization: A Prospective Comparative Study in Patients With Predominantly Mild Primary Hyperparathyroidism," *Surgery*, 1997, 121(6):601-5.

Doppman JL, Skarulis MC, Chen CC, et al, "Parathyroid Adenomas in the Aortopulmonary Window," *Radiology*, 1996, 201(2):317-8.

Gallowitsch HJ, Mikosch P, Kresnik E, et al, "Technetium 99m Tetrofosmin Parathyroid Imaging. Results With Double-Phase Study and SPECT in Primary and Secondary Hyperparathyroidism," *Invest Radiol*, 1997, 32(8):459-65.

Kipper MS, LaBarbera JJ, Krohn LD, et al, "Localization of a Parathyroid Adenoma by the Addition of Pinhole Imaging to Tc-99m Sestamibi Dual-Phase Scintigraphy. Report of a Case and Review of Experience," *Clin Nucl Med*, 1997, 22(2):73-5.

Light VL, McHenry CR, Jarjoura D, et al, "Prospective Comparison of Dual-Phase Technetium 99m Sestamibi Scintigraphy and High Resolution Ultrasonography in the Evaluation of Abnormal Parathyroid Glands," *Am Surg*, 1996, 62(7):562-7.

Malhotra A, Silver CE, Deshpande V, et al, "Preoperative Parathyroid Localization With Sestamibi," *Am J Surg*, 1996, 176(6):637-40.

McHenry CR, Lee K, Saadey J, et al, "Parathyroid Localization With Technetium 99m Sestamibi: A Prospective Evaluation," *J Am Coll Surg*, 1996, 183(1):25-30.

Miller DL, Doppman JL, Shawker TH, et al, "Localization of Parathyroid Adenomas in Patients Who Have Undergone Surgery. Part I. Noninvasive Imaging Methods," *Radiology*, 1987, 162(1 Pt 1):133-7.

Neumann DR, Esselstyn CB Jr, Kim EY, et al, "Preliminary Experience With Double-Phase SPECT Using Tc-99m Sestamibi in Patients With Hyperparathyroidism," *Clin Nucl Med*, 1997, 22(4):217-21.

Seymour R, Rees J, Sharma AK, et al, "Paget's Disease of the Sternum Simulating an Ectopic Adenoma on Parathyroid Scintigraphy," *Clin Nucl Med*, 1997, 22(9):621-4.

Song AU, Phillips TE, Edmond CV, et al, "Success of Preoperative Imaging and Unilateral Neck Exploration for Primary Hyperparathyroidism," *Otolaryngol Head Neck Surg*, 1999, 121(4):393-7.

Takebayashi S, Hidai H, Chiba T, et al, "Hyperfunctional Parathyroid Glands With 99m Tc MIBI Scan: Semiquantitative Analysis Correlated With Histologic Findings," *J Nucl Med*, 1999, 40(11):1792-7.

- **Parathyroid Scintigraphy** *see* Parathyroid Scan *on page 459*
- **Parotid Scan** *see* Salivary Gland Scan *on page 465*
- **Perchlorate Discharge Test** *see* Thyroid Uptake *on page 471*
- **Perfusion Lung Scan** *see* Lung Scan, Perfusion *on page 453*
- **Perfusion-Ventilation Scan** *see* Lung Scan, Perfusion *on page 453*
- **Phlebothrombogram, Radionuclide** *see* Venogram, Radionuclide *on page 472*
- **Plasma/Blood Volume** *see* Blood Volume *on page 439*
- **Plasma Volume Measurement** *see* Blood Volume *on page 439*
- **Pulmonary Scan** *see* Lung Scan, Perfusion *on page 453*
- **PYP Cardiac Scan** *see* Myocardial Infarction Scan *on page 456*
- **Pyrophosphate Cardiac Scan** *see* Myocardial Infarction Scan *on page 456*
- **Quantitative Perfusion Lung Scan** *see* Lung Scan, Perfusion *on page 453*
- **Quantitative Ventilation Lung Scan** *see* Lung Scan, Ventilation *on page 454*
- **Radioactive Iodine Uptake** *see* Thyroid Uptake *on page 471*
- **Radioactive Renogram** *see* Renal Scan *on page 463*
- **Radioactive Venogram** *see* Venogram, Radionuclide *on page 472*
- **Radioactive Vitamin B_{12} Absorption Test, With or Without Intrinsic Factor** *see* Schilling Test *on page 466*
- **Radioiodine Thyroid Uptake and/or Scan** *see* Thyroid Uptake *on page 471*
- **Radioisotope Hepatic Scan** *see* Liver and Spleen Scan *on page 452*
- **Radioisotope Liver-Lung Scan** *see* Radioisotope Liver-Lung Scan for Subdiaphragmatic Abscesses *on page 461*

Radioisotope Liver-Lung Scan for Subdiaphragmatic Abscesses

Synonyms Lung-Liver Scan for Subdiaphragmatic Abscesses; Radioisotope Liver-Lung Scan

Procedure Commonly Includes The patient receives intravenous injections of technetium-99m (^{99m}Tc) macroaggregated albumin (MAA) and ^{99m}Tc sulfur colloid to localize the lungs and liver. Multiple images are acquired centered over the right hemidiaphragm to detect any abnormal spaces or loculations between the right lung and liver.

Indications Liver-lung imaging may be helpful in the detection of subdiaphragmatic abscesses and in differentiating between lung and liver lesions adjacent to the diaphragm.

Patient Preparation The patient should have all RIA blood work performed, or at least drawn, prior to injection of any radioactive material. The patient does not need to be fasting or NPO for this procedure.

Special Instructions Requisition must state the current patient diagnosis in order to select the most appropriate radiopharmaceutical and/or imaging technique.

Duration of Procedure: 1 hour
Radiopharmaceutical: ^{99m}Tc MAA and ^{99m}Tc sulfur colloid

Technique The application of single-photon emission tomography (SPECT) techniques may contribute significantly to the diagnostic accuracy of this imaging study.

Turnaround Time A written report will be sent to the patient's chart and/or to the referring physician.

Causes for Rejection Barium radiographic procedures within 24 hours prior to isotope. Other recent Nuclear Medicine procedure may interfere. If uncertain, call the Nuclear Medicine Department.

Limitations This study may also be able to delineate a left sided subdiaphragmatic abscess. It is most useful in detecting space occupying lesions between the top of the liver and the right hemidiaphragm.

Additional Information Abdominal CT scanning and radionuclide procedures using gallium-67 or indium-111 leukocytes have largely replaced this procedure.

References

Chau WK and Chan SC, "Sonographic Diagnosis of a Small Fistulous Communication Between a Subphrenic Abscess and a Perforated Duodenal Ulcer," *J Clin Ultrasound*, 2000, 28(3):153-6.

Conway JH, Nyquiest AC, and Goldson E, "Posterior Mediastinal Abscess Caused by Invasive Group A *Streptococcus* Infection," *Pediatr Infect Dis J*, 1996, 15(6):547-9.

Domjan JM, Tung KT, and Johnson C, "Bare Area Abscess: Imaging Findings and Potential Communication With the Mediastinum," *Br J Radiol*, 1997, 70(835):754-7.

Gallowitsch HJ, Mikosch P, Kresnik E, et al, "Thyroglobulin and Low-Dose Iodine-131 and Technetium-99m-Tetrofosmin Whole-Body Scintigraphy in Differentiated Thyroid Carcinoma," *J Nucl Med*, 1998, 39(5):870-5.

Halvorsen RA Jr, Foster WL Jr, Wilkinson RH Jr, et al, "Hepatic Abscess: Sensitivity of Imaging Tests and Clinical Findings," *Gastrointest Radiol*, 1988, 13(2):135-41.

Oppenheim BE, Wellman HN, and Hoffer PB, "Liver Imaging," *Diagnostic Nuclear Medicine*, Gottschalk A, Hoffer PB, and Potchen EJ, eds, Baltimore, MD: Williams & Wilkins, 1988, 549-50.

Sangar VK, Gini A, Fuentes RT, et al, "Diagnosis of a Liver Abscess With Gallium-67 and Radiocolloid Tomography," *Clin Nucl Med*, 1989, 14(6):443-5.

Uemoto S, Inomata Y, Egawa H, et al, "Effects of Hypoxemia on Early Postoperative Course of Liver Transplantation in Pediatric Patients With Intrapulmonary Shunting," *Transplantation*, 1997, 63(3):407-14.

Yen TC, Tsai MF, and Tzen KY, "Biliary and Liver Abscesses Demonstrated With Tc-99m DISIDA and Ga-67 Imaging," *Clin Nucl Med*, 1998, 23(12):853-4.

♦ **Radionuclide Angiography** *see* Cardiac Blood Pool Scan, EKG-Gated *on page 442*

♦ **Radionuclide Angiography, Stress** *see* Cardiac Blood Pool Scan, EKG-Gated *on page 442*

♦ **Radionuclide Bone Scan** *see* Bone Scan *on page 440*

♦ **Radionuclide Cineangiography** *see* Cardiac Blood Pool Scan, First Pass *on page 443*

♦ **Radionuclide Cisternography** *see* Cisternogram *on page 445*

♦ **Radionuclide Liver Scan** *see* Liver and Spleen Scan *on page 452*
♦ **Radionuclide Perfusion Lung Scan** *see* Lung Scan, Perfusion *on page 453*
♦ **Radionuclide Ventilation Lung Scan** *see* Lung Scan, Ventilation *on page 454*
♦ **Radionuclide Ventriculogram** *see* Cardiac Blood Pool Scan, EKG-Gated *on page 442*
♦ **Radionuclide Ventriculogram, First Pass** *see* Cardiac Blood Pool Scan, First Pass *on page 443*
♦ **RAI Uptake and/or Scan** *see* Thyroid Uptake *on page 471*
♦ **RBC Survival Test** *see* Chromium-51 Red Cell Survival *on page 444*
♦ **Red Blood Cell Sequestration** *see* Chromium-51 Red Cell Survival *on page 444*
♦ **Red Cell Mass** *see* Blood Volume *on page 439*
♦ **Red Cell Mass** *see* Red Cell Volume *on page 462*
♦ **Red Cell Mass Measurement** *see* Blood Volume *on page 439*
♦ **Red Cell Survival** *see* Chromium-51 Red Cell Survival *on page 444*

Red Cell Volume

Related Information

Blood Volume *on page 439*

Synonyms Chromium-Labeled Red Cell Volume; Red Cell Mass

Procedure Commonly Includes Determination of red cell volume is a nonimaging procedure in which the patient receives an intravenous injection of a known volume of his red cells which are labeled with a known amount of chromium (^{51}Cr). A sample of the patient's blood is drawn after equilibration of the radiolabeled cells and the circulating red cell volume can then be calculated.

Indications Red cell volume measurement is helpful in the differential diagnosis of polycythemia. The procedure is also helpful in monitoring the effects of some antineoplastic drugs. Red cell volume measurement is routinely combined with plasma volume measurements to determine total blood volume (see Blood Volume *on page 439*).

Contraindications

- patient actively bleeding
- edema

Patient Preparation The patient should have all RIA blood work performed, or at least drawn, prior to injection of any radioactive material. The patient does not need to be fasting or NPO for this procedure. Other blood samples should not be taken during this procedure. Nor should transfusions of blood products be given.

Special Instructions Requisition must state the current patient diagnosis in order to select the most appropriate radiopharmaceutical and/or imaging technique. Also include the patient's accurate height and weight.

Duration of Procedure: 2-3 hours
Radiopharmaceutical: Chromium-51 chromate for RBC label

Turnaround Time A written report will be sent to the patient's chart and/or to the referring physician.

Causes for Rejection Other recent Nuclear Medicine procedure may interfere. If uncertain, call the Nuclear Medicine Department.

Normal Findings Normal RBC and blood volumes are a function of the size and sex of the patient. Expected volumes are estimated based on body surface area. Measured volumes are compared to the expected results and normally can vary ±20%. Obese patients may have volumes somewhat less than expected.

Limitations The procedure is technically difficult with multiple laboratory steps which tend to introduce errors.

Additional Information The assessment of anemia and polycythemia (assessment of whether or not one of these conditions truly exists) depends foremost upon a reliable and direct determination of red cell volume. RBC count, Hgb level, and Hct provide only concentration parameters, the measured number or amount relative to the solution in which it exists. In a number of clinical situations (eg, acute blood loss) the RBC count, Hgb, and Hct will not indicate the actual decrease or increase in circulating red cell mass. In the majority of clinical situations CBC components (RBC count, etc) do correlate with RBC volume. Due to technical complexity (resulting in high cost and prolonged turnaround time), CBC is usually used, especially for follow-up or monitoring situations, even though RBC mass study would provide a more meaningful result. Nevertheless, some clinical situations (eg, polycythemia, complicated fluid, and electrolyte management problems) will benefit from at least initial red cell volume determination.

References

Bhargava KK, Palestro CJ, Camaya MV, et al, "Radionuclide Analysis of Drug-Induced Blood-Pool Changes in Liver and Other Organs," *J Nucl Med*, 2000, 41(3):474-9.

Campbell WW, Beard JL, Joseph LJ, et al, "Chromium Picolinate Supplementation and Resistive Training by Older Men: Effects on Iron-Status and Hematologic Indexes," *Am J Clin Nutr*, 1997, 66(4):944-9.

Dawry FP, "Splenic Sequestration of Red Blood Cells: A Computerized Approach Using Two Radionuclides," *J Nucl Med Tech*, 1988, 16:185-6.

Leslie WD, Dupont JO, and Peterdy AE, "Effect of Obesity on Red Cell Mass Results," *J Nucl Med*, 1999, 40(3):422-8.

Mock DM, Lankford GL, Widness JA, et al, "Measurement of Circulating Red Cell Volume Using Biotin-Labeled Red Cells," *Transfusion*, 1999, 39(2):149-55.

Ohki S, Kunimoto F, Isa Y, et al, "Accuracy of Carboxyhemoglobin Dilution Method for the Measurement of Circulating Blood Volume," *Can J Anaesth*, 2000, 47(2):150-4.

Orth VH, Rehm M, Thiel M, et al, "First Clinical Implications of Perioperative Red Cell Volume Measurement," *Anesth Analg*, 1998, 87(6):1234-8.

Pollycove M and Tono M, "Blood Volume," *Diagnostic Nuclear Medicine*, 2nd ed, Gottschalk A, Hoffer PB, and Potchen EJ, eds, Baltimore, MD: Williams & Wilkins, 1988, 690-8.

Srivastava SC and Chervu LR, "Radionuclide-Labeled Red Blood Cells: Current Status and Future Prospects," *Semin Nucl Med*, 1984, 14(2):68-82.

Renal Scan

Related Information

Angiogram, Radionuclide *on page 437*

Synonyms Kidney Scan; Radioactive Renogram; Renal Scintigraphy; Renogram

Applies to Diuretic Renal Scan; Hippuran Scan; Triple Phase Renal Scan (Renogram, Renal Flow and Scan)

Procedure Commonly Includes The patient receives an intravenous injection of the appropriate renal radiopharmaceutical (see following table). Initial rapid sequence images are acquired to assess renal perfusion if a technetium-99m (^{99m}Tc) compound is used. Sequential static images are then acquired for the next 30-45 minutes to evaluate renal cortical uptake, excretion, and parenchymal clearance. Delayed images may be required to evaluate patients with obstruction or renal insufficiency.

Radiopharmaceuticals for Renal Imaging

Isotope	Compound	Physiology	Measurement
^{99m}Tc	DMSA	Cortical binding	Renal function; cortical imaging
	DTPA	Glomerular filtration	Renal perfusion and function; quantitative GFR
	Glucoheptonate	Cortical binding	Renal perfusion and function; cortical imaging
	Mertiatide (MAG_3)	Effective renal plasma flow	Renal function; quantitative ERPF
^{123}I ^{131}I	Hippuran	Effective renal plasma flow	Renal function; quantitative ERPF

^{99m}Tc DTPA or glucoheptonate can be given in sufficient dose (10-15 mCi) to accurately assess renal arterial perfusion.

^{123}I hippuran provides better image resolution and technical statistical information than the higher energy ^{131}I form.

Indications Renal imaging is an accurate technique for evaluating multiple parameters of renal function to compare and correlate with the anatomic information gained by ultrasound or other radiographic procedures. With computer acquisition of images, differential estimates of left and right kidney

(Continued)

Renal Scan *(Continued)*

contributions to glomerular filtration rate and effective renal plasma flow can be calculated. With the use of diuretic stimulation during the functional phase, it is possible to differentiate between anatomic obstruction and nonobstructive residual dilatation from previous hydronephrosis. By using one of the cortical imaging agents (^{99m}Tc GHA or DMSA) high resolution delayed images of isotope activity in the renal cortex can be obtained. These help in evaluating suspected renal masses, scarring, cysts, infarcts, or cortical irregularities such as a column of Bertin. Renal perfusion imaging after an oral dose of captopril has recently been demonstrated to be a useful screening test for renovascular hypertension.

Patient Preparation The patient should have all RIA blood work performed, or at least drawn, prior to the injection of any radioactive material. The patient does not need to be fasting or NPO for this procedure. In fact, fluid intake should be encouraged during the 2 hours prior to renal imaging unless the patient has a restricted fluid intake for other reasons.

Special Instructions Requisition must state the current patient diagnosis in order to select the most appropriate radiopharmaceutical and/or imaging technique.

Duration of Procedure: 1 to 1½ hours
Radiopharmaceutical: See table.

Turnaround Time A written report will be sent to the patient's chart and/or to the referring physician.

Causes for Rejection Other recent Nuclear Medicine procedure may interfere. If uncertain, call the Nuclear Medicine Department.

Normal Findings Prompt symmetric bilateral perfusion; good early cortical accumulation bilaterally with visualization of the collecting systems by 3-5 minutes postinjection; rapid excretion into the bladder with no delay to indicate a partial or complete obstruction

Limitations At serum creatinine levels >3 mg/dL, renal insufficiency will produce apparent decreases in renal perfusion and function. Hippuran and MAG-3 may be the better radiopharmaceutical choices for imaging in these cases.

References

Bagni B, Orsolon P, Fattori A, et al, "Renal SPECT With Tc-99m DMSA in Children With Upper Urinary Tract Infections Using a Triple-Headed Gamma Camera," *Clin Nucl Med*, 1997, 22(12):838-43.

Conway JJ, "The Role of Scintigraphy in Urinary Tract Infection," *Semin Nucl Med*, 1988, 18(4):308-19.

Craig JC, Irwig LM, Howman-Giles RB, et al, "Variability in the Interpretation of Dimercaptosuccinic Acid Scintigraphy After Urinary Tract Infection in Children," *J Nucl Med*, 1998, 39(8):1428-32.

Dunn EK, Distant DA, and Strashun AM, "Tc-99m MAG3 Evaluation of Recipients With Dual Adult Cadaveric Renal Allografts. Simultaneous Transplantation of Both Kidneys From Marginal Donors," *Clin Nucl Med*, 1999, 24(8):547-52.

Eshima D, Fritzberg AR, and Taylor A Jr, "^{99m}Tc Renal Tubular Function Agents: Current Status," *Semin Nucl Med*, 1990, 20(1):28-40.

Fabrizio MD, Chancellor MB, Rivas DA, et al, "The Role of Renal Scintigraphy in the Evaluation of Spinal Cord Injury Patients With Presumed Urosepsis," *J Urol*, 1996, 156(5):1730-4.

Fine EJ and Sarkar S, "Differential Diagnosis and Management of Renovascular Hypertension Through Nuclear Medicine Techniques," *Semin Nucl Med*, 1989, 19(2):101-15.

Lantsberg S, Rachinsky I, Lupu L, et al, "Unilateral Acute Renal Cortical Necrosis: Correlative Imaging," *Clin Nucl Med*, 2000, 25(3):184-6.

Loutfi I, Al-Zaabi K, and Elgazzar AH, "Tc-99m DMSA Renal Scan in First-Time Versus Recurrent Urinary Tract Infection-Yield and Patterns of Abnormalities," *Clin Nucl Med*, 1999, 24(12):931-5.

Majd M and Rushton HG, "Renal Cortical Scintigraphy in the Diagnosis of Acute Pyelonephritis," *Semin Nucl Med*, 1992, 22(2):98-111.

Nally JV Jr and Black HR, "State-of-the-Art Review: Captopril Renography - Pathophysiological Considerations and Clinical Observations," *Semin Nucl Med*, 1992, 22(2):85-97.

Poropat M, Batinic D, Basic M, et al, "Tc-99m DTPA Renal Scintigraphy Using Deconvolution Analysis With six Functional Images of the Mean Time to Evaluate Acute Pyelonephritis," *Clin Nucl Med*, 1999, 24(2):120-4.

Powsner RA, Edelstein RA, Jaffe T, et al, "Diagnosis of Postoperative Urinary Ascites Using Renal Scintigraphy," *Clin Nucl Med*, 1997, 22(8):523-5.

Tulchinsky M, Dietrich TJ, Eggli DF, et al, "Technetium-99m-MAG3 Scintigraphy in Acute Renal Failure After Transplantation: A Marker of Viability and Prognosis," *J Nucl Med*, 1997, 38(3):475-8.

van Jaarsveld BC, Krijnen P, Derkx FH, et al, "The Place of Renal Scintigraphy in the Diagnosis of Renal Artery Stenosis. Fifteen Years of Clinical Experience," *Arch Intern Med*, 1997, 157(11):1226-34.

Yen TC, Tzen KY, Lin WY, et al, "Identification of new Renal Scarring in Repeated Episodes of Acute Pyelonephritis Using Tc-99m DMSA Renal SPECT," *Clin Nucl Med*, 1998, 23(12):828-31.

♦ **Renal Scintigraphy** *see* Renal Scan *on page 463*

♦ **Renogram** *see* Renal Scan *on page 463*

♦ **Rest Thallium Scan** *see* Myocardial Perfusion Scan *on page 457*

♦ **Rose Bengal Liver Scan** *see* Biliary Scan *on page 438*

Salivary Gland Scan

Synonyms Parotid Scan

Procedure Commonly Includes The patient receives an intravenous injection of technetium-99m (^{99m}Tc) pertechnetate which is taken up and secreted by the salivary glands. Immediate magnified images of the glands are acquired. Repeat images are acquired after the patient ingests lemon juice to stimulate salivary secretion.

Indications This procedure is helpful in the differential diagnosis of dry mouth conditions (eg, Sjögren syndrome, salivary duct obstructions, and other parotid conditions such as asymmetric hypertrophy and mass lesions, especially Warthin's tumors).

Patient Preparation The patient does not need to be fasting or NPO for this procedure. The patient should have all RIA blood work performed, or at least drawn, prior to the injection of any radioactive material.

Special Instructions Requisition must state the current patient diagnosis in order to select the most appropriate radiopharmaceutical and/or imaging technique.

Duration of Procedure: 1 hour

Radiopharmaceutical: ^{99m}Tc pertechnetate

Turnaround Time A written report will be sent to the patient's chart and/or to the referring physician.

Causes for Rejection Other recent Nuclear Medicine procedure may interfere. If uncertain, call the Nuclear Medicine Department.

Limitations The procedure will not definitely differentiate benign lesions from malignant ones.

Additional Information Computer acquisition of scintigraphic data is acquired over time and analysis is performed which is useful for determining salivary flow kinetics. Conditions in which this would be useful are in the diagnosis of Sjögren syndrome, obstruction with calculi, and sialadenitis.

References

Arbab AS, Koizumi K, Hiraike S, et al, "Will Thallium-201 Replace Gallium-67 in Salivary Gland Scintigraphy?" *J Nucl Med*, 1996, 37(11):1819-23.

Aung W, Yamada I, Umehara I, et al, "Sjögren Syndrome: Comparison of Assessments With Quantitative Salivary Gland Scintigraphy and Contrast Sialography," *J Nucl Med*, 2000, 41(2):257-62.

Azaz B, Regev E, Casap N, et al, "Sialolithectomy Done With a CO_2 Laser: Clinical and Scintigraphic Results," *J Oral Maxillofac Surg*, 1996, 54(12):1479.

Bongers V, De Klerk JM, van Den Biezenbos AR, et al, "Value of Technetium-99-m Pertechnetate Imaging in the Differential of Salivary Gland Lesions," *Ann Otol Rhinol Laryngol*, 1997, 106(5):432-4.

Choi DS, Na DG, Byun HS, et al, "Salivary Gland Tumors: Evaluation With Two-Phase Helical CT," *Radiology*, 2000, 214(1):231-6.

Copely DJ and Smith R, "Salivary Scintigraphy: Unilateral Increased Activity," *Semin Nucl Med*, 1986, 16(3):222-3.

Hermann GA, Vivino FB, Shnier D, et al, "Diagnostic Accuracy of Salivary Scintigraphic Indices in Xerostomic Populations," *Clin Nucl Med*, 1999, 24(3):167-72.

Hermann GA, Vivino FB, Shnier D, et al, "Variability of Quantitative Scintigraphic Salivary Indices in Normal Subjects," *J Nucl Med*, 1998, 39(7):1260-3.

Murata Y, Yamada I, Umehara I, et al, "Diagnostic Accuracy of Technetium-99m-Pertechnetate Scintigraphy With Lemon Juice Stimulation to Evaluate Warthin's Tumor," *J Nucl Med*, 1998, 39(1):43-6.

Peterson MK and Butler RR Jr, "Warthin's Tumor Demonstrated With Tc-99m Pertechnetate SPECT and CT," *Clin Nucl Med*, 1998, 23(4):244-7.

Shih WJ, Stipp V, Magoun S, et al, "Medullary Thyroid Carcinoma Imaged by Tc-99m MIBI SPECT and Tl-201 Chloride/Tc-99m Pertechnetate Subtraction SPECT," *Clin Nucl Med*, 1996, 21(3):213-7.

Umehara I, Yamada I, Murata Y, et al, "Quantitative Evaluation of Salivary Gland Scintigraphy in Sjögren Syndrome," *J Nucl Med*, 1999, 40(1):64-9.

Schilling Test

Synonyms Radioactive Vitamin B_{12} Absorption Test, With or Without Intrinsic Factor; Schilling Test, Stages 1 and 2; Vitamin B_{12} Absorption Test

Procedure Commonly Includes The patient ingests an oral dose of radiolabeled vitamin B_{12}. An intramuscular injection of nonradioactive vitamin B_{12} is then given which is rapidly absorbed and saturates any available hepatic binding sites. The radiolabeled vitamin B_{12}, once absorbed in the terminal ileum, is then promptly excreted in the urine. The patient's urine is collected for a 24-hour period and the percent of the original dose present in the urine is calculated.

Indications The Schilling test measures the patient's ability to absorb vitamin B_{12} from the intestinal tract and to excrete absorbed vitamin into the urine. The stage 1 test employs radiolabeled vitamin B_{12} alone (see table). If abnormal, stage 2, radiolabeled vitamin B_{12} with intrinsic factor is performed. These tests are useful for evaluating any macrocytic anemia to detect pernicious anemia. It helps in the differentiation of intrinsic factor deficiency from other causes of vitamin B_{12} malabsorption. In inflammatory bowel disease the Schilling test helps to determine the presence and severity of involvement in the distal small bowel. On rare occasions, a stage 3 test may be useful. This employs vitamin B_{12} alone but after a 7-10 day course of oral tetracycline. This serves to distinguish bacterial overgrowth in the small bowel from other causes of vitamin B_{12} malabsorption.

Schilling Test

Stage	Content	Application
I	Vitamin B_{12}	Screening test for normal absorption vs malabsorption of vitamin
II	Vitamin B_{12} + intrinsic factor	Differentiates conditions of intrinsic factor deficiency (eg, congenital or postgastrectomy) from other causes of malabsorption
III	Vitamin B_{12} after P.O. tetracycline course	Differentiates syndrome of bacterial overgrowth from other causes of malabsorption

Patient Preparation The patient should have all RIA blood work performed, or at least drawn, prior to injection of any radioactive material. Also, any measurement of serum vitamin B_{12} and folate should be drawn before beginning this test. The patient must be fasting overnight and should remain fasting for an hour after receiving the oral dose of radiolabeled vitamin B_{12}. The patient will be instructed to collect all urine for 24 hours. In some departments, a 48-hour collection is routine (ie, two sequential 24-hour collections). An incomplete urine collection will invalidate the test results.

Special Instructions Requisition must state the current patient diagnosis in order to select the most appropriate radiopharmaceutical and/or imaging technique.

Duration of Procedure: 24-48 hours

Radiopharmaceutical: Cobalt-57 labeled vitamin B_{12}

Turnaround Time A written report will be sent to the patient's chart and/or to the referring physician following submission of urine specimen.

Specimen 24-hour urine collection

Causes for Rejection Other recent Nuclear Medicine procedure may interfere. If uncertain, call the Nuclear Medicine Department.

Normal Findings The normal stage 1 result is an excretion >10% of the originally administered oral dose into the urine within 24 hours. A result <10% excretion should be followed by a stage 2 test. Normalization of excretion in stage 2 confirms a lack of intrinsic factor as the cause of malabsorption. An incomplete urine collection, even the loss of a single specimen in the 24-hour collection, may give an artifactually low result.

Limitations The test without intrinsic factor must be completed before testing with intrinsic factor. If other isotope tests are to be performed, schedule the

Schilling tests first. The presence of renal dysfunction, pancreatic insufficiency, myxedema, liver disease, or any other condition resulting in the decreased absorption of B_{12} from the GI tract, its concentration in the liver, or its excretion in the urine may result in abnormal values. This procedure presumes normal renal function. In renal insufficiency or in elderly males with possible prostatic hypertrophy and high bladder residual volumes, urine collections are sometimes continued for 48-72 hours.

References

Cohen MB, "Vitamin B_{12} Deficiency," *Semin Nucl Med*, 1981, 11(3):226-7.

Fish MB, "Measurement of Gastrointestinal Absorption of Vitamin B_{12}," *Diagnostic Nuclear Medicine*, Gottschalk A, Hoffer PB, and Potchen EJ, eds, Baltimore, MD: Williams & Wilkins, 1988, 699-706.

Lake-Bakaar G, Elsakr M, Hagag N, et al, "Changes in Parietal Cell Structure and Function in HIV Disease," *Dig Dis Sci*, 1996, 41(7):1398-408.

Lindgren A, Swolin B, Nilsson O, et al, "Serum Methylmalonic Acid and Total Homocysteine in Patients With Suspected Cobalamin Deficiency: A Clinical Study Based on Gastrointestinal Histopathological Findings," *Am J Hematol*, 1997, 56(4):230-8.

Markle HV, "Cobalamin," *Crit Rev Clin Lab Sci*, 1996, 33(4):247-356.

Pannek J, Haupt G, Schulze H, et al, "Influence of Continent Ileal Urinary Diversion on Vitamin B_{12} Absorption," *J Urol*, 1996, 155(4):1206-8.

Penix LP, "Ischemic Strokes Secondary to Vitamin B_{12} Deficiency-Induced Hyperhomocystinemia," *Neurology*, 1998, 51(2):622-4.

Rhode BM, Arseneau P, Cooper BA, et al, "Vitamin B_{12} Deficiency After Gastric Surgery for Obesity," *Am J Clin Nutr*, 1996, 63(1):103-9.

Snow CF, "Laboratory Diagnosis of Vitamin B_{12} and Folate Deficiency: A Guide for the Primary Care Physician," *Arch Intern Med*, 1999, 159(12):1289-98.

Zittoun J and Zittoun R, "Modern Clinical Testing Strategies in Cobalamin and Folate Deficiency," *Semin Hematol*, 1999, 36(1):35-46.

Zuckier LS, Stabin M, Krynycki BR, et al, "Effect of Prior Radiopharmaceutical Administration on Schilling Test Performance: Analysis and Recommendations," *J Nucl Med*, 1996, 37(12):1995-9.

- ♦ **Schilling Test, Stages 1 and 2** *see* Schilling Test *on page 466*
- ♦ **Scrotal Scan** *see* Testicular Scan *on page 467*
- ♦ **Selenium-75 Parathyroid Scan** *see* Parathyroid Scan *on page 459*
- ♦ **Sestamibi Scan** *see* Myocardial Perfusion Scan *on page 457*
- ♦ **Soft Tissue Scan** *see* Gallium Scan, Abscess and/or Tumor *on page 447*
- ♦ **Spleen Scan** *see* Liver and Spleen Scan *on page 452*
- ♦ **Splenic Sequestration Study** *see* Chromium-51 Red Cell Survival *on page 444*
- ♦ **Stress Gated Study** *see* Cardiac Blood Pool Scan, EKG-Gated *on page 442*
- ♦ **Stress Thallium Scan** *see* Myocardial Perfusion Scan *on page 457*
- ♦ **Superior Venacavagram** *see* Angiogram, Radionuclide *on page 437*
- ♦ **Survival of Red Blood Cells** *see* Chromium-51 Red Cell Survival *on page 444*
- ♦ **Technetium Thyroid Scan** *see* Thyroid Scan *on page 469*

Testicular Scan

Synonyms Scrotal Scan; Testicular Torsion Scan

Procedure Commonly Includes The patient receives an intravenous injection of technetium-99m (^{99m}Tc) pertechnetate. Dynamic serial perfusion images of the scrotal and perineal area are acquired to assess testicular blood flow. Additional static images are also acquired.

Indications The primary use of testicular imaging is the differentiation between testicular torsion and epididymitis in cases of acute scrotal pain. Other conditions such as hematoma, abscess, tumor, hydrocele, and spermatocele may be detected but the procedure is less accurate for these conditions.

Patient Preparation The patient should have all RIA blood work performed, or at least drawn, prior to the injection of any radioactive material. The patient does not need to be fasting or NPO for this procedure.

Special Instructions Requisition must state the current patient diagnosis in order to select the most appropriate radiopharmaceutical and/or imaging technique.

Duration of Procedure: 30 minutes
Radiopharmaceutical: ^{99m}Tc pertechnetate
(Continued)

Testicular Scan *(Continued)*

Turnaround Time A written report will be sent to the patient's chart and/or to the referring physician.

Normal Findings Homogenous and symmetric distribution of activity in the testes with no focal decreases or increases.

References

Barloon TJ, Weissman AM, and Kahn D, "Diagnostic Imaging of Patients With Acute Scrotal Pain," *Am Fam Physician*, 1996, 53(5):1734-50.

Burgher SW, "Acute Scrotal Pain," *Emerg Med Clin North Am*, 1998, 16(4):781-809.

Connolly LP, Treves St, Davis RT, et al, "Pediatric Applications of Pinhole Magnification Imaging," *J Nucl Med*, 1999, 40(11):1896-901.

Hawtrey CE, "Assessment of Acute Scrotal Symptoms and Findings. A Clinician's Dilemma" *Urol Clin North Am*, 1998, 25(4):715-23.

Lowry PA, Pjura GA, Kim EE, et al, "Radionuclide Imaging of the Lower Genitourinary Tract," *Diagnostic Nuclear Medicine*, Gottschalk A, Hoffer PB, and Potchen EJ, eds, Baltimore, MD: Williams & Wilkins, 1988, 973-84.

Lutzker LG and Zuckier LS, "Testicular Scanning and Other Applications of Radionuclide Imaging of the Genital Tract," *Semin Nucl Med*, 1990, 20(2):159-88.

Paltiel HJ, Connolly LP, Atala A, et al, "Acute Scrotal Symptoms in Boys With an Indeterminate Clinical Presentation: Comparison of Color Doppler Sonography and Scintigraphy," *Radiology*, 1998, 207(1):223-31.

Yildiz A, Baltaoglu I, Ozdemir A, et al, "Changing Imaging Patterns After Testicular Torsion Demonstrated by Serial Scintigraphic Studies," *Clin Nucl Med*, 1999, 24(11):888-9.

- **Testicular Torsion Scan** *see* Testicular Scan *on page 467*
- **Tetrofosmin Scan** *see* Myocardial Perfusion Scan *on page 457*
- **Thallium-201 Scan** *see* Myocardial Perfusion Scan *on page 457*
- **Thallium Scan, Rest Only** *see* Myocardial Perfusion Scan *on page 457*
- **Thallium Stress Test** *see* Myocardial Perfusion Scan *on page 457*
- **Three-Phase Bone Scan** *see* Bone Scan *on page 440*
- **Thrombophlebogram, Radionuclide** *see* Venogram, Radionuclide *on page 472*

Thyroid Metastatic Survey, Iodine-131

Related Information

Thyroid Scan *on page 469*

Synonyms ^{131}I Body Scan; ^{131}I Metastatic Survey; ^{131}I Neck and Chest Survey; ^{131}I Whole Body Survey

Procedure Commonly Includes The patient receives an oral dose of iodine-131 sodium iodide which localizes in residual thyroid tissue or in iodine-avid metastatic sites from thyroid carcinoma. Images of the neck, thorax, and other body areas are acquired at 24-72 hours later.

Indications Radioiodine surveys are used to delineate residual thyroid tissue after surgical procedures for thyroid carcinoma and to detect regional or distant metastases.

Patient Preparation The patient should have all RIA blood work performed, or at least drawn, prior to injection of any radioactive material. The patient should be fasting (NPO) for 4 hours prior to receiving the oral dose. The patient should avoid ingesting iodine-containing foods or medications for at least 2 weeks prior to the procedure. Any thyroid hormone medications should also be discontinued for at least 2 weeks (T_3) or 4 weeks (T_4). An alternative method employing pretreatment with intramuscular synthetic TSH injections rather than thyroid hormone withdrawal may be selected in patients for whom medication withdrawal is contraindicated.

Special Instructions Requisition must state the current patient diagnosis in order to select the most appropriate radiopharmaceutical and/or imaging technique. Special instructions for this procedure will be discussed with the patient by Nuclear Medicine personnel.

Duration of Procedure: 1-2 hours

Radiopharmaceutical: Iodine-131 sodium iodide. Under certain conditions, other radiopharmaceuticals (eg, thallium-201 thallous chloride) may be employed.

Turnaround Time A written report will be sent to the patient's chart and/or to the referring physician.

Normal Findings There may be normal uptake of radioiodine in residual remnants of tissue after partial or near-total thyroidectomy. There is also excretion of iodine by the salivary glands, stomach, and kidneys/bladder.

Limitations Administration of iodine-containing foods and medications as well as radiographic contrast media will suppress radioiodine uptake in thyroid or metastatic tissue. Iodine-containing compounds and foods interfere with any tests using radioactive iodine. The following exogenous iodine sources may suppress uptake measurements or scans for the time indicated:

- iodine compounds (Lugol's, tincture, potassium iodide, kelp): 1-2 weeks
- seafood, Ovaltine®, vitamin pills, Ornade®, Combid® cough syrups: 3-5 days
- Diodrast, Hypaque®, Renografin® (ie, intravenous pyelograms, CT with contrast and arteriograms): 4-6 weeks
- lipiodol (ie, bronchograms), Oragrafin® (ie, gallbladder exams), Pantopaque® (ie, myelograms): at least 6 months
- antithyroid drugs (ie, propylthiouracil, Tapazole®): 7 days
- thyroid hormone (ie, desiccated thyroid, thyroxine): 4 weeks
- tri-iodothyronine (Cytomel®): 10-12 day

Call the Nuclear Medicine Department for further information.

Residual functioning thyroid tissue will usually prevent sufficient uptake in metastatic sites to allow visualization. Thus, residual tissue must be ablated with high-dose radioiodine before adequate later investigation for metastases can be undertaken.

References

Aktay R, Rezai K, Seabold JE, et al, "Four- to Twenty-Four-Hour Uptake Ratio: An Index of Rapid Iodine-131 Turnover in Hyperthyroidism," *J Nucl Med*, 1996, 37(11):1815-9.

Chung JK, Lee YJ, Jeong JM, et al, "Clinical Significance of Hepatic Visualization on Iodine-131 Whole-Body Scan in Patients With Thyroid Carcinoma," *J Nucl Med*, 1997, 38(8):1191-5.

Garcia-Sanchis L, Lopez-Aznar D, Oltra A, et al, "Metastatic Follicular Thyroid Carcinoma to the Kidney: A Case Report," *Clin Nucl Med*, 1999, 24(1):48-50.

Harder W, Lind P, Molnar M, et al, "Thallium-201 Uptake With Negative Iodine-131 Scintigraphy and Serum Thyroglobulin in Metastatic Oxyphilic Papillary Thyroid Carcinoma," *J Nucl Med*, 1998, 39(2):236-8.

Lorberboym M and Mechanick JI, "Accelerated Thyrotoxicosis Induced by Iodinated Contrast Media in Metastatic Differentiated Thyroid Carcinoma," *J Nucl Med*, 1996, 37(9):1532-5.

Lorberboym M, Murthy S, Mechanick JI, et al, "Thallium-201 and Iodine-131 Scintigraphy in Differentiated Thyroid Carcinoma," *J Nucl Med*, 1996, 37(9):1487-91.

Menzel C, Grünwald F, Schomburg A, et al, ""High-Dose" Radioiodine Therapy in Advanced Differentiated Thyroid Carcinoma," *J Nucl Med*, 1996, 37(9):1496-503.

Ringel MD and Ladenson PW, "Diagnostic Accuracy of 131I Scanning With Recombinant Human Thyrotropin Versus Thyroid Hormone Withdrawal in a Patient With Metastatic Thyroid Carcinoma and Hypopituitarism," *J Clin Endocrinol Metab*, 1996, 81(5):1724-5.

Tsuchimochi S, Nakajo M, Hino Y, et al, "Separation of I-131-Positive Juxtagastric Metastatic Thyroid Carcinoma From the Stomach by Simultaneous Dual-Isotope Imaging With I-131 and Tc-99m Pertechnetate," *Clin Nucl Med*, 1999, 24(9):704-5.

Thyroid Scan

Related Information

Thyroid Metastatic Survey, Iodine-131 *on page 468*

Synonyms Iodine Thyroid Scan; Technetium Thyroid Scan; Thyroid Scan and Uptake; Thyroid Scintigraphy

Applies to Thyroid Uptake and Thyroid Scanning

Procedure Commonly Includes The patient receives an intravenous injection of technetium-99m (^{99m}Tc) pertechnetate which is trapped like iodide in the thyroid gland. Images of the thyroid are acquired beginning 20-40 minutes after injection. If radioactive iodine is employed, the dose of either iodine-131 or iodine-123 is given orally and images are acquired at 6 or 24 hours. Either ^{99m}Tc or iodine scans are often combined with radioiodine uptake measurements.

Indications Thyroid imaging is useful in evaluating the location, approximate size, anatomy, and functional status of the thyroid gland. This is especially helpful for thyroid nodules, multinodular goiter, thyroiditis, and possible ectopic thyroid tissue (eg, lingual or mediastinal).

Patient Preparation The patient should have all RIA blood work performed, or at least drawn, prior to injection of any radioactive material. Patients should be fasting for at least 2 hours before receiving oral radioiodine. There are no

(Continued)

Thyroid Scan *(Continued)*

special preparations for ^{99m}Tc scans. Any recently ingested iodine or radiographic procedures using iodinated contrast may suppress radioiodine or ^{99m}Tc localization in the thyroid gland. Refer to Limitations.

Special Instructions Requisition must state the current patient diagnosis in order to select the most appropriate radiopharmaceutical and/or imaging technique.

Duration of Procedure: 30 minutes to 1 hour

Radiopharmaceutical: ^{99m}Tc pertechnetate, iodine-131 or iodine-123 sodium iodide

Turnaround Time A written report will be sent to the patient's chart and/or to the referring physician.

Causes for Rejection Other recent Nuclear Medicine procedure may interfere. If uncertain, call the Nuclear Medicine Department. Recent radiographic procedure using iodinated contrast.

Normal Findings Homogeneous and symmetric distribution of activity throughout the thyroid gland

Limitations Iodine-containing compounds and foods interfere with any tests using radioactive iodine. The following exogenous iodine sources may suppress uptake measurements or scans for the time indicated:

- iodine compounds (Lugol's, tincture, potassium iodide, kelp): 1-2 weeks.
- seafood, Ovaltine®, vitamin pills, Ornade®, Combid® cough syrups: 3-5 days
- Diodrast, Hypaque®, Renografin® (ie, intravenous pyelograms, CT with contrast and arteriograms): 4-6 weeks
- lipiodol (ie, bronchograms), Oragrafin® (ie, gallbladder exams), Pantopaque® (ie, myelograms): at least 6 months
- antithyroid drugs (ie, propylthiouracil, Tapazole®): 7 days
- thyroid hormone (ie, desiccated thyroid, thyroxine): 4 weeks
- tri-iodothyronine (Cytomel®): 10-12 days

Call the Nuclear Medicine Department for further information.

Additional Information A variation of thyroid scanning is performed for detection of metastases from primary thyroid carcinoma. See Thyroid Metastatic Survey, Iodine-131 *on page 468*.

References

Alonso O, Lago G, Mut F, et al, "Thyroid Imaging With Tc-99m MIBI in Patients With Solitary Cold Single Nodules on Pertechnetate Imaging," *Clin Nucl Med*, 1996, 21(5):363-7.

Alonso O, Mut F, Lago G, et al, "Double-Phase Scanning of the Thyroid Gland With Tc-99m MIBI in a Patients With a Malignant Nodule: A Case of Tracer Redistribution?" *Clin Nucl Med*, 1997, 22(6):413-4.

Apostolopoulos DJ, Houstoulaki E, Giannakenas C, et al, "Technetium-99m-Tetrofosmin for Parathyroid Scintigraphy: Comparison to Thallium-Technetium Scanning," *J Nucl Med*, 1998, 39(8):1433-41.

Billotey C, Sarfati E, Aurengo A, et al, "Advantages of SPECT in Technetium-99m-Sestamibi Parathyroid Scintigraphy," *J Nucl Med*, 1996, 37(11):1773-8.

Fjeld JG, "Attribution of Use of Perchlorate in Parathyroid Scintigraphy," *J Nucl Med*, 1999, 40(10):1769.

Ishimura E, Okamura T, Masaki H, et al, "Amyloid Goiter: Radiological Study in a Case Presenting Hypothyroidism," *Horm Metab Res*, 1996, 28(1):27-31.

Kresnick E, Gallowitsch HJ, Mikosch P, et al, "Technetium-99m-MIBI Scintigraphy of Thyroid Nodules in an Endemic Goiter Area," *J Nucl Med*, 1997, 38(1):62-5.

Leslie WK, Riese KT, Guzman R, et al, "Technetium-99m-Pertechnetate Uptake by Intrathyroidal Parathyroid Adenoma," *J Nucl Med*, 1996, 37(5):861-2.

McHenry CR, Lee K, Saadey J, et al, "Parathyroid Localization With Technetium-99m-Sestamibi: A Prospective Evaluation," *J Am Coll Surg*, 1996, 183(1):25-30.

Vattimo A, Bertelli P, Cintorino M, et al, "Hurthle Cell Tumor Dwelling in hot Thyroid Nodules: Preoperative Detection With Technetium-99m-MIBI Dual-Phase Scintigraphy," *J Nucl Med*, 1998, 39(5):822-5.

♦ **Thyroid Scan and Uptake** *see* Thyroid Scan *on page 469*

♦ **Thyroid Scintigraphy** *see* Thyroid Scan *on page 469*

♦ **Thyroid Suppression Test** *see* Thyroid Uptake *on page 471*

♦ **Thyroid TSH Stimulation Test** *see* Thyroid Uptake *on page 471*

Thyroid Uptake

Synonyms Radioactive Iodine Uptake; Radioiodine Thyroid Uptake and/or Scan; RAI Uptake and/or Scan; Thyroid Uptake and Scan; Uptake and Scan, 6- and/or 24-Hour

Applies to Perchlorate Discharge Test; Thyroid Suppression Test; Thyroid TSH Stimulation Test; Thyroid Uptake and Thyroid Scanning

Procedure Commonly Includes A small oral dose of radioiodine is administered to the patient. A calculation of uptake by the thyroid gland is made at 4-6 hours and/or at 24 hours by measuring the radioactivity present in the anterior neck over the gland. This procedure usually involves a thyroid scan also.

Indications The thyroid uptake directly measures the ability of the thyroid gland to trap and organify circulating iodide. Uptake measurements accurately detect and quantify the effects of thyroid disease. Uptake values are used in conjunction with measurement of circulating thyroid hormone levels to differentiate primary and secondary causes of these conditions. They are also used to plan therapy for thyroid disorders, especially therapy involving larger doses of radioiodine. Serial uptake measurements are helpful in long-term management and follow-up of patients.

Patient Preparation The patient should have all RIA blood work performed, or at least drawn, prior to injection of any radioactive material. Patients should be fasting for at least 2 hours before receiving the oral radioiodine dose. They may resume their normal diet 1 hour after the dose is given but should avoid iodine ingestion in food or medications for the duration of the procedure. Any recently ingested iodine or radiographic procedures using iodinated contrast may suppress uptake measurements. Refer to Limitations. Thyroid suppression, thyroid stimulation, and perchlorate discharge tests involve measurement of baseline thyroid uptake, then pharmacologic intervention, then repeat uptake measurement. Call the Nuclear Medicine Department for consultation when ordering these tests.

Special Instructions Requisition must state the current patient diagnosis in order to select the most appropriate radiopharmaceutical and/or imaging technique.

Duration of Procedure: 24 hours

Radiopharmaceutical: Iodine-131 or iodine-123 sodium iodide

Turnaround Time A written report will be sent to the patient's chart and/or to the referring physician at the completion of the procedure.

Causes for Rejection Other recent Nuclear Medicine procedure may interfere. If uncertain, call the Nuclear Medicine Department.

Normal Findings Normal values cover a wide range and are somewhat dependent on local variations in dietary iodine consumption by the population and technical differences between laboratories. An approximate normal range is 5% to 15% at 4-6 hours and 10% to 30% at 24 hours. Normal ranges have gradually decreased in the last 50 years due to progressive increases in dietary iodine sources.

Limitations Iodine-containing compounds and foods interfere with any tests using radioactive iodine. The following exogenous iodine sources may suppress uptake measurements or scans for the time indicated:

- iodine compounds (Lugol's, tincture, potassium iodide, kelp): 1-2 weeks
- seafood, Ovaltine®, vitamin pills, Ornade®, Combid® cough syrups: 3-5 days
- Diodrast, Hypaque®, Renografin® (ie, intravenous pyelograms, CT with contrast and arteriograms): 4-6 weeks
- lipiodol (ie, bronchograms), Oragrafin® (ie, gallbladder exams), Pantopaque® (ie, myelograms): at least 6 months
- antithyroid drugs (ie, propylthiouracil, Tapazole®): 7 days
- thyroid hormone (ie, desiccated thyroid, thyroxine): 4 weeks
- tri-iodothyronine (Cytomel®): 10-12 days

Call the Nuclear Medicine Department for further information.

Additional Information If iodine-131 treatment of hyperthyroidism is anticipated at a future date, notify the Nuclear Medicine Department when making appointment for uptake and scan. See table.

(Continued)

Thyroid Uptake *(Continued)*

Special Tests of Thyroid Function

Test	Intervention	Use
Thyroid suppression	24-hour uptake; triiodothyronine (T_3) 24 μg/day orally for 8 days; uptake repeated	Assess borderline hyperthyroidism, autonomy of functioning nodules or diffuse enlargement
Thyroid stimulation	24-hour uptake; thyroid stimulating hormone (TSH) 10 IU/day for 3 days; uptake repeated	Differentiate between primary vs secondary hypothyroidism; identify thyroid tissue (by scanning) suppressed by autonomously functioning nodules
Perchlorate discharge	2-hour uptake; potassium perchlorate 1 g orally; uptake repeated hourly for 2 hours	Measures dissociation between trapping and organification of iodide: congenital or acquired defects

These interventions are approximate and may vary in individual departments.

References

Anderson BG and Powsner RA, "Stability of Values for Thyroid Radioiodine Uptake," *J Nucl Med*, 1996, 37(5):805-6.

Farahati J, Bier D, Scheubeck M, et al, "Effect of Specific Activity on Cardiac Uptake of Iodine-123-MIBG," *J Nucl Med*, 1997, 38(3):447-51.

Ross DS, "Syndromes of Thyrotoxicosis With Low Radioactive Iodine Uptake," *Endocrinol Metab Clin North Am*, 1998, 27(1):169-85.

Roti E, Minelli R, Giuberti T, et al, "Multiple Changes in Thyroid Function in Patient's With Chronic Active HCV Hepatitis Treated With Recombinant Interferon-Alpha," *Am J Med*, 1996, 101(5):482-7.

Slatosky J, Shipton B, and Wahba H, "Thyroiditis: Differential Diagnosis and Management," *Am Fam Physician*, 2000, 61(4):1047-52, 1054.

Vemulakonda US, Atkins FB, and Ziessman HA, "Therapy Dose Calculation in Grave's Disease Using Early I-123 Uptake Measurements," *Clin Nucl Med*, 1996, 21(2):102-5.

♦ **Thyroid Uptake and Scan** *see* Thyroid Uptake *on page 471*

♦ **Thyroid Uptake and Thyroid Scanning** *see* Thyroid Scan *on page 469*

♦ **Thyroid Uptake and Thyroid Scanning** *see* Thyroid Uptake *on page 471*

♦ **Total Blood Volume** *see* Blood Volume *on page 439*

♦ **Triple Phase Renal Scan (Renogram, Renal Flow and Scan)** *see* Renal Scan *on page 463*

♦ **Uptake and Scan, 6- and/or 24-Hour** *see* Thyroid Uptake *on page 471*

♦ **Vascular Dynamic Study** *see* Angiogram, Radionuclide *on page 437*

♦ **Vascular Flow Study** *see* Angiogram, Radionuclide *on page 437*

♦ **VCU** *see* Voiding Cystourethrogram, Radionuclide *on page 473*

♦ **VCUG** *see* Voiding Cystourethrogram, Radionuclide *on page 473*

Venogram, Radionuclide

Related Information

Cardiac Blood Pool Scan, EKG-Gated *on page 442*

Synonyms Isotope Venogram; Lower Extremity Venogram, Radionuclide; Phlebothrombogram, Radionuclide; Radioactive Venogram; Thrombophlebogram, Radionuclide

Procedure Commonly Includes The patient receives an intravenous injection by one of the following techniques:

- via a vein in the dorsum of each foot with rapid sequence image acquisition of the venous structures of the lower extremities during and immediately following injection; the radiopharmaceutical is usually technetium-99m (^{99m}Tc) MAA and the procedure is usually performed as part of a perfusion lung scan.
- via an arm vein with static images of the lower extremities acquired at equilibrium; the radiopharmaceutical is usually ^{99m}Tc pertechnetate to radiolabel circulating RBC (See Cardiac Blood Pool Scan, EKG-Gated *on page 442*.)

Indications Radionuclide venography is used as a screening test for detecting deep vein thrombosis of the lower extremities. It can be performed in patients who are allergic to iodinated radiographic contrast media.

Patient Preparation The patient does not need to be fasting or NPO for this procedure. The patient should have all RIA blood work performed, or at least drawn, prior to the injection of any radioactive material.

Special Instructions Requisition must state the current patient diagnosis in order to select the most appropriate radiopharmaceutical and/or imaging technique.

Duration of Procedure: 1 hour

Radiopharmaceutical: ^{99m}Tc labeled RBC or ^{99m}Tc MAA

Turnaround Time A written report will be sent to the patient's chart and/or to the referring physician.

Causes for Rejection Other recent Nuclear Medicine procedure may interfere. If uncertain, call the Nuclear Medicine Department.

Normal Findings Symmetric visualization of deep and superficial large venous structures in the lower extremities

Limitations Radionuclide venograms have less specificity and less sensitivity than radiographic contrast venograms. It can be difficult to differentiate acute thrombosis from patients with chronic changes due to previous thrombotic disease.

References

Dalsing MC, Raju S, Wakefield TW, et al, "A Multicenter, Phase I Evaluation of Cryopreserved Venous Valve Allografts for the Treatment of Chronic Deep Venous Insufficiency," *J Vasc Surg*, 1999, 30(5):854-64.

Graf O, Boland GW, Kaufman JA, et al, "Anatomic Variants of Mesenteric Veins: Depiction With Helical CT Venography," *AJR Am J Roentgenol*, 1997, 168(5):1209-13.

Katz MG, Khazin V, Steinmetz A, et al, "Distribution of Cerebral Flow Using Retrograde Versus Antegrade Cerebral Perfusion," *Ann Thorac Surg*, 1999, 67(4):1065-9.

Laissy JP, Cinqualbre A, Loshkajian A, et al, "Assessment of Deep Venous Thrombosis in the Lower Limbs and Pelvis: MR Venography Versus Duplex Doppler Sonography," *AJR Am J Roentgenol*, 1996, 167(4):971-5.

Leclerc JR, Wolfson C, Arzoumanian A, et al, "Technetium-99m Red Blood Cell Venography in Patients With Clinically Suspected Deep Vein Thrombosis: A Prospective Study," *J Nucl Med*, 1988, 29(9):1498-506.

Menegazzo D, Laissy JP, Durrbach A, et al, "Hemodialysis Access Fistula Creation: Preoperative Assessment With MR Venography and Comparison With Conventional Venography," *Radiology*, 1998, 209(3):723-8.

Ozsvath RR, Casey SO, Lustrin ES, et al, "Cerebral Venography: Comparison of CT and MR Projection Venography," *AJR Am J Roentgenol*, 1997, 169(6):1699-707.

Raju S, Fountain T, Neglen P, et al, "Axial Transformation of the Profunda Femoris Vein," *J Vasc Surg*, 1998, 27(4):651-9.

Rudavsky AZ, "Radionuclide Angiography in the Evaluation of Arterial and Venous Grafts," *Semin Nucl Med*, 1988, 18(3):261-8.

Screaton NJ, Gillard JH, Berman LH, et al, "Duplicated Superficial Femoral Veins: A Source of Error in the Sonographic Investigation of Deep Vein Thrombosis," *Radiology*, 1998, 206(2):397-401.

Westrich GH, Allen ML, Tarantino SJ, et al, "Ultrasound Screening for Deep Venous Thrombosis After Total Knee Arthroplasty. 2-Year Reassessment," *Clin Orthop*, 1998, (356):125-33.

Wildberger JE, Vorwerk D, Kilbinger M, et al, "Bedside Testing (SimpliRED) in the Diagnosis of Deep Vein Thrombosis. Evaluation of 250 Patients," *Invest Radiol*, 1998, 33(4):232-5.

♦ **Ventilation Lung Scan** *see* Lung Scan, Ventilation *on page 454*

♦ **Ventilation-Perfusion Lung Scan** *see* Lung Scan, Perfusion *on page 453*

♦ **Ventilation-Perfusion Lung Scan** *see* Lung Scan, Ventilation *on page 454*

♦ **Vitamin B_{12} Absorption Test** *see* Schilling Test *on page 466*

Voiding Cystourethrogram, Radionuclide

Synonyms Bladder Reflux Study; VCU; VCUG

Procedure Commonly Includes The patient must have an indwelling urinary bladder catheter in place. A dose of technetium-99m (^{99m}Tc) pertechnetate is instilled into the bladder along with a maximally tolerated volume of sterile normal saline solution via the catheter. Sequential static images of the bladder and ureters are acquired during the filling, postfilling, voiding, and postvoiding phases to detect retrograde vesicoureteral reflux from the bladder and/or abnormally high postvoid residual volume.

(Continued)

Voiding Cystourethrogram, Radionuclide *(Continued)*

Indications The radionuclide VCUG is a useful procedure for the detection and follow-up of pediatric patients with bladder reflux causing recurrent urinary tract infections. The radionuclide study is more sensitive than a radiographic contrast VCUG and imparts only approximately 10% of the radiation dose. However, a contrast VCUG is often recommended at the time of diagnosis of reflux to better delineate any anatomic abnormalities. The radionuclide procedure is then used as the primary follow-up technique for these patients, many of whom will outgrow their reflux and not require surgical intervention.

Patient Preparation The patient does not need to be fasting or NPO for this procedure. The patient should have all RIA blood work performed, or at least drawn, prior to the injection of any radioactive material.

Special Instructions Requisition must state the current patient diagnosis in order to select the most appropriate radiopharmaceutical and/or imaging technique.

Duration of Procedure: 30 minutes
Radiopharmaceutical: ^{99m}Tc pertechnetate

Turnaround Time A written report will be sent to the patient's chart and/or to the referring physician.

Causes for Rejection Other recent Nuclear Medicine procedure may interfere. If uncertain, call the Nuclear Medicine Department.

Normal Findings Normal bladder activity which clears upon voiding with no reflux into ureters or significant bladder residual volume

Limitations The radionuclide VCUG had less anatomic resolution than the radiographic contrast technique but is more sensitive and has a lower radiation exposure to the patient.

References

Cilento BG Jr, Bauer SB, Retik AB, et al, "Urachal Anomalies: Defining the Best Diagnostic Modality," *Urology*, 1998, 52(1):120-2.

Corrales JG and Elder JS, "Segmental Multicystic Kidney and Ipsilateral Duplication Anomalies," *J Urol*, 1997, 157(1):267.

Dremsek PA, Gindi K, Voitl P, et al, "Renal Pyelectasis in Fetuses and Neonates: Diagnostic Value of Renal Pelvis Diameter in Pre- and Postnatal Sonographic Screening," *AJR Am J Roentgenol*, 1997, 168(4):1017-9.

Fielding JR, Lee JH, Dubeau CE, et al, "Voiding Cystourethrography Findings in Elderly Women With Urge Incontinence," *J Urol*, 2000, 163(4):1216-8.

Glazier DB, Whang MI, Geffner SR, et al, "Evaluation of Voiding Cystourethrography Prior to Renal Transplantation," *Transplantation*, 1996, 62(12):1762-5.

Hellerstein S, "Urinary Tract Infections in Children: Why They Occur and How to Prevent Them," *Am Fam Physician*, 1998, 57(10):2440-6, 2452-4.

Mesrobian HG, Zacharias A, Balcom AH, et al, "Ten Years of Experience With Isolated Urachal Anomalies in Children," *J Urol*, 1997, 158(3 Pt 2):1316-8.

Puri P, Cascio S, Lakshmandass G, et al, "Urinary Tract Infection and Renal Damage in Sibling Vesicoureteral Reflux," *J Urol*, 1998, 160(3 Pt 2):1028-30, 1038.

Shandera KC, Rozanski TA, and Jaffers G, "The Necessity of Voiding Cystourethrogram in the Pretransplant Urologic Evaluation," *Urology*, 1996, 47(2):198-200.

Strife JL, Bissett GS, Kirks DR, et al, "Nuclear Cystography and Renal Sonography: Findings in Girls With Urinary Tract Infections," *AJR Am J Roentgenol*, 1989, 153(1):115-9.

Sty JR and Wells RG, "Radionuclide Cystography," *Nucl Med Ann*, 1990, 223-38.

Summerville DA and Treves ST, "Radionuclide Detection of Vesicoureteral Reflux," *Current Concepts Diagn Nucl Med*, 1986, 3:4-9.

- ♦ **V/Q Scan** *see* Lung Scan, Perfusion *on page 453*
- ♦ **Wall Motion Study** *see* Cardiac Blood Pool Scan, EKG-Gated *on page 442*
- ♦ **WBC Scan** *see* Indium Leukocyte Scan *on page 450*
- ♦ **White Blood Cell Scan** *see* Indium Leukocyte Scan *on page 450*
- ♦ **Whole Body Bone Scan** *see* Bone Scan *on page 440*
- ♦ **Xenon Lung Scan** *see* Lung Scan, Ventilation *on page 454*

ULTRASOUND

- ♦ **Penile Ultrasound** *see* Ultrasound, Penile Duplex *on page 500*
- ♦ **Percutaneous Nephrostomy** *see* Ultrasound, Nephrostomy, Guided *on page 494*
- ♦ **Peripheral Arteries and Veins Ultrasound** *see* Ultrasound, Peripheral Arteries and Veins *on page 501*
- ♦ **Popliteal Ultrasound** *see* Ultrasound, Peripheral Arteries and Veins *on page 501*
- ♦ **Pregnancy, Complete Sonogram** *see* Ultrasound, OB, Limited *on page 496*
- ♦ **Pregnancy, Echo** *see* Ultrasound, OB, Limited *on page 496*
- ♦ **Prostate Ultrasound** *see* Ultrasound, Prostate *on page 501*
- ♦ **Radiotherapy Plan Ultrasound** *see* Ultrasound, Radiotherapy Plan *on page 502*
- ♦ **RADS** *see* Ultrasound, Renal Artery *on page 503*
- ♦ **Renal Artery Duplex Scanning** *see* Ultrasound, Renal Artery *on page 503*
- ♦ **Renal Artery Ultrasound** *see* Ultrasound, Renal Artery *on page 503*
- ♦ **Renal Biopsy Ultrasound** *see* Ultrasound, Kidney Biopsy *on page 491*
- ♦ **Renal Cyst Puncture Ultrasound** *see* Ultrasound, Kidney Cyst Puncture *on page 492*
- ♦ **Renal Transplant Ultrasound** *see* Ultrasound, Renal Transplant *on page 503*
- ♦ **Renal Ultrasound** *see* Ultrasound, Kidneys *on page 493*
- ♦ **RUQ** *see* Ultrasound, Hepatic *on page 488*
- ♦ **Spleen Ultrasound** *see* Ultrasound, Spleen *on page 505*
- ♦ **Superficial Soft Tissue Mass Ultrasound** *see* Ultrasound, Soft Tissue Mass *on page 504*
- ♦ **Testicular Ultrasound** *see* Ultrasound, Testicular *on page 506*
- ♦ **Thoracentesis Ultrasound** *see* Ultrasound, Thoracentesis *on page 506*
- ♦ **Thyroid Ultrasound** *see* Ultrasound, Thyroid *on page 507*
- ♦ **Transrectal Ultrasound** *see* Ultrasound, Endorectal *on page 485*
- ♦ **Transvaginal Ultrasound** *see* Ultrasound, Transvaginal *on page 509*

Ultrasound, Abdomen

Synonyms Abdomen Ultrasound

Applies to Follow-up Ultrasound Abdomen; Follow-up Ultrasound Retroperitoneal; Ultrasound Retroperitoneal

Procedure Commonly Includes Liver, spleen, gallbladder, pancreas, and biliary tree

Indications Presence of neoplasms, cystic lesions, enlarged lymph nodes, bile ducts, abdominal abscesses, pancreatic mass or pseudocysts, gallbladder calculi, or any malignancies

Contraindications

- open wound or incision overlying examination area
- recent barium study

Patient Preparation The patient should not have had a barium study within the 3 days prior to study. The examinations may be up to 1 hour each. An emergency exam or an unpredictably long preceding exam may result in additional delay. **Note**: Ultrasound exam is to be scheduled before endoscopy, endoscopic retrograde cholangiopancreatography, colonoscopy, or a barium study. If barium study was done, bowel preparation is needed before doing ultrasound examination. **No** barium studies should have been done for **at least** 2 days preceding exam. NPO after midnight before day of examination.

Special Instructions All outpatient examinations are by appointment only. All inpatients are placed on the daily schedule as time permits and are performed as scheduled. Nonemergent examinations are given secondary priority and therefore may not be able to be performed the same day scheduled. Patients will generally be asked to stay after the examination until films are reviewed by the radiologist. Instruct the patient that ultrasound uses sound waves to image the different organs. There is **no** radiation involved, therefore, it is not harmful to the patient.

Equipment Standard B-mode real time ultrasonic imager with 2-5 MHz transducer

Technique A gel is applied to the skin and a handheld transducer is swept across the abdomen to image the appropriate organs. Sound waves are used for the imaging and no radiation exposure is present. Images are recorded on x-ray film.

Data Acquired Transverse, sagittal, and oblique images of upper abdominal organs

Turnaround Time A typed report will generally be issued within 36 hours. A preliminary verbal report generally can be given to the referring physician on request.

Causes for Rejection Bowel gas, barium, eating or drinking, unresponsive or poorly responsive patient, open wound(s) overlying area of study

Normal Findings Absence of abnormal masses, fluid collections, enlarged structures, or calcifications

Additional Information Request for this study will result in imaging of liver, gallbladder, pancreas, and spleen. Individual study of any of these organs can be ordered as a specific examination (eg, gallbladder, ultrasound). Solid and cystic abnormalities of each of these organs may be detected as well as adenopathy or retroperitoneal masses. It is not uncommon to be unable to visualize the pancreas and/or retroperitoneum in its entirety due to overlying bowel gas. Common abnormalities detected by this modality include cholelithiasis, biliary tree dilatation, primary carcinomas of liver, gallbladder, and pancreas as well as metastatic disease to any organ studied. Ascites is also readily detected as well as inflammatory masses or collections.

References

Ballard RB, Rozycki GS, Newman PG, et al, "An Algorithm to Reduce the Incidence of False-Negative FAST Examinations in Patients at High Risk for Occult Injury. Focused Assessment for the Sonographic Examination of the Trauma Patient," *J Am Coll Surg*, 1999, 189(2):145-50.

Bernardino ME, "The Liver: Anatomy and Examination Techniques," *Lippindiology*, Taveras JT and Ferrucci JT, eds, Philadelphia, PA: Lippincott Williams & Wilkins, 1988.

Chao HC and Kong MS, "Sonographic Diagnosis of Mesenteric Hematoma," *J Clin Ultrasound*, 1999, 27(5):284-6.

Cooperberg PL and Rowley VA, "Abdominal Sonographic Examination Technique," *Radiology*, Taveras JT and Ferrucci JT, eds, Philadelphia, PA: Lippincott Williams & Wilkins, 1988.

Fisher AJ, Paulson EK, Sheafor DH, et al, "Small Lymph Nodes of the Abdomen, Pelvis, and Retroperitoneum: Usefulness of Sonographically Guided Biopsy," *Radiology*, 1997, 205(1):185-90.

Frezza EE, Solis RL, Silich RJ, et al, "Competency-Based Instruction to Improve the Surgical Resident Technique and Accuracy of the Trauma Ultrasound," *Am J Surg*, 1999, 65(9):884-8.

Gardeil F, Greene R, Stuart B, et al, "Subcutaneous Fat in the Fetal Abdomen as a Predictor of Growth Restriction," *Obstet Gynecol*, 1999, 94(2):209-12.

Goldberg BB, *Abdominal Ultrasonography*, New York, NY: John Wiley and Sons Inc, 1984.

Memel DS, Dodd GD 3rd, and Esola CC, "Efficacy of Sonography as a Guidance Technique for Biopsy of Abdominal, Pelvic, and Retroperitoneal Lymph Nodes," *AJR Am J Roentgenol*, 1996, 167(4):957-62.

Netzer P, Binek J, Hammer B, et al, "Utility of Abdominal Sonography in Patients With Idiopathic Deep Vein Thrombosis," *J Clin Ultrasound*, 1999, 27(4):177-81.

Petrikovsky BM, Oleschuk C, Lesser M, et al, "Prediction of Fetal Macrosomia Using Sonographically Measured Abdominal Subcutaneous Tissue Thickness," *J Clin Ultrasound*, 1997, 25(7):378-82.

Tous F and Busto M, "Assessment of Abdominal Sonography in the Diagnosis of Tumors of the Gastroduodenal Tract," *J Clin Ultrasound*, 1997, 25(5):243-7.

Ultrasound, Abscess Drainage, Guided

Synonyms Aspiration, Ultrasound Guided; Drainage, Ultrasound Guided

Procedure Commonly Includes The location of abnormal fluid collections and insertion of needle and/or drain into the collection.

Indications Diagnostic aspiration of fluid, therapeutic drainage of fluid

Contraindications

- inadequate access by ultrasound
- bleeding diathesis

Patient Preparation NPO for 2 hours prior to examination. Referring physician may desire pretreatment with prophylactic I.V. antibiotics.

Aftercare Check physician order sheet. Monitor vital signs in department for 1-hour postprocedure.

Special Instructions Inpatients only. All procedures are scheduled after consultation with a radiologist. All inpatients are placed on an on call

(Continued)

Ultrasound, Abscess Drainage, Guided *(Continued)*

schedule. After hours, approval is given by the radiologist on call. Recent (less than 2 weeks) PT and PTT results should be available at the time of the procedure.

Complications Hemorrhage, sepsis

Equipment Standard B-mode real time ultrasonic imager with 2-5 MHz transducer and biopsy guides if desired. Appropriate aspiration needle (18- to 22-gauge) and drain (5-11 F).

Technique A gel is applied to the skin and a handheld transducer is swept across the area of interest to image the appropriate organs. Sound waves are used for the imaging and no radiation exposure is present. An appropriate access route is chosen and a needle is placed into the abnormal collection. Local anesthesia as well as I.V. analgesia may be given. Images are recorded on x-ray film.

Turnaround Time A typed report will generally be issued within 36 hours. A preliminary verbal report generally can be given to the referring physician on request.

Specimen Fluid aspirated from abnormal collection

Container Aerobic and anaerobic culture containers

Storage Instructions Culture containers should be sent immediately to the Bacteriology Laboratory.

Causes for Rejection Contamination of cutaneous entry site, needle traversing bowel, patient unable to remain motionless during the procedure

Limitations Fluid unable to be obtained due to inadequate access or increased viscosity

Additional Information If therapeutic, this procedure may preclude the need for surgery.

References

Cardinal E, Chhem RK, and Beauregard CG, "Ultrasound-Guided Interventional Procedures in the Musculoskeletal System," *Radiol Clin North Am*, 1998, 36(3):597-604.

Chang KJ and Wiersema MJ, "Endoscopic Ultrasound-Guided Fine-Needle Aspiration Biopsy and Interventional Endoscopic Ultrasonography. Emerging Technologies," *Gastrointest Endosc Clin N Am*, 1997, 7(2):221-35.

Collado A, Palou J, Garcia-Penit J, et al, "Ultrasound-Guided Needle Aspiration in Prostatic Abscess," *Urology*, 1999, 53(3):548-52.

Fornage BD, "Sonographically Guided Needle Biopsy of Nonpalpable Breast Lesions," *J Clin Ultrasound*, 1999, 27(7):385-98.

Heneghan JP, Everts RJ, and Nelson RC, "Multiple Fluid Collections: CT- or US-Guided Aspiration - Evaluation of Microbiologic Results and Implications for Clinical Practice," *Radiology*, 1999, 212(3):669-72.

Hook GW and Ikeda DM, "Treatment of Breast Abscesses With US-Guided Percutaneous Needle Drainage Without Indwelling Catheter Placement," *Radiology*, 1999, 213(2):579-82.

McGahan JP, Brown B, Jones CD, et al, "Pelvic Abscesses: Transvaginal US-Guided Drainage With the Trocar Method," *Radiology*, 1996, 200(2):579-81.

Mueller PR and Van Sonnenberg EV, "Abscesses and Fluid Collections: Detection and Drainage," *Radiology*, Taveras JT and Ferrucci JT, eds, Philadelphia, PA: Lippincott Williams & Wilkins, 1988.

Rajak CL, Gupta S, Jain S, et al, "Percutaneous Treatment of Liver Abscesses: Needle Aspiration Versus Catheter Drainage," *AJR Am J Roentgenol*, 1998, 170(4):1035-9.

Rifkin MD and Goldberg BB, "Aspiration and Biopsy Techniques," *Abdominal Ultrasonography*, 2nd ed, Goldberg BB, ed, New York, NY: John Wiley and Sons Inc, 1984.

Sivarajasingam V, Sharma V, Crean SJ, et al, "Ultrasound-Guided Needle Aspiration of Lateral Masticator Space Abscess," *Oral Surg Oral Med Oral Pathol Oral Radiol Endod*, 1999, 88(5):616-9.

Sperling DC, Needleman L, Eschelman DJ, et al, "Deep Pelvic Abscesses: Transperineal US-Guided Drainage," *Radiology*, 1998, 208(1):111-5.

Staren ED and O'Neill TP, "Ultrasound-Guided Needle Biopsy of the Breast," *Surgery*, 1999, 126(4):629-34.

Takashima S, Sone S, Nomura N, et al, "Nonpalpable Lymph Nodes of the Neck: Assessment With US and US-Guided Fine-Needle Aspiration Biopsy," *J Clin Ultrasound*, 1997, 25(6):283-92.

Ultrasound, Amniocentesis

Synonyms Amniocentesis Ultrasound

Procedure Commonly Includes Locating appropriate puncture site for amniocentesis and subsequent performance of amniocentesis under direct visualization.

Indications Used in the last two trimesters of pregnancy to determine postmaturation, deformities, Rh incompatibility, amniotic fluid bilirubin level, amniotic fluid L/S ratio, amniotic fluid α-fetoprotein level, and genetic malformations

Contraindications
- inadequate amount of fluid
- anterior placenta
- presence of fetal vertex or trunk in needle path

Patient Preparation The examination may be long, up to 1 hour including waiting time. An emergency examination or an unpredictably long preceding examination may result in additional delay. **Note**: Each Rh-negative unsensitized woman whose husband is not known to be Rh-negative should receive Rh immune globulin.

Special Instructions The patient is brought to Radiology and the procedure is performed by a radiologist or obstetrician with the aid of ultrasound. The patient is required to stay in the hospital for a few hours for precautionary measures.

Complications Pain, amnionitis (infection), abortion, hemorrhage, trauma to fetus, rupture of membranes, placental or subchorionic hematoma, Rh sensitization, premature labor, abruptio placenta, maternal death

Equipment Standard B-mode real time ultrasonic imager with 2-5 MHz transducer. Biopsy guide if desired; 20- or 22-gauge spinal needle.

Technique Under ultrasound guidance, an appropriate location is found to insert a small needle into the amniotic fluid. The skin is marked appropriately and prepared for placement of the needle using sterile technique. Needle is placed and amniotic fluid aspirated.

Data Acquired Images of area to be sampled

Turnaround Time A typed report will generally be issued within 36 hours. A preliminary verbal report generally can be given to the referring physician on request.

Specimen Amniotic fluid

Causes for Rejection Patient unable to tolerate exam

Normal Findings Successful aspiration of adequate amount of amniotic fluid

Limitations Amniotic fluid not obtainable due to placenta location or lack of suitable puncture site, little or no amniotic fluid available for amniocentesis

References

Guariglia L and Rosata P, "Isolated Mild Fetal Pyelectasis Detected by Transvaginal Sonography in Advanced Maternal Age," *Obstet Gynecol*, 1998, 92(5):833-6.

Hendrix NW and Chauhan SP, "Sonographic Examination of Twins. From First Trimester to Delivery of Second Fetus," *Obstet Gynecol Clin North Am*, 1998, 25(3):609-21.

Lennon CA and Gray DL, "Sensitivity and Specificity of Ultrasound for the Detection of Neural Tube and Ventral Wall Defects in a High-Risk Population," *Obstet Gynecol*, 1999, 94(4):562-6.

Maher JE, Kleinman GE, Lile W, et al, "The Construction and Utility of an Amniocentesis Trainer," *Am J Obstet Gynecol*, 1998, 179(5):1225-7.

Malone FD, Marino T, Bianchi DW, et al, "Isolated Clubfoot Diagnosed Prenatally: Is Karotyping Indicated?" *Obstet Gynecol*, 2000, 95(3):437-40.

Platt LO, Hill LM, DeVore GR, et al, "Amniocentesis: Current Concepts and Techniques," *The Principles and Practice of Ultrasonography in Obstetrics Gynecology*, Sanders and James, eds, Norwalk, CT: Appleton-Century-Crofts, 1985.

Smith JF Jr, Bergmann M, Gildersleeve R, et al, "A Simple Model for Learning Stereotactic Skills in Ultrasound-Guided Amniocentesis," *Obstet Gynecol*, 1998, 92(2):303-5.

Vintzileos AM, Campbell WA, Rodis JF, et al, "The Use of Second-Trimester Genetic Sonogram in Guiding Clinical Management of Patients at Increased Risk for Fetal Trisomy 21," *Obstet Gynecol*, 1996, 87(6):948-52.

Ultrasound, Aorta

Synonyms Aorta Ultrasound

Procedure Commonly Includes Abdominal aorta and proximal iliac arteries

Indications Determine the presence and size of aortic aneurysms

Contraindications Recent barium study

Patient Preparation The patient is held NPO at midnight. Please inform all patients that the examinations may be up to 1 hour including waiting time. An emergency exam or an unpredictably long preceding exam may result in additional delay. **Note**: Ultrasound exam is to be scheduled before endoscopy, endoscopic retrograde cholangiopancreatography, colonoscopy, or a barium study. If a barium study was done, bowel preparation is needed before

(Continued)

Ultrasound, Aorta *(Continued)*

doing ultrasound examination. **No** barium studies should have been done for **at least** 2 days preceding exam.

Special Instructions All outpatient exams are by appointment only. All inpatients are placed on a daily schedule and called for exam in order of priority. After hours, approval is given by the radiologist on call. Instruct the patient that ultrasound uses sound waves to image the different organs. There is **no** radiation involved, therefore, it is not harmful to the patient. The patient may be asked to wait until the films are checked to make sure more are not necessary.

Equipment Standard B-mode real time ultrasonic imager with 2-5 MHz transducer

Technique A gel is applied to the skin and a handheld transducer is swept across the aorta to image the appropriate organs. Sound waves are used for the imaging and no radiation exposure is present. Images are recorded on x-ray film.

Data Acquired Transverse and longitudinal images of abdominal aorta and bifurcation

Turnaround Time A typed report will be generated within 36 hours. A preliminary verbal report will be given to the referring physician upon request.

Causes for Rejection Bowel gas, barium, eating or drinking

Normal Findings ≤3 cm maximal transverse diameter

Critical Values Maximal transverse diameter >3 cm

Additional Information Ultrasound is a useful modality to evaluate for presence of an abdominal aortic aneurysm, particularly involving the distal aorta. Evaluation of the proximal abdominal aorta may be problematic due to overlying bowel gas.

References

Buck T, Gorge G, Hunold P, et al, "Three-Dimensional Imaging in Aortic Disease by Lighthouse Transesophageal Echocardiography Using Intravascular Ultrasound Catheters. Comparison to Three-Dimensional Transesophageal Echocardiography and Three-Dimensional Intra-aortic Ultrasound Imaging," *J Am Soc Echocardiogr*, 1998, 11(3):243-58.

Erturk H, Erden A, Yurdakul M, et al, "Pseudoaneurysm of the Abdominal Aorta Diagnosed by Color Duplex Doppler Sonography," *J Clin Ultrasound*, 1999, 27(4):202-5.

Evangelista A, Garcia-del-Castillo H, Gonzalez-Alujas T, et al, "Diagnosis of Ascending Aortic Dissection by Transesophageal Echocardiography: Utility of M-Mode in Recognizing Artifacts," *J Am Coll Cardiol*, 1996, 27(1):102-7.

Fox AD, Witeley MS, Murphy P, et al, "Comparison of Magnetic Resonance Imaging Measurements of Abdominal Aortic Aneurysms With Measurements Obtained by Other Imaging Techniques and Intraoperative Measurements: Possible Implications for Endovascular Grafting," *J Vasc Surg*, 1996, 24(4):632-8.

Gooding GA, "B-Mode and Duplex Examination of the Aorta, Iliac Arteries and Portal Vein," *Introduction to Vascular Ultrasonography*, Zweibel WJ, ed, New York, NY: Grune and Stratton Inc, 1986.

Kronzon I, Tunick PA, Rosen R, et al, "Ultrasound Evaluation of Endovascular Repair of Abdominal Aortic Aneurysms," *J Am Soc Echocardiogr*, 1998, 11(4):377-80.

Sato DT, Goff CD, Gregory RT, et al, "Endoleak After Aortic Stent Graft Repair: Diagnosis by Color Duplex Ultrasound Scan Versus Computed Tomography Scan," *J Vasc Surg*, 1998, 28(4):657-63.

Uflacker R, Horn J, Phillips G, et al, "Intravascular Sonography in the Assessment of Traumatic Injury of the Thoracic Aorta," *AJR Am J Roentgenol*, 1999, 173(3):665-70.

Vaduganathan P, Ewton A, Nagueh SF, et al, "Pathologic Correlates of Aortic Plaques, Thrombi and Mobile "Aortic Debris" Imaged *In Vivo* With Transesophageal Echocardiography," *J Am Coll Cardiol*, 1997, 30(2):357-63.

van Essen JA, Gussenhoven EJ, van der Lugt A, et al, "Accurate Assessment of Abdominal Aortic Aneurysm With Intravascular Ultrasound Scanning: Validation With Computed Tomographic Angiography," *J Vasc Surg*, 1999, 29(4):631-8.

van Essen JA, van der Lugt A, Gussenhoven EJ, et al, "Intravascular Ultrasonography Allows Accurate Assessment of Abdominal Aortic Aneurysm: An *In Vitro* Validation Study," *J Vasc Surg*, 1998, 27(2):347-53.

♦ **Ultrasound Aspiration** *see* Ultrasound, Biopsy Localization *on page 480*

Ultrasound, Biopsy Localization

Synonyms Biopsy Localization Ultrasound; Ultrasound Aspiration; Ultrasound Localization

Procedure Commonly Includes Localization of abnormal mass followed by biopsy under direct visualization.

Indications Cyst localization, organ or lesion biopsy or aspiration

Contraindications Bleeding diathesis

Patient Preparation NPO for 2 hours prior to examination. The procedure may take up to several hours depending on the complexity of any given individual case. PT and PTT are performed within 48 hours prior to procedure.

Aftercare Check physician order sheet. Monitor vital signs in department for 3 hours if patient is an outpatient, 1 hour iF patient is an inpatient.

Special Instructions All outpatient exams are by appointment only. All procedures are scheduled after consultation with radiologist. All inpatients are placed on a daily schedule and called for in order of priority. After hours, approval is given by the radiologist on call. Recent PT and PTT results should be available at time of procedure.

Complications Bleeding, infection

Equipment Standard B-mode real time ultrasonic imager with biopsy guide, 2-5 MHz transducer, aspiration or cutting type biopsy needle (18- to 22-gauge).

Technique A gel is applied to the skin and a handheld transducer is swept across the area of interest to image the appropriate organs. Sound waves are used for the imaging and no radiation exposure is present. An appropriate access route is chosen and a needle is placed into the abnormal collection. Local anesthesia as well as I.V. analgesia may be given. Images are recorded on x-ray film.

Data Acquired Tissue and/or fluid samples, images of area and/or organ biopsied

Turnaround Time A typed report will generally be issued within 36 hours. A preliminary verbal report generally can be given to the referring physician on request.

Specimen Fluid and/or tissue

Container Sterile saline, sterile slides for cytology, fixative for core tissue samples, culture tubes, tubes for chemistry evaluation

Sampling Time Immediate

Storage Instructions Samples should immediately be sent to the appropriate laboratory (ie, cytology, pathology, bacteriology).

Causes for Rejection Contamination by nonsterile object

Limitations Insufficient material for analysis, patient unable to remain still, lesion unable to be visualized secondary to overlying bowel gas

Additional Information Many abnormal masses in the abdomen are approachable by the percutaneous route. Exploratory laparotomy may be avoided and this procedure can be performed on an outpatient basis.

References

Arya S, Nagarkatti DG, Dudhat SB, et al, "Soft Tissue Sarcomas: Ultrasonographic Evaluation of Local Recurrences," *Clin Radiol*, 2000, 55(3):193-7.

Cleverly JR, Jackson AR, and Bateman AC, "Preoperative Localization of Breast Microcalcification Using High-Frequency Ultrasound," *Clin Radiol*, 1997, 52(12):924-6.

Naas K and O'Neill WC, "Bedside Renal Biopsy: Ultrasound Guidance by the Nephrologist," *Am J Kidney Dis*, 1999, 34(5):955-9.

Parker SH, Kercher JM, and Dennis MA, "Sonographically Guided Mammotome Extraction of Retained Localization Wire," *AJR AM J Roentgenol*, 1999, 173(4):903-4.

Rifkin MD and Goldberg BB, "Aspiration and Biopsy Techniques," *Abdominal Ultrasonography*, 2nd ed, Goldberg BB, ed, New York, NY: John Wiley and Sons Inc, 1984.

Rozycki GC, "Surgeon-Performed Ultrasound: Its Use in Clinical Practice," *Ann Surg*, 1998, 228(1):16-28.

Ultrasound, Breast

Synonyms Breast Ultrasound

Procedure Commonly Includes Specific area of breast which contains a mammographic abnormality.

Indications To differentiate solid from cystic lesions in the breast

Patient Preparation The examination may be long, up to 1 hour including waiting time. An emergency examination or an unpredictably long preceding examination may result in additional delay.

Special Instructions A recent mammogram **must** accompany the patient or be available at examination time. All outpatient examinations are by appointment only. All inpatients are placed on the daily schedule as time permits and are performed as scheduled. Nonemergent examinations are given secondary

(Continued)

Ultrasound, Breast *(Continued)*

priority and therefore may not be able to be performed the same day scheduled. Patients will generally be asked to stay after the examination until films are reviewed by the radiologist. All outpatients are by appointment only.

Equipment Standard B-mode ultrasonic imager with 5-10 MHz transducer

Technique A gel is applied to the skin and a handheld transducer is swept across the breast(s) showing breast tissue. Sound waves are used for the imaging and no radiation exposure is present. Images are recorded on x-ray film.

Data Acquired Sagittal, transverse, and oblique images of portions of the breast(s)

Turnaround Time A typed report will generally be issued within 36 hours. A preliminary verbal report generally can be given to the referring physician on request.

Normal Findings Solid breast tissue without focal mass or cyst

Limitations Patient unable to remain sitting quietly or obese patient

Additional Information This study is most useful in the determination of whether a mammographic abnormality is a simple cyst or a solid mass. If found not to be a simple cyst, malignancy cannot be excluded.

References

Baker JA, Soo MS, and Mengoni P, "Sonographically Guided Percutaneous Interventions of the Breast Using a Steerable Ultrasound Beam," *AJR AM J Roentgenol*, 1999, 172(1):157-9.

Birdwell RL, Ikeda DM, Jeffrey SS, et al, "Preliminary Experience With Power Doppler Imaging of Solid Breast Masses," *AJR Am J Roentgenol*, 1997, 169(3):703-7.

Cox BA, Kelly KM, Ko P, et al, "Ultrasound Characteristics of Breast Carcinoma," *Am Surg*, 1998, 64:934-8.

Fornage BD, "Sonographically Guided Needle Biopsy of Nonpalpable Breast Lesions," *J Clin Ultrasound*, 1999, 27(7):385-98.

Hieken TJ and Velasco JM, "A Prospective Analysis of Office-Based Breast Ultrasound," *Arch Surg*, 1998, 133(5):504-7.

Kopans DB, "Other Breast Imaging Modalities," *Radiology*, Taveras JT and Ferrucci JT, eds, Philadelphia, PA: Lippincott Williams & Wilkins, 1988.

Okamoto H, Ogawara T, and Inoue S, et al, "Clinical Management of Nonpalpable or Small Breast Masses by Find-Needle Aspiration Biopsy (FNAB) Under Ultrasound Guidance," *J Surg Oncol*, 1998, 67(4):246-50.

Raza S and Braum JK, "Solid Breast Lesions: Evaluation With Power Doppler US," *Radiology*, 1997, 203(1):164-8.

Rozycki GS, "Surgeon-Performed Ultrasound: Its Use in Clinical Practice," *Ann Surg*, 1998, 228(1):16-28.

Sahin-Akyar G and Sumer H, "Color Doppler Ultrasound and Spectral Analysis of Tumor Vessels in the Differential Diagnosis of Solid Breast Masses," *Invest Radiol*, 1996, 31(2):72-9.

Schiller VL, Karlen L, and Brenner RJ, "Pseudoaneurysm of the Breast: The Use of Color Doppler Sonography," *AJR Am J Roentgenol*, 1998, 170(4):1112.

Schroeder RJ, Maeurer J, Vogl TJ, et al, "D-Galactose-Based Signal-Enhanced Color Doppler Sonography of Breast Tumors and Tumorlike Lesions," *Invest Radiol*, 1999, 34(2):109-15.

Schutze B, Marx C, Fleck M, et al, "Diagnostic Evaluation of Sonographically Visualized Breast Lesions by Using a New Clinical Amplitude/Velocity Reference Imaging Technique (CARI Sonography)," *Invest Radiol*, 1998, 33(6):341-7.

Staren ED and Fine R, "Breast Ultrasound for Surgeons," *Am Surg*, 1996, 62(2):108-12.

Ultrasound, Chest Wall

Synonyms Chest Wall Ultrasound

Procedure Commonly Includes Specific portion of the chest wall.

Indications Measurement of distance between anterior surface to chest wall prior to radiation therapy, check for pleural effusions

Contraindications Open wound or incision overlying examination area

Patient Preparation The examination may be long, up to 1 hour including waiting time. An emergency examination or an unpredictably long preceding examination may result in additional delay.

Special Instructions All outpatient examinations are by appointment only. All inpatients are placed on the daily schedule as time permits and are performed as scheduled. Nonemergent examinations are given secondary priority and therefore may not be able to be performed the same day scheduled. Patients will generally be asked to stay after the examination until films are reviewed by the radiologist.

Equipment Standard ultrasonic imager with high frequency transducer (5-10 MHz)

Technique A gel is applied to the skin and a handheld transducer is swept across the area of interest to image the appropriate organs. Sound waves are used for the imaging and no radiation exposure is present. Images are recorded on x-ray film.

Data Acquired Transverse, longitudinal, and oblique images of the chest wall with measurements of chest wall thickness

Turnaround Time A typed report will generally be issued within 36 hours. A preliminary verbal report generally can be given to the referring physician on request.

Additional Information Study is generally performed prior to radiation therapy and to identify loculated pleural effusions.

References

Petrikovsky BM, Schneider EP, Klein VR, et al, "Fetal Breasts in Normal and Down Syndrome Fetuses," *J Clin Ultrasound* 1996, 24(9):507-11.

Rozycki GS, "Surgeon-Performed Ultrasound: Its Use in Clinical Practice," *Ann Surg*, 1998, 228(1):16-28.

Spettell CM, Levin DC, Rao VM, et al, "Practice Patterns of Radiologists and Nonradiologists: Nationwide Medicare Data on the Performance of Chest and Skeletal Radiography and Abdominal and Pelvic Sonography," *AJR Am J Roentgenol*, 1998, 171(1):3-5.

Ultrasound, Duplex Carotid

Synonyms Carotid Ultrasound

Procedure Commonly Includes Examination of the carotid arteries to look for plaque, stenosis, or occlusion in the common, internal, or external carotid arteries

Indications Checking the carotid arteries for plaque formation, stenosis, or occlusion; asymptomatic bruit, TIA, stroke, confirm the presence of subclavian steal

Contraindications

- presence of indwelling catheter of any kind
- presence of a fresh incision site

Patient Preparation The examination may be long, up to 1 hour including waiting time. An emergency examination or an unpredictably long preceding examination may result in additional delay.

Equipment Standard B-mode real time ultrasonic images with Doppler capabilities, 7-10 MHz transducer

Technique A gel is applied to the sides of the neck and a handheld transducer is swept over the area of the carotid arteries. Sound waves are used for the imaging and no radiation exposure is present. Images are recorded on x-ray film.

Data Acquired Transverse and longitudinal images of common carotid, internal, and external carotid arteries; quantitative Doppler flow parameters throughout visualized vessels

Turnaround Time A typed report will generally be issued within 36 hours. A preliminary verbal report generally can be given to the referring physician on request.

Causes for Rejection Inability of patient to hold head still, high bifurcation of carotid artery. If carotid bifurcation is located past the angle of the jaw, visualization may not be possible.

Normal Findings Absence of stenosis or occlusion of common carotid artery or branches

Critical Values Fifty percent or greater stenosis of studied vessel is considered hemodynamically significant

Additional Information Duplex carotid ultrasound is a very useful means of noninvasively screening for atherosclerotic disease of the carotid arteries. Both the severity of plaque formation as well as an estimate of the degree of stenosis is reliably obtained. When significant disease is detected, angiography should be performed to fully evaluate the extent of disease. This examination is useful in the serial evaluation of patients to rule out progressive disease.

References

Abu Rahma AF, Pollack JA, Robinson PA, et al, "The Reliability of Color Duplex Ultrasound in Diagnosing Total Carotid Artery Occlusion," *Am J Surg*, 1997, 174(2):185-7.

Arnold JA, Modaresi KB, Thomas N, et al, "Carotid Plaque Characterization by Duplex Scanning: Observer Error May Undermine Current Clinical Trials," *Stroke*, 1999, 30(1):61-5.

(Continued)

Ultrasound, Duplex Carotid *(Continued)*

Baumgartner RW, Arnold M, Gonner F, et al, "Contrast-Enhanced Transcranial Color-Coded Duplex Sonography in Ischemic Cerebrovascular Disease," *Stroke*, 1997, 28(12):2473-8.

Baumgartner RW, Mattle HP, and Schroth G, "Assessment of ≥60% and <50% Intracranial Stenoses by Transcranial Color-Coded and Duplex Sonography," *Stroke*, 1999, 31(1):87-92.

Carpenter JP, Lexa FJ, and Davis JT, et al, "Determination of Duplex Doppler Ultrasound Criteria Appropriate to the North Symptomatic Carotid Endarterectomy Trial," *Stroke*, 1996, 27(4):695-9.

Chen YW, Jeng JS, Liu HM, "Carotid and Transcranial Color-Coded Duplex Sonography in Different Types of Carotid-Cavernous Fistula," *Stroke*, 2000, 31(3):701-6.

Dagirmanjian A, Davis DA, Rothfus WE, et al, "Detection of Clinically Silent Intracranial Emboli Ipsilateral to Internal Carotid Occlusions During Cerebral Angiography," *AJR Am J Roentgenol*, 2000, 174(2):367-9.

Delcker A, Diener HC, and Wilhelm H, et al, "Source of Cerebral Microembolic Signals in Occlusion of the Internal Cartoid Artery," *J Neurol*, 1997, 244(5):312-7.

Droste DW, Jurgens R, Nabavi DG, et al, "Echocontrast-Enhanced Ultrasound of Extracranial Internal Cartoid Artery High-Grade Stenosis and Occlusion," *Stroke*, 1999, 30(11):2302-6.

Droste DW, Jurgens R, Weber S, et al, "Benefit of Echocontrast-Enhanced Transcranial Color-Coded Duplex Ultrasound in the Assessment of Intracranial Collateral Pathways," *Stroke*, 2000, 31(4):920-3.

Gerriets T, Seidel G, Fiss I, et al, "Contrast-Enhanced Transcranial Color-Coded Duplex Sonography: Efficiency and Validity," *Neurology*, 1999, 52(6):1133-7.

Kemeny V, Droste DW, Nabavi DG, et al, "Collateralization of an Occluded Internal Carotid Artery via a vas Vasorum," *Stroke*, 1998, 29(2):521-3.

Kuntz KM, Polak JF, Wittemore AD, et al, "Duplex Ultrasound Criteria for the Identification of Carotid Stenosis Should Be Laboratory Specific," *Stroke*, 1997, 28(3):597-602.

Link J, Brossman J, Penselin V, et al, "Common Carotid Artery Bifurcation: Preliminary Results of CT Angiography and Color-Coded Duplex Sonography Compared With Digital Subtraction Angiography," *AJR Am J Roentgenol*, 1997, 168(2):361-5.

Patel ST, Kuntz KM, and Kent KC, "Is Routine Duplex Ultrasound Surveillance After Carotid Endarterectomy Cost-Effective?", *Surgery*, 1998, 124(2):343-51.

Plicher DB and Ricci MA, "Vascular Ultrasound," *Surg Clin North Am*, 1998, 78(2):273-93.

Turkenburg JL, van Oostayen JA, and Bollen WL, "Role of Carotid Sonography as a First Examination in the Evaluation of Patients With Transient Ischemic Attacks and Strokes: Benefit in Relation to Age," *J Clin Ultrasound*, 1999, 27(2):65-9.

van Everdingen KJ, van der Grond J, and Kappelle JL, "Overestimation of a Stenosis in the Internal Carotid Artery by Duplex Sonography Caused by an Increase in Volume Flow," *J Vasc Surg*, 1998, 27(3):479-85.

Wain RA, Lyon RT, Veith FJ, et al, "Accuracy of Duplex Ultrasound in Evaluating Carotid Artery Anatomy Before Endarterectomy," *J Vasc Surg*, 1998, 27(2):235-42.

Ultrasound, Duplex Hepatic Vessels

Synonyms Color Doppler Ultrasound

Applies to Colorflow, Liver; Duplex Colorflow Ultrasound Liver

Procedure Commonly Includes Hepatic, portal, and IVC blood flow

Indications Evaluation of hepatic blood vessels, abnormal hepatic vessels, intrahepatic masses

Patient Preparation The examination may be long, up to 1 hour including waiting time. An emergency examination or an unpredictably long preceding examination may result in additional delay.

Special Instructions All outpatient examinations are by appointment only. All inpatients are placed on the daily schedule as time permits and are performed as scheduled. Nonemergent examinations are given secondary priority and therefore may not be able to be performed the same day scheduled. Patients will generally be asked to stay after the examination until films are reviewed by the radiologist.

Equipment Standard B-mode real time ultrasonic imager with colorflow Doppler capabilities and a 3-5 MHz transducer.

Technique A gel is applied to the skin and a handheld transducer is swept across the area of interest to image the appropriate organs. Sound waves are used for the imaging and no radiation exposure is present. Images are recorded on x-ray film.

Data Acquired Longitudinal, transverse, and oblique images with Doppler flow parameters

Turnaround Time A typed report will generally be issued within 36 hours. A preliminary verbal report generally can be given to the referring physician on request.

Additional Information Examination is valuable in evaluating portal and hepatic venous flow. Hepatic arterial flow and flow within the IVC are also studied. The procedure is often performed to evaluate porto-systemic venous shunts and for presence of Budd-Chiari syndrome, cavernous transformation of the IVC, tumor thrombus in the IVC.

References

Hosten N, Puls R, Lemke AJ, et al, "Contrast-Enhanced Power Doppler Sonography: Improved Detection of Characteristic Flow Patterns in Focal Liver Lesions," *J Clin Ultrasound*, 1999, 27(3):107-15.

Leen E, Anderson JR, Robertson J, et al, "Doppler Index Perfusion in the Detection of Hepatic Metastases Secondary to Gastric Carcinoma," *Am J Surg*, 1997, 173(2):99-102.

Paulson EK, Kliewer MA, Frederick MG, et al, "Hepatic Artery: Variability in Measurement of Resistive Index and Systolic Acceleration Time in Healthy Volunteers," *Radiology*, 1996, 200(3):725-9.

Platt JF, Yutzy GG, Bude RO, et al, "Use of Doppler Sonography for Revealing Hepatic Artery Stenosis in Liver Transplant Recipients," *AJR Am J Roentgenol*, 1997, 168(2):473-6.

Rozycki GS, "Surgeon-Performed Ultrasound: Its Use in Clinical Practice," *Ann Surg*, 1998, 228(1):16-28.

Someda H, Moriyasu F, Hamato N, et al, "Change in Hepatic Arterial Hemodynamics Induced by Hepatocellular Carcinoma Detected With Doppler Sonography," *J Clin Ultrasound*, 1997, 25(7):359-65.

Walsh KM, Leen E, MacSween RN, et al, "Hepatic Blood Flow Changes in Chronic Hepatitis C Measure By Duplex Color Sonography: Relationship to Histological Features," *Dig Dis Sci*, 1998, 43(12):2584-90.

Ultrasound, Duplex Upper Extremity

Procedure Commonly Includes Peripheral masses

Indications Evaluation of vascular lesions of any extremity or vascularity of a lesion

Patient Preparation Examinations may be long, lasting up to 1 hour including waiting time. An emergency examination or an unpredictably long preceding examination may result in additional delay.

Special Instructions All outpatient examinations are by appointment only. All inpatients are placed on the daily schedule as time permits and are performed as scheduled. Nonemergent examinations are given secondary priority and therefore may not be able to be performed the same day scheduled. Patients will generally be asked to stay after the examination until films are reviewed by the radiologist.

Equipment Standard B-mode real time ultrasonic imager with 5-10 MHz, Doppler, and colorflow capability

Technique A gel is applied to the skin and a handheld transducer is swept across the area of interest to image the appropriate organs. Sound waves are used for the imaging and no radiation exposure is present. Images are recorded on x-ray film.

Data Acquired Longitudinal and transverse images of vessels studied with Doppler flow parameters

Turnaround Time A typed report will generally be issued within 36 hours. A preliminary verbal report generally can be given to the referring physician on request.

Additional Information Study may be useful in evaluating the vascularity of a mass lesion. Useful in evaluating for hemangioma, AVM, pseudoaneurysm.

References

Bast SC, Perry JR, Poppiti R, et al, "Upper Extremity Blood Flow in Collegiate and High School Baseball Pitchers. A Preliminary Report," *Am J Sports Med*, 1996, 24(6):847-51.

Jackson MR, Brengman ML, and Rick NM, et al, "Delayed Presentation of 50 Years After a World War II Vascular Injury With Intraoperative Localization By Duplex Ultrasound of a Traumatic False Aneurysm," *J Trauma*, 1997, 43(1):159-61.

Passman MA, Criado E, Farber MA, et al, "Efficacy of Color Flow Duplex Imaging for Proximal Upper Extremity Venous Ouflow Obstruction in Hemodialysis Patients," *J Vasc Surg*, 1998, 28(5):869-75.

Rozycki GS, "Surgeon-Performed Ultrasound: Its Use in Clinical Practice," *Ann Surg*, 1998, 228(1):16-28.

Silva MB Jr, Hobson RW 2nd, Pappas PJ, et al, "A Strategy for Increasing Use of Autogenous Hemodialysis Access Procedures: Impact of Preoperative Noninvasive Evaluation," *J Vasc Surg*, 1998, 27(2):302-7.

Ultrasound, Endorectal

Related Information

Ultrasound, Prostate *on page 501*

Synonyms Endorectal Ultrasound; EUS; Transrectal Ultrasound

(Continued)

Ultrasound, Endorectal *(Continued)*

Procedure Commonly Includes Placement of an EUS probe into the rectum for transrectal images

Indications EUS is used to stage rectal tumors, determine the integrity of the sphincter mechanism in incontinent patients, and to assess the extent and location of anorectal sepsis.

Patient Preparation A single Fleet® enema is given approximately 1 hour prior to the procedure. No sedation is required for this examination, and minimal, if any, discomfort is associated with EUS.

Equipment The most widely used EUS system is the Bruel and Kjaer scanner type 3535 with a hand-held rotating endoprobe, type 1850. The probe is 24 cm in length. A 7-10 MHz transducer can be inserted onto the end of the probe and rotated at 4-6 cycles/second, emitting soundwaves into the tissue. The end of the probe is covered with either a latex balloon or plastic cap that is filled with degassed water to maintain acoustic coupling between the transducer and the tissue.

Technique The patient is placed in either the lithotomy or left lateral position. When one is imaging rectal tumors, proctoscopy should be done first to locate the lesion. A specially designed, commercially available proctoscope that is 2 cm wide permits passage of the EUS probe down its shaft. Scanning should actually be started several cm above the lesion because metastatic lymph nodes, if present, are usually located above or at the level of the lesion rather than below. Once the probe is at the desired location, the balloon is inflated with a minimum of 30 mL of degassed water and the probe is gradually withdrawn caudally.

Data Acquired Circumferential images of the anal anatomy are recorded on x-ray film.

Normal Findings Absence of abnormal masses, fluid collections, enlarged lymph nodes, or calcifications

Additional Information For staging of rectal tumors, EUS has advantages over CT and MRI. First, the EUS probe is placed in close proximity to the area of interest, and the resolution and imaging quality are thus greatly enhanced. Second, the EUS unit is a small and portable, allowing its use in the office setting, in the operating room, and at the patient's bedside. Third, it is a relatively low-cost procedure. Fourth, because minimal preparation is needed, no pain is caused, no sedation is required, and the examination is fast. Finally, because the surgeon can use it promptly during the initial consultation with the patient and incorporate the information gained immediately into the treatment plan, care is expedited.

References

Chin JL, Downey DB, Mulligan M, et al, "Three-dimensional Transrectal Ultrasound Guided Cryoablation for Localized Prostate Cancer in Nonsurgical Candidates: A Feasibility Study and Report of Early Results," *J Urol*, 1998, 159(3):910-4.

Gualdi GF, Casciani E, Guadalaxara A, et al, "Local Staging of Rectal Cancer With Transrectal Ultrasound and Endorectal Magnetic Resonance Imaging: Comparison With Histologic Findings," *Dis Colon Rectum*, 2000, 43(3):338-45.

Hunerbein M, Below C, and Schlag PM, "Three-Dimensional Endorectal Ultrasonography for Staging of Obstructing Rectal Cancer," *Dis Colon Rectum*, 1996, 39(6):636-42.

Hunerbein M, Dohmoto M, Haensch W, et al, "Evaluation and Biopsy of Recurrent Rectal Cancer Using Three-Dimensional Endosonography," *Dis Colon Rectum*, 1996, 39(12):1373-8.

Matthews GJ, Motta J, and Fracehia JA, "The Accuracy of Transrectal Ultrasound Prostate Volume Estimation: Clinical Correlations," *J Clin Ultrasound*, 1996, 24(9):501-5.

Oberwalder M, Tschmelitsch J, Conrad F, et al, "Endosonographic Image of a Retrorectal Bowel Duplication: Report of a Case," *Dis Colon Rectum*, 1998, 41(6):802-3.

Parivar F, Hricak H, Shinohara K, et al, "Detection of Locally Recurrent Prostate Cancer After Cryosurgery: Evaluation by Transrectal Ultrasound, Magnetic Resonance Imaging, and Three-Dimensional Proton Magnetic Resonance Spectroscopy," *Urology*, 1996, 48(4):594-9.

Rozycki GS, "Surgeon-Performed Ultrasound: Its Use in Clinical Practice," *Ann Surg*, 1998, 228(1):16-28.

Saclarides TJ, "Endorectal Ultrasound," *Surg Clin North Am*, 1998, 78(2):237-49.

Zagoria RJ, Schlarb CA, Ott DJ, et al, "Assessment of Rectal Tumor Infiltration Utilizing Endorectal MR Imaging and Comparison With Endoscopic Rectal Sonography," 1997, 64(4):312-7.

Ultrasound, Extremity

Synonyms Extremity Ultrasound

Procedure Commonly Includes Specific area of an extremity

Indications Diagnosis of popliteal aneurysms, Baker's cyst, hematoma

Contraindications Open wound or incision overlying examination area

Patient Preparation No patient preparation is necessary. Examinations may be long, 30 minutes to 1 hour each. An emergency exam or an unpredictably long preceding exam may necessitate waiting on the part of the next patient.

Special Instructions All outpatient examinations are by appointment only. All inpatients are placed on the daily schedule as time permits and are performed as scheduled. Nonemergent examinations are given secondary priority and therefore may not be able to be performed the same day scheduled. Patients will generally be asked to stay after the examination until films are reviewed by the radiologist. Instruct the patient that ultrasound uses sound waves to image the different organs. There is **no** radiation involved, therefore, it is not harmful to the patient.

Equipment Standard B-mode ultrasonic imager with 5-10 MHz transducer

Technique A gel is applied to the skin and a handheld transducer is swept across the area of interest to image the appropriate organs. Sound waves are used for the imaging and no radiation exposure is present. Images are recorded on x-ray film.

Data Acquired Longitudinal, transverse, and oblique images of the area of interest are obtained.

Turnaround Time A typed report will generally be issued within 36 hours. A preliminary verbal report generally can be given to the referring physician on request.

Additional Information This examination is most valuable to evaluate for the presence of abnormal fluid collections. If present, it can determine if the fluid collection is simple or complex in nature.

References

Bardo DM, Applegate KE, Goske MJ, et al, "Superficial Venous Thrombosis Presenting As a Painful Popliteal Fossa Mass in a Child," *J Clin Ultrasound*, 1998, 26(9):470-3.

Do DD, Braunschweig M, Baumgartner I, et al, "Adventitial Cystic Disease of the Popliteal Artery: Percutaneous US-Guided Aspiration," *Radiology*, 1997, 203(3):743-6.

Drescher MJ and Smally AJ, "Thrombophlebitis and Pseudothrombophlebitis in the ED," *Am J Emerg Med*, 1997, 15(7):683-5.

Hertzberg BS, Kliewer MA, De Long DM, et al, "Sonographic Estimates of Vein Size in the Lower Extremities: Subjective Assessment Compared With Direct Measurement," *J Clin Ultrasound*, 1998, 26(3):113-7.

Koppensteiner R, Katzenschlager R, Ahmadi A, et al, "Demonstration of Cystic Adventitial Disease by Intravascular Ultrasound Imaging," *J Vasc Surg*, 1996, 23(3):534-6.

Mouratidis B and Antonio G, "Sonographic Diagnosis of Subcapsular Liver Hematoma Mimicking Tumor in a Neonate," *J Clin Ultrasound*, 2000, 28(1):53-7.

Trottier SJ, Todi S, and Veremakis C, "Validation of an Inexpensive B-Mode Ultrasound Device for Detection of Deep Vein Thrombosis," *Chest*, 1996, 110(6):1547-50.

Ultrasound, Gallbladder

Related Information

Oral Cholecystogram, Gallbladder Series *on page 362*

Synonyms Gallbladder Ultrasound

Procedure Commonly Includes Gallbladder and biliary tree

Indications Cholelithiasis, cholecystitis, neoplasms, lesions, polyps, or ductal obstruction

Contraindications

- open wound or incision overlying examination area
- recent barium study

Patient Preparation The patient should be on a low fat diet the night before the examination with NPO for 10 hours prior to the examination. No laxatives are given the day of the examination. No barium studies should have been performed on the patient for **at least** 2 days preceding the examination. Endoscopy, ERCP, colonoscopy, and abdominal CT should be performed after this examination. Nuclear Medicine studies may be ordered prior to the examination. The examination may be long, up to 1 hour including waiting time. An emergency examination or an unpredictably long preceding examination may result in additional delay. **Note**: Ultrasound exam to be scheduled before a barium study. If barium study was done, bowel preparation is needed before doing ultrasound examination.

(Continued)

Ultrasound, Gallbladder *(Continued)*

Special Instructions All outpatient examinations are by appointment only. All inpatients are placed on the daily schedule as time permits and are performed as scheduled. Nonemergent examinations are given secondary priority and therefore may not be able to be performed the same day scheduled. Patients will generally be asked to stay after the examination until films are reviewed by the radiologist.

Equipment Standard B-mode real time ultrasonic imager with 2-5 MHz transducer.

Technique A gel is applied to the skin and a handheld transducer is swept across the area of interest to image the appropriate organs. Sound waves are used for the imaging and no radiation exposure is present. Images are recorded on x-ray film.

Data Acquired Longitudinal, transverse, and oblique views of the gallbladder; longitudinal image of common bile duct

Turnaround Time A typed report will generally be issued within 36 hours. A preliminary verbal report generally can be given to the referring physician on request.

Causes for Rejection Gas, barium, oral ingestion of food or fluids, obesity

Normal Findings Absence of cholelithiasis

Critical Values Common bile duct ≤6 mm prior to cholecystectomy, ≤11 mm after cholecystectomy

Additional Information This is a very sensitive examination for evaluation of the presence of gallstones as well as biliary tree dilatation. Additionally, soft tissue masses and abnormal collections can be detected.

References

Ballard RB, Rozycki GS, Knudson MM, et al, "The Surgeon's Use of Ultrasound in the Acute Setting," *Surg Clin North Am*, 1998, 78(2):337-64.

Bernardino ME, "The Liver: Anatomy and Examination Techniques," *Radiology*, Taveras JT and Ferrucci JT, eds, Philadelphia, PA: Lippincott Williams & Wilkins, 1988.

Cooperberg PL and Rowley VA, "Abdominal Sonographic Examination Technique," *Radiology*, Taveras JT and Ferrucci JT, eds, Philadelphia, PA: Lippincott Williams & Wilkins, 1988.

Fujita N, Noda Y, Kobayashi G, et al, "Diagnosis of the Depth of Invasion of Gallbladder Carcinoma by EUS," *Gastrointest Endosc*, 1999, 50(5):659-63.

Goldberg BB, *Abdominal Ultrasonography*, New York, NY: John Wiley and Sons Inc, 1984.

Henderson SO, Sung J, and Mandavia D, "Serial Abdominal Ultrasound in the Setting of Trauma," *J Emerg Med*, 2000, 18(1):79-81.

Muguruma N, Okamura S, Okahisa T, et al, "Endoscopic Sonography in the Diagnosis of Xanthogranulomatous Cholecystitis," *J Clin Ultrasound*, 1999, 27(6):347-50.

Olcott EW, Jeffrey RB Jr, and Jain KA, "Power Versus Color Doppler Sonography of the Normal Cystic Artery: Implications for Patients With Acute Cholecystitis," *Am J Roentgenol*, 1997, 168(3):703-5.

Pauletzki J, Sackmann M, Holl J, et al, "Evaluation of Gallbladder Volume and Emptying With a Novel Three-Dimensional Ultrasound System: Comparison With the Sum-of-Cylinders and the Ellipsoid Methods," *J Clin Ultrasound*, 1996, 24(6):277-85.

Shirahama M, Onohara S, Miyamoto Y, et al, "Incisional Hernia of Gallbladder in a Patient With Gallbladder Carcinoma: Sonographic Demonstration," *J Clin Ultrasound*, 1997, 25(7):398-400.

Soyer P, Brouland JP, Boudiaf M, et al, "Color Velocity Imaging and Power Doppler Sonography of the Gallbladder Wall: A New Look at Sonographic Diagnosis of Acute Cholecystitis," *Am J Roentgenol*, 1998, 171(1):183-8.

Uggowitzer M, Kugler C, Schramayer G, et al, "Sonography of Acute Cholecystitis: Comparison of Color and Power Doppler Sonography in Detecting a Hypervascularized Gallbladder Wall," *Am J Roentgenol*, 1997, 168(3):707-12.

Ultrasound, Hepatic

Synonyms Hepatic Ultrasound; Liver Ultrasound; RUQ

Procedure Commonly Includes Liver, biliary tract, gallbladder, right kidney (limited)

Indications To evaluate for the presence of hepatitis, malignancies, cysts, biliary obstruction

Patient Preparation Ultrasound examination should be performed before endoscopy, ERCP, colonoscopy, barium studies, and abdominal CT. Nuclear Medicine studies may be performed first. NPO after midnight. The examination may be long, up to 1 hour including waiting time. An emergency examination or an unpredictably long preceding examination may result in additional delay.

Special Instructions All outpatient examinations are by appointment only. All inpatients are placed on the daily schedule as time permits and are performed as scheduled. Nonemergent examinations are given secondary priority and therefore may not be able to be performed the same day scheduled. Patients will generally be asked to stay after the examination until films are reviewed by the radiologist.

Equipment Standard B-mode ultrasonic imager 2-5 MHz transducer

Technique A gel is applied to the skin and a handheld transducer is swept across the area of interest to image the appropriate organs. Sound waves are used for the imaging and no radiation exposure is present. Images are recorded on x-ray film.

Data Acquired Longitudinal, transverse, and oblique images of the liver; limited images of the gallbladder and right kidney

Turnaround Time A typed report will generally be issued within 36 hours. A preliminary verbal report generally can be given to the referring physician on request.

Causes for Rejection Gas, barium, oral ingestion of food

Additional Information This examination is useful to evaluate for the presence of hepatic mass lesions, cysts or other collections, calcifications or biliary tree dilatations. Diffuse hepatic parenchymal disease may be detected as well.

References

Abbitt PL, "Ultrasonography. Update on Liver Technique," *Radiol Clin North Am*, 1998, 36(2):299-307.

Gabata T, Matsui O, Kadoya M, et al, "Aberrant Gastric Venous Drainage in a Focal Spared Area of Segment IV in Fatty Liver: Demonstration With Color Doppler Sonography," *Radiology*, 1997, 203(2):461-3.

Gorka W, Kagalwalla A, McParland BJ, et al, "Diagnostic Value of Doppler Ultrasound in the Assessment of Liver Cirrhosis in Children: Histopathological Correlation," *J Clin Ultrasound*, 1996, 24(6):287-95.

Kliewer MA, Sheafor DH, Paulson EK, et al, "Percutaneous Liver Biopsy: A Cost-Benefit Analysis Comparing Sonographic and CT Guidance," *Am J Roentgenol*, 1999, 173(5):1199-202.

Koito K, Namieno T, and Morita K, "Differential Diagnosis of Small Hepatocellular Carcinoma and Adenomatous Hyperplasia With Power Doppler Sonography," *Am J Roentgenol*, 1998, 170(1):157-61.

Larcos G, Sorokopud H, Berry G, et al, "Sonographic Screening for Hepatocellular Carcinoma in Patients With Chronic Hepatitis or Cirrhosis: An Evaluation," *Am J Roentgenol*, 1998, 171(2):433-5.

Mouratidis B and Antonio G, "Sonographic Diagnosis of Subcapsular Liver Hematoma Mimicking Tumor in a Neonate," *J Clin Ultrasound*, 2000, 28(1):53-7.

Platt JF, Yutzy GG, Bude RO, et al, "Use of Doppler Sonography for Revealing Hepatic Artery Stenosis in Liver Transplant Recipients," *Am J Roentgenol*, 1997, 168(2):473-6.

Rhim H and Dodd GD III, "Radiofrequency Thermal Ablation of Liver Tumors," *J Clin Ultrasound*, 1999, 27(5):221-9.

Rozycki GS, "Surgeon-Performed Ultrasound: Its Use in Clinical Practice," *Ann Surg*, 1999, 228(1):16-28.

Rozycki GS, Ochsner MG, Feliciano DV, et al, "Early Detection of Hemoperitoneum by Ultrasound Examination of the Right Upper Quadrant: A Multicenter Study," *J Trauma*, 1998, 45(5):878-83.

Shapiro RS, Stancato-Pasik A, Glajchen N, et al, "Color Doppler Applications in Hepatic Imaging," *Clin Imaging*, 1998, 22(4):272-9.

Ultrasound, Intraoperative Real Time Scanning

Synonyms Intraoperative Ultrasound; IOUS; Laparoscopic Ultrasound; LUS

Procedure Commonly Includes Scanning of organs (eg, brain, spinal cord, kidney, liver, gallbladder, biliary tree, pancreas) with a specialized transducer head during surgery or laparoscopy and obtaining real time images

Indications Localization of tumors, stones, and cystic masses, as well as tumor staging during surgery

Special Instructions Study scheduled after consultation with radiologist.

Equipment Standard B-mode real time ultrasonic imager with 5-10 MHz transducer.

Technique A handheld transducer is swept across the area of interest to image the appropriate organs. Sound waves are used for the imaging and no radiation exposure is present. Images are recorded on x-ray film.

Turnaround Time A typed report will generally be issued within 36 hours. A preliminary verbal report generally can be given to the referring physician on request.

(Continued)

Ultrasound, Intraoperative Real Time Scanning *(Continued)*

References

Barbot DJ, Marks JH, Feld RI, et al, "Improved Staging of Liver Tumors Using Laparoscopic Intraoperative Ultrasound," *J Surg Oncol*, 1997, 64(1):63-7.

Bowerman RA, McCracken S, Silver TM, et al, "Abdominal and Miscellaneous Applications of Intraoperative Ultrasound," *Radiol Clin North Am*, 1985, 23(1):107-19.

Brunt LM, Bennett HF, Teefey SA, et al, "Laparoscopic Ultrasound Imaging of Adrenal Tumors During Laparoscopic Adrenalectomy," *Am J Surg*, 1999, 178(6):490-5.

Heniford BT, Iannitti DA, Hale J, et al, "The Role of Intraoperative Ultrasonography During Laparoscopic Adrenalectomy," *Surgery*, 1997, 122(6):1068-73, discussion 1073-4.

Knake JE, Bowerman RA, Silver TM, et al, "Neurosurgical Applications of Intraoperative Ultrasound," *Radiol Clin North Am*, 1985, 23(1):73-90.

Kolecki R and Schirmer B, "Intraoperative and Laparoscopic Ultrasound," *Surg Clin North Am*, 1998, 78(2):251-71.

Letterie GS, "Ultrasound Guidance During Endoscopic Procedures," *Obstet Gynecol Clin North Am*, 1999, 26(1):63-82.

Machi J and Sigel B, "Operative Ultrasound in General Surgery," *Am J Surg*, 1996, 172(1):15-20.

Machi J, Tateishi T, Oishi AJ, et al, "Laparoscopic Ultrasonography Versus Operative Cholangiography During Laparoscopic Cholecystectomy: Review of the Literature and a Comparison With Open Intraoperative Ultrasonography," *J Am Coll Surg*, 1999, 188(4):360-7.

Ohtani T, Kawai C, Shirai Y, et al, "Intraoperative Ultrasonography Versus Cholangiography During Laparoscopic Cholecystectomy: A Prospective Comparative Study," *J Am Coll Surg*, 1997, 185(3):274-82.

Rahusen FD, Cuesta MA, Borgstein PJ, et al, "Selection of Patients for Resection of Colorectal Metastases to the Liver Using Diagnostic Laparoscopy and Laparoscopic Ultrasonography," *Ann Surg*, 1999, 230(1):31-7.

Santambrogio R, Montorsi M, Bianchi P, et al, "Common Bile Duct Exploration and Laparoscopic Cholecystectomy: Role of Intraoperative Ultrasonography," *J Am Coll Surg*, 1997, 185(1):40-8.

Zhang W, Niu HO, Su ZX, et al, "Intraoperative Ultrasound-Guided Transhepatic Lithotomy. A New Alternative Surgical Procedure for the Management of Residual Hepatic Stones," *Arch Surg*, 1997, 132(3):300-3.

Ultrasound, Intravascular

Synonyms Endoluminal Ultrasonography; Intravascular Ultrasound; IVUS

Procedure Commonly Includes Application of conventional ultrasound technology to catheter-based delivery systems for the evaluation of normal and abnormal vascular anatomy from an endoluminal position. IVUS can provide information in addition to that obtained by conventional imaging techniques such as contrast angiography, CT, MRI, and transcutaneous ultrasonograpy.

Indications Plaque characterization and morphology; evaluation of stenosis cross-sectional area; assessment of balloon angioplasty; evaluation of vessel dissections and flaps; assessing effects of intravascular stents and deployment of endovascular prostheses

Contraindications

Left heart catheterization

- severe congestive heart failure
- advanced renal insufficiency
- severe peripheral vascular disease
- history of cholesterol embolization

Right heart catheterization

- tricuspid valve prosthesis
- right-sided intracardiac mass

Patient Preparation Patients must have a written and properly identified consultation from a cardiologist recorded in the chart prior to the procedure. The consultant's note should state indications for the procedure and evaluation of risk to the patient.

Left heart catheterization: CBC, BUN, creatinine, chest x-ray, and electrocardiogram should be recorded in the chart the day before the test. A serum potassium should also be ordered the day before the test on all patients receiving diuretics; if the Judkin's technique will be used, shave the patient's iliofemoral areas the day before the procedure; two units of blood may be on call in the Blood Bank. The requesting physician may need to obtain a signed procedure permit for the invasive diagnostic test. Patients younger than 18 years of age must have a parent or legal guardian sign the permit. Patients receiving digitalis should be given their usual dose the morning of the catheterization. A sedative such as midazolam should be given on call from the Cardiac Catheterization Laboratory. For AM patients, omit breakfast on the day of the test. For PM patients, juice and coffee may be given at breakfast time. The patient's weight is obtained on the day of the procedure and recorded in the chart. All patients are sent to the laboratory on a stretcher wearing a hospital gown and regular slippers.

Aftercare Right heart catheterization (including HIS bundle electrograms): Remove dressing after 4 hours. Check for hematoma or bleeding at catheter insertion site twice in 1 hour. If a cutdown was performed, remove the sutures in 5-7 days.

Left heart catheterization (including coronary angiograms): Check the patient's heart rate, blood pressure, arterial puncture site, and distal pulses four times at 15-minute intervals, then four times at 30-minute intervals, then four times at 1-hour intervals. If the femoral approach has been used, enforce absolute bedrest for 6 hours.

Equipment A specialized multiple-element, phased-array, catheter-tip transducer (10-30 MHz) capable of producing 360° transmural images via an IVUS probe ranging from 3.5-6.2 French in diameter. The catheter has a "sidesaddle" or over-the-wire configuration, allowing the IVUS probe to advance along a guidewire.

Data Acquired Circumferential images of the vascular endolumen

Normal Findings Good understanding of normal and abnormal vascular anatomy is required to interpret IVUS images. Absence of plaque or vessel dissection is normal. Nondiseased vessels have a three-layer appearance of muscular arteries, with the echolucent media being between the more echodense intima and adventitia.

Additional Information Accurate assessment of IVUS images relies on the use of appropriate frequency catheters in various locations to determine the factors being investigated.

References

Blessing E, Hausmann D, Sturm M, et al, "Intravascular Ultrasound and Stent Implantation: Intraobserver and Interobserver Variability," *Am Heart J*, 1999, 137(2):368-71.

Gorge G, Ge J, and Erbel R, "Role of Intravascular Ultrasound in the Evaluation of Mechanisms of Coronary Interventions and Restenosis," *Am J Cardiol*, 1998, 81(12A):91G-5G.

Moussa I, Moses J, Di Mario C, et al, "Does the Specific Intravascular Ultrasound Criterion Used to Optimize Stent Expansion Have an Impact on the Probability of Stent Restenosis?" *Am J Cardiol*, 1999, 83(7):1012-7.

Muller-Hulsbeck S, Schwarzenberg H, Hutzelmann A, et al, "Intravascular Ultrasound Evaluation of Peripheral Arterial Stent-Grafts," *Invest Radiol*, 2000, 35(2):97-104.

Wilson EP and White RA, "Intravascular Ultrasound," *Surg Clin North Am*, 1998, 78(4):561-74.

Ultrasound, Kidney Biopsy

Related Information

Kidney Biopsy *on page 126*

Synonyms Kidney Biopsy Ultrasound; Renal Biopsy Ultrasound

Procedure Commonly Includes Use of real time ultrasound imaging to direct biopsy of renal mass

Indications Provide tissue sample or fluid sample for diagnostic purposes

Contraindications Coagulopathy

Patient Preparation The examination may be long, up to 1 hour including waiting time. An emergency examination or an unpredictably long preceding examination may result in additional delay.

Aftercare Check physician order sheet. Monitor vital signs in department for 1 hour postprocedure.

Special Instructions All outpatient examinations are by appointment only. All inpatients are placed on the daily schedule as time permits and are performed as scheduled. Nonemergent examinations are given secondary priority and therefore may not be able to be performed the same day scheduled. Patients will generally be asked to stay after the examination until films are reviewed by the radiologist.

Complications Hemorrhage, infection

Equipment Standard B-mode real time ultrasonic imager with 2-5 MHz transducer.

(Continued)

Ultrasound, Kidney Biopsy *(Continued)*

Technique A gel is applied to the skin and a handheld transducer is swept across the area of interest to image the appropriate organs. Sound waves are used for the imaging and no radiation exposure is present. Images are recorded on x-ray film.

Turnaround Time A typed report will generally be issued within 36 hours. A preliminary verbal report generally can be given to the referring physician on request.

Specimen Fluid and/or tissue

Container Sterile saline, sterile slides for cytology, fixative for core tissue samples, culture tubes, tubes for chemistry evaluation

Sampling Time Immediate

Storage Instructions Samples should immediately be sent to the appropriate laboratory (ie, cytology, pathology, bacteriology).

Causes for Rejection Obesity, inability to suspend respiration or lie motionless, inability to locate good access to site

References

Chau WK and Chan SC, "Improved Sonographic Visualization by Fluid Challenge Method of Renal Lithiasis in the Nondilated Collecting System. Experience in Seven Cases," *Clin Imaging*, 1997, 21(4):276-83.

Cost GA, Merguerian PA, Cheerasarn SP, et al, "Sonographic Renal Parenchymal and Pelvicaliceal Areas: New Quantitative Parameters for Renal Sonographic Followup," *J Urol*, 1996, 156(2 Pt 2):725-9.

Gottlieb RH, Voci SL, Cholewinski SP, et al, "Sonography: A Useful Tool to Detect the Mechanical Cause of Renal Transplant Dysfunction," *J Clin Ultrasound*, 1999, 27(6):325-33.

Gupta S, Gulati M, and Suri S, "Ultrasound-Guided Percutaneous Nephrostomy in Nondilated Pelvicaliceal System," *J Clin Ultrasound*, 1998, 26(3):177-9.

Khajehdehi P, Junaid SM, Salinas-Madrigal L, et al, "Percutaneous Renal Biopsy in the 1990s: Safety, Value, and Implications for Early Hospital Discharge," *Am J Kidney Dis*, 1999, 34(1):92-7.

Levine E, "Acquired Cystic Kidney Disease," *Radiol Clin North Am*, 1996, 34(5):947-64.

Nass K and O'Neill WC, "Bedside Renal Biopsy: Ultrasound Guidance by the Nephrologist," *Am J Kidney Dis*, 1999, 34(5):955-9.

Platt JF, Rubin JM, and Ellis JH, "Lupus Nephritis: Predictive Value of Conventional and Doppler US and Comparison With Serologic and Biopsy Parameters," *Radiology*, 1997, 203(1):82-6.

Richter F, Kasabian NG, Irwin RJ Jr, et al, "Accuracy of Diagnosis by Guided Biopsy of Renal Mass Lesions Classified Indeterminate by Imaging Studies," *Urology*, 2000, 55(3):348-52.

Rifkin MD and Goldberg BB, "Aspiration and Biopsy Techniques," *Abdominal Ultrasonography*, 2nd ed, Goldberg BB, ed, New York, NY: John Wiley and Sons Inc, 1984.

Roy C, Tuchmann C, Pfleger D, et al, "Potential Role of Duplex Doppler Sonography in Acute Renal Colic," *J Clin Ultrasound*, 1998, 26(9):427-32.

Sheih CP, Li YW, Liao YJ, et al, "Diagnosing the Combination of Renal Dysgenesis, Gartner's Duct Cyst and Ipsilateral Mullerian Duct Obstruction," *J Urol*, 1998, 159(1):217-21.

Zhou Q, Cardoza JD, and Barth R, "Prenatal Sonography of Congenital Renal Malformations," *Am J Roentgenol*, 1999, 173(5):1371-6.

Ultrasound, Kidney Cyst Puncture

Synonyms Kidney Cyst Puncture Ultrasound; Renal Cyst Puncture Ultrasound

Procedure Commonly Includes Use of real time ultrasound imaging to direct aspiration of renal cyst

Indications Provide fluid or tissue sample for diagnostic purposes

Contraindications

- inadequate access by ultrasound
- bleeding diathesis

Patient Preparation The examination may be long, up to 1 hour including waiting time. An emergency examination or an unpredictably long preceding examination may result in additional delay.

Aftercare Follow physician's orders

Special Instructions All outpatient examinations are by appointment only. All inpatients are placed on the daily schedule as time permits and are performed as scheduled. Nonemergent examinations are given secondary priority and therefore may not be able to be performed the same day scheduled. Patients will generally be asked to stay after the examination until films are reviewed by the radiologist.

Complications Hemorrhage, infection

Equipment Standard B-mode real time ultrasonic imager with 2-5 MHz transducer.

Technique A gel is applied to the skin and a handheld transducer is swept across the area of interest to image the appropriate organs. Sound waves are used for the imaging and no radiation exposure is present. Images are recorded on x-ray film. Following sterile preparation of the skin and use of local anesthesia, a small (20- to 22-gauge) needle is introduced into the suspected cyst under real time ultrasonic visualization.

Data Acquired A sample of fluid and/or tissue is obtained for analysis.

Turnaround Time A typed report will generally be issued within 36 hours. A preliminary verbal report generally can be given to the referring physician on request.

Specimen Fluid and/or tissue

Container Sterile saline, sterile slides for cytology, fixative for core tissue samples, culture tubes, tubes for chemistry evaluation

Sampling Time Immediate

Storage Instructions Samples should immediately be sent to the appropriate laboratory (ie, cytology, pathology, bacteriology).

Causes for Rejection Obesity, inability to suspend respiration or lie motionless, inability to locate good access to site

References

Chau WK and Chan SC, "Improved Sonographic Visualization by Fluid Challenge Method of Renal Lithiasis in the Nondilated Collecting System. Experience in Seven Cases" *Clin Imaging*, 1997, 21(4):276-83.

Cost GA, Merguerian PA, Cheerasarn SP, et al, "Sonographic Renal Parenchymal and Pelvicaliceal Areas: New Quantitative Parameters for Renal Sonographic Followup," *J Urol*, 1996, 156(2 Pt 2):725-9.

Docimo SG and Silver RI, "Renal Ultrasonography in Newborns With Prenatally Detected Hydronephrosis: Why Wait?" *J Urol*, 1997, 157(4):1387-9.

Gill B, Bennett RT, Barnhard Y, et al, "Can Fetal Renal Artery Doppler Studies Predict Postnatal Renal Function in Morphologically Abnormal Kidneys? A Preliminary Report," *J Urol*, 1996, 156(1):190-2.

Gottlieb RH, Voci SL, Cholewinski SP, et al, "Sonography: A Useful Tool to Detect the Mechanical Causes of Renal Transplant Dysfunction," *J Clin Ultrasound*, 1999, 27(6):325-33.

Gupta S, Gulati M, and Suri S, "Ultrasound-Guided Percutaneous Nephrostomy in Nondilated Pelvicaliceal System," *J Clin Ultrasound*, 1998, 26(3):177-9.

Khajehdehi P, Junaid SM, Salinas-Madrigal L, et al, "Percutaneous Renal Biopsy in the 1990s: Safety, Value, and Implications for Early Hospital Discharge," *Am J Kidney Dis*, 1999, 34(1):92-7.

Levine E, "Acquired Cystic Kidney Disease," *Radiol Clin North Am*, 1996, 34(5):947-64.

Nass K and O'Neill WC, "Bedside Renal Biopsy: Ultrasound Guidance by the Nephrologist," *Am J Kidney Dis*, 1999, 34(5):955-9.

Platt JF, Rubin JM, and Ellis JH, "Lupus Nephritis: Predictive Value of Conventional and Doppler US and Comparison With Serologic and Biopsy Parameters," *Radiology*, 1997, 203(1):82-6.

Richter F, Kasabian NG, Irwin RJ Jr, et al, "Accuracy of Diagnosis by Guided Biopsy of Renal Mass Lesions Classified Indeterminate by Imaging Studies," *Urology*, 2000, 55(3):348-52.

Roy C, Tuchmann C, Pfleger D, et al, "Potential Role of Duplex Doppler Sonography in Acute Renal Colic," *J Clin Ultrasound*, 1998, 26(9):427-32.

Sheih CP, Li YW, Liao YJ, et al, "Diagnosing the Combination of Renal Dysgenesis, Gartner's Duct Cyst, and Ipsilateral Mullerian Duct Obstruction," *J Urol*, 1998, 159(1):217-21.

Zhou Q, Cardoza JD, and Barth R, "Prenatal Sonography of Congenital Renal Malformations," *AJR Am J Roentgenol*, 1999, 173(5):1371-6.

Ultrasound, Kidneys

Synonyms Kidneys Ultrasound; Renal Ultrasound

Procedure Commonly Includes Kidneys

Indications Evaluation of cysts and neoplasms, calcifications, abscess, and hydronephrosis and hydroureter

Patient Preparation The examination may be long, up to 1 hour including waiting time. An emergency examination or an unpredictably long preceding examination may result in additional delay. **Note**: Ultrasound exam to be scheduled before a barium study. If barium study was done, bowel preparation is needed before doing ultrasound examination.

Special Instructions All outpatient examinations are by appointment only. All inpatients are placed on the daily schedule as time permits and are performed as scheduled. Nonemergent examinations are given secondary priority and therefore may not be able to be performed the same day scheduled. Patients will generally be asked to stay after the examination until films are reviewed by the radiologist.

(Continued)

Ultrasound, Kidneys *(Continued)*

Equipment Standard B-mode real time ultrasonic imager with 2-5 MHz transducer.

Technique A gel is applied to the skin and a handheld transducer is swept across the area of interest to image the appropriate organs. Sound waves are used for the imaging and no radiation exposure is present. Images are recorded on x-ray film.

Data Acquired Longitudinal and transverse images of each kidney

Turnaround Time A typed report will generally be issued within 36 hours. A preliminary verbal report generally can be given to the referring physician on request.

Causes for Rejection Patient unable to cooperate with positioning and respiratory maneuvers; bowel gas, barium, obesity

Additional Information Rapid, sensitive evaluation for the presence of hydronephrosis. Useful in confirming the cystic nature of lesions. Detection of hydroureter is often problematic.

References

Chau WK and Chan SC, "Improved Sonographic Visualization by Fluid Challenge Method of Renal Lithiasis in the Nondilated Collecting System," *Clin Imaging*, 1997, 21(4):276-83.

Cost GA, Merguerian PA, Cheerasam SP, et al, "Sonographic Renal Parenchymal and Pelvicaliceal Areas: New Quantitative Parameters for Renal Sonographic Followup," *J Urol*, 1996, 156(2 Pt 2):725-9.

Docimo SG and Silver RI, "Renal Ultrasonography in Newborns With Prenatally Detected Hydronephrosis: Why Wait?" *J Urol*, 1997, 157(4):1387-9.

Gill B, Bennett RT, Barnhard Y, et al, "Can Fetal Renal Artery Doppler Studies Predict Postnatal Renal Function in Morphologically Abnormal Kidneys? A Preliminary Report," *J Urol*, 1996, 156(1):190-2.

Gottlieb RH, Voci SL, Cholewinski SP, et al, "Sonography: A Useful Tool to Detect the Mechanical Causes of Renal Transplant Dysfunction," *J Clin Ultrasound*, 1999, 27(6):325-33.

Gupta S, Gulati M, and Suri S, "Ultrasound-Guided Percutaneous Nephrostomy in Nondilated Pelvicaliceal System," *J Clin Ultrasound*, 1998, 26(3):177-9.

Khajehdehi P, Junaid SM, Salinas-Madrigal L, et al, "Percutaneous Renal Biopsy in the 1990s: Safety, Value, and Implications for Early Hospital Discharge," *Am J Kidney Dis*, 1999, 34(1):92-7.

Levine E, "Acquired Cystic Kidney Disease," *Radiol Clin North Am*, 1996, 34(5):947-64.

Nass K and O'Neill WC, "Bedside Renal Biopsy: Ultrasound Guidance by the Nephrologist," *Am J Kidney Dis*, 1999, 34(5):955-9.

Platt JF, Rubin JM, and Ellis JH, "Lupus Nephritis: Predictive Value of Conventional and Doppler US and Comparison With Serologic and Biopsy Parameters," *Radiology*, 1997, 203(1):82-6.

Richter F, Kasabian NG, Irwin RJ Jr, et al, "Accuracy of Diagnosis by Guided Biopsy of Renal Mass Lesions Classified Indeterminate by Imaging Studies," *Urology*, 2000, 55(3):348-52.

Roy C, Tuchmann C, Pfleger D, et al, "Potential Role of Duplex Doppler Sonography in Acute Renal Colic," *J Clin Ultrasound*, 1998, 26(9):427-32.

Sheih CP, Li YW, Liao YJ, et al, "Diagnosing the Combination of Renal Dysgenesis, Gartner's Duct Cyst and Ipsilateral Mullerian Duct Obstruction," *J Urol*, 1998, 159(1):217-21.

Zhou Q, Cardoza JD, and Barth R, "Prenatal Sonography of Congenital Renal Malformations," *AJR Am J Roentgenol*, 1999, 173(5):1371-6.

♦ **Ultrasound Localization** *see* Ultrasound, Biopsy Localization *on page 480*

Ultrasound, Nephrostomy, Guided

Applies to Nephrostomy; Percutaneous Nephrostomy

Procedure Commonly Includes Use of real time ultrasound imaging to direct placement of a nephrostomy tube into the dilated renal collecting system

Indications Hydronephrosis

Contraindications

- inadequate access by ultrasound
- bleeding diathesis

Patient Preparation The procedure may be long, up to several hours including waiting time. An emergency examination or an unpredictably long preceding examination may result in additional delay.

Special Instructions All procedures performed after consultation with radiologist. All inpatients are placed on the daily schedule as time permits and performed as scheduled. Nonemergent examinations are given secondary priority and therefore may not be able to be performed the same day scheduled.

Complications Hemorrhage, sepsis

Equipment Standard B-mode real time ultrasonic imager with 2-5 MHz transducer and biopsy guide if desired. Appropriate percutaneous nephrostomy kit.

Technique A gel is applied to the skin and a handheld transducer is swept across the area of interest to image the appropriate organs. Sound waves are used for the imaging and no radiation exposure is present. An appropriate access route is chosen and a needle is placed into the renal collecting system under sterile conditions. Local anesthesia and I.V. analgesia are given. The needle is exchanged for nephrostomy catheter. Images are recorded on x-ray film.

Turnaround Time A typed report will generally be issued within 36 hours. A preliminary verbal report generally can be given to the referring physician on request.

Specimen Urine, infected urine

Container Aerobic and anaerobic culture containers

Storage Instructions Culture containers should be sent immediately to the Bacteriology Laboratory.

Causes for Rejection Patient unable to remain motionless during study

Additional Information Procedure allows decompression of obstructed kidney without surgery.

References

Blazer S, Zimmer EZ, Blumenfeld Z, et al, "Natural History of Fetal Simple Renal Cysts Detected in Early Pregnancy," *J Urol*, 1999, 162(3 Pt 1):812-4.

Gupta S, Gulati M, and Suri S, "Ultrasound-Guided Percutaneous Nephrostomy in Nondilated Pelvicaliceal System," *J Clin Ultrasound*, 1998, 26(3):177-9.

Khajehdehi P, Junaid SM, Salinas-Madrigal L, et al, "Percutaneous Renal Biopsy in the 1990s: Safety, Value, and Implications for Early Hospital Discharge," *Am J Kidney Dis*, 1999, 34(1):92-7.

Levine E, "Acquired Cystic Kidney Disease," *Radiol Clin North Am*, 1996, 34(5):947-64.

Nass K and O'Neill WC, "Bedside Renal Biopsy: Ultrasound Guidance by the Nephrologist," *Am J Kidney Dis*, 1999, 34(5):955-9.

Platt JF, Rubin JM, and Ellis JH, "Lupus Nephritis: Predictive Value of Conventional and Doppler US and Comparison With Serologic and Biopsy Parameters," *Radiology*, 1997, 203(1):82-6.

Richter F, Kasabian NG, Irwin RJ Jr, et al, "Accuracy of Diagnosis by Guided Biopsy of Renal Mass Lesions Classified Indeterminate by Imaging Studies," *Urology*, 2000, 55(3):348-52.

Rifkin MD and Goldberg BB, "Aspiration and Biopsy Techniques," *Abdominal Ultrasonography*, 2nd ed, Goldberg BB, ed, New York, NY: John Wiley and Sons Inc, 1984.

Sheih CP, Li YW, Liao YJ, et al, "Diagnosing the Combination of Renal Dysgenesis, Gartner's Duct Cyst, and Ipsilateral Mullerian Duct Obstruction," *J Urol*, 1998, 159(1):217-21.

Ultrasound, OB, Complete

Procedure Commonly Includes Examination of the fetus for viability, placenta localization, measurements of the fetus to determine fetal age and weight, and examination of the maternal pelvis to rule out masses. This study also includes the evaluation of the fetal cerebral ventricles, urinary bladder, kidneys, stomach, spinal and umbilical cord.

Indications Evaluate for total age and viability, IUGR, placenta position, amount of amniotic fluid and presence of certain anomalies.

Patient Preparation The examination may be long, up to 1 hour including waiting time. An emergency examination or an unpredictably long preceding examination may result in additional delay. The patient must have a full urinary bladder at the time of study. The patient should drink 32 oz of water 1½-1 hour prior to the study.

Special Instructions All outpatient examinations are by appointment only. All inpatients are placed on the daily schedule as time permits and are performed as scheduled. Nonemergent examinations are given secondary priority and therefore may not be able to be performed the same day scheduled. Patients will generally be asked to stay after the examination until films are reviewed by the radiologist.

Equipment Standard B-mode real time ultrasonic imager with 2-5 MHz transducer.

Technique A gel is applied to the skin and a handheld transducer is swept across the uterus to image the appropriate organs. Sound waves are used for the imaging and no radiation exposure is present. Images are recorded on x-ray film.

Data Acquired Transverse, longitudinal, and oblique images of the uterus, placenta, and fetus(es). Biparietal diameter (BPD), abdominal circumference

(Continued)

Ultrasound, OB, Complete *(Continued)*

(AC), and femur length (FL) are reported in the second through the third trimesters with estimated gestational age (GA) and fetal weight reported. First trimester, gestational sac size, and/or crown to rump length are reported. Survey of cerebral ventricles, urinary bladder, stomach, kidneys, spine, and umbilical cord insertion site into fetus is performed. Fetal age and viability, position of the placenta, and the amount of amniotic fluid are determined.

Turnaround Time A typed report will generally be issued within 36 hours. A preliminary verbal report generally can be given to the referring physician on request.

Additional Information When evaluating for intrauterine growth retardation, patient should have two ultrasound exams approximately 4-6 weeks apart. Growth retardation cannot be diagnosed on the basis of one exam. This examination is valuable in evaluating for the presence of fetal structural abnormalities, detection of intrauterine growth retardation, and fetal gestational age. Placenta previa and abruptio placenta may be detected.

References

Bofill JA and Sharp GH, "Obstetric Sonography. Who to Scan, When to Scan, and by Whom," *Obstet Gynecol Clin North Am*, 1998, 25(3):465-78.

Fleischer AC and James AE, "Obstetric Sonography: Normal Pregnancy and Anatomical Variants," *Radiology*, Taveras JT and Ferrucci JT, eds, Philadelphia, PA: Lippincott Williams & Wilkins, 1988.

Lennon CA and Gray DL, "Sensitivity and Specificity of Ultrasound for the Detection of Neural Tube and Ventral Wall Defects in a High-Risk Population," *Obstet Gynecol*, 1999, 94(4):562-6.

Magriples U and Copel JA, "Accurate Detection of Anomalies by Routine Ultrasonography in an Indigent Clinic Population," *Am J Obstet Gynecol*, 1998, 179(4):978-81.

Oyelese KO, Turner M, Lees C, et al, "Vasa Previa: An Avoidable Obstetric Tragedy," *Obstet Gynecol Surv*, 1999, 54(2):138-45.

Platt LO, Hill LM, DeVore GR, et al, "Amniocentesis: Current Concepts and Techniques," *The Principles and Practice of Ultrasonography in Obstetrics Gynecology*, Sanders and James, eds, Norwalk, CT: Appleton-Century-Crofts, 1985.

Timor-Tritch IE and Monteagudo A, "Scanning Techniques in Obstetrics and Gynecology," *Clin Obstet Gynecol*, 1996, 39(1):167-74.

Ultrasound, OB, Limited

Synonyms Fetal Age; Gestational Age; Pregnancy, Complete Sonogram; Pregnancy, Echo

Procedure Commonly Includes Examination of the fetus for viability and well being, placenta localization, measurements of the fetus to determine fetal age, and examination of the maternal pelvis to rule out masses

Indications Diagnosis of pregnancy, fetal age, placenta localization, multiple pregnancies, fetal position, amniotic fluid, fetal anomalies, fetal viability, growth retardation

Patient Preparation The examination may be long, up to 1 hour including waiting time. An emergency examination or an unpredictably long preceding examination may result in additional delay. The patient must have a full urinary bladder at the time of study. The patient should drink 32 oz of water 1½-1 hour prior to the study.

Special Instructions All outpatient examinations are by appointment only. All inpatients are placed on the daily schedule as time permits and are performed as scheduled. Nonemergent examinations are given secondary priority and therefore may not be able to be performed the same day scheduled. Patients will generally be asked to stay after the examination until films are reviewed by the radiologist.

Equipment Standard B-mode real time ultrasonic imager with 2-5 MHz transducer.

Technique A gel is applied to the skin and a handheld transducer is swept across the area of interest to image the appropriate organs. Sound waves are used for the imaging and no radiation exposure is present. Images are recorded on x-ray film.

Data Acquired Transverse, longitudinal, and oblique images of the uterus, placenta, and fetus(es). Biparietal diameter (BPD), abdominal circumference (AC), and femur length (FL) are reported in the second through the third trimesters with estimated gestational age (GA) reported. First trimester, gestational sac size, and/or crown to rump length are reported. Survey of cerebral ventricles, urinary bladder, stomach, kidneys, spine, and umbilical cord insertion site into fetus is **not** performed. Fetal age and viability, position of the placenta, and the amount of amniotic fluid are determined.

Turnaround Time A typed report will generally be issued within 36 hours. A preliminary verbal report generally can be given to the referring physician on request.

Limitations The patient not having a full bladder

Additional Information When evaluating for intrauterine growth retardation, patient should have two ultrasound exams approximately 4-6 weeks apart. Growth retardation cannot be diagnosed on basis of one exam.

References

Bofill JA and Sharp GH, "Obstetric Sonography. Who to Scan, When to Scan, and by Whom," *Obstet Gynecol Clin North Am*, 1998, 25(3):465-78.

Fleischer AC and James AE, "Obstetric Sonography: Normal Pregnancy and Anatomical Variants," *Radiology*, Taveras JT and Ferrucci JT, eds, Philadelphia, PA: Lippincott Williams & Wilkins, 1988.

Lennon CA and Gray DL, "Sensitivity and Specificity of Ultrasound for the Detection of Neural Tube and Ventral Wall Defects in a High-Risk Population," *Obstet Gynecol*, 1999, 94(4):562-6.

Magriples U and Copel JA, "Accurate Detection of Anomalies by Routine Ultrasonography in an Indigent Clinic Population," *Am J Obstet Gynecol*, 1998, 179(4):978-81.

Oyelese KO, Turner M, Lees C, et al, "Vasa Previa: An Avoidable Obstetric Tragedy," *Obstet Gynecol Surv*, 1999, 54(2):138-45.

Platt LO, Hill LM, DeVore GR, et al, "Amniocentesis: Current Concepts and Techniques," *The Principles and Practice of Ultrasonography in Obstetrics Gynecology*, Sanders and James, eds, Norwalk, CT: Appleton-Century-Crofts, 1985.

Timor-Tritch IE and Monteagudo A, "Scanning Techniques in Obstetrics and Gynecology," *Clin Obstet Gynecol*, 1996, 39(1):167-74.

Ultrasound, Pancreas

Synonyms Pancreas Ultrasound

Procedure Commonly Includes Pancreas, biliary tree, and gallbladder

Indications Evaluate pancreatic size and shape, presence of neoplasm, cystic lesions, pseudocyst, pancreatitis

Contraindications

- open wound or incision overlying examination area (routine study)
- recent barium study

Patient Preparation The patient should not have had a barium study within the 3 days prior to study. The examinations may be up to 1 hour each. An emergency exam or an unpredictably long preceding exam may result in additional delay. NPO after midnight before day of examination.

Special Instructions All outpatient examinations are by appointment only. All inpatients are placed on the daily schedule as time permits and are performed as scheduled. Nonemergent examinations are given secondary priority and therefore may not be able to be performed the same day scheduled. Patients will generally be asked to stay after the examination until films are reviewed by the radiologist.

Equipment Standard B-mode real time ultrasonic imager with 2-5 MHz transducer.

Technique A gel is applied to the skin and a handheld transducer is swept across the area of interest to image the appropriate organs. Sound waves are used for the imaging and no radiation exposure is present. Images are recorded on x-ray film.

Turnaround Time A typed report will generally be issued within 36 hours. A preliminary verbal report generally can be given to the referring physician on request.

Causes for Rejection Gas, barium, oral ingestion of food, body habitus, rib artifacts

Additional Information Request for this study results in study of the pancreas with limited evaluation of other nearby organs.

References

Bender GN, Case B, Tsuchida A, et al, "Using Sector Endoluminal Ultrasound to Identify the Normal Pancreas When Axial Computed Tomography Is Falsely Positive," *Invest Radiol*, 1999, 34(1):71-4.

Catalano MF, Lahoti S, Geenan JE, et al, "Dynamic Imaging of the Pancreas Using Real-Time Endoscopic Ultrasonography With Secretin Stimulation," *Gastrointest Endosc*, 1998, 48(6):580-7.

(Continued)

Ultrasound, Pancreas *(Continued)*

Catalano MF, Lahoti S, Geenan JE, et al, "Prospective Evaluation of Endoscopic Ultrasonography, Endoscopic Retrograde Pancreatography, and Secretin Test in the Diagnosis of Chronic Pancreatitis," *Gastrointest Endosc*, 1998, 48(1):11-7.

Cooperberg PL and Rowley VA, "Abdominal Sonographic Examination Technique," *Radiology*, Taveras JT and Ferrucci JT, eds, Philadelphia, PA: Lippincott Williams & Wilkins, 1988.

Di Stasi M, Lencioni R, Solmi L, et al, "Ultrasound-Guided Fine Needle Biopsy of Pancreatic Masses: Results of a Multicenter Study," *Am J Gastroenterol*, 1998, 93(8):1329-33.

Frazee RC, Singh H, and Erickson RA, "Endoscopic Ultrasound for Peripancreatic Masses," *Am J Surg*, 1997, 174(6):596-8.

Goldberg BB, *Abdominal Ultrasonography*, New York, NY: John Wiley and Sons Inc, 1984.

Gress F, Ikenberry S, Sherman S, et al, "Endoscopic Ultrasound-Directed Pancreatography," *Gastrointest Endosc*, 1996, 44(6):736-9.

Inui K, Nakazawa S, Yoshino J, et al, "Endoluminal Ultrasonography for Pancreatic Diseases," *Gastroenterol Clin North Am*, 1999, 28(3):771-81.

Lewis JD, Faigel DO, Morris JB, et al, "Splenic Vein Thrombosis Secondary to Focal Pancreatitis Diagnosed by Endoscopic Ultrasonography," *J Clin Gastroenterol*, 1998, 26(1):54-6.

Siegel MJ and Sivit CJ, "Pancreatic Emergencies," *Radiol Clin North Am*, 1997, 35(4):815-30, 814.

Yassa NA, Yang J, Stein S, et al, "Gray-Scale and Color-Flow Sonography of Pancreatic Ductal Adenocarcinoma," *J Clin Ultrasound*, 1997, 25(9):473-80.

Ultrasound, Parathyroids

Synonyms Parathyroids Ultrasound

Procedure Commonly Includes Parathyroid glands

Indications Evaluation of parathyroid size as well as abnormal masses

Patient Preparation The examination may be long, up to 1 hour including waiting time. An emergency examination or an unpredictably long preceding examination may result in additional delay.

Special Instructions All outpatient examinations are by appointment only. All inpatients are placed on the daily schedule as time permits and are performed as scheduled. Nonemergent examinations are given secondary priority and therefore may not be able to be performed the same day scheduled. Patients will generally be asked to stay after the examination until films are reviewed by the radiologist.

Equipment Standard B-mode real time ultrasonic imager with 7.5-10 MHz transducer.

Technique A gel is applied to the skin and a handheld transducer is swept across the area of interest to image the appropriate organs. Sound waves are used for the imaging and no radiation exposure is present. Images are recorded on x-ray film.

Data Acquired Longitudinal, sagittal, and oblique images of parathyroid glands

Turnaround Time A typed report will generally be issued within 36 hours. A preliminary verbal report generally can be given to the referring physician on request.

Causes for Rejection Overlying thyroid pathology

Additional Information Patients referred for this examination should have a proven diagnosis of hyperparathyroidism. This test is used to define the anatomy of the parathyroids and not to assess function. It most often is performed in the preoperative evaluation of a patient with hyperparathyroidism.

References

Becker D, Blair HF, Becker W, et al, "Thyroid Autonomy With Color-Coded Image-Directed Doppler Sonography: Internal Hypervascularization for the Recognition of Autonomous Adenomas," *J Clin Ultrasound*, 1997, 25(2):63-9.

Butch RJ, Simeone JF, and Mueller PR, "Thyroid and Parathyroid Ultrasonography," *Radiol Clin North Am*, 1985, 23(1):57-71.

Cho YS, Lee HK, Ahn IM, et al, "Sonographically Guided Ethanol Sclerotherapy for Benign Thyroid Cysts: Results in 22 Patients," *AJR Am J Roentgenol*, 2000, 174(1):213-6.

Erdem S, Bashekim C, Kizilkaya E, et al, "Clinical Application of Tc-99m Tetrofosmin Scintigraphy in Patients With Cold Thyroid Nodules. Comparison With Color Doppler Sonography," *Clin Nucl Med*, 1997, 22(2):76-9.

Frasoldati A, Pesenti M, Toschi E, et al, "Detection and Diagnosis of Parathyroid Incidentaloma During Thyroid Sonography," *J Clin Ultrasound*, 1999, 27(9):492-8.

Gailloud P, Khan HG, Khaw N, et al, "The Supraisthmic Anastomotic Arch: A Potential Pitfall in Doppler Sonography of the Thyroid Gland," *AJR Am J Roentgenol*, 1998, 170(2):497-8.

Gallowitsch HJ, Mikosch P, Kresnik E, et al, "Technetium 99m Tetrofosmin Parathyroid Imaging. Results With Double-Phase Study and SPECT in Primary and Secondary Hyperparathyroidism," *Invest Radiol*, 1997, 32(8):459-65.

Koslin DB, Adama J, Andersen P, et al, "Preoperative Evaluation of Patients With Primary Hyperparathyroidism: Role of High-Resolution Ultrasound," *Laryngoscope*, 1997, 107(9):1249-53.

Lane MJ, Desser TS, Weigel RJ, et al, "Use of Color and Power Doppler Sonography to Identify Feeding Arteries Associated With Parathyroid Adenomas," *AJR Am J Roentgenol*, 1998, 171(3):819-23.

Mizokami T, Okamura K, Sato K, et al, "Localized Painful Giant-Cell Thyroiditis Without Inflammatory Signs in a Euthyroid Patient Followed by Serial Sonography," *J Clin Ultrasound*, 1998, 26(6):329-32.

Profanter C, Klinger A, Strolz S, et al, "Surgical Therapy for Primary Hyperparathyroidism in Patients With Previous Thyroid Surgery," *Am J Surg*, 1999, 178(5):374-6.

Rozycki GS, "Surgeon-Performed Ultrasound: Its Use in Clinical Practice," *Ann Surg*, 1998, 228(1):16-28.

Simeone JF, "Ultrasound Examination of the Thyroid and Parathyroid," *Radiology*, Taveras JT and Ferrucci JT, eds, Philadelphia, PA: Lippincott Williams & Wilkins, 1988.

Takashima S, Takayama F, Wang Q, et al, "Thyroid Metastasis From Rectal Carcinoma Coexisting With Hashimoto's Thyroiditis: Gray-Scale and Power Doppler Sonographic Findings," *J Clin Ultrasound*, 1998, 26(7):361-5.

Taki S, Kakuda K, Kakuma K, et al, "Thyroid Nodules: Evaluation With US-Guided Core Biopsy With an Automated Biopsy gun," *Radiology*, 1997, 202(3):874-7.

Tessler FN and Tublin ME, "Thyroid Sonography: Current Applications and Future Directions," *AJR Am J Roentgenol*, 1999, 173(2):437-43.

Ultrasound, Pelvis

Synonyms Lower Abdomen Ultrasound; Pelvis Ultrasound

Procedure Commonly Includes Uterus, fallopian tubes, ovaries, bilateral adnexa, appendix region

Indications Pelvic masses and abscess, uterus size, IUD localization, and pregnancy diagnosis. Ectopic pregnancy, dermoid cyst, pelvic inflammatory disease, ovarian cyst, fibroid tumor, and bladder tumor.

Patient Preparation Instruct patient to drink four 8 oz glasses of water 45 minutes prior to exam and not to empty bladder. The examination may be long, up to 1 hour including waiting time. An emergency examination or an unpredictably long preceding examination may result in additional delay. No barium studies should have been performed on the patient for **at least** 2 days preceding exam. **Note:** Ultrasound exam is to be scheduled before a barium study. If barium study was done, bowel preparation is needed before doing ultrasound examination.

Special Instructions All outpatient examinations are by appointment only. All inpatients are placed on the daily schedule as time permits and are performed as scheduled. Nonemergent examinations are given secondary priority and therefore may not be able to be performed the same day scheduled. Patients will generally be asked to stay after the examination until films are reviewed by the radiologist.

Equipment Standard B-mode real time ultrasonic imager with 2-5 MHz transducer.

Technique A gel is applied to the skin and a handheld transducer is swept across the area of interest to image the appropriate organs. Sound waves are used for the imaging and no radiation exposure is present. Images are recorded on x-ray film.

Data Acquired Longitudinal, transverse, and oblique images

Turnaround Time A typed report will generally be issued within 36 hours. A preliminary verbal report generally can be given to the referring physician on request.

Causes for Rejection Bowel gas, barium, patient not having full bladder, patient scheduled for barium studies and/or IVP

Additional Information This study is valuable for the detection of ovarian cysts and neoplasms, uterine abnormalities, presence of abnormal collections such as abscess and endometrioma. May aid in the diagnosis of ectopic pregnancy.

References

Desser TS, Jeffrey RB Jr, Lane MJ, et al, "Tissue Harmonic Imaging: Utility in Abdominal and Pelvic Sonography," *J Clin Ultrasound*, 1999, 27(3):135-42.

Estroff JA, "Emergency Obstetric and Gynecologic Ultrasound," *Radiol Clin North Am*, 1997, 35(4):921-57.

(Continued)

Ultrasound, Pelvis *(Continued)*

Fisher AJ, Paulson Ek, Sheafor DH, et al, "Small Lymph Nodes of the Abdomen, Pelvis, and Retroperitoneum: Usefulness of Sonographically Guided Biopsy," *Radiology*, 1997, 205(1):185-90.

Forstner R, Kalbhen CL, Filly RA, et al, "Abdominopelvic MR Imaging in the Nonobstetric Evaluation of Pregnant Patients," *AJR Am J Roentgenol*, 1996, 166(5):1139-44.

Hall DA and Hann LE, "Gynecologic Radiology: Benign Disorders," *Radiology*, Taveras JT and Ferrucci JT, eds, Philadelphia, PA: Lippincott Williams & Wilkins, 1988.

Jain KA and Gerscovich EO, "Sonographic Spectrum of Pelvic Vascular Malformations in Women," *J Clin Ultrasound*, 1999, 27(9):523-30.

Khalife S, Falcone T, Hemmings R, et al, "Diagnostic Accuracy of Transvaginal Ultrasound in Detecting Free Pelvic Fluid," *J Reprod Med*, 1998, 43(9):795-8.

Lang FC, "Ectopic Pregnancy," *Radiology*, Taveras JT and Ferrucci JT, eds, Philadelphia, PA: Lippincott Williams & Wilkins, 1988.

Memel DS, Dodd GD 3rd, and Esola CC, "Efficacy of Sonography as a Guidance Technique for Biopsy of Abdominal, Pelvic, and Retroperitoneal Lymph Nodes," *AJR Am J Roentgenol*, 1996, 167(4):957-62.

Shih CH, "Effect of Emergence Physician-Performed Pelvic Sonography on Length of Stay in the Emergency Department," *Ann Emerg Med*, 1997, 29(3):348-51.

Sperling DC, Needleman L, Eschelman DJ, et al, "Deep Pelvic Abscesses: Transperineal US-Guided Drainage," *Radiology*, 1998, 208(1):111-5.

Vural M, Kacar S, Kosar U, et al, "Symptomatic Wandering Accessory Spleen in the Pelvis: Sonographic Findings," *J Clin Ultrasound*, 1999, 27(9):534-6.

Zornoza J, "Gynecologic Radiology: Malignant," *Radiology*, Taveras JT and Ferrucci JT, eds, Philadelphia, PA: Lippincott Williams & Wilkins, 1988.

Zornoza J, "The Pelvis: Anatomy and Examination Techniques," *Radiology*, Taveras JT and Ferrucci JT, eds, Philadelphia, PA: Lippincott Williams & Wilkins, 1988.

Ultrasound, Penile Duplex

Related Information

Penile Blood Flow *on page 290*

Synonyms Penile Ultrasound

Procedure Commonly Includes Penis

Indications Primary impotence, vasculogenic impotence

Patient Preparation The examination may be long, up to 1 hour including waiting time. An emergency examination or an unpredictably long preceding examination may result in additional delay.

Special Instructions Examinations scheduled after consultation with radiologist. All outpatient examinations are by appointment only. All inpatients are placed on the daily schedule as time permits and are performed as scheduled. Nonemergent examinations are given secondary priority and therefore may not be able to be performed the same day scheduled. Patients will generally be asked to stay after the examination until films are reviewed by the radiologist.

Equipment Standard B-mode real time ultrasonic imager with Doppler capability with 7.5-10 MHz transducer

Technique A gel is applied to the skin and a handheld transducer is swept across the area of interest to image the appropriate organs. Sound waves are used for the imaging and no radiation exposure is present. Images are recorded on x-ray film.

Data Acquired Doppler flow data of major penile vessels

Turnaround Time A typed report will generally be issued within 36 hours. A preliminary verbal report generally can be given to the referring physician on request.

Additional Information Examination may be valuable in the evaluation of impotence of vascular origin.

References

Chiou RK, Alberts GL, Pomeroy BD, et al, "Study of Cavernosal Arterial Anatomy Using Color and Power Doppler Sonography: Impact on Hemodynamic Parameter Measurement," *J Urol*, 1999, 162(2):358-60.

Chung WS, Park YY, and Kwon SW, "The Impact of Aging on Penile Hemodynamics in Normal Responders to Pharmacological Injection: A Doppler Sonographic Study," *J Urol*, 1997, 157(6):2129-31.

Levine LA and Coogan CL, "Penile Vascular Assessment Using Color Duplex Sonography in Men With Peyronie's Disease," *J Urol*, 1996, 155(4):1270-3.

Mancini M, Bartolini M, Maggi M, et al, "The Presence of Arterial Anatomical Variations can Affect the Results of Duplex Sonographic Evaluation of Penile Vessels in Impotent Patients," *J Urol*, 1996, 155(6):1919-23.

Rozycki GS, "Surgeon-Performed Ultrasound: Its Use in Clinical Practice," *Ann Surg*, 1998, 228(1):16-28.

Sattar AA, Wery D, Golzarian J, et al, "Correlation of Nocturnal Penile Tumescence Monitoring Duplex Ultrasonography and Infusion Cavernosometry for the Diagnosis of Erectile Dysfunction," *J Urol*, 1996, 155(4):1274-6.

Tam PY, Keller T, Poppiti R, et al, "Hemodynamic Effects on Transurethral Alprostadil Measured by Color Duplex Ultrasonography in Men With Erectile Dysfunction," *J Urol*, 1998, 160(4):1321-4.

Ultrasound, Peripheral Arteries and Veins

Synonyms Iliac Arteries Ultrasound; Peripheral Arteries and Veins Ultrasound; Popliteal Ultrasound

Procedure Commonly Includes Peripheral arteries and/or veins

Indications Determine aneurysm, cysts, pseudoaneurysm, deep vein thrombosis (DVT), arterial insufficiency

Patient Preparation The examination may be long, up to 1 hour including waiting time. An emergency examination or an unpredictably long preceding examination may result in additional delay.

Special Instructions Specific vessels of interest to be studied as well as location must be specified. All outpatient examinations are by appointment only. All inpatients are placed on the daily schedule as time permits and are performed as scheduled. Nonemergent examinations are given secondary priority and therefore may not be able to be performed the same day scheduled. Patients will generally be asked to stay after the examination until films are reviewed by the radiologist.

Equipment Standard B-mode real time ultrasonic imager with Doppler capability with 5-10 MHz transducer

Technique A gel is applied to the skin and a handheld transducer is swept across the area of interest to image the appropriate organs. Sound waves are used for the imaging and no radiation exposure is present. Images are recorded on x-ray film.

Turnaround Time A typed report will generally be issued within 36 hours. A preliminary verbal report generally can be given to the referring physician on request.

Normal Findings Presence of appropriate flow, compressibility of venous structures

Additional Information Examination is valuable in the detection of pseudoaneurysms, aneurysms, arterial insufficiency, and deep venous thrombosis (DVT)

References

Bimbaum Y, Fishbein MC, Luo H, et al, "Regional Remodeling of Atherosclerotic Arteries: A Major Determinant of Clinical Manifestations of Disease," *J Am Coll Cardiol*, 1997, 30(5):1149-64.

Keyes LE, Frazee BW, Snoey ER, et al, "Ultrasound-Guided Brachial and Basilic Vein Cannulation in Emergency Department Patients With Difficult Intravenous Access," *Ann Emerg Med*, 1999, 34(6):711-4.

Libertiny G and Hands L, "Lower Limb Deep Vein Flow in Patients With Peripheral Vascular Disease," *J Vasc Surg*, 1999, 29(6):1065-70.

Sofocleous CT, Schur I, Cooper SG, et al, "Sonographically Guided Placement of Peripherally Inserted Central Venous Catheters: Review of 355 Procedures," *AJR Am J Roentgenol*, 1998, 170(6):1613-6.

Ultrasound, Prostate

Synonyms Prostate Ultrasound

Procedure Commonly Includes Prostate, seminal vesicles

Indications Evaluate for the presence of a prostatic lesion

Contraindications Recent rectosigmoid surgery

Patient Preparation The patient should not void 1 hour prior to examination. A cleansing enema should be given to patient 2 hours prior to examination. The patient must not have had recent rectosigmoid surgery.

Special Instructions All outpatient examinations are by appointment only. All inpatients are placed on the daily schedule as time permits and are performed as scheduled. Nonemergent examinations are given secondary priority and therefore may not be able to be performed the same day scheduled. Patients will generally be asked to stay after the examination until films are reviewed by the radiologist.

(Continued)

Ultrasound, Prostate *(Continued)*

Equipment Standard B-mode real time ultrasonic imager with 2-5 MHz transrectal transducer.

Technique A cylindrical transrectal ultrasound transducer is inserted into the rectum. The transducer is then gently rocked back and forth to obtain needed images.

Data Acquired Sagittal and transverse images of prostate and seminal vesicles

Turnaround Time A typed report will generally be issued within 36 hours. A preliminary verbal report generally can be given to the referring physician on request.

Additional Information This examination may be useful in the detection of prostatic carcinoma.

References

Bree RL, "The Role of Color Doppler and Staging Biopsies in Prostate Cancer Detection," *Urology*, 1997, 49(3A Suppl):31-4.

Connolly JA, Shinohara K, Presti JC Jr, et al, "Local Recurrence After Radical Prostatectomy: Characteristics in Size, Location, and Relationship to Prostate-Specific Antigen and Surgical Margins," *Urology*, 1996, 47(2):225-31.

Koch WF, Ezz el Din K, de Wildt MJ, et al, "The Outcome of Renal Ultrasound in the Assessment of 556 Consecutive Patients With Benign Prostatic Hyperplasia," *J Urol*, 1996, 155(1):186-9.

Lavoipierre AM, Snow RM, Frydenberg M, et al, "Prostatic Cancer: Role of Color Doppler Imaging in Transrectal Sonography," *AJR Am J Roentgenol*, 1998, 171(1):205-10.

Matthew GJ, Motta J, and Fracehia JA, "The Accuracy of Transrectal Ultrasound Prostate Volume Estimation: Clinical Correlations," *J Clin Ultrasound*, 1996, 24(9):501-5.

Ochiai A and Kojima M, "Correlation of Ultrasound-Estimated Bladder Weight With Ultrasound Appearance of the Prostate and Postvoid Residual Urine in Men With Lower Urinary Tract Symptoms," *Urology*, 1998, 51(5):722-9.

Terris MK, Afzal N, and Kabalin JN, "Correlation of Transrectal Ultrasound Measurements of Prostate and Transition Zone Size With Symptom Score, Bother Score, Urinary Flow Rate, and Post-Void Residual Volume," *Urology*, 1998, 52(3):462-6.

Terris MK, Hammerer PG, and Nickas ME, "Comparison of Ultrasound Imaging in Patients Undergoing Transperineal and Transrectal Prostate Ultrasound," *Urology*, 1998, 52(6):1070-2.

Tewari A, Indudhara R, Shinohara K, et al, "Comparison of Transrectal Ultrasound Prostatic Volume Estimation With Magnetic Resonance Imaging Volume Estimation and Surgical Specimen Weight in Patients With Benign Prostatic Hyperplasia," *J Clin Ultrasound*, 1996, 24(4):169-74.

Ukimura O, Kojima M, Inui E, et al, "A Statistical Study of the American Urological Association Symptom Index for Benign Prostatic Hyperplasia in Participants of Mass Screening Program for Prostatic Diseases Using Transrectal Sonography," *J Urol*, 1996, 156(5):1673-8.

Ultrasound, Radiotherapy Plan

Synonyms Radiotherapy Plan Ultrasound

Procedure Commonly Includes Specific anatomic area per request

Indications Measurement of distance between anterior surface to chest wall, mark boundaries of tumor for radiotherapist, measure distance to tumor and dimensions of therapy site

Equipment Standard B-mode real time ultrasonic imager with 5-7 MHz transducer.

Technique A gel is applied to the skin and a handheld transducer is swept across the area of interest to image the appropriate organs. Sound waves are used for the imaging and no radiation exposure is present. Images are recorded on x-ray film.

Turnaround Time A typed report will generally be issued within 36 hours. A preliminary verbal report generally can be given to the referring physician on request.

Causes for Rejection Bowel gas, barium, body habitus on patients with abdominal tumors

Additional Information Examination is limited to demarcating appropriate field used in radiotherapy.

References

Arya S, Nagarkatti DG, Dudhat SB, et al, "Soft Tissue Sarcomas: Ultrasonographic Evaluation of Local Recurrences," *Clin Radiol*, 2000, 55(3):193-7.

Carmody BJ, Arora S, Avena R, et al, "Accelerated Carotid Artery Disease After High-Dose Head and Neck Radiotherapy: Is There a Role for Routine Carotid Duplex Surveillance?" *J Vasc Surg*, 1999, 30(6):1045-51.

Cheng SW, Wu LL, Ting AC, et al, "Irradiation-Induced Extracranial Carotid Stenosis With Head and Neck Malignancies," *Am J Surg*, 1999, 178(4):323-8.

Ho S, Lau WY, and Leung WT, "Ultrasound Guided Internal Radiotherapy Using Yttrium-90 Glass Microspheres for Liver Malignancies," *J Nucl Med*, 1997, 38(7):1169-70.

Isenberg G, Chak A, Canto MI, et al, "Endoscopic Ultrasound in Restaging of Esophageal Cancer After Neoadjuvant Chemoradiation," *Gastrointest Endosc*, 1998, 48(2):158-63.

Lattanzi J, McNeeley S, Hanlon A, et al, "Ultrasound-Based Stereotactic Guidance of Precision Conformal External Beam Radiation Therapy in Clinically Localized Prostate Cancer," *Urology*, 2000, 55(1):73-8.

Lohnert M, Doniec JM, Kovacs G, et al, "New Method of Radiotherapy for Anal Cancer With Three-Dimensional Tumor Reconstruction Based on Endoanal Ultrasound and Ultrasound-Guided Afterloading Therapy," *Dis Colon Rectum*, 1998, 41(2)169-76.

Rozycki GS, "Surgeon-Performed Ultrasound: Its Use in Clinical Practice," *Ann Surg*, 1998, 228(1):16-28.

Tian JH, Xu BX, Zhang JM, et al, "Ultrasound-Guided Internal Radiotherapy Using Yttrium-90-Glass Microspheres for liver Malignancies," *J Nucl Med*, 1996, 37(6):958-63.

Ultrasound, Renal Artery

Synonyms RADS; Renal Artery Duplex Scanning; Renal Artery Ultrasound

Procedure Commonly Includes Ultrasound of the renal arteries to look for plaque, stenosis, or occlusion

Indications Evaluate patients with malignant or accelerated hypertension, young patients with hypertension, presence of a flank bruit, decreased serum potassium of unknown cause, and azotemia

Patient Preparation The procedure is performed on the patient after overnight fasting and takes 1-1½ hours to complete.

Equipment Standard B-mode real time ultrasonic imager with Doppler capabilities, 2.5-3.0 MHz transducer

Technique The patient is in the supine position with a pillow under the head. A gel is applied to the skin and a handheld transducer is swept across the area of interest to image the appropriate vasculature.

Data Acquired Longitudinal, transverse, and oblique images with Doppler flow parameters

Turnaround Time A typed report will generally be issued within 36 hours. A preliminary verbal report generally can be given to the referring physician on request.

Normal Findings Absence of stenosis or occlusion of renal arteries

Additional Information Flow velocities are recorded for the aorta as well as the renal arteries. Renal-aortic ratio (RAR) is the accepted criterion for the diagnosis of renal artery stenosis. RAR >3.5 is abnormal and indicates >60% diameter-reducing stenosis.

References

Brunt LM, Bennett HF, Teefey SA, et al, "Laparoscopic Ultrasound Imaging of Adrenal Tumors During Laparoscopic Adrenalectomy," *Am J Surg*, 1999, 178(6):490-5.

Elbeery JR, Brown PM, and Chitwood WR Jr, "Intraoperative MIDCABG Arteriography Via the Left Radial Artery: A Comparison With Doppler Ultrasound for Assessment of Graft Patency," *Ann Thorac Surg*, 1998, 66(1):51-5.

Gill B, Bennett RT, Barnhard Y, et al, "Can Fetal Renal Artery Doppler Studies Predict Postnatal Renal Function in Morphologically Abnormal Kidneys? A Preliminary Report," *J Urol*, 1996, 156(1):190-2.

Gottlieb RH, Voci SL, Cholewinski SP, et al, "Sonography: A Useful Tool to Detect the Mechanical Causes of Renal Transplant Dysfunction," *J Clin Ultrasound*, 1999, 27(6):325-33.

Koo CK, Rodger S, and Baxter GM, "Extra-Renal Pseudoaneurysm: An Uncommon Complication Following Renal Transplantation," *Clin Radiol*, 1999, 54(11):755-8.

Loubeyre P, Cahen R, Grozel F, et al, "Transplant Renal Artery Stenosis. Evaluation of Diagnosis With Magnetic Resonance Angiography Compared With Color Duplex Sonography and Arteriography," *Transplantation*, 1996, 62(4):446-50.

Pilcher DB and Ricci MA, "Vascular Ultrasound," *Surg Clin North Am*, 1998, 78(2):273-93.

Sakarya ME, Arslan H, and Unal O, "The Role of Power Doppler Sonography in the Prenatal Evaluation of Fetal Renal Vasculature," *Clin Imaging*, 1999, 23(1):32-4.

Zimmermann P and Ranta T, "Doppler Assessment of the Maternal Interlobar Renal and Uterine Arteries in Mid-Pregnancy in Women at Low and High Risk for Pregnancy-Induced Hypertension," *J Clin Ultrasound*, 1998, 26(5):239-45.

Ultrasound, Renal Transplant

Synonyms Renal Transplant Ultrasound

Procedure Commonly Includes Renal transplant

Patient Preparation The examination may be long, up to 1 hour including waiting time. An emergency examination or an unpredictably long preceding examination may result in additional delay.

(Continued)

Ultrasound, Renal Transplant *(Continued)*

Special Instructions All outpatient examinations are by appointment only. All inpatients are placed on the daily schedule as time permits and are performed as scheduled. Nonemergent examinations are given secondary priority and therefore may not be able to be performed the same day scheduled. Patients will generally be asked to stay after the examination until films are reviewed by the radiologist.

Equipment Standard B-mode real time ultrasonic imager with Doppler capability with 2-5 MHz transducer

Technique A gel is applied to the skin and a handheld transducer is swept across the area of interest to image the appropriate organs. Sound waves are used for the imaging and no radiation exposure is present. Images are recorded on x-ray film.

Turnaround Time A typed report will generally be issued within 36 hours. A preliminary verbal report generally can be given to the referring physician on request.

Additional Information Detection of perirenal fluid collections such as abscess urinoma or lymphocele. Doppler parameters are obtained to evaluate perfusion.

References

Akiyama T, Ikegami M, Hara Y, et al, "Hemodynamic Study of Renal Transplant Chronic Rejection Using Power Doppler Sonography," *Transplant Proc*, 1996, 28(3):1458-60.

Elbeery JR, Brown PM, and Chitwood WR Jr, "Intraoperative MIDCABG Arteriography Via the Left Radial Artery: A Comparison With Doppler Ultrasound for Assessment of Graft Patency," *Ann Thorac Surg*, 1998, 66(1):51-5.

Ferraresso M, Raiteri M, Bellapi A, et al, "Use of a Newly Developed Ultrasound Contrast Medium for Color Doppler Evaluation in Kidney Transplantation," *Transplant Proc*, 1999, 31(1-2):1354-6.

Gottlieb RH, Voci SL, Cholewinski SP, et al, "Sonography: A Useful Tool to Detect the Mechanical Causes of Renal Transplant Dysfunction," *J Clin Ultrasound*, 1999, 27(6):325-33.

Koo CK, Rodger S, and Baxter GM, "Extra-Renal Pseudoaneurysm: An Uncommon Complication Following Renal Transplantation," *Clin Radiol*, 1999, 54(11):755-8.

Loubeyre P, Cahen R, Grozel F, et al, "Transplant Renal Artery Stenosis. Evaluation of Diagnosis With Magnetic Resonance Angiography Compared With Color Duplex Sonography and Arteriography," *Transplantation*, 1996, 62(4):446-50.

Martinoli C, Crespi G, Bertolotto M, et al, "Interlobular Vasculature In Renal Transplants: A Power Doppler US Study With MR Correlation," *Radiology*, 1996, 200(1):111-7.

Mazuecos A, Garcia T, Alonso F, et al, "Value of Reversed Diastolic Flow in Doppler Sonography of Renal Transplant," *Transplant Proc*, 1997, 29(1-2):167-8.

Rifkin MD, Needleman L, Pasto ME, et al, "Evaluation of Renal Transplant Rejection by Duplex Doppler Examination: Value of the Resistive Index," *AJR Am J Roentgenol*, 1987, 148(4):759-62.

Sakarya ME, Arslan H, and Unal O, "The Role of Power Doppler Sonography in the Prenatal Evaluation of Fetal Renal Vasculature," *Clin Imaging*, 1999, 23(1):32-4.

Salgado O, Garcia R, Rincon O, et al, "Acute Tubular Necrosis in Renal Transplantation Evaluated by Color Duplex Sonography," *Transplant Proc*, 1996, 28(6):3337-9.

Trillaud H, Merville P, Tran Le Linh P, et al, "Color Doppler Sonography in Early Renal Transplantation Follow-up: Resistive Index Measurements Versus Power Doppler Sonography," *AJR Am J Roentgenol*, 1998, 171(6):1611-5.

Zimmermann P and Ranta T, "Doppler Assessment of the Maternal Interlobar Renal and Uterine Arteries in Mid-Pregnancy in Women at Low and High Risk for Pregnancy-Induced Hypertension," *J Clin Ultrasound*, 1998, 26(5):239-45.

♦ **Ultrasound Retroperitoneal** *see* Ultrasound, Abdomen *on page 476*

Ultrasound, Soft Tissue Mass

Synonyms Superficial Soft Tissue Mass Ultrasound

Procedure Commonly Includes Soft tissue mass

Indications Evaluate for the presence of mass, determine if a mass is solid or cystic, determine size of a mass

Patient Preparation The examination may be long, up to 1 hour including waiting time. An emergency examination or an unpredictably long preceding examination may result in additional delay.

Special Instructions All outpatient examinations are by appointment only. All inpatients are placed on the daily schedule as time permits and are performed as scheduled. Nonemergent examinations are given secondary priority and therefore may not be able to be performed the same day scheduled. Patients will generally be asked to stay after the examination until films are reviewed by the radiologist.

Equipment Standard B-mode real time ultrasonic imager with 2-7 MHz transducer.

Technique A gel is applied to the skin and a handheld transducer is swept across the area of interest to image the appropriate organs. Sound waves are used for the imaging and no radiation exposure is present. Images are recorded on x-ray film.

Turnaround Time A typed report will generally be issued within 36 hours. A preliminary verbal report generally can be given to the referring physician on request.

Additional Information This examination is useful in determining the size of peripheral masses. The examination will determine if the mass is solid, cystic, or complex.

References

Adler RS, Bell Ds, Bamber JC, et al, "Evaluation of Soft-Tissue Masses Using Segmented Color Doppler Velocity Images: Preliminary Observations," *AJR Am J Roentgenol*, 1999, 172(3):781-8.

Bond CD, Hennrikus WL, and Della Maggiore ED, "Prospective Evaluation of Newborn Soft-Tissue Hip "Clicks" With Ultrasound," *J Pediatr Orthop*, 1997, 17(2):199-201.

Dubois J, Patriquin HB, Garel L, et al, "Soft-Tissue Hemangiomas in Infants and Children Using Doppler Sonography," *AJR Am J Roentgenol*, 1998, 171(1):247-52.

Jacobson JA, "Musculoskeletal Sonography and MR Imaging. A Role for Both Imaging Methods," *Radiol Clin North Am*, 1999, 37(4):713-35.

Kubota A, Imano M, Yonekura T, et al, "Infantile Myofibromatosis of the Triceps Detected by Prenatal Sonography," *J Clin Ultrasound*, 1999, 27(3):147-50.

Liberman L, Bonaccio E, Hamele-Bena D, et al, "Benign and Malignant Phyllodes Tumors: Mammographic and Sonographic Findings," *Radiology*, 1996, 198(1):121-4.

Pinette MG, Pan YQ, Pinette SG, et al, "Prenatal Diagnosis of Fetal Bladder and Cloacal Exstrophy by Ultrasound. A Report of Three Cases," *J Reprod Med*, 1996, 41(2):132-4.

Van der Woude HJ and Vanderschueren G, "Ultrasound in Musculoskeletal Tumors With Emphasis on Its Role in Tumor Follow-up," *Radiol Clin North Am*, 1999, 37(4):753-66.

Ultrasound, Spleen

Synonyms Spleen Ultrasound

Procedure Commonly Includes Spleen, left kidney (limited)

Indications Determines size, presence of calcifications, infarction, trauma, mass, cysts

Patient Preparation All patients should be NPO for 12 hours prior to the exam. Examination should be performed prior to endoscopy, ERCP, barium studies, colonoscopy. The examination may be long, up to 1 hour including waiting time. An emergency examination or an unpredictably long preceding examination may result in additional delay.

Special Instructions All outpatient examinations are by appointment only. All inpatients are placed on the daily schedule as time permits and are performed as scheduled. Nonemergent examinations are given secondary priority and therefore may not be able to be performed the same day scheduled. Patients will generally be asked to stay after the examination until films are reviewed by the radiologist.

Equipment Standard B-mode real time ultrasonic imager with 2-5 MHz transducer.

Technique A gel is applied to the skin and a handheld transducer is swept across the area of interest to image the appropriate organs. Sound waves are used for the imaging and no radiation exposure is present. Images are recorded on x-ray film.

Turnaround Time A typed report will generally be issued within 36 hours. A preliminary verbal report generally can be given to the referring physician on request.

Causes for Rejection Gas, barium, oral ingestion of food, body habitus, rib artifacts

Additional Information This examination is most useful in evaluating for the presence of abnormal splenic collections or masses. Approximate size can also be determined.

References

Bolognesi M, Sacerdoti D, Merkel C, et al, "Splenic Doppler Impedance Indices: Influence of Different Portal Hemodynamic Conditions," *Hepatology*, 1996, 23(5):1035-40.

Ferrozzi F, Bova D, and De Chiara F, "Hemangioendothelioma of the Spleen: Imaging Findings at Color Doppler, US, and CT," *Clin Imaging*, 1999, 23(2):111-4.

(Continued)

Ultrasound, Spleen *(Continued)*

Forsberg F, Goldberg BB, Liu JB, et al, "Tissue-Specific US Contrast Agent for Evaluation of Hepatic and Splenic Parenchyma," *Radiology*, 1999, 210(1):125-32.

Goldberg BB, *Abdominal Ultrasonography*, New York, NY: John Wiley and Sons Inc, 1984.

Keogan MT, Freed KS, Paulson EK, et al, "Imaging-Guided Percutaneous Biopsy of Focal Splenic Lesions: Update on Safety and Effectiveness," *AJR Am J Roentgenol*, 1999, 172(4):933-7.

Koda M, Hosyo K, Murawaki Y, et al, "The Wandering Spleen With Collateral Vessels Containing Gastric Varices: Color Doppler Ultrasound Imaging," *J Clin Ultrasound*, 1996, 24(9):528-32.

Vural M, Kacar S, Kosar U, et al, "Symptomatic Wandering Accessory Spleen in the Pelvis: Sonographic Findings," *J Clin Ultrasound*, 1999, 27(9):534-6.

Ultrasound, Testicular

Synonyms Testicular Ultrasound

Procedure Commonly Includes Evaluation of scrotal contents

Indications Lesions, enlargement, epididymitis, torsion

Patient Preparation The examination may be long, up to 1 hour including waiting time. An emergency examination or an unpredictably long preceding examination may result in additional delay.

Special Instructions All outpatient examinations are by appointment only. All inpatients are placed on the daily schedule as time permits and are performed as scheduled. Nonemergent examinations are given secondary priority and therefore may not be able to be performed the same day scheduled. Patients will generally be asked to stay after the examination until films are reviewed by the radiologist.

Equipment Standard B-mode real time ultrasonic imager with 7-10 MHz transducer.

Technique A gel is applied to the skin and a handheld transducer is swept across the testicles to image the appropriate organs. Sound waves are used for the imaging and no radiation exposure is present. Images are recorded on x-ray film.

Turnaround Time A typed report will generally be issued within 36 hours. A preliminary verbal report generally can be given to the referring physician on request.

Causes for Rejection Lack of patient cooperation, unable to hold still for exam

Additional Information Very useful examination for detecting occult malignancies of the testicle. Other lesions seen include spermatocele, varicocele, hydrocele, hematocele, infarct, orchitis, and epididymitis

References

Baker La, Sigman D, Mathews RI, et al, "An Analysis of Clinical Outcomes Using Color Doppler Testicular Ultrasound for Testicular Torsion," *Pediatrics*, 2000, 105(3 Pt 1):604-7.

Bree RL and Hoang DT, "Scrotal Ultrasound," *Radiol Clin North Am*, 1996, 34(6):1183-205.

Hendrikx AJ, Dang CL, Vroegindeweij D, et al, "B-Mode and Colour-Flow Duplex Ultrasonography: A Useful Adjunct in Diagnosing Scrotal Diseases?" *Br J Urol*, 1997, 79(1):58-65.

Herbener TE, "Ultrasound in the Assessment of the Acute Scrotum," *J Clin Ultrasound*, 1996, 24(8):405-21.

Holloway BJ, Belcher HE, Letourneau JG, et al, "Scrotal Sonography: A Valuable Tool in the Evaluation of Complications Following Inguinal Hernia Repair," *J Clin Ultrasound*, 1998, 26(7):341-4.

Horstman WG, "Scrotal Imaging," *Urol Clin North Am*, 1997, 24(3):653-71.

Krone KD and Carroll BA, "Scrotal Ultrasound," *Radiol Clin North Am*, 1985, 23(1):121-39.

Luker GD and Siegel MJ, "Scrotal US in Pediatric Patients: Comparison of Power and Standard Color Doppler US," *Radiology*, 1996, 198(2):381-5.

Pierik FH, Dohle GR, van Muiswinkel JM, et al, "Is Routine Scrotal Ultrasound Advantageous in Infertile Men?" *J Urol*, 1999, 162(5):1618-20.

Ultrasound, Thoracentesis

Related Information

Thoracentesis *on page 263*

Synonyms Thoracentesis Ultrasound

Procedure Commonly Includes Use of real time ultrasound to find suitable puncture site for thoracentesis and perform thoracentesis

Indications Provide a suitable site for thoracentesis

Patient Preparation The examination may be long, up to 1 hour including waiting time. An emergency examination or an unpredictably long preceding examination may result in additional delay.

Aftercare Check physician order sheet. Chest x-rays on inspiration and expiration are routine to rule out a pneumothorax.

Special Instructions All outpatient examinations are by appointment only. All inpatients are placed on the daily schedule as time permits and are performed as scheduled. Nonemergent examinations are given secondary priority and therefore may not be able to be performed the same day scheduled. Patients will generally be asked to stay after the examination until films are reviewed by the radiologist.

Equipment Standard B-mode real time ultrasonic imager with 7-10 MHz transducer.

Technique A gel is applied to the skin and a handheld transducer is swept across the area of interest to image the appropriate organs. Sound waves are used for the imaging and no radiation exposure is present. Images are recorded on x-ray film.

Turnaround Time A typed report will generally be issued within 36 hours. A preliminary verbal report generally can be given to the referring physician on request.

Causes for Rejection Lack of suitable puncture site

References

Ballard RB, Rozycki GS, Knudson MM, et al, "The Surgeon's Use of Ultrasound in the Acute Setting," *Surg Clin North Am*, 1998, 78(2):337-64.

Colt HG, Brewer N, and Barbur E, "Evaluation of Patient-Related and Procedure-Related Factors Contributing to Pneumothorax Following Thoracentesis," *Chest*, 1999, 116(1):134-8.

Gervais DA, Petersein A, Lee MJ, et al, "US-Guided Thoracentesis: Requirement for Post-procedure Chest Radiography in Patients Who Receive Mechanical Ventilation Versus Patients Who Breathe Spontaneously," *Radiology*, 1997, 204(2):503-6.

Keske U, "Ultrasound-Aided Thoracentesis in Intensive Care Patients," *Intensive Care Med*, 1999, 25(9):896-7.

Lichtenstein D, Hulot JS, Rabiller A, et al, "Feasibility and Safety of Ultrasound-Aided Thoracentesis in Mechanically Ventilated Patients," *Intensive Care Med*, 1999, 25(9):955-8.

Neff CC and Van Sonnenberg E, "Percutaneous Drainage of Pleural Collections," *Radiology*, Taveras JT and Ferrucci JT, eds, Philadelphia, PA: Lippincott Williams & Wilkins, 1988.

Petersen S, Freitag M, Albert W, et al, "Ultrasound-Guided Thoracentesis in Surgical Intensive Care Patients," *Intensive Care Med*, 1999, 25(9):1029.

Zironi G, Piscaglia F, Gainai S, et al, "Intrahepatic Artery Pseudoaneurysm: A Possible Complication of Blind Thoracentesis," *J Clin Ultrasound*, 1999, 27(3):151-5.

Ultrasound, Thyroid

Synonyms Thyroid Ultrasound

Procedure Commonly Includes Thyroid gland

Indications Prove whether a palpable mass is a simple cyst; enlarged thyroid

Contraindications Patient unable to lay supine with head hyperextended

Patient Preparation The examination may be long, up to 1 hour including waiting time. An emergency examination or an unpredictably long preceding examination may result in additional delay. **Note**: Ultrasound exam to be scheduled before a barium study. If barium study was done, bowel preparation is needed before doing ultrasound examination.

Special Instructions All outpatient examinations are by appointment only. All inpatients are placed on the daily schedule as time permits and are performed as scheduled. Nonemergent examinations are given secondary priority and therefore may not be able to be performed the same day scheduled. Patients will generally be asked to stay after the examination until films are reviewed by the radiologist.

Equipment Standard B-mode real time ultrasonic imager with 5-10 MHz transducer.

Technique A gel is applied to the skin and a handheld transducer is swept across the area of interest to image the appropriate organs. Sound waves are used for the imaging and no radiation exposure is present. Images are recorded on x-ray film.

Turnaround Time A typed report will generally be issued within 36 hours. A preliminary verbal report generally can be given to the referring physician on request.

Limitations The patient has to have palpable mass and a cold spot on the Nuclear Medicine thyroid scan. Thyroid exams will not be done without a previous Nuclear Medicine scan unless the referring physician has consulted a radiologist.

(Continued)

Ultrasound, Thyroid *(Continued)*

Additional Information If patient is pregnant, then Nuclear Medicine thyroid scan is not a prerequisite. Physician should consult a radiologist before ordering exam if patient is pregnant.

References

Becker D, Bair HJ, Becker W, et al, "Thyroid Autonomy With Color-Coded Image-Directed Doppler Sonography: Internal Hypervascularization for the Recognition of Autonomous Adenomas," *J Clin Ultrasound*, 1997, 25(2):63-9.

Butch RJ, Simeone JF, and Mueller PR, "Thyroid and Parathyroid Ultrasonography," *Radiol Clin North Am*, 1985, 23(1)57-71.

Cho YS, Lee HK, Ahn IM, et al, "Sonographically Guided Ethanol Sclerotherapy for Benign Thyroid Cysts: Results in 22 Patients," *AJR Am J Roentgenol*, 2000, 174(1):213-6.

Erdem S, Bashekim C, Kizilkaya E, et al, "Clinical Application of Tc-99m Tetrofosmin Scintigraphy in Patients With Cold Thyroid Nodules. Comparison With Color Doppler Sonography," *Clin Nucl Med*, 1997, 22(2):76-9.

Frasoldati A, Pesenti M, Toschi E, et al, "Detection and Diagnosis of Parathyroid Incidentaloma During Thyroid Sonography," *J Clin Ultrasound*, 1999, 27(9):492-8.

Gailloud P, Khan HG, Khaw N, et al, "The Supraisthmic Anastomotic Arch: A Potential Pitfall in Doppler Sonography of the Thyroid Gland," *AJR AM J Roentgenol*, 1998, 170(2):497-8.

Gallowitsch HJ, Mikosch P, Kresnik E, et al, "Technetium 99m Tetrofosmin Parathyroid Imaging. Results With Double-Phase Study and SPECT in Primary and Secondary Hyperparathyroidism," *Invest Radiol*, 1997, 32(8):459-65.

Koslin DB, Adams J, Andersen P, et al, "Preoperative Evaluation of Patients With Primary Hyperparathyroidism: Role of High-Resolution Ultrasound," *Laryngoscope*, 1997, 107(9):1249-53.

Lane MJ, Desser TS, Weigel RJ, et al, "Use of Color and Power Doppler Sonography to Identify Feeding Arteries Associated With Parathyroid Adenomas," *AJR Am J Roentgenol*, 1998, 171(3):819-23.

Mizokami T, Okamura K, Sato K, et al, "Localized Painful Giant-Cell Thyroiditis Without Inflammatory Signs in a Euthyroid Patient Followed by Serial Sonography," *J Clin Ultrasound*, 1998, 26(6):329-32.

Profanter C, Klinger A, Strolz S, et al, "Surgical Therapy for Primary Hyperparathyroidism in Patients With Previous Thyroid Surgery," *Am J Surg*, 1999, 178(5):374-6.

Rozycki GS, "Surgeon-Performed Ultrasound: Its Use in Clinical Practice," *Ann Surg*, 1998, 228(1):16-28.

Simeone JF, "Ultrasound Examination of the Thyroid and Parathyroid," *Radiology*, Taveras JT and Ferrucci JT, eds, Philadelphia, PA: Lippincott Williams & Wilkins, 1988.

Takashima S, Takayama F, Wang Q, et al, "Thyroid Metastasis From Rectal Carcinoma Coexisting With Hashimoto's Thyroiditis: Gray-Scale and Power Doppler Sonographic Findings," *J Clin Ultrasound*, 1998, 26(7):361-5.

Taki S, Kakuda K, Kakuma K, et al, "Thyroid Nodules: Evaluation With US-Guided Core Biopsy With an Automated Biopsy Gun," *Radiology*, 1997, 202(3):874-7.

Tessler FN and Tublin ME, "Thyroid Sonography: Current Applications and Future Directions," *AJR Am J Roentgenol*, 1999, 173(2):437-43.

Ultrasound, Transcranial Doppler

Procedure Commonly Includes Intracranial common carotid arteries, anterior cerebral, posterior cerebral, middle cerebral, anterior and posterior communicating arteries, vertebral and basilar arteries

Indications Evaluate velocity of (blood flow) in intracranial arteries, evaluation of presence of vasospasm intracranial arterial stenosis

Patient Preparation The examination may be long, up to 1 hour including waiting time. An emergency examination or an unpredictably long preceding examination may result in additional delay.

Special Instructions All outpatient examinations are by appointment only. All inpatients are placed on the daily schedule as time permits and are performed as scheduled. Nonemergent examinations are given secondary priority and therefore may not be able to be performed the same day scheduled. Patients will generally be asked to stay after the examination until films are reviewed by the radiologist.

Equipment Pulsed Doppler transcranial ultrasound unit with 2 MHz transducer

Technique A gel is applied to the skin and a handheld transducer is swept across the area of interest to obtain flow velocity data. Sound waves are used for the imaging and no radiation exposure is present.

Turnaround Time A typed report will generally be issued within 36 hours. A preliminary verbal report generally can be given to the referring physician on request.

Additional Information Relatively new device to evaluate the intracranial circulation. May be of value to detect stenosis, occlusion, spasm, and vascular steals.

References

Arnolds BJ and von Reutern GM, "Transcranial Doppler Sonography. Examination Technique and Normal Reference Values," *Ultrasound Med Biol*, 1986, 12(2):115-23.

Droste DW, Hansberg T, Kemeny V, et al, "Oxygen Inhalation Can Differentiate Gaseous From Nongaseous Microemboli Detected by Transcranial Doppler Ultrasound," *Stroke*, 1997, 28(12):2453-6.

Droste DW, Jurgens R, Weber S, et al, "Benefit of Echocontrast-Enhanced Transcranial Color-Coded Duplex Ultrasound in the Assessment of Intracranial Collateral Pathways," *Stroke*, 2000, 31(4):920-3.

Hennerici M, Rautenberg W, Sitzer G, et al, "Transcranial Doppler Ultrasound for the Assessment of Intracranial Arterial Flow Velocity. Part I. Examination Technique and Normal Values," *Surg Neurol*, 1987, 27(5):439-48.

Hoksbergen AW, Legemate DA, Ubbink DT, et al, "Success Rate of Transcranial Color-Coded Duplex Ultrasonography in Visualizing the Basal Cerebral Arteries in Vascular Patients Over 60 Years of Age," *Stroke*, 1999, 30(7):1450-5.

Lennard N, Smith J, Dumville J, et al, "Prevention of Postoperative Thrombotic Stroke After Carotid Endarterectomy: The Role of Transcranial Doppler Ultrasound," *J Vasc Surg*, 1997, 26(4):579-84.

Nosan DK, Gomez CR, Boyd JH, et al, "Intraoperative Transcranial Doppler Ultrasound in Head and Neck Surgery: A Preliminary Report," *Am J Otolaryngol*, 1998, 19(4):223-7.

Poulin MJ, Syed RJ, and Robbins PA, "Assessments of Flow by Transcranial Doppler Ultrasound in the Middle Cerebral Artery During Exercise in Humans," *J Appl Physiol*, 1999, 86(5):1632-7.

Ringelstein EB, Droste DW, Babikian VL, et al, "Consensus on Microembolus Detection by TCD. International Consensus Group on Microembolus Detection," *Stroke*, 1998, 29(3):725-9.

Valdueza JM, Schmierer K, Mehraein S, et al, "Assessment of Normal Flow Velocity in Basal Cerebral Veins. A Transcranial Doppler Ultrasound Study," *Stroke*, 1996, 27(7):1221-5.

Wardlaw JM, Offin R, Teasdale GM, et al, "Is Routine Transcranial Doppler Ultrasound Monitoring Useful in the Management of Subarachnoid Hemorrhage?" *J Neurosurg*, 1998, 88(2):272-6.

Wilterdink JL, Feldmann E, Furie KL, et al, "Transcranial Doppler Ultrasound Battery Reliably Identifies Severre Internal Carotid Artery Stenosis," *Stroke*, 1997, 28(1):133-6.

Ultrasound, Transvaginal

Synonyms Transvaginal Ultrasound

Procedure Commonly Includes Uterus, ovaries, adnexa

Indications Pelvic masses and abscess, uterus size, IUD localization and pregnancy diagnosis; ectopic pregnancy, dermoid cyst, pelvic inflammatory disease, ovarian cyst, fibroid tumor, and bladder tumor

Patient Preparation The examination may be long, up to 1 hour including waiting time. An emergency examination or an unpredictably long preceding examination may result in additional delay.

Special Instructions All outpatient examinations are by appointment only. All inpatients are placed on the daily schedule as time permits and are performed as scheduled. Nonemergent examinations are given secondary priority and therefore may not be able to be performed the same day scheduled. Patients will generally be asked to stay after the examination until films are reviewed by the radiologist.

Equipment Standard B-mode real time ultrasonic imager with 3-5 MHz transvaginal transducer.

Technique A gel is applied to the skin and a handheld transducer is placed into the vagina to image the pelvis. Sound waves are used for the imaging and no radiation exposure is present. Images are recorded on x-ray film.

Data Acquired Coronal, sagittal images of uterus and adnexa

Turnaround Time A typed report will generally be issued within 36 hours. A preliminary verbal report generally can be given to the referring physician on request.

References

Alcazar JL, Laparte C, Jurado M, et al, "The Role of Transvaginal Ultrasonography Combined With Color Velocity Imaging and Pulsed Doppler in the Diagnosis of Endometrioma," *Fertil Steril*, 1997, 67(3):487-91.

Ayida G, Kennedy S, Barlow D, et al, "Contrast Sonography for Uterine Cavity Assessment: A Comparison of Conventional Two-Dimensional With Three-Dimensional Transvaginal Ultrasound; A Pilot Study," *Fertil Steril*, 1996, 66(5):848-50.

Barnhart KT, Simhan H, and Kamelle SA, "Diagnostic Accuracy of Ultrasound Above and Below the Beta-hCG Discriminatory Zone," *Obstet Gynecol*, 1999, 94(4):583-7.

Blaas HG, Eik-Nes SH, Berg S, et al, "*In-Vivo* Three-Dimensional Ultrasound Reconstructions of Embryos and Early Fetuses," *Lancet*, 1998, 352(9135):1182-6.

(Continued)

Ultrasound, Transvaginal *(Continued)*

Chen KH and Konchak P, "Use of Transvaginal Color Doppler Ultrasound to Diagnose Vasa Previa," *J Am Osteopath Assoc*, 1998, 98(2):116-7.

Crane JM, Van den Hof M, Armson BA, et al, "Transvaginal Ultrasound in the Prediction of Preterm Delivery: Singleton and Twin Gestations," *Obstet Gynecol*, 1997, 90(3):357-63.

Khalife S, Falcone T, Hemmings R, et al, "Diagnostic Accuracy of Transvaginal Ultrasound in Detecting Free Pelvic Fluid," *J Reprod Med*, 1998, 43(9):795-8.

Lee A, Sator M, Kratochwil A, et al, "Endometrial Volume Change During Spontaneous Menstrual Cycles: Volumetry by Transvaginal Three-Dimensional Ultrasound," *Fertil Steril*, 1997, 68(5):831-5.

Newman PG and Rozycki GS, "The History of Ultrasound," *Surg Clin North Am*, 1998, 78(2):179-95.

Zalar RW Jr, "Transvaginal Ultrasound and Preterm Prelabor: A Nonrandomized Intervention Study," *Obstet Gynecol*, 1996, 88(1):20-3.

Ultrasound, Urinary Bladder

Synonyms Urinary Bladder Ultrasound

Procedure Commonly Includes Urinary bladder, prostate (limited)

Indications Bladder neoplasm, bladder calculi, foreign bodies, prostate hypertrophy, bladder carcinoma

Patient Preparation Outpatient: Instruct patient to drink 16 oz of fluid 1 hour prior to exam and not to empty bladder. Inpatient: Ultrasound will notify the floor when to instruct the patient to drink 16 oz of fluid. The examination may be long, up to 1 hour including waiting time. An emergency examination or an unpredictably long preceding examination may result in additional delay.

Special Instructions All outpatient examinations are by appointment only. All inpatients are placed on the daily schedule as time permits and are performed as scheduled. Nonemergent examinations are given secondary priority and therefore may not be able to be performed the same day scheduled. Patients will generally be asked to stay after the examination until films are reviewed by the radiologist.

Equipment Standard B-mode real time ultrasonic imager with 2-5 MHz transducer.

Technique A gel is applied to the skin and a handheld transducer is swept across the area of interest to image the appropriate organs. Sound waves are used for the imaging and no radiation exposure is present. Images are recorded on x-ray film.

Turnaround Time A typed report will generally be issued within 36 hours. A preliminary verbal report generally can be given to the referring physician on request.

References

Bih LI, Ho CC, Tsai SJ, et al, "Bladder Shape Impact on the Accuracy of Ultrasonic Estimation of Bladder Volume," *Arch Phys Med Rehabil*, 1998, 79(12):1553-6.

Hiraoka M, Hori C, Tsukahara H, et al, "Voiding Function Study With Ultrasound in Male and Female Neonates," *Kidney Int*, 1999, 55(5):1920-6.

Oak SN, Kulkarni B, and Chaubal N, "Color Flow Doppler Sonography: A Reliable Alternative to Voiding Cystourethrogram in the Diagnosis of Vesicoureteral Reflux in Children," *Urology*, 1999, 53(6):1211-4.

Schenider P, Birner P, Gendo A, et al, "Bladder Volume Determination: Portable 3-D Versus Stationary 2-D Ultrasound Device," *Arch Phys Med Rehabil*, 2000, 81(1):18-21.

Simforoosh N, Dadkhah F, Hosseini SY, et al, "Accuracy of Residual Urine Measurement in men: Comparison Between Real-Time Ultrasonography and Catheterization," *J Urol*, 1997, 158(1):59-61.

♦ **Urinary Bladder Ultrasound** *see* Ultrasound, Urinary Bladder *on page 510*

ACRONYMS AND ABBREVIATIONS GLOSSARY

ACRONYMS AND ABBREVIATIONS GLOSSARY

a . . . atto (10^{-18})
A . . . apical; artery
A_1 . . . blood group antigen
A_1AT . . . alpha$_1$ antitrypsin
A_2 . . . aortic second sound; blood group antigen
aa . . . of each (ana)
aaa . . . androgenic anabolic agent; aromatic amino acid
AAA . . . abdominal aortic aneurysm; acquired aplastic anemia; acute anxiety attack
AAAAA . . . aphasia, agnosia, apraxia, agraphia, and alexia
AAB . . . action against burns; aminoazobenzene
AABB . . . American Association of Blood Banks
AABCC . . . alertness (consciousness), airway, breathing, circulation, and cervical spine
AAC . . . antibiotic associated colitis
AACC . . . American Association of Clinical Chemistry
AACSH . . . adrenal androgen corticotropic stimulation hormone
AAE . . . acute allergic encephalitis; annuloaortic ectasia
AaG . . . alveolar arterial gradient
AAGS . . . adult adrenogenital syndrome
AAIN . . . acute allergic intestinal nephritis
AAL . . . anterior axillary line
AAMS . . . acute aseptic meningitis syndrome
AAN . . . analgesic abuse nephropathy; analgesic associated nephropathy
AAO . . . amino acid oxidase; awake to alert and oriented
$(A\text{-}a)O_2$ . . . alveolar-arterial oxygen gradient
AAP . . . American Academy of Pediatrics
AAPC . . . antibiotic-associated pseudomembranous colitis
AAPCC . . . American Association of Poison Control Centers
$A\text{-}aP_{CO2}$ . . . alveolar-arterial carbon dioxide difference
AAPF . . . antiarteriosclerosis polysaccharide factor
AAPM . . . antibiotic-associated pseudomembranous colitis
AAR . . . active avoidance reaction; acute articular rheumatism; antigen-antiglobulin reaction; Australia antigen radioimmunoassay
AAS . . . acute abdominal series; atomic absorption spectrometry
AASH . . . adrenal androgen stimulating hormone
AASP . . . acute atrophic spinal paralysis; ascending aorta synchronized pulsation
AAT . . . alpha antitrypsin
AAU . . . acute anterior uveitis
AAVV . . . accumulated alveolar ventilatory volume
Ab . . . antibody
AB . . . abdominal; abort; antibiotic
A&B . . . apnea and bradycardia
A/B . . . acid-base ratio; apnea and bradycardia
ABA . . . abscissic acid; allergic bronchopulmonary aspergillosis; antibacterial activity
ABB . . . Albright-Butler-Bloomberg (syndrome)
ABC . . . avidin-biotin complex
ABD . . . after bronchodilator; aged, blind, and disabled; aggressive behavioral disturbance; average body dose
ABE . . . acute bacterial endocarditis
ABG . . . arterial blood gas
ABL . . . abetalipoprotein
ABLB . . . alternate binaural loudness balance
ABMT . . . autologous bone marrow transplantation
ABO . . . ABO blood group
ABPA . . . allergic bronchopulmonary aspergillosis
ABR . . . auditory brainstem response

ABS . . . alkylbenzene sulfonate
ac . . . before meals (ante cibum)
Ac . . . actinium
AC . . . air conduction; alternating current
ACA . . acute cerebellar ataxia; anticardiolipin antibody; Du Pont chemistry analyzer
ACC . . . amylase creatinine clearance
ACD . . . acid-citrate-dextrose
ACE . . . angiotensin converting enzyme
AChR . . . acetylcholine receptor antibody
ACL . . . anterior cruciate ligament
ACLS . . . advanced cardiac life support
ACOG . . . American College of Obstetrics and Gynecology
ACOP . . . . Adriamycin (doxorubicin), cyclophosphamide, Oncovin (vincristine), and prednisone
ACOPP . . . . . . Adriamycin (doxorubicin), cyclophosphamide, Oncovin (vincristine), prednisone, and procarbazine
AcP . . . acid phosphatase
ACPA . . . anticytoplasmic antibodies
ACT . . . activated clotting time
ACTH . . . adrenocorticotropic hormone
ACTN . . . adrenocorticotropin
ACV . . . acyclovir; amifostine, cisplatin, and vinblastine
ACVB . . . aortocoronary venous bypass
ACVD . . . acute cardiovascular disease
ad . . . right ear; up to (ad)
AD . . . admitting diagnosis; atopic dermatitis
a.d. . . . alternating days
ADA . . . adenosine deaminase
ADA# . . . American Diabetes Association diet number
ADAS . . . Alzheimer Disease Assessment Scale
ADC . . . Aid to Dependent Children
ADCC . . . antibody-dependent cell-mediated cytotoxicity
ADCONFU . . . . Adriamycin (doxorubicin), cyclophosphamide, Oncovin (vincristine), and 5-fluorouracil
ADD . . . attention deficit disorder
ADDH . . . attention deficit disorder with hyperactivity
ADH . . . alcohol dehydrogenase; antidiuretic hormone
ADHD . . . attention deficit hyperactive disorder
ADIC . . . . . . Adriamycin (doxorubicin) and dimethyltriazenylimidazole carboxamide (dacarbazine)
ADL . . . active daily living
ad lib . . . as desired (ad libitum)
ADM . . . admission
ADME . . . absorption, distribution, metabolism, and excretion
ADNase . . . anti-DNAse
ADO . . . adolescent medicine
ADP . . . adenosine 5-diphosphate
ADR . . . acceptable dental remedies; acute dystonic reaction; Adriamycin; adverse drug reaction
ADRs . . . adverse drug reactions
ADT . . . adenosine triphosphate; alternate-day treatment
AED . . . anticonvulsant drugs
AEP . . . . acute edematous pancreatitis; auditory evoked potential; average evoked potential
AER . . . . acoustic evoked response; agranular endoplasmic reticulum; auditory evoked response; average evoked response
AES . . . adult emergency service; antiembolic stockings
AF . . . acid-fast; amniotic fluid; aortic flow; artrial fibrillation; atrial flutter
AFB . . . acid-fast bacillus; aortofemoral bypass; aspirated foreign body
AFBG . . . aortofemoral bypass graft
AFC . . . adult foster care
AFCI . . . acute focal cerebral ischemia
AFDC . . . Aid to Families with Dependent Children
AFEB . . . afebrile
aff . . . afferent
AF/F . . . atrial fibrillation and/or flutter
AFib . . . atrial fibrillation
AFL . . . atrial flutter
AFND . . . acute febrile neutrophilic dermatosis
AFO . . . ankle-foot orthrosis
aFP, AFP . . . alpha-fetoprotein
AFRD . . . acute febrile respiratory disease

AFRI . . . acute febrile respiratory illness
AFS . . . acid-fast smear
Ag . . . antigen; silver
AG . . . abdominal girth
A/G . . . albumin/globulin ratio
AGA . . . accelerated growth area; appropriate for gestational age; average for gestational age
AGF . . . angle of greatest flexion
agit . . . shake
agit ante us. . . . shake before using
agit bene . . . shake well
AGN . . . acute glomerular nephritis
$AgNO_3$ . . . silver nitrate
AGS . . . adrenogenital syndrome
AH . . . antihyaluronidase
A-H . . . atrial-His
AHA . . acquired hemolytic anemia; acute hemolytic anemia; autoimmune hemolytic anemia
AHBC . . . hepatitis B core antibody
AHC . . . acute hemorrhagic conjunctivitis; acute hemorrhagic cystitis
AHE . . . acute hemorrhagic encephalomyelitis
AHF . . . acute heart failure; antihemophilic factor (factor VIII)
AHFS . . . American Hospital Formulary Service
AHG . . . antihemophilic globulin
AHLE . . . acute hemorrhagic leukoencephalitis
AHP . . . acute hemorrhagic pancreatitis
AHT . . . antihyaluronidase titer
AI . . accidental injury; allergy index; aortic insufficiency; artificial insemination; atrial insufficiency
AICC . . . anti-inhibitor coagulant complex
AID . . . acquired immunodeficiency disease; acute infectious disease
AIDS . . . acquired immunodeficiency syndrome
AIDS-KS . . . acquired immunodeficiency syndrome with Kaposi sarcoma
AIHA . . . autoimmune hemolytic anemia
AIHD . . . acquired immune hemolytic disease
AIMS . . abnormal involuntary movement scale; arthritis impact measurement scale
AIP . . . acute intermittent porphyria; average intravascular pressure
AJ . . . ankle jerk
AJR . . . abnormal jugular reflex
AK . . . adenylate kinase; above the knee
A/K . . . above knee (amputation)
AKA . . . above knee (amputation); all known allergies; also known as
AK amp . . . above knee amputation
AKP . . . alkaline phosphatase
Al . . . aluminum
AL . . . acute leukemia; arterial line
ALA . . . aminolevulinic acid
ALAC . . . antibiotic-loaded acrylic cement
ALAD . . . abnormal left axis deviation
alb . . . albumin
ALF . . . acute liver failure
ALFT . . . abnormal liver function test
A-line . . . arterial catheter; arterial line
alk . . . alkaline
AlkP . . . alkaline phosphatase
alk phos, alk p'tase . . . alkaline phosphates
all. . . . allergic/allergy
ALL . . . acute lymphoblastic leukemia; acute lymphocytic leukemia
ALMI . . . anterior lateral myocardial infarction
ALO . . . average lymphocyte output
$Al(OH)_3$ . . . aluminum hydroxide
ALOMAD . . . Adriamycin (doxorubicin), Leukeran (chlorambucil), Oncovin (vincristine), methotrexate, actinomycin D, and dacarbazine
ALOS . . . average length of stay
AlP, ALP . . . alkaline phosphatase
AlPI . . . alkaline phosphatase isoenzymes
ALS . . acute lateral sclerosis; advanced life support; amyotrophic lateral sclerosis; antilymphocyte serum
ALT . . . alanine aminotransferase
ALT/AST . . . ratio of serum alanine aminotransferase to serum aspartate aminotransferase
Am . . . americium

AM . . . acute myelofibrosis; alveolar mucosa; morning
a.m. . . . before noon
AMA . . . against medical advice; American Medical Association; antimitrochondrial antibody
amb, AMB . . . ambulate/ambulatory
AMBL . . . acute myeloblastic leukemia
ambul . . . ambulate/ambulatory
AMegL, AMEGL . . . acute megakaryoblastic leukemia
AMI . . . acute myocardial infarction
AML . . . acute myeloblastic leukemia; acute myelogenous leukemia
AMOL . . . acute monoblastic/monocytic leukemia
AMP . . . adenosine monophosphate
AMPS . . . acid mucopolysaccharide
AMPT . . . alpha-methyl-p-tyrosine
AMS . . . acute mountain sickness; altered mental status
AMT . . . acute miliary tuberculosis
AN . . acanthosis nigricans; anorexia nervosa; aseptic necrosis; avascular necrosis
ANA . . . antinuclear antibody
ANC . . . absolute neutrophil count
ANCA . . . antineutrophil cytoplasmic antibodies
ANDA . . . Abbreviated New Drug Application
ANF . . . antinuclear factor
ANLL . . . acute nonlymphocytic leukemia
ANOVA . . . analysis of variance
ANP . . . atrial natriuretic peptide
anti-TB . . . antituberculosis
ant. pit. . . . anterior pituitary
ant. prand . . . before parturition
AO . . . abdominal aorta; aortic opening
A&O . . . alert and oriented
AOD . . . adult-onset diabetes
AODA . . . alcohol and other drug abuse
AODM . . . adult onset diabetes mellitus
aort sten . . . aortic stenosis
AOS . . . acridine orange staining
AOV . . . aortic value
AP . . . acid phosphatase; adolescent psychiatry; antepartum; anteroposterior; appendectomy; appendicitis; assessment and plans
ap . . . before dinner; prior to
A-P . . . anterior-posterior
A&P . . . anterior and posterior; assessment and plans
A/P . . . ascites-plasma (ratio)
APACHE . . . acute physiology and chronic health evaluation (systems)
APAP . . . acetaminophen
APB . . . atrial premature beat
APCA . . . antiparetial cell antibody
APCD . . . adult polycystic kidney disease
APD . . . acute polycystic disease; adult polycystic disease
APE . . . doxorubicin (Adriamycin), cisplatin (Platinol), and etoposide
APGAR . . appearance, pulse, grimace, activity, and respiration (score of newborn physical status)
aph . . . aphasia
APhA . . . American Pharmaceutical Association
APKD . . . adult polycystic kidney disease
APP . . . alum-precipitating pyridine
APSAC . . . anisoylated plasminogen streptokinase activator complex
APTT . . . activated partial thromboplastin time
APUD . . . amine precursor uptake and decarboxylation
aq . . . water (aqua)
aq ad . . . add water
Ar . . . argon
AR . . . aortic regurgitation; apical-radial (pulse)
A-R, A/R . . . apical-radial (pulse)
ARA . . . antireticulin antibody
araC-Hu . . . arabinosylcytosine (cytarabine) and hydroxyurea
ARC . . . acquired immunodeficiency syndrome-related complex
ARD . . . antimicrobial removal device; acute respiratory distress
ARDS . . . adult respiratory distress syndrome
ARF . . . acute renal failure
ARF/CRF . . . acute renal failure/chronic renal failure
ARLD . . . alcohol-related liver disease
ARM . . . artificial rupture of membranes

ARN . . . . acute renal/retinal necrosis
AROM . . . . active range of motion; artificial rupture of membranes
Ars . . . . arylsulfatase
ART . . . . arterial line
ARV . . . . AIDS-associated retrovirus; AIDS-related virus; anterior right ventricular (wall)
as . . . . left ear
As . . . . arsenic
AS . . . . anal sphincter; ankylosing spondylitis; aortic stenosis; atrial septum; atrial stenosis
AsA . . . . arylsulfatase A
ASA . . . . acetylsalicylic acid
ASAP . . . . as soon as possible
ASAT . . . . aspartate aminotransferase
AsB . . . . arylsulfatase B
ASCP . . . . American Society of Clinical Pathologists
ASCVD . . . . arteriosclerotic cardiovascular disease
ASD . . . . Alzheimer senile dementia; atrial septal defect
ASDH . . . . acute subdural hematoma
ASHD . . . . arteriosclerotic/atherosclerotic heart disease; atrial septal heart disease
ASHP . . . . American Society of Health-System Pharmacists
ASK . . . . antistreptokinase
ASKA . . . . antiskeletal antibody
ASLO . . . . antistreptolysin O
ASLT . . . . antistreptolysin test
ASMA . . . . antismooth muscle antibody
ASO . . . . antistreptolysin O; arterioselerosis obliterans
asp . . . . aspirate
ASP . . . . ankylosing spondylitis
ASS . . . . acute serum sickness
AST . . . . antistreptolysin titer; aspartate aminotransferase
ASVD . . . . arteriosclerotic vascular disease
At . . . . astatine
AT, A-T . . . . ataxia-telangiectasia
ATB . . . . atrial tachycardia with block; atypical tuberculosis
at. fib, At Fib . . . . atrial fibrillation
ATG . . . . antithymocyte globulin
AT-III . . . . antithrombin III
ATL . . . . adult T-cell leukemia
ATLL . . . . adult T-cell leukemia/lymphoma
ATLS . . . . advanced trauma life support
ATLV . . . . adult T-cell leukemia virus
ATN . . . . acute tubular necrosis
ATP . . . . adenosine triphosphate
ATPase . . . . adenosine triphosphatase
ATR . . . . Achilles tendon reflex
atr fib., ATR FIB . . . . atrial fibrillation
ATS . . . . American Thoracic Society
au . . . . each ear (auris utro)
Au . . . . gold
^{198}Au . . . . radioisotope of gold
AU . . . . both ears together
AUB . . . . abnormal uterine bleeding
AUC . . . . area under the curve
aud, AUD . . . . arthritis of unknown diagnosis
AUGIB . . . . acute upper gastrointestinal bleeding
AUL . . . . acute undifferentiated leukemia
aur fib., AUR FIB . . . . auricular fibrillation
AUS . . . . acute urethral syndrome
A-V . . . . arteriovenous; atrioventricular; audiovisual
AVA . . . . availability
AVB . . . . atrioventricular block
AVE . . . . aortic valve echocardiogram
AVH . . . . acute viral hepatitis
AVHB . . . . atrioventricular heart block
AVHD . . . . acquired valvular heart disease
AVM . . . . arteriovenous malformation
AVP . . . . aqueous vasopressin; arginine vasopressin
AVR . . . . accelerated ventricular rhythm; aortic valve replacement
AVSS . . . . afebrile, vital signs stable
A&W . . . . alive and well
Ax . . . . axillary

AZA-CR . . . azacitidine
AZT . . . zidovudine
B . . . boron
Ba . . . barium
BA . . . Bachelor of Arts
B&A . . . brisk and active
BAC . . . blood alcohol concentration
BACON . . . bleomycin, Adriamycin (doxorubicin), CCNU (lomustine), Oncovin (vincristine), and nitrogen mustard (mechlorethamine)
BACOP . . . bleomycin, Adriamycin (doxorubicin), cyclophosphamide, Oncovin (vincristine), and prednisone
BACT bischloroethylnitrosourea, arabinosylcytosine, Cytoxan (cyclophosphamide), and 6-thioguanine; bleomycin, Adriamycin (doxorubicin), Cytoxan (cyclophosphamide), and tamoxifen citrate
BaE, BAE . . . barium enema
BaEn . . . barium enema
BAEP . . . brainstem auditory evoked potential
BAER . . . brainstem auditory evoked response
BAL . . . bronchoalveolar lavage
B ALL . . . B-cell acute lymphoblastic leukemia
BAN . . . British approved name
BAND . . . band neutrophil (stab)
BAO . . . basal acid output
BAP . . . bleomycin, Adriamycin (doxorubicin), and prednisone
BAVP . . . balloon aortic valvuloplasty
BB . . . Blood Bank
BBB . . . blood-brain barrier; bundle-branch block
BBBB . . . bilateral bundle-branch block
BBC . . . basal cell carcinoma
BBF . . . bronchial blood flow
BBPRL . . . big big prolactin
BBT . . . basal body temperature
BB to MM . . . belly button to medial malleolus
B Bx . . . breast biopsy
BC . . . bone conduction
B&C . . . bed and chair
B-CAVE . . . bleomycin, CCNU (lomustine), Adriamycin (doxorubicin), and Velban (vinblastine)
BCC . . . basal cell carcinoma
BCCa . . . basal cell carcinoma
BCD . . . basal cell dysplasia; bleomycin, cyclophosphamide, and dactinomycin
BCE . . . basal cell epithelioma
BCG . . . bacillus Calmette-Guérin
BCH . . . basal cell hyperplasia/hypoplasia
BCLL . . . B-cell chronic lymphocytic leukemia
BCLS . . . basic cardiac life support (system)
BCM . . . bovine cervical mucus
BCNU . . . carmustine
BCP . . . birth control pills; blood cell profile
BCPs . . . birth control pills
bcr . . . breakpoint cluster region
bd . . . twice a day (bis in die)
BD . . . bronchodilators
BDH-V . . . BCNU (carmustine), hydroxyurea, dacarbazine, and vincristine
BDM . . . black divorced male
B-DOPA . . . bleomycin, dacarbazine, Oncovin (vincristine), prednisone, and Adriamycin (doxorubicin)
Be . . . beryllium
BE . . . bacterial endocarditis; barium enema; below-elbow (amputation)
B/E . . . below-elbow (amputation)
BEA . . . below-elbow amputation
BEC . . . bacterial endocarditis
BEI . . . butanol-extractable iodine
benzodiazepine-GABA . . . gamma-aminobutyric acid
BEP . . . brainstem evoked potential
BERA . . . brainstem evoked response auditory
BF, B/F . . . black female
BFH . . . benign familial hematuria
BFS . . . blood fasting sugar
BFT . . . bentonite flocculation test
BFW . . . Bartlett-Farling-Wimbaly brush
BG . . . baby girl

B-G . . . . Bender-Gestalt (test)
BGC . . . . basal-ganglion calcification
BGL . . . . blood glucose level
BGlu . . . . blood glucose
BGP . . . . bone GLA protein
BHAT . . . . beta-blocker heart attack trial
BHB . . . . beta-hydroxybutyrate
BHD . . . . BCNU (carmustine), hydroxyurea, and dacarbazine
BHI . . . . brain heart infusion
BHT . . . . butylated hydroxytoluene
Bi . . . . bismuth
bid, BID . . . . twice a day (bis in die)
BIP . . . . blood pressure
BJ . . . . Bence Jones; biceps jerk; bone and joint
Bk . . . . berkelium
BK . . . . below knee
B/K . . . . below-knee (amputation)
BKA . . . . below-knee amputation
BKTT . . . . below-knee to toe (cast)
BKWC . . . . below-knee walking cast
BKWP . . . . below-knee walking plaster
Bl . . . . black
BLEO . . . . bleomycin
BLEO-MOPP . . bleomycin, mechlorethamine, Oncovin (vincristine), and prednisone
blk . . . . black
BLL . . . . below lower limit; bilateral lower lobe; brows, lids, and lashes
Bl Obs . . . . bladder observation
bl pr, BL PR . . . . blood pressure
BLS . . . . basic life support
BM . . . . black male; bone marrow; bowel movement; breast milk
B/M . . . . black male
BMA . . . . bone marrow arrest; bone marrow aspirate
BMD . . . . bone mineral density
BMJ . . . . bones, muscles, joints
BML . . . . bone marrow lymphocytosis
BMMA . . . . Bone Mass Measurement Act
BMR . . . . basal metabolic rate
BMT . . . . bone marrow transplantation
BNB . . . . blood-nerve barrier
BNC . . . . bladder neck contracture
BNO . . . . bladder neck obstruction
BNR . . . . bladder neck resection/retraction
B&O . . . . belladonna and opium
BOLD . . . . bleomycin, Oncovin (vincristine), lomustine, and dacarbazine
BOM . . . . bilateral otitis media
BOMA . . . . bilateral otitis media, acute
BOO . . . . bladder outlet obstruction
BOP . . . . bleomycin, Oncovin (vincristine), and prednisone
BOPAM . . . bleomycin, Oncovin (vincristine), prednisone, Adriamycin (doxorubicin), and methotrexate
BP . . . . back pressure; blood pressure
B/P . . . . blood pressure
BPD . . . . biparietal diameter
BPH . . . . benign prostatic hyperplasia
bpm . . . . beats per minute
BPO . . . . bilateral partial oophorectomy
BPPP . . . . bilateral pedal pulses present
BPR . . . . blood per rectum
BPs . . . . blood pressure, systolic
BPS . . . . . . beats per secone; bilateral partial salpingectomy; breaths per second
BPT . . . . benign paroxysmal torticollis
BPV . . . . benign paroxysmal vertigo
Br . . . . bromine; bromide
BR . . . . bathroom; bedrest
BrdU 5-bromodeoxyuridine
BrM . . . . breast milk
BRO . . . . bromocriptine; bronchoscopy
broch . . . . bronchoscopy
BRP . . . . bathroom privileges
BRR . . . . baroreceptor reflex response
BRU . . . . bromide urine
BS . . . . Bachelor of Science; blood sugar; bowel sounds; breath sounds

bsa, BSA — body surface area
BSEP — brainstem evoked potential
BSN — bowel sounds normal
BSNA — bowel sounds normal and active
BSO — bilateral salpingo-oophorectomy; bilateral serous otitis
BSOM — bilateral serous otitis media
BSP — bromsulfophthalein
BSR — basal skin resistance; blood sedimentation
BT — breast tumor
BTG — beta thromboglobulin
BTL — bilateral tubal ligation
BTPS — body temperature, ambient pressure, and saturated with water vapor (gas)
BTS — bradycardia-tachycardia syndrome
BU — bethesda units
BUN — blood urea nitrogen
BVAP — BCNU (carmustine), vincristine, Adriamycin (doxorubicin), and prednisone
BVL — bilateral vas ligation
BVP — blood volume pulse
bw, BW — birth weight; bite-wing (radiograph); body water; body weight
BWA — bed wetter admission
BWS — battered woman syndrome
BWt — birth weight
bx, BX — biopsy
bz, BZ — benzodiazepine
BZD, BZDZ — benzodiazepine
c — with (cum)
C — carbon
C_2 — s[illegible] vertebra
Ca — calcium
CA — cancer antigen; caproic acid; cardiac arrest; chronological age; Cocaine Anonymous
C&A — conscious and alert
CA 15-3 — tumor marker antigen
CA 19-9 — tumor marker antigen
CA 50 — tumor marker antigen
CA 125 — tumor marker antigen
CAA — computer-aided assessment; computer-assisted assessment
CAAT — computer-assisted axial tomography
CAB — coronary artery bypass
CABG — coronary artery bypass graft
CABGS — coronary artery bypass graft surgery
CABS — coronary artery bypass surgery
CAC — circulating anticoagulant
CaCl — calcium chloride
$CaCO_3$ — calcium carbonate
CACX — cancer of cervix
Cad — cadaver
CAD — cadaver; computer-assisted diagnosis; coronary artery disease; cyclophosphamide, Adriamycin (doxorubicin), and dacarbazine; cytosine arabinoside and daunorubicin
CaEDTA — calcium disodium edetate
CAF — cyclophosphamide, Adriamycin (doxorubicin), and fluorouracil
CAFP — cyclophosphamide, Adriamycin (doxorubicin), fluorouracil, and prednisone
CAFVP — cyclophosphamide, Adriamycin (doxorubicin), fluorouracil, vincristine, and prednisone
CAG — cholangiogram; coronary angiogram/angiography
CAH — chronic active hepatitis; chronic aggressive hepatitis; combined atrial hypertrophy
CAHD — coronary arteriosclerotic heart disease; coronary atherosclerotic heart disease
CALD — chronic active liver disease
CALGB — cancer and leukemia group B
cALL — common null cell acute lymphocytic leukemia
CALLA — common acute lymphoblastic leukemia antigen
CAMB — cyclophosphamide, Adriamycin (doxorubicin), methotrexate, and bleomycin
CAMEO — cyclophosphamide, Adriamycin (doxorubicin), methotrexate, etoposide, and Oncovin (vincristine)
CAMF — cyclophosphamide, Adriamycin (doxorubicin), methotrexate, and fluorouracil
cAMP — cyclic AMP
CAMP — cyclophosphamide, Adriamycin (doxorubicin), methotrexate, and procarbazine

Can . . . . . cancer antigen
CAO . . . . . chronic airway obstruction
Ca_{o2} . . . . . arterial oxygen concentration
CAOD . . . . . coronary artery occlusive disease
CAOM . . . . . chronic adhesive otitis media
CAP . . . . . cancer of prostate; community-acquired pneumonia; cyclophosphamide, Adriamycin (doxorubicin), and Platino (cisplatin); cyclophosphamide, Adriamycin (doxorubicin), and prednisone
CAPD . . . . . chronic ambulatory peritoneal dialysis
CAS . . . . . carotid artery stenosis; coronary artery spasm
CASA . . . . . computer-assisted semen analysis
CAST . . . . . cardiac arrhythmia suppression trial
CAT . . computed axial tomography; cytosine arabinoside, Adriamycin (doxorubicin), and thioguanine
CATT . . . . . calcium tolerance test
CAV . . . . . cyclophosphamide, Adriamycin (doxorubicin), and vincristine
CAVB . . . . . complete atrioventricular block
CAVC . . . . . common arterioventricular canal
CAVD . . . . . complete atrioventricular dissociation; completion, arithmetic problems, vocabulary, following directions (battery)
CAVDH . . . . . continuous arteriovenous hemodialysis; continuous arteriovenous hemofiltration (with) dialysis
CAVE . . . . . CCNU (lomustine), Adriamycin (doxorubicin), and vinblastine
CAVH . . . . . continuous arteriovenous hemofiltration
CAVP . . . cyclophosphamide, Adriamycin (doxorubicin), vincristine, and prednisone
CAV-P-VP . . . . . cyclophosphamide, Adriamycin (doxorubicin), vincristine, Platino (cisplatin), and VP16-213 (etoposide)
CB . . . . . chair and bed; chest-back
C&B . . . . . chair and bed
C-B, C/B . . . . . chest-back
CBA . . . . . chronic bronchitis and asthma
CBAT . . . . . Coag battery; Coulter battery
CBBB . . . . . complete bundle-branch block
CBC . . . . . complete blood count
CBCN . . . . . carbenicillin
CBD . . . . . common bile duct
CBDC . . . . . chronic bullous disease of childhood
CBDE . . . . . common bile duct ligation
CBE . . . . . clinical breast examination
CBF . . capillary blood flow; cerebral blood flow; coronary blood flow; cortical blood flow
CBFS . . . . . cerebral blood flow studies
CBFV . . . . . cerebral blood flow velocity
CBG . . . . . capillary blood gases; coronary bypass graft
CBH . . . . . chronic benign hepatitis
CBI . . . . . continuous bladder irrigation
CBIL . . . . . conjugated bilirubin
CBL . . . . . circulating blood lymphocytes
CBPPA . . cyclophosphamide, bleomycin, procarbazine, prednisone, and Adriamycin (doxorubicin)
CBPS . . . . . coronary bypass surgery
CBS . . . . . chronic brain syndrome
CBT circulating blood volume; cyclophosphamide, BCNU (carmustine), and VP16-213 (etoposide); computerized body tomography
CBVD . . . . . cerebrovascular disease
CC . . . . . chief complaint; closing capacity; colony count
C&C . . . . . cold and clammy
C/C . . . . . chief complaint
CCB . . . . . calcium channel blocker
CCH . . . . . chronic cholestatic hepatitis
CCI . . . . . chronic coronary insufficiency; corrected count increment
CCK . . . . . cholecystokinin
CCK-OP . . . . . cholecystokinin-octapeptide
CCL . . . . . carcinoma cell line
CCMS . . . . . clean-catch midstream (urine)
CCMSU . . . . . clean-catch midstream urine
CCMSUA . . . . . clean-catch midstream urinalysis
C_{cr} . . . . . creatinine clearance
CC&S . . . . . cornea, conjunctiva, and sclera
CCU . . . . . cardiac care unit; coronary care unit
CCUA . . . . . clean catch urinalysis
CCV . . . . . CCNU (lomustine), cyclophosphamide, and vincristine

CCVB . . . . CCNU (lomustine), cyclophosphamide, vincristine, and bleomycin
CCVD . . . . chronic cerebrovascular disease
CCVPP . . . . . CCNU (lomustine), cyclophosphamide, vinblastine, procarbazine, and prednisone
Cd . . . . cadmium
C&D . . . . curettage and desiccation
CDA . . . . congenital dyserythropoietic anemia
CDC . . . . carboplatin, doxorubicin, and cyclophosphamide; Centers for Disease Control
CDDP . . . . cis-diaminedichloroplatinum
CDP . . . . . chlordiazepoxide; continuous distending pressure; cytidine diphosphate
CDU . . . . cumulative dose unit
CDX . . . . chlordiazepoxide
CDZ . . . . chlordiazepoxide
Ce . . . . cerium
C&E . . . . consultation and examination
CEA . . . . carcinoembryonic antigen
CEBV . . . . chronic Epstein-Barr virus
CERD . . . . chronic end-stage renal disease
CES . . . . conjugated estrogenic substances
CEV . . . . cyclophosphamide, etoposide, and vincristine
C&F . . . . curettage and fulguration
Cf . . . . californium
CF . . . . cardiac failure; caucasian female; complement fixation; cystic fibrosis
CFCL . . . . continuous flow centrifugation leukapheresis
CFL . . . . cisplatin, fluorouracil, and leucovorin calcium
CFM . . . . cyclophosphamide, fluorouracil, and citoxantrone
CFU . . . . colony forming units
CG . . . . chorionic gonadotropin
CGB . . . . chronic gastrointestinal (tract) bleeding
CGH . . . . chorionic gonadotropic hormone
CGL . . . . chronic granulocytic leukemia
CH . . . . case history; congenital hypothyroidism
CHA . . . . chronic hemolytic anemia
CHAM-OCA . . . . . cyclophosphamide, hydroxyurea, actinomycin D (dactinomycin), methotrexate, Oncovin (vincristine), citrovorum factor (leucovorin), and Adriamycin (doxorubicin)
CHAP . . . . cyclophosphamide, hexamethylmelamine, Adriamycin (doxorubicin), and Platino (cisplatin)
CHBHA . . . . congenital Heinz body hemolytic anemia
CHD . . Chediak-Higashi disease; congenital heart disease; congenital hip disease/dysplasia; congestive heart disease; coronary/cyanotic heart disease; cyclophosphamide, hexamethylmelamine, cisplatin
CHF . . . . . congenital hepatic fibrosis; congestive heart failure; cyclophosphamide, hexamethylmelamine, and 5-fluorouracil
CHI . . . . closed head injury
CHO . . . . cyclophosphamide, hydroxydaunorubicin, and Oncovin (vincristine)
CHOP . . . . cyclophosphamide, hydroxydaunorubicin, Oncovin (vincristine), and prednisone
CHOR . . . . . . cyclophosphamide, hydroxydaunorubicin, Oncovin (vincristine), and radiation
CHS . . . . central hypoventilation syndrome
CHT . . . . closed head trauma
CI . . cardiac index; cardiac insufficiency; color index; confidence intervals; coronary insufficiency
CIBD . . . . chronic inflammatory bowel disease
CIC . . . . circulating immune complexes
cic-DDP . . . . cis-diaminedichloroplatinum
CIE . . . . counterimmunoelectrophoresis
CIF . . . . clone-inhibiting factor
CIHD . . . . chronic ischemic heart disease
CIN . . . . cervical intraepithelial neoplasia; chronic interstitial nephritis
CIP . . . . cellular immunocompetence profile
CIPD . . . . chronic inflammatory polyradiculoneuropathy, demyelinating
circ & sen . . . . circulation and sensation
CIRR . . . . cirrhosis
CISCA . . . . cisplatin, cyclophosphamide, and Adriamycin (doxorubicin)
CIVII . . . . continuous intravenous insulin infusion
CIXU . . . . constant infusion excretory urogram
CJD . . . . Creutzfeldt-Jakob disease
CJS . . . . Creutzfeldt-Jakob syndrome
CK . . . . creatine kinase

CK-ISO . . . creatine kinase isoenzyme
Cl . . . chlorine
CL . . . cirrhosis of liver
Cla . . . clarithromycin
CLA . . . certified laboratory assistant
CLBB . . . complete left bundle-branch block
CLD . . . chronic liver disease
CLL . . . cholesterol-lowering lipid; chronic lymphocytic leukemia
CLO . . . cod liver oil
CLS . . . clinical laboratory scientist
CLSL . . . chronic lymphosarcoma (cell) leukemia
cm . . . centimeter
Cm . . . curium
cm^2 . . . square centimeter
cm^3 . . . cubic centimeter
CM . . . caucasian male; contrast media; culture media
C&M . . . cocaine and morphine
C/M . . . counts per minute
CMA . . . chronic metabolic acidosis; cow's milk allergy
C_{max} . . . maximum concentration of drug
CMB . . . carbolic methylene blue
CMBBT . . . cervical mucous basal body temperature
CMC . . . carboxymethylcellulose; cyclophosphamide, methotrexate, and CCNU (lomustine)
CMF . . . cyclophosphamide, methotrexate, and fluorouracil
CMFH . . . cyclophosphamide, methotrexate, fluorouracil, and hydroxyurea
CMFP . . . cyclophosphamide, methotrexate, fluorouracil, prednisone
CMF-TAM . . . cyclophosphamide, methotrexate, fluorouracil, and tamoxifen
CMFV . . . cyclophosphamide, methotrexate, fluorouracil, and vincristine
CMFVP . . . cyclophosphamide, methotrexate, fluorouracil, vincristine, and prednisone
CMG . . . congenital myasthenia gravis; cystometrogram
CMI . . . carbohydrate metabolism index; cell-mediated immunity
c/min . . . cycles per minute
C_{min} . . . minimum concentration of ddrug
CML . . . cell-mediated lymphocytotoxicity/lympholysis; cell-mediated lysis; chronic myelogenous leukemia
CMM . . . cell-mediated mutagenesis
CMML . . . chronic myelomonocytic leukemia
C-MOPP . . . cyclophosphamide, mechlorethamine, Oncovin (vincristine), procarbazine, and prednisone
CMP . . . cardiomyopathy; cervical mucus penetration
CMP-FX . . . complement fixation
CMPT . . . cervical mucous penetration test
CMSUA . . . clean, midstream urinalysis
CMV . . . cisplatin, methotrexate, and vinblastine; cytomegalovirus
CMVIG . . . cytomegalovirus immune globulin
CMV-IGIV . . . cytomegalovirus immune globulin intravenous
CMVS . . . culture midvoid specimen
CN . . . caudate nucleus; congenital nephrosis; cyanogen
CNDC . . . chronic nonspecific diarrhea of childhood
CNF . . . cyclophosphamide, Novantrone (mitoxantrone), and fluorouracil
CNHD . . . congenital nonspherocytic hemolytic disease
CNP . . . cranial nerve palsy
CNS . . . central nervous system; coagulase negative staph
CNSHA . . . congenital nonspherocytic hemolytic anemia
Co . . . cobalt
c/o . . . check out
^{57}Co . . . radioisotope of cobalt
^{58}Co . . . radioisotope of cobalt
^{60}Co . . . radioisotope of cobalt
CO . . . carbon monoxide; cardiac output
CO_2 . . . carbon dioxide
CO_3 . . . carbonate
C/O . . . check out; complaint of
CoA . . . coenzyme A
COAD . . . chronic obstructive airway/arterial disease
coag . . . coagulation
COAG . . . chronic open angle glaucoma
COAP . . . cyclophosphamide, Oncovin (vincristine), arabinosylcytosine, and prednisone

COB . . . . chronic obstructive bronchitis; cisplatin, Oncovin (vincristine), and bleomycin; coordination of benefits
COBRA . . . . Consolidated Omnibus Budget Reconciliation Act
COBS . . . . chronic organic brain syndrome
COBT . . . . chronic obstruction of biliary tract
COC . . . . combined oral contraceptive
COD . . . . cause of death
COEPS . . . . cortical origination extrapyramidal system
COHb . . . . carboxyhemoglobin
COLD . . . . chronic obstructive lung disease
COM . . . . chronic otitis media; cyclophosphamide, Oncovin (vincristine), and methotrexate; cyclophosphamide, Oncovin (vincristine), and methyl-CCNU (semustine)
COMA . . . . cyclophosphamide, Oncovin (vincristine), methotrexate, and arabinosylcytosine
COMB . . cyclophosphamide, Oncovin (vincristine), methyl-CCNU (semustine), and bleomycin
COMLA . . cyclophosphamide, Oncovin (vincristine), methotrexate, leucovorin, and arabinosylcytosine
COMP . . . cyclophosphamide, Oncovin (vincristine), methotrexate, and prednisone
COMS . . . . chronic organic mental syndrome
COMT . . . . catechol-o-methyltransferase
CONPADRI I . . cyclophosphamide, Oncovin (vincristine), L-phenylalanine mustard, and Adriamycin (doxorubicin)
CONPADRI II . . . . CONPADRI I plus high dose methotrexate
CONPADRI III . . . . CONPADRI I plus intensified doxorubicin
COP . . . . capillary osmotic pressure; chronic obstructive pulmonary; cyclophosphamide, Oncovin (vincristine), and prednisone
COPA . . . . . . cyclophosphamide, Oncovin (vincristine), prednisone, and Adriamycin (doxorubicin)
COP-BLAM . . . . . cyclophosphamide, Oncovin (vincristine), prednisone, bleomycin, Adriamycin (doxorubicin), and Matulane (procarbazine)
COPD . . . . chronic obstructive pulmonary disease
COPE . . . . chronic obstructive pulmonary emphysema
COPP . . . . cyclophosphamide, Oncovin (vincristine), procarbazine, and prednisone
CORD . . . . chronic obstructive respiratory disease
COT . . . . continuous oxygen therapy
COTX . . . . cast removed, take x-ray
CP . . cardiac pacing; cardiac performance; cardiopulmonary; cerebral palsy; chest pain; cyclophosphamide and prednisone
C&P . . . . . . compensation and pension; complete and pain-free (range of motion); cystoscopy and pyelogram
C/P . . . . cardiopulmonary; cholesterol-phospholipid
CPA . . . . carotid phonoangiography; cyclophosphamide
CPAP . . . . continuous positive airway pressure
CPB . . . . cardiopulmonary bypass
CPBV . . . . cardiopulmonary blood volume
CPCS . . . . clinical pharmacokinetics consulting service
CPD . . . childhood polycystic disease; chronic peritoneal dialysis; citrate phosphate dextrose; cyst disease protein
CPDA . . . . citrate phosphate dextrose adenine
CPE . . . . chronic pulmonary emphysema; cytopathogenic effects
CPH . . . . chronic persistent hepatitis
CPI . . . . coronary prognostic index
CPIP . . . . chronic pulmonary insufficiency of prematurity
CPK . . . . creatine phosphokinase
CPK-2 . . . . creatine phosphokinase MB fraction
CPK-BB . . . . creatine phosphokinase BB fraction
CPKD . . . . childhood polycystic kidney disease
CPK-MB . . . . creatine phosphokinase of muscle band
cpm, CPM . . . . counts per minute
CPmax . . . . peak (maximum) serum concentration
CPmin . . . . trough (minimum) serum concentration
CPMS . . . . chronic progressive multiple sclerosis
CPP . . . . cerebral perfusion pressure
CPPB . . . . continuous positive pressure breathing
CPPD . . calcium pyrophosphate dihydrate; chest percussion and postural drainage
CPR . . cardiac and pulmonary rehabilitation; cardiopulmonary resuscitation; cortisol production rate
cps . . . . counts per second; cycles per second
CPS . . . . . cardioplegic perfusion solution; cardiopulmonary support; characters per second; Compendium of Pharmaceuticals and Specialties

CPT . . . chest physiotherapy
CPUE . . . chest pain of unknown etiology
CQA . . . concurrent quality assurance
Cr . . . chromium
^{51}Cr . . . radioisotope of chromium
C&R . . . cardiac and respiratory; convalescence and rehabilitation; cystoscopy and retrograde
CRA . . . central retinal artery
CRAMS . . . circulation, respiration, abdomen, motor, and speech
CRAO . . . central retinal artery occlusion
CRD . . . childhood rheumatic disease; chronic renal disease; chronic respiratory disease
Cre . . . creatinine
creat . . . creatinine
CRF . . chronic renal failure; chronic respiratory failure; corticotropin releasing factor
crit, Crit . . . hematocrit
CRL . . . crown rump length
CRM . . . cross-reacting material
CROP . . . cyclophosphamide, rubidazone, Oncovin (vincristine), and prednisone
CRP . . . C-reactive protein
CRPD . . . chronic restrictive pulmonary disease
CRS . . . catheter related sepsis
CRST . . . calcinosis, Raynaud phenomenon, sclerodactylia, telangiectasis
CRT . . . cadaver renal transplant; cardiac resuscitation team; cathode ray tube
CRTX . . . cast removed, take x-ray
CRU . . . cardiac rehabilitation unit; clinical research unit
CRV . . . central retinal vein
CRVF . . . congestive right ventricular failure
CRVO . . . central retinal vein occlusion
c/s . . . cycles per second
Cs . . . cesium
CS . . . cesarean section; coronary sclerosis
C/S . . . cesarean section; culture and sensitivity
C&S . . . cough and sneeze; culture and sensitivity; culture and susceptibility
C-S . . . cervical spine
CsA . . . cyclosporin A
CS&CC . . . culture, sensitivity, and colony count
C sect . . . cesarean section
CSF . . . cerebrospinal fluid; colony-stimulated factor
CSII . . . continuous subcutaneous insulin infusion
CSIIP . . . continuous subcutaneous insulin infusion pump
CSNS . . . carotid sinus nerve stimulation
CSO . . . copied standing orders
CSOM . . . chronic serous/suppurative otitis media
CSP . . . carotid sinus pressure; chemistry screening profile
CSR . . . corrected sedimentation rate
CSS . . carotid sinus stimulation; carotid sinus syndrome; coronary sinus stimulation
CST . . . cardiac stress test; cavernous sinus thrombosis; convulsive shock therapy
CSUF . . . continuous slow ultrafiltration
CT . . . cardiac tamponade; circulation time; clotting time; computerized tomography
C/T . . . compression to traction ratio; crossmatch to transfusion ratio
CTA . . . clear to auscultation; Committee on Thrombolytic Agents; computed tomoangiography
CTAB . . . cetyltrimethylammonium bromide
CTAP . . . computed tomography during arterial portography
CTAT . . . computed transaxial tomography
CTD . . . carpal tunnel decompression; chest tube drainage; congenital thymic dysplasia; connective tissue disease
CT&DB . . . cough, turn, and deep breath
CTDW . . . continues to do well
C/TG . . . cholesterol-triglyceride
CTGA . . . complete transposition of great arteries
CTM . . . *Chlamydia* transport media
C&TN BLE . . . color and temperature normal, both lower extremities
CTP . . . comprehensive treatment plan
C-TPN . . . cyclic total parenteral nutrition
CTPP . . . cerebral tissue perfusion pressure
CTPVO . . . chronic thrombotic pulmonary vascular obstruction
CTS . . . carpal tunnel syndrome
CTT . . . computerized transaxial tomography
CTUWSD . . . chest tube under water-seal drainage
CTV . . . cervical and thoracic vertebrae

CTX ... cytoxan
Cu ... copper
CU ... cardiac unit; cause unknown
CUC ... chronic ulcerative colitis
CUE ... cumulative urinary excretion
CV ... cardiovascular; cervical vertebra; coefficient of variation; conjugata vera
CVA ... cardiovascular accident; cerebrovascular accident; cyclophosphamide, vincristine, and Adriamycin (doxorubicin)
CVA-BMP ... cyclophosphamide, Oncovin (vincristine), Adriamycin (doxorubicin), BCNU (carmustine), methotrexate, and procarbazine
CVB ... CCNU (lomustine), vinblastine, and bleomycin
CVC ... central venous catheter
CVD ... cardiovascular disease; cerebrovascular disease; cerebrovascular disorder; collagen vascular disease
CVE ... cerebrovascular evaluation
CVEB ... cisplatin, vinblastine, etoposide, and bleomycin
CVF ... cardiovascular failure; central visual field; cervicovaginal fluid
CVHD ... chronic valvular heart disease
CVI ... cardiovascular insufficiency; cerebral vascular insufficiency; continuous venous infusion
CVM ... cyclophosphamide, vincristine, and methotrexate
CVO ... central vein occlusion
CVOD ... cerebrovascular obstructive disease
CVP ... cardiac valve procedure; cardioventricular pacing; central venous pressure; cyclophosphamide, vincristine, and prednisone
CVPP ... cyclophosphamide, vincristine, prednisone, and procarbazine
CVR ... cardiovascular-renal (disease); cardiovascular resistance
CVRD ... cardiovascular-renal disease
CVS ... cardiovascular system; clean voided specimen
c/w, C/W ... compatible/consistent with
CW ... cardiac work
CWI ... cardiac work index
CWOP ... childbirth without pain
CWP ... childbirth without pain
CWS ... chest wall stimulation
Cx ... cervical; cervix
CXR ... chest x-ray
CXTX ... cervical traction
CyADIC ... cyclophosphamide, Adriamycin (doxorubicin), and DIC (dacarbazine)
CYT ... cyclophosphamide
Cy-VA-DIC ... cyclophosphamide, Oncovin (vincristine), Adriamycin (doxorubicin), DTIC (dacarbazine)
d ... day
1/d ... daily, one per day
2/d ... twice a day
D_5W ... 5% dextrose in water solution
DA ... dopamine; ductus arteriosus
DAB ... days after birth
DALA ... delta aminolevulinic acid
D and C ... dilation and curettage
DAP ... Adriamycin (doxorubicin) and Platino (cisplatin)
DAT ... daunorubicin, arabinosylcytosine, and thioguanine; direct antiglobulin test
DAW ... dispense as written
db ... decibel
DB ... deep breath
D/B ... date of birth
DB&C ... deep breathing and coughing
DBE ... deep breathing exercise
DBF ... disturbed bowel function
DBI ... development at birth index
DBP ... diastolic blood pressure
DBS ... deep brain stimulation; diminished breath sounds
d/c ... discontinue
DC ... daily census; daunorubicin and cytarabine; dilation and curettage; direct current
D&C ... dilation and curettage
D/C ... diarrhea/constipation discharge; discontinue
DCAG ... double coronary artery graft
DC&B ... dilation, curettage, and biopsy
DCBE ... double contrast barium enema
DCBF ... dynamic cardiac blood flow
DCCMP ... daunomycin, cyclocytidine, 6-mercaptopurine, and prednisone

DCG — dynamic electrocardiogram
DCH — delayed and cutaneous hypersensitivity
DCMP — daunomycin, cytarabine, 6-mercaptopurine, and prednisone
DCPM — daunomycin, cytarabine, prednisone, and mercaptopurine
DCS — decompression sickness
DCSA — double-contrast shoulder arthrography
DCx — double convex
DD — differential diagnosis; discharge diagnosis
D&D — diarrhea and dehydration
D/D — differential diagnosis
dDAVP, DDAVP — deamino-8-d-arginine vasopressin (desmopressin acetate)
DDD — degenerative disc disease
DDI — dideoxyinosine; dressing dry and intact
DDP — diaminedichloroplatinum
DDS — damaged disk syndrome; diaminodiphenylsulfone
DDT — dichloro-diphenyltrichloroethane
DDVP — dimethyldichlorovinyl phosphate (dichlorvos)
DDx, DDX — differential diagnosis
D&E — diet and elimination
DEA — Drug Enforcement Agency
DEAE — diethylaminoethyl
DEC — deceased
DED — date of expected delivery
DER — dermatome evoked response; disulfiram-ethanol reaction
DEXA — dual energy x-ray absorptiometry
DF — decapacitation factor (sperm); decayed and filled (permanent teeth); diastolic filling
DFA — diet for age; direct fluorescent antibody
DFMO — difluoromethylornithine
DFMR — daily fetal movement
DFP — diastolic filling period; diisopropylfluorophosphonate
dg — decigram
DGE — delayed gastric emptying
DGI — disseminated gonococcal infection
DGM — diffuse glomerulonephritis
DGS — diabetic glomerulosclerosis
DH — daily habits; dermatitis herpetiformis
DHA — dehydroepiandrosterone
DHAD — dihydroxybisaminoanthraquinone dihydrochloride
DHCA — deep hypothermia and circulatory arrest
DHEA — dehydroepiandrosterone
DHEA-S — dehydroepiandrosterone sulfate
DHF — dengue hemorrhagic fever
DHFS — dengue hemorrhagic fever shock (syndrome)
DHL — diffuse histiocytic lymphoma
DHR — delayed hypersensitivity reaction
DHS — delayed hypersensitivity; duration of hospital stay
DHST — delayed hypersensitivity test
DHT — dihydrotestosterone
DI — date of injury; diabetes insipidus; dispensing information; dyspnea index
D&I — debridement and irrigation; dry and intact
DIAGNO — differential diagnosis
DIC — disseminated intravascular coagulation
DIDMOAD — diabetes insipidus, diabetes mellitus, optic atrophy, and deafness (syndrome)
dif — differential (blood count)
diff — difference; differential
Diff — differential (blood count)
DIFF — differential (blood count)
diff diag — differential diagnosis
DIFP — diffuse interstitial; fibrosing pneumonitis
dig, dig. — digitalis
DIG — digitalis; digitoxin; digoxin
dig. tox — digitalis toxicity
DIH — died in hospital
DILD — diffuse interstitial lung
DILE — drug-induced lupus erythematosus
DIMOAD — diabetes insipidus, diabetes mellitus, optic atrophy, and deafness (syndrome)
DIP — desquamative interstitial pneumonia/pneumonitis; dichlorophenolindophenol
DIPC — diffuse interstitial pulmonary calcification
diph — diphtheria

diph-tox . . . diphtheria toxoid
DIRD . . . drug-induced renal disease
DISIDA . . . diisopropyl-iminodiacetic acid
DIVA . . . digital intravenous angiography
DIVBC . . . disseminated intravascular blood coagulation
DIVC . . . disseminated intravascular coagulation
DJD . . . degenerative joint disease
DK . . . diabetic ketoacidosis
DKA . . . diabetic ketoacidosis; did not keep appointment
DKB . . . deep knee bends
DKP . . . dibasic potassium phosphate
dL . . . deciliter
D-L . . . Donath-Landsteiner
DLB . . . diffuse and lymphoblastic; direct laryngoscopy and bronchoscopy
DLC . . . differential leukocyte count; double-lumen catheter
DLCO . . . diffusing capacity of the lung for carbon monoxide
DLE . . . discoid lupus erythematosus
DLF . . . digoxin-like factors
DLS . . . daily living skills
DLV . . . defective leukemia virus
DLWD . . . diffuse lymphocytic, well differentiated
dm . . . decimeter
DM . . . diabetes mellitus; diabetic mother; diastolic murmur
DMAARD . . . delayed-mechanism-of-action antirheumatic drug
DMARD . . . disease-modifying antirheumatic drug
DMC . . . dactinomycin, methotrexate, and cyclophosphamide
DME . . . degenerative myoclonus epilepsy
DMF . . . decayed, missing, and filled (teeth)
DMKA . . . diabetes mellitus ketoacidosis
DML . . . diffuse mixed lymphoma
DMO . . . dimethyloxazolidinedione
DMOOC . . . diabetes mellitus out of control
DMS . . . delayed microembolism syndrome; delayed muscle soreness
DMSO . . . dimethylsulfoxide
D,M,V,P . . . disk, macula, vessels, periphery
D&N . . . distance and near (vision)
D/N . . . dextrose/nitrogen ratio
DNA . . . deoxyribonucleic acid
DNase . . . deoxyribonuclease
DNBT . . . dinitroblue
DND . . . died of natural death
DNI . . . do not intubate
DNKA . . . did not keep appointment
DNL . . . diffuse nodular lymphoma; disseminated necrotizing leukoencephalopathy
DNP . . . deoxyribonucleoprotein
DNPH . . . dinitrophenylhydrazine
DNS . . . do not substitute
DNT . . . did not test
DO . . . doctor's orders
D/O . . . disorder
DOA . . . date of admission; date of arrival; dead on arrival
DOA-DRA . . . dead on arrival despite resuscitative attempts
DOAP . . . daunorubicin, Oncovin (vincristine), araC (cytarabine), and prednisone
DOB . . . date of birth
DOC . . . date of conception; deoxycorticosterone; diabetes out of control; died of other causes; diet of choice; drug of choice
DOD . . . date of death; date of discharge; died of disease
DOE . . . date of examination; dyspnea on exertion
DOES . . . disorders of excessive sleepiness
DOI . . . date of injury; died of injuries
DOL . . . day of life (followed by number)
DOOC . . . diabetes out of control
dos . . . dose (dosis)
DOS . . . day of surgery
DOSS . . . diocytl sodium sulfosuccinate
DOT . . . date of transcription; date of transfer; died on (operating) table
DP . . . deep pulse; dental prosthodontics; diastolic pressure
DPE . . . dipivalyl epinephrine
DPFR . . . diastolic pressure-flow relationship
DPG . . . diphosphoglycerate
DPGN . . . diffuse proliferative glomerulonephritis
DPH . . . diphenhydramine; diphenylhydantoin

DPJ . . . . . dementia paralytica juvenilis
DPL . . . . . diagnostic peritoneal lavage
DPN . . . . . dermatosis papalosa nigra; diabetic polyneuropathy
DPPC . . . . . dipalmitoylphosphatidylcholine
DPT . . . . . diphtheria toxoid, pertussis vaccine, tetanus toxoid
DPTP . . . . . diphtheria, pertussis, tetanus, poliomyelitis (vaccines)
DPTPM . . . . . diphtheria, pertussis, tetanus, poliomyelitis, measles (vaccines)
DPU . . . . . delayed pressure urticaria
DPUD . . . . . duodenal peptic ulcer disease
DQ . . . . . developmental quotient
dr . . . . . diabetic retinopathy
Dr . . . . . doctor
DR . . . . . diabetic retinopathy; donor related
DRE . . . . . digital rectal examination
DRG . . . . . diagnostic related group(s)
DRR . . . . . dorsal root reflex
D&S . . . . . dermatology and syphilology; dilation and suction
D/S . . . . . dextrose and sodium chloride; dextrose/saline
DSA . . . . . digital subtraction angiography
DSC . . . . . decussation superior cerebellar; differential scanning colorimeter
DSCG . . . . . disodium cromoglycate
DSD . . . . . discharge summary dictated; dry sterile dressing
DSDB . . . . . direct self-destructive behavior
ds-DNA . . . . . double-stranded DNA
DSE . . . . . digital subtraction echocardiogram
DSF . . . . . disulfiram
DSM . . . . . Diagnostic and Statistical Manual (of Mental Disorders)
DSP . . . . . decreased sensory perception
DST . . . . . dexamethasone suppression test
Dt . . . . . duration of tetany
DT . . . . . delirium tremons; duration tetany; dye test
D&T . . . . . diagnosis and treatment
D/T . . . . . date of treatment; deaths/total (ratio)
dtd . . . . . let such doses be given (dentur tales doses)
DTH . . . . . delayed-type hypersensitivity
DTM . . . . . dermatophyte test medium
DTO . . . . . deodorized opium tincture
DTP . . . . . diphtheria-tetanus pertussis; distal tingling on percussion
DTR . . . . . deep tendon reflex
DTs, DT's . . . . . delirium tremens
dU . . . . . deoxyuridine
DU . . . . . decubitus ulcer; diabetic urine; diagnosis undetermined; diffuse and undifferentiated; duodenal ulcer
DUI . . . . . driving under the influence
DUID . . . . . driving under the influence of drugs
DUL . . . . . diffuse undifferentiated lymphoma
DUR . . . . . Drug Usage Review
DV . . . . . deep vein
D&V . . . . . diarrhea and vomiting
DVA . . . . . desacetylvinblastine amide (vindesine)
DVLP . . . . . daunomycin, vincristine, L-asparaginase, and prednisone
DVPA . . . . . daunorubicin, vincristine, prednisone, and L-asparaginase
DVPL-ASP . . . . . daunorubicin, vincristine, prednisone, and L-asparaginase
DVR . . . . . double valve replacement
DVT . . . . . deep vein thrombosis
dw . . . . . dry weight
DWD . . . . . died with disease
DWDL . . . . . diffuse well-differentiated lymphocytic (lymphoma)
DWI . . . . . driving while intoxicated; driving while impaired
Dx . . . . . diagnosis
DXA . . . . . dual x-ray absorptiometry
DXR . . . . . deep x-ray
DXT . . . . . deep x-ray therapy
Dy . . . . . dysprosium
dysp . . . . . dyspnea
DZAPO . . . . daunorubicin, azacytidine, araC (cytarabine), prednisone, and Oncovin (vincristine)
DZT . . . . . dizygotic twins
E . . . . . exa (10^{18})
EA . . . . . early antigen
E&A . . . . . evaluate and advise
EAC . . . . . external auditory canal

EACA . . . . epsilon-aminocaproic acid
EAHF . . . . eczema, asthma, and hay fever (complex)
EAR . . . . electroencephalographic
EB . . . . Epstein-Barr
E-B . . . . Epstein-Barr (virus)
EBA . . . . epidermolysis bullosa acquisita/atrophicans
EBAB . . . . equal breath sounds bilaterally
EBEA . . . . Epstein-Barr early antigen
EBL . . . . erythroblastic leukemia; estimated blood loss
EBNA . . . . Epstein-Barr nuclear antigen
EBS . . . . epidermolysis bullosa simplex
EBV . . . . Epstein-Barr virus
EBVCA . . . . Epstein-Barr virus, capsid antigen
EBVEA . . . . Epstein-Barr virus, early antigen
EBVNA . . . . Epstein-Barr virus, nuclear antigen
EC . . . . *Escherichia coli*; extracellular
ECA . . . . external carotid artery
E-CABG . . . . endarterectomy and coronary artery bypass grafting
ECBV . . . . effective circulating blood volume
ECC . . . . edema, clubbing, and cyanosis; embryonal cell carcinoma; endocervical curettage
ECG . . . . electrocardiogram
Echo . . . . echocardiogram; echoencephalogram
ECHO . . . . echocardiogram; etoposide, cyclophosphamide, hydroxydaunomycin (Adriamycin), and Oncovin (vincristine); ultrasound
ECPR . . . . external cardiopulmonary resuscitation
ECT . . . . electroconvulsive therapy; emission computed tomography
ECV . . . . extracellular volume
ECVD . . . . extracellular volume of distribution
ECVE . . . . extracellular volume expansion
ECW . . . . extracellular water
EDTA . . . . ethylenediaminetetraacetic acid
EDWITH . . . . end-diastolic wall thickness
EDX . . . . electrodiagnosis
EE, E&E . . . . eyes and ears
E-E . . . . end to end (anastomosis); erythema-edema (reaction)
EECG . . . . electroencephalogram/electroencephalography
EEE . . . . edema, erythema, and exudate
EEEP . . . . end-expiratory esophageal pressure
EEG . . . . electroencephalogram
EEGA . . . . electroencephalographic audiometry
EENT . . . . eyes, ears, nose, throat
EEP . . . . end-expiratory pressure
EF . . . . ejection fraction; extended-field
EFA . . . . essential fatty acids
EFM . . . . external fetal monitoring
EFV . . . . extracellular fluid volume
EFVC . . . . expiratory flow-volume curve
EF/WM . . . . ejection fraction/wall motion
eg . . . . example
EGA . . . . estimated gestational age
EGC . . . . early gastric cancer
EGD . . . . esophagogastroduodenoscopy
EGFR . . . . epidermal growth factor receptor
EH . . . . enlarged heart; essential hypertension
EHBD . . . . extrahepatic bile duct
EHBF . . . . estimated hepatic blood flow; extrahepatic blood flow
EHDP . . . . ethanehydroxydiphosphonic acid
EHEC . . . . enterohemorrhagic *E. coli*
EHL . . . . electrohydraulic lithotripsy
EHO . . . . extrahepatic obstruction
EIA . . . . enzyme immunoassay
EID . . . . electroimmunodiffusion
EIEC . . . . enteroinvasive *E. coli*
EJ . . . . ejection (fraction); external jugular
EKG . . . . electrocardiogram
ELISA . . . . enzyme-linked immunosorbent assay
ELOS . . . . estimated length of stay
ELT . . . . euoglobulin lysis time
EM . . . . electron microscopy
E&M . . . . endocrine and metabolic
E/M . . . . electron microscopy

EMA . . . endomysial antibody
EMC . . . electron microscopy; encephalomyocarditis
EMC&R . . . emergency medical care and rescue
EMCV . . . encephalomyocarditis
EMG . . . electromyelogram; electromyogram
E-MICR . . . electron microscopy
EMIT . . . enzyme-multiplied immunoassay technique
EMM . . . erythema multiforme major
EMR . . . electromagnetic radiation; empty, measure, and record
EMS . . . early morning specimen; early morning stiffness; electrical muscle stimulation; eosinophil myalgia syndrome
ENA . . . extractable nuclear antigen
ENG . . . electronystagmography
ENL . . . erythema nodosum leprosum
ENT . . . ear, nose, and throat
EO . . . ethylene oxide
EOG . . . electro-oculogram
EOJ . . . extrahepatic obstructive jaundice
eos . . . eosinophil
EP . . . ectopic pregnancy; electrophoresis; electrophysiologic
EPA . . . Environmental Protection Agency
EPBI . . . exercise penile-brachial index
EPEC . . . enteropathogenic *E. coli*
EPEG . . . etoposide
EPF . . . early pregnancy factor
EPIS . . . episiotomy
EPP . . . erythropoietic protoporphyria
EPS . . . electrophysiologic studies; extrapyramidal side effect; extrapyramidal symptom; extrapyramidal syndrome
EPSEs . . . extrapyramidal side effects
EPT . . . early pregnancy test; Eidetic Parents Test; endoscopic papillotomy
Eq . . . equivalent
Er . . . erbium
ER . . . emergency room; estrogen receptors
ER+ . . . estrogen receptor-positive
E&R . . . equal and reactive; examination and report
ERA . . . estrogen receptor assay; evoked response audiometry
ERC . . . (pupils) equal, reactive and contracting
ERCP . . . endoscopic retrograde cholangiopancreatography
ERE . . . external rotation in extension
ERF . . . external rotation in flexion
ERG . . . electroretinogram
ERPF . . . effective renal plasma flow
ERT . . . estrogen replacement therapy; external radiation therapy
ERV . . . expiratory reserve volume
Es . . . Einsteinium
ES . . . electrical stimulation
ESA . . . end-to-side anastomosis
ESAP . . . evoked sensory (nerve) action potention
ESB . . . electrical stimulation of brain
ESLD . . . end-stage liver disease
ESP . . . extrasensory perception
ESR . . . erythrocyte sedimentation rate
ESRD . . . end-stage renal disease
ESRF . . . end-stage renal failure
ESRS . . . extra pyramidal symptom rating scale
EST . . . electroshock therapy
et . . . and (et)
ETA . . . endotracheal aspirates; estimated time of arrival
ETD . . . eustachian tube dysfunction
ETEC . . . enterotoxigenic *E. coli*
ETO . . . estimated time of ovulation; eustachian tube obstruction
EtOH . . . ethyl alcohol
ETOX . . . ethylene oxide
ETS-2 . . . Educational Testing Service; electrical transcranial stimulation;
ETT . . . extrathyroidal thyroxine
EU . . . Ehrlich unit
EUL . . . expected upper limit
EUP . . . extrauterine pregnancy
EUS . . . endorectal ultrasound
EVI . . . endocardial, vascular, and interstitial

EVR . . . evoked visual response
EVS . . . endoscopic variceal sclerosis
EW . . . emergency ward
EWT . . . erupted wisdom teeth
ExEF . . . ejection fraction during exercise
Ez . . . eczema
f . . . femto (10^{-15})
F . . . fluorine
FA . . . false aneurysm; fatty acid; filterable agent; fluorescent antibody
F/A . . . fetus active
FAA . . . folic acid antagonist; formaldehyde, acetic acid, and alcohol (solution)
FAB . . . French-American-British
FAC . . . femoral arterial cannulation; fluorouracil, Adriamycin (doxorubicin), and cyclophosphamide
FAC-LEV . . . fluorouracil, Adriamycin (doxorubicin), cyclophosphamide, and levamisole
FACP . . . Fellow of the American College of Physicians; ftorafur, Adriamycin (doxorubicin), cyclophosphamide, and platinol (cisplatin)
FACS . . fluorouracil, Adriamycin (doxorubicin), cyclophosphamide, and streptozocin
FAD . . . familial Alzheimer dementia; familial autonomic dysfunction; flavin adenine dinucleotide
FAM . . . fluorouracil, Adriamycin (doxorubicin), and mitomycin C
FAMA . . . fluorescent antibody to membrane antigen
FAME . . . fluorouracil, Adriamycin (doxorubicin), and methyl CCNU (semustine)
FAMMM . . . familiar atypical multiple mole melanoma (syndrome)
FAM-S . . . fluorouracil, Adriamycin (doxorubicin), mitomycin C, and streptozocin
FANA . . . fluorescent antinuclear antibody
FAS . . . fetal alcohol syndrome
FB . . . finger breadths; foreign bodies
F/B . . . forward bending
FBA . . . fecal bile acid
FBC . . . full blood count; functional bactericidal concentration
FBCOD . . . foreign body of the cornea, oculus dexter (right eye)
FBCOS . . . foreign body of the cornea, oculus sinister (left eye)
FBD . . . fibrocystic breast disease
FBG . . . fasting blood glucose
FBH . . . familiar benign hypercalcemia
FBHH . . . familiar benign hypocalciuric hypercalcemia
FBL . . . fetal blood loss
FBM . . . fetal breathing movement
FBP . . . femoral blood pressure; fibrin breakdown product
FBS . . . fasting blood sugar
FBSS . . . failed back surgery syndrome
FBW . . . fasting blood work
Fc . . . portion of antibody molecule bound by membrane receptors
F&C . . . foam and condom
F/C . . . fever and chills
FCDB . . . fibrocystic disease of breast
FCE . . . fluorouracil, cisplatin, and etoposide
F-CL . . . fluorouracil and calcium leucovorin
FCSNVD . . . fever, chills, sweating, nausea, vomiting, and diarrhea
FCVD . . . fracture complete and varus deformity
FD . . . food and drug
F&D . . . fixed and dilated
F/D . . . fracture/dislocation
FDA . . . Federal Drug Administration
FDBL . . . fecal daily blood loss
FD&C . . . Food, Drug, and Cosmetic (Act)
FDP . . . fibrin degradation product; fructose diphosphate
Fe . . . iron
FEC . . . fluorouracil, etoposide, and cisplatin; forced expiratory capacity
$FeCl_3$ . . . ferric chloride
FEF . . . forced expiratory flow
FEFV . . . forced expiratory flow volume
FENa . . . fractional excretion of sodium (Na)
FEP . . . free erythrocyte protoporphyrin
FER . . . flexion, extension, and rotation
FES . . . functional electrical stimulation
FETI . . . fluorescent energy transfer immunoassay
Fe/TIBC . . . iron saturation of serum transferrin
FEUO . . . for external use only
FEV . . . forced expiratory volume

FEVB .... frequency ectopic ventricular beat
FEV_t .... forced expiratory volume
FEV_t/VC .... ratio of one-second forced expiratory volume to vital capacity
FF .... fat-free (diet); filtration fraction; force fluids
F&F .... fixes and follows
FFA .... free fatty acids
FFB .... flexible fiberoptic bronchoscopy
FFD .... fat-free diet
FFDCA .... Food, Drug, and Cosmetic (Act)
FFP .... fresh frozen plasma
FFROM .... full, free range of motion
FFS .... fat-free solid; fat-free supper
FFW .... fat-free weight
fg .... femtogram
FGF .... father's grandfather
FGM .... father's grandmother
FGS .... focal glomerular sclerosis
FGT .... female genital tract
FH .... familial hypercholesterolemia; family history
FHA .... familial hypoplastic anemia
FHD .... family history of diabetes
FHH .... familial hypocalciuric hypercalcemia; family history of hirsutism
FHIP .... family health insurance plan
FHMI .... family history of mental illness
FHP .... family history positive
FHR .... fetal heart rate; fetal heart rhythm
FHS .... fetal heart sounds
FH_x .... family history
FIC .... functional inhibitory concentration
FID .... father in delivery
FIF .... forced inspiratory flow
FIH .... fat-induced hyperglycemia
FIL .... father-in-law
FIS .... forced inspiratory spirogram
FITC .... fluorescein isothiocyanate
FIUO .... for internal use only
FIV .... forced inspiratory volume in one second
FIVC .... forced inspiratory vital capacity
FJRM .... full joint range of movement/motion
fL .... femtoliter; fluid
FI_{O2} .... force inspiratory oxygen; fraction of inspired oxygen
FL .... full liquids (diet)
FLA .... left frontal anterior (position of fetus)
FLC .... fatty liver cell
FLD .... fatty liver disease
FLGA .... full-term, large for gestational age
FLKS .... fatty liver and kidney syndrome
FLP .... left frontal posterior (position of fetus)
FLS .... fatty liver syndrome
FLU A .... influenza A virus
Fm .... fermium
FM .... face mask
F&M .... firm and midline (uterus)
FMC .... fetal movement count
FMDV .... foot-and-mouth disease virus
FME .... foot-mouth extraction
FMEN .... familial multiple endocrine neoplasia
FMH .... family medical history
fmol .... femtomole
FMULC .... free monoclonal urinary light chains
FMV .... fluorouracil, methyl-CCNU (semustine), and vincristine
FMX .... full-mouth x-ray
FN .... facial nerve; false-negative
F-N .... finger-to-nose (coordination test)
FNA .... fine needle aspiration
FNA-B .... fine needle aspiration biopsy
FNF .... femoral neck fracture; finger-nose-finger (coordination test)
FOB .... father of baby; fiberoptic bronchoscopy
FOC .... father of child
FOD .... free of disease
FOOB .... fell out of bed
FOOSH .... fell on outstretched hand

FOS .... fiberoptic sigmoidoscopy
fp .... forearm pronated
FP .... false-positive; forearm pronated
F-P .... femoral popliteal
FPB .... femoral popliteal bypass
FPIA .... fluorescence polarization immunoassay
FPVB .... demoral-popliteal vein bypass
Fr .... francium
FR .... failure rate
F&R .... force and rhythm (of pulse)
FRA .... fluorescent rabies antibody
FrBB, FRBB .... fracture of both bones
FRC .... frozen red cells; functional residual capacity
FRF .... follicle-stimulating hormone-releasing factor
FRH .... follicle-stimulating hormone-releasing hormone
FRM .... full range of motion
FROM .... full range of motion
FS .... frozen section
F&S .... full and soft (diet)
FSB .... fetal scalp blood
FSBM .... full-strength breast milk
FSG .... focal sclerosing glomerulonephritis; focal segmental glomerulosclerosis
FSGA .... full-term, small for gestational age
FSGHS .... focal segmental glomerular hyalinosis and sclerosing
FSGN .... focal sclerosing glomerulonephritis
FSGS .... focal segmental glomerulosclerosis
FSH .... follicle stimulating hormone
FSH/LR-RH .... follicle-stimulating hormone and luteinizing hormone-releasing hormone
FSH-RF .... follicle-stimulating hormone-releasing factor
FSH-RH .... follicle-stimulating hormone-releasing hormone
FSI .... foam stability index
FSL .... fasting serum level
FSP .... familial spastic paraplegia; fibrin split products
ft .... make (fiat, fiant)
FT .... free thyroxine; full-term
FT_3I .... free triiodothyronine index
FTA .... fluorescent treponemal antibody
FTA-ABS .... fluorescent treponemal antibody absorption
FTD .... failure to descend
FTI .... free thyroxine index
FTN .... finger-to-nose (coordination test)
FTNB .... full-term newborn
FTND .... full-term normal delivery
FTP .... failure to progress (in labor)
FTT .... failure to thrive; fat tolerance test
FU .... fluorouracil; follow-up
5-FU 5-fluorouracil
F&U .... flanks and upper quadrants
F/U .... follow-up
FUDR .... floxuridine; fluorodeoxyuridine
FUDR-MP .... floxuridine monophosphate
FUE .... fever of unknown etiology
FUO .... fever of unknown/undetermined origin
FUOV .... follow-up office visit
FUR .... fluorouracil riboside; fluorouridine
FURAM .... ftorafur, Adriamycin (doxorubicin), and mitomycin
FVC .... forced vital capacity
FVE .... forced volume, expiratory
FVH .... focal vascular headache
FVIC .... forced inspiratory vital capacity
FVL .... femoral vein ligation
Fx .... fracture
FX .... factor X
FxBB .... fracture of both bones
g .... gram
G+ .... gram-positive
G- .... gram-negative
G-6-PD .... glucose 6-phosphate dehydrogenase
Ga .... gallium
GABA .... gamma-aminobutyric acid
GAD .... generalized anxiety disorder

GAL .... galactosemia
G and D .... growth and development
GAS .... gastric acid secretion
GAW .... airway conductance
GAZT .... glucuronide derivative of azidothymidine
GB .... gallbladder
G&B .... good and bad
GBD .... gallbladder disease
GBM .... glomerular basement membrane
GBS .... gallbladder series; gastric bypass surgery
GC .... geriatric chair; gonococcus; gonorrhea culture; gas chromatography
G+C .... gram-positive cocci
GCA .... gastric cancerous area; giant cell arteritis
GC/MS .... gas chromatography/mass spectrometry
G-CSF .... granulocyte colony-stimulating factors
GCSF .... granulocyte cell-stimulating factor
GCU .... gonococcal urethritis
GCV .... ganciclovir
Gd .... gadolinium
G&D .... growth and development
g/dL .... gram percent
gdw .... gram dry weight
Ge .... germanium
GE .... gastroesophageal
GEN/ENDO .... general anesthesia with endotracheal intubation
GER .... gastroesophageal reflux
GEU .... gestation, extrauterine
GF .... gastric fistula; gastric fluid
GFM .... good fetal movement
GFR .... glomerular filtration rate
GFS .... global focal sclerosis
GGCT .... ground glass clotting time
GGT .... gamma-glutamyltransferase
GH .... growth hormone
GHB .... glycohemoglobin
GHD .... growth hormone deficiency
GH-RH .... growth hormone-releasing hormone
GH-RIF .... growth hormone release-inhibiting factor
GH-RIH .... growth hormone release-inhibiting hormone
GI .... gastrointestinal; glucose intolerance; good impression
GIB .... gastrointestinal bleeding
GIFT .... gamete intrafallopian
GIH .... gastric inhibitory hormone
GIP .... gastric inhibitory polypeptide
GIS .... gastrointestinal series
GIT .... gastrointestinal tract
GITT .... gastrointestinal transit time; glucose-insulin tolerance test
GK .... galactokinase
GL .... gastric lavage
GLC .... gas-liquid chromatography
GM .... gastric mucosa; geometric mean; grand mal; grandmother
GM+ .... gram-positive
GM- .... gram-negative
GM-CFU .... granulocyte-macrophage colony-forming unit
GMS .... Grocott-Gomori methenamine-silver
Gn .... gonadotropin
GN .... gonococcus
G/N .... glucose/nitrogen (ratio in urine)
GNR .... gram-negative rod
GnRH .... gonadotropin releasing hormone
GO .... gonorrhea
GOT .... glutamic-oxaloacetic transaminase
GP .... glycoprotein
GPD .... glucose-6-phosphate dehydrogenase
GPK .... guinea pig kidney
GPR .... gram-positive rod
GPT .... glutamic-pyruvic transaminase
GPUT .... galactose phosphate uridyl transferase
gr+ .... gram-positive
GR .... glutathione reductase
G+R .... gram-positive rod
G-R .... gram-negative rod

GR-FR . . . grandfather
GR-MO . . . grandmother
GrP . . . gram-positive
G/S . . . glucose and saline
GSA65 . . . gross virus antigen
GSD . . . glycogen storage disease
GSH . . . glutathione; growth stimulating hormone
GSR . . . galvanic skin response; generalized Schwartzman reaction
GSSR . . . generalized Sandarelli-Shwartzman reaction
GSW . . . gunshot wound
GSWA . . . gunshot wound to abdomen
GT . . . gait training; gamma-glutamyltransferase
GTB . . . gastrointestinal tract bleeding
GTP . . . glutamyl transpeptidase
GTT . . . glucose tolerance test
gtt(s) . . . drop(s) (gutta)
GU . . . genitourinary; gastric ulcer; gonococcal urethritis
GVHD . . . graft-versus-host disease
GVHR . . . graft-versus-host reaction
GWA . . . gunshot wound of abdomen
GWT . . . gunshot wound of the throat
GXT . . . graded exercise test
gyn . . . gynecological
h . . . hour (hora)
H . . . hydrogen
Ha . . . hahnium
HA . . . headache; hemagglutination; hemolytic anemia
H/A . . . headache
HAA . . . hepatitis-associated antigen
HABA . . . hydroxybenzeneazobenzoic acid
HAI . . . hemagglutination inhibition
HAM . . . hexamethylmelamine, Adriamycin (doxorubicin), and melphalan; hypoparathyroidism, Addison disease, and mucocutaneous candidiasis (syndrome)
HANE . . . hereditary angioneurotic edema
HASCHD . . . hypertensive arteriosclerotic heart disease
HASCVD . . . hypertensive arteriosclerotic cardiovascular disease
HASHD . . . hypertensive arteriosclerotic heart disease
HAV . . . hepatitis A virus
HAVAB . . . hepatitis A virus antibody
Hb . . . hemoglobin
HBAb . . . hepatitis B antibody
HBAg . . . hepatitis B antigen
HB_c . . . hepatitis B core
HBD . . . hydroxybutric dehydrogenase
HBDH . . . hydroxybutyrate dehydrogenase
HB_eAg . . . hepatitis B e antigen
HBF . . . hepatic blood flow
HBO . . . hyperbaric oxygen (therapy); hyperbaric oxygenation
HBOT . . . hyperbaric oxygenation
HBP . . . high blood pressure
HB_sAg . . . hepatitis B surface antigen
HBV . . . hepatitis B vaccine; hepatitis B virus
HBW . . . high birth weight
HC . . . homocystinuria
HCAP . . . handicapped
H-CAP . . . hexamethylmelamine, cyclophosphamide, Adriamycin (doxorubicin), and Platinol (cisplatin)
HCFA . . . Health Care Financing Administration
HCFSH . . . human chorionic follicle-stimulating hormone
hCG . . . human chorionic gonadotropin
HCl . . . hydrochloric acid
HCL . . . hairy-cell leukemia
HCO_3 . . . bicarbonate
H'crit . . . hematocrit
HCS . . . human chorionic somatomammotropin
Hct, HCT . . . hematocrit
HD . . . Hodgkin disease
HDL . . . high density lipoprotein
HDLC . . . high density lipoprotein cholesterol
HDLs . . . high density lipoproteins
HDMP . . . high-dose methylprednisolone

HDMTX . . . . . high-dose methotrexate
HDMTX-CF . . . . . high-dose methotrexate and citrovorum factor
HDMTX/LV . . . . . high-dose methotrexate and leucovorin
HDN . . . . . hemolytic disease of the newborn
HDP . . . . . hydroxydimethylpyrimidine
He . . . . . helium
HEENT . . . . . head, ears, eyes, nose. and throat
HEG . . . . . hemorrhagic erosive gastritis
hemat . . . . . hematocrit
HEMPAS . . . . . here. erythroblastic multinuclearity with positive acidified serum
hep . . . . . hepatitis
HEp . . . . . human epithelial cells
HES . . . . . acute hypereosinophilic syndrome
Hf . . . . . hafnium
HFHL . . . . . high-frequency hearing loss
HFI . . . . . hereditary fructose intolerance
Hg . . . . . mercury
^{197}Hg . . . . . radioisotope of mercury
^{203}Hg . . . . . radioisotope of mercury
HG . . . . . herpes gestationis
HGA . . . . . homogentisic acid
Hgb . . . . . hemoglobin
hGG, HGG . . . . . human gamma globulin
HGH . . . . . human growth hormone
HGPRT . . . . . hypoxanthine guanine phosphoribosyl transferase
Hgt . . . . . height
H/H . . . . . hemoglobin and hematocrit
HHC . . . . . home health care
HHD . . . . . hypertensive heart disease
HHH . . . . . hyperornithinemia, hyperammonemia-homocitrullinuria
HHM . . . . . humoral hypercalcemia of malignancy
HHS . . . . . (Department of) Health and Human Services
HHT . . . . . head holter traction
HI . . . . . head injury; hydriodic acid
HIAA . . . . . hydroxyindoleacetic acid
HIB . . . . . *Haemophilus influenzae* B
HIDA . . . . . acetanilidoiminodiacetic acid
HIP . . . . . humoral immunocompetence profile
HIT . . . . . heparin-induced thrombocytopenia
HITB . . . . . *Haemophilus influenzae* type B (meningitis)
HIV . . . . . human immunodeficiency virus
HK . . . . . hexokinase
H-K . . . . . hand-to-knee (test); heel to knee (test)
HKAHO . . . . . hip-knee-ankle-foot orthosis
HKAO . . . . . hip-knee-ankle orthosis
HKO . . . . . hip-knee orthosis (splint)
HKS . . . . . hip-knee-shin (test)
HL . . . . . half-life (of radioactive element); hearing level; Hickman line
H&L . . . . . heart and lungs
H/L . . . . . heparin lock
HLA . . histocompatibility leukocyte antigen; histocompatibility locus antigen; human leukocyte antigen
HLK . . . . . heart, liver, and kidneys
H&L OK . . . . . heart and lungs normal
HLT . . . . . heart-lung transplantation
HLV . . . . . herpes-like virus
HMB . . . . . homatropine methylbromide
HME . . . . . heat, massage, and exercise
HMETSC . . . . . heavy metal screen
HMG-CoA . . . . . hepatic hydroxymethylglutaryl coenzyme A
HMM . . . . . hexamethylmelamine
HMO . . . . . Health Maintenance Organization
HMS . . . . . hexose monophosphate shunt
HMT . . . . . hematocrit
HMW . . . . . high molecular weight
HMWK . . . . . high molecular weight kininogen
HMX . . . . . heat, massage, and exercise
HN . . . . . head nurse
H&N . . . . . head and neck
HNS . . . . . head and neck surgery
HNV . . . . . has not voided
Ho . . . . . holmium

HO . . . . . house officer
H/O . . . . . history of
HOA . . . . . hip osteoarthritis
HOB . . . . . head of bed
HOB UPSOB . . . . . head of bed up for shortness of breath
HOH . . . . . hard of hearing
HOP . . . . . high oxygen pressure; hydroxydaunomycin (doxorubicin), Oncovin (vincristine), and prednisone
hor . . . . . (L. *hora somni* hour of sleep) at bedtime
hor som . . . . . (L. *hora somni* hour of sleep) at bedtime
HP . . . . . hot packs
H&P . . . . . history and physical
HPE . . . . . history and physical examination
hpf . . . . . high power field
HPFH . . . . . hereditary persistence of fetal hemoglobin
HPI . . . . . history of present illness
HPL . . . . . human placental lactogen
HPLC . . . . . high-performance liquid chromatography
HPN . . . . . home parenteral nutrition
HPP . . . . . human pancreatic polypeptide
HPPA . . . . . hydroxyphenylpyruvic acid
HPPH . . . . . hydroxyphenyl-phenylhydantoin
HPT . . . . . hyperparathyroidism
hPTH . . . . . human parathyroid hormone
HPV . . . . . *Haemophilus pertussis* vaccine; human papillomavirus
HR . . . . . heart rate; hospital record
H&R . . . . . hysterectomy and radiation
HRA . . . . . health risk appraisal
HRANA . . . . . histone reactive ANA
HRCT . . . . . high resolution CT
HRL . . . . . head rotation (to) left
HRLM . . . . . high resolution light microscopy
HRR . . . . . head rotation (to) right
HRs . . . . . Hamilton Rating Scale
hs . . . . . at bedtime (hora somni)
HS . . . . . half strength; herpes simplex; hereditary spherocytosis
HSA . . . . . human serum albumin
h som . . . . . (L. *hora somni* hour of sleep) at bedtime
HSV . . . . . herpes simplex virus
HSVE . . . . . herpes simplex virus encephalitis
ht . . . . . height
HT . . . . . hypertension; hypodermic tablet
H&T . . . . . hospitalization and treatment
3-HT . . . . . 3-hydroxytyramine (dopamine)
5-HT . . . . . 5-hydroxytyramine (serotonin)
HTK . . . . . heel to knee (test)
HTLV . . . . . human T-lymphotropic virus
HTN . . . . . hypertension
HTP . . . . . hydroxytrytophan
HTVD . . . . . hypertensive vascular disease
HUS . . . . . hemolytic-uremic syndrome; hyaluronidase unit for semen
HV . . . . . herpes virus
H&V . . . . . hemigastrectomy and vagotomy
H-V . . . . . His-ventricular
HVA . . . . . homovanillic acid
HVLP . . . . . high volume, low pressure
Hx . . . . . history
HXM . . . . . hexamethylmelamine
Hz . . . . . hertz
I . . . . . indeterminate; intermediate; iodine
^{125}I . . . . . radioisotope of iodide
^{131}I . . . . . radioisotope of iodide
Ia . . . . . antigen
I&A . . . . . irrigation and aspiration
IAA . . . . . indole acetic acid
I-3-AA . . . . . indole-3-acetic acid
IABC . . . . . intra-aortic balloon catheter; intra-aortic balloon counterpulsation
IABCP . . . . . intra-aortic balloon counterpulsation
IABP . . . . . intra-aortic balloon pump
IACB . . . . . intra-aortic counterpulsation balloon
IADH . . . . . inappropriate antidiuretic hormone
IADHS . . . . . inappropriate antidiuretic hormone syndrome

IAO . . . immediately after onset
IARF . . . ischemic acute renal failure
IAT . . . indirect antiglobulin test
Ib . . . a glycoprotein
IBBBB . . . incomplete bilateral bundle-branch
IBC . . . iron binding capacity
IBD . . . infectious bowel disease; inflammatory bowel disease; irritable bowel disease; ischemic bowel disease
IBP . . . intra-aortic balloon pumping
IBW . . . ideal body weight
IC . . . immune complexes; inspiratory capacity
ICA . . . internal carotid artery
ICD . . . immune complex disease; isocitrate dehydrogenase
ICDH . . . isocitrate dehydrogenase
ICF . . . intracellular fluid
ICG . . . indocyanine green
ICH . . . intracranial hemorrhage; intracranial hypertension
ICN . . . intensive care neonatal
ICS . . . intercostal space
ICSH . . . interstitial cell stimulating hormone
ICT . . . indirect Coombs' test
ICU . . . intensive care unit
ICVH . . . ischemic cerebrovascular headache
ID . . . identification; immunodiffusion; infectious disease; intradermal(ly)
I&D . . . incision and drainage
IDA . . . iron deficiency anemia; image display and analysis
IDAT . . . indirect antiglobulin test
IDC . . . idiopathic dilated cardiomyopathy
IDDF . . . investigational drug data form
IDDM . . . insulin dependent diabetes mellitus
IDDS . . . implantable drug delivery system; investigational drug data sheet
IDL . . . intermediate-density lipoprotein
IDM . . . idiopathic disease of myocardium; intermediate-dose methotrexate
IDVC . . . indwelling venous catheter
I&E . . . internal and external
I/E . . . inspiratory/expiratory
IEF . . . isoelectric focusing
IEM . . . inborn errors of metabolism
IEP . . . immunoelectrophoresis
IF . . . immunofluorescence; inspiratory force; interstitial fluid; intrinsic factor
IFA . . . indirect fluorescent antibody
IFCPC . . . Internal Federation of Cervical Pathology and Colposcopy
IFIX . . . immunofixation
IFLrA . . . recombinant human leukocyte interferon A
IFOS . . . ifosfamide
IFX . . . ifosfamide
Ig . . . immunoglobulin
IGH . . . idiopathic growth hormone
IGIM . . . immune globulin intramuscular
IGT . . . impaired glucose tolerance
IHA . . . indirect hemagglutination
IHSS . . . idiopathic hypertrophic subaortic stenosis
IIb-IIIa . . . glycoproteins found on platelet membranes
IIF . . . indirect immunofluorescence
II-para . . . secudipara (second pregnancy)
III-para . . . tertipara (third pregnancy)
IK . . . immobilized knee
I.M. . . . intramuscular
IMAC . . . ifosfamide, mesna uroprotection, Adriamycin (doxorubicin), and cisplatin
IMD . . . inherited metabolic disorders
IMIG . . . intramuscular immunoglobulin
IMP . . . impression
IMV . . . inferior mesenteric vein; intermittent mandatory ventilation
In . . . indium
INB . . . ischemic necrosis (of) bone
IND . . . investigational new drug
Inh . . . inhaler
INH . . . isonicotinic acid hydrazide; isoniazid
INK . . . injury not known
INR . . . international normalized ratio
I and O . . . intake and output
I&O . . . in and out; intake and output

IOF . . . . . intraocular fluid
IOFNA . . . . . intraoperative fine needle aspiration
IOH . . . . . idiopathic orthostatic hypotension
IOL . . . . . intraocular lens
IOLI . . . . . intraocular lens implantation
IOP . . . . . intraocular pressure
IOT . . . . . intraocular tension
IOUS . . . . . intraoperative ultrasound
IOV . . . . . initial office visit
IP . . . . . intraperitoneal(ly)
I-PAO . . . . . insulin induced peak acid output
I-para . . . . . primipara (first pregnancy)
IPCD . . . . . infantile polycystic disease
IPF . . . . . idiopathic pulmonary fibrosis
IPG . . . . . impedence phlebograph
IPPB . . . . . intermittent positive pressure breathing
Ir . . . . . iridium
IR . . . . . infrared
I&R . . . . . insertion and removal
IRB . . . . . institutional review board
IRBBB . . . . . incomplete right bundle-branch block
IRBC . . . . . immature red blood cell
IRDS . . . . . infant respiratory distress syndrome
IRG . . . . . immunoreactive glucose
IRGH . . . . . immunoreactive growth hormone
IRI . . . . . immunoreactive insulin
IRMA . . . . . immunoradiometric assay
IRT . . . . . immunoreactive trypsinogen
ISADH . . . . . inappropriate secretion of antidiuretic hormone
ISD . . . . . isosorbide dinitrate
ISDN . . . . . isosorbide dinitrate
ISE . . . . . ion-selective electrode
ISF . . . . . interstitial fluid
ISFV . . . . . interstitial fluid volume
ISI . . . . . infarct size index
ISS . . . . . Injury Severity Scale
IT . . . . . inhalation therapy; intrathecal(ly)
ITCP . . . . . immunogenic thrombocytopenic purpura
ITP
. . . . idiopathic thrombocytopenic purpura; immunogenic thrombocytopenic purpura
ITT . . . . . identical twins (raised) together; insulin tolerance test; iron tolerance test
IU . . . . . International unit
IUD . . . . . intrauterine death; intrauterine device
IUGR . . . . . intrauterine growth retardation
IUP . . . . . intrauterine pregnancy
IUPC . . . . . intrauterine pressure catheter
IUPD . . . . . intrauterine pregnancy, delivered
IUT . . . . . intrauterine transfusion
I.V. . . . . . intravenous
IVAC . . . . . I.V. infusion control device
IVAD . . . . . implanted vascular access device
IVB . . . . . intraventricular block
IVBAT . . . . . intravascular bronchoalveolar tumor
IVBC . . . . . intravascular blood coagulation
IVC . . . . . inferior vena cava; intravenous cholangiography
IVCP . . . . . inferior vena cava pressure
IVCT . . . . . inferior vena cave thrombosis
IVDU . . . . . intravenous drug (use)
IVH . . . . . intravenous hyperalimentation; intraventricular hemorrhage
IVIG . . . . . intravenous immune globulin; intravenous immunoglobulin
IVN . . . . . intravenous nutrition
IVP . . . . . intravenous push; intravenous pyelogram
IVPB . . . . . intravenous piggyback
IVSA . . . . . intravenous digital subtraction angiography
IVSD . . . . . intraventricular septal defect
IVUS . . . . . intravascular coronary ultrasound
IVV . . . . . influenza virus vaccine
IWMI . . . . . inferior wall myocardial infarct(ion)
JA . . . . . juvenile atrophy
JD . . . . . juvenile-onset diabetes
JDM . . . . . juvenile-onset diabetes mellitus
JF . . . . . joint fluid

JJ .... jaw jerk
JOD .... juvenile-onset diabetes
JODM .... juvenile-onset diabetes mellitus
JOMAC .... judgment, orientation, memory, abstraction, and calculation
JOMACI .... judgment, orientation, memory, abstraction, and calculation intact
JPB .... junctional premature beat
JRA .... juvenile rheumatoid arthritis
JVD .... jugular-venous distension
JVP .... jugular-venous pressure; jugular vein/venous pulse
k .... kilo (10^3)
K .... potassium
KA .... alkaline phosphatase
KAFO .... knee-ankle-foot orthosis
KAO .... knee-ankle orthosis
K-B .... Kleihauer-Betke
kcal .... kilocalorie
KCl .... potassium chloride
KCN .... potassium cyanide
KDA .... known drug allergies
kg .... kilogram
KGS .... ketogenic steroids
kL .... kiloliter
km .... kilometer
KO .... keep open
KOH .... potassium hydroxide
Kr .... krypton
KS .... ketosteroids; Kaposi sarcoma
KS/OI .... Kaposi sarcoma and opportunistic infections
KU .... Karmen units
KUB .... kidney and urinary bladder
KUS .... kidney(s), ureter(s), and spleen
KVO .... keep vein open
KW .... Keith-Wagener
L .... left; liter; lumbar
L_2 .... second lumbar vertebra
La .... lanthanum
LA .... latex agglutination; left atrium; local anesthetic
L&A .... light and accommodation
LAD .... left anterior descending (artery)
LAH .... left atrial hypertrophy
LAHB .... left anterior hemiblock
LAI .... labioincisal
LAO .... left anterior oblique
Lap .... laparotomy
LAP .. laparoscopy; left atrial pressure; leucine aminopeptidase; leukocyte alkaline phosphatase
LASA .... lipid-associated sialic acid
LATS .... long-acting thyroid stimulating hormone
LATS-P .... long-acting thyroid-stimulation-protector
LB .... left bundle
L&B .... left and below
LBA .... left basal artery
LBB .... left breast biopsy; left bundle-branch
LBBB .... left bundle-branch block
LBBsB .... left bundle-branch system block
LBBX .... left biopsy examination
LBCD .... left border (of) cardiac dullness
LBM .... lean body mass
LBO .... large bowel obstruction
LBP .... low back pain; low blood pressure
LBV .... left brachial vein
LBW .... lean body weight; low birth weight
LBWI .... low birth weight infant
LC .... lethal concentration
LCBF .... local cerebral blood flow
LCI .... lung clearance index
LCIS .... lobular carcinoma *in situ*
LCM .... lymphocytic choriomeningitis
LCO .... low cardiac output
LCOS .... low cardiac output syndrome
LCS .... left coronary sinus; Leydig cell stimulation
LD .... labor and delivery; lactate dehydrogenase; lethal dose; light difference

L&D .... labor and delivery
LD_1 .... lactate dehydrogenase fraction 1
LDH .... lactate dehydrogenase
LDHI .... LDH isoenzymes
LDL .... low density lipoprotein
LDLC .... low density lipoprotein cholesterol
LDLs .... low density lipoproteins
LDT .... lactate dehydrogenase total
LDV .... lactate dehydrogenase virus
Le .... Lewis antigen
LE .... left ear; left eye; lens extraction; lower extremity; lupus erythematosus
LEA .... lower extremity arterial
LEEP .... loop electrosurgical excisional procedure
LEM .... lateral eye movement
LES .... lower esophageal sphincter
LETZ .... loop excision of transformation
LLETZ .... large loop excision of transformation
LEV .... lower extremity venous
LFA .... left femoral artery
LFC .... left frontal craniotomy
LFD .... lactose-free diet
LFT .... liver function test
LGV .... lymphogranuloma venereum
LH .... luteinizing hormone
LHA .... left hepatic artery
LHF .... left heart failure
LHP .... left hemiparesis; left hemiplegia
LHRF .... luteinizing hormone releasing factor
LHRH .... luteinizing hormone releasing hormone
LHV .... left ventricular hypertrophy
Li .... lithium
LIC .... left iliac crest
LIO .... left inferior oblique
LISS .... low ionic strength saline
L-J .... Löwenstein-Jensen
LKM .... liver/kidney microsomes
LKS .... liver, kidneys, spleen
LKSB .... liver, kidneys, spleen, (and) bladder
LKS non.pal. .... liver, kidneys, (and) spleen not palpable
LLA .... lupus-like anticoagulant
LLDH .... liver lactate dehydrogenase
LLL .... left lower lobe
LLLE .... lower lid, left eye
LLN .... limit of normal
LLQ .... left lower quadrant
LLRE .... lower lid, right eye
LLSB .... left lower scapular border; left lower sternal border
LLT .... left lateral thigh
LM .... light microscopy
LMD .... left main disease
LMF .... left middle finger
LMN .... lower motor neuron
LMP .... last menstrual period
LMW .... low molecular weight
LMWH .... low molecular weight heparin
LOA .... leave of absence; left occipital anterior
LOC .... laxative of choice
LOM .... left otitis media; limitation of motion
LOP .... leave on pass
LOS .... length of stay; loss of sight; lower (o)esophageal sphincter
LOSP .... lower (o)esophageal sphincter pressure
LP .... light perception; lumbar puncture
LPC .... leukocyte-poor cells (leukocyte depleted)
lpf .... low power field
LPHB .... left posterior hemiblock
LPIH .... left posterior-inferior hemiblock
LPO .... left posterior oblique
LP&P .... light perception and projection
LPRBC .... leukocyte-poor red blood cells
LQTS .... long QT syndrome
L&R .... left and right
L/R .... left-to-right (ratio)

LRC . . . Lipid Research Clinic
LRH . . . luteinizing releasing hormone
L&S . . . liver and spleen
L/S . . . lecithin/sphingomyelin ratio
LSD . . . lysergic acid diethylamide
LSG . . . labial salivary gland
LSN . . . left substantia nigra; left sympathetic nerve
LSO . . . lateral superior olive (of brain); left salpingo-oophorectomy
LSVC . . . left superior vena cava
LTC . . . long-term care
LTCPs . . . L-tryptophan-containing products
LTE . . . leukotriene E
LTGA . . . left transposition (of) great artery
LTT . . . lactose tolerance test; limited treadmill test; lymphocyte transformation test
Lu . . . lutetium
L&U . . . lower and upper (extremities)
LUL . . . left upper lobe
LUQ . . . left upper quadrant
LUS . . . laparoscopic ultrasound
LV . . . lung volume
LVET . . . left ventricular ejection time
LVH . . . left ventricular hypertrophy
LVOT . . . left ventricular outflow tract
LVW . . . lateral vaginal wall
L&W . . . living and well
Lw . . . lawrencium
Lytes . . . electrolytes
m . . . meter; milli (10^{-3})
M . . . mega (10^{6}); mix (misce)
M-2 . . . vincristine, carmustine, cyclophosphamide, melphalan, and prednisone
m^2 . . . square meter
m^3 . . . cubic meter
MA . . . Master of Arts
mA . . . milliampere
M/A . . . mood and/or affect
MA-1 . . . a type of respirator
MAA . . . microaggregatedalbumin
MABOP . . . Mustargen (nitrogen mustard), Adriamycin (doxorubicin), bleomycin, Oncovin (vincristine), and prednisone
MABP . . . mean arterial blood pressure
MACC . . . methotrexate, Adriamycin (doxorubicin), cyclophosphamide, and CCNU (lomustine)
MAI . . . *Mycobacterium avium-intracellulare*
MAO . . . maximal acid output; monoamine oxidase
MAP . . . mitomycin, Adriamycin (doxorubicin), and cisplatin
MAR . . . medication administration record; mixed antiglobulin reaction
MAT . . . multifocal atrial tachycardia
MB . . . a fraction of creatine kinase
MBA . . . Master of Business Administration
M-BACOD . . . methotrexate, bleomycin, Adriamycin (doxorubicin), cyclophosphamide, Oncovin (vincristine), and dexamethasone
MBC . . . methotrexate, bleomycin, and cisplatin; minimum bactericidal concentration; maximum breathing capacity
MB-CK . . . creatinine kinase isoenzyme containing M and B subunits
MBD . . . maximum bactericidal dilution; methotrexate, bleomycin, and diaminedichloroplatinum (cisplatin)
MBE . . . may be elevated
MBG . . . mean blood glucose
MBP . . . myelin basic protein
mc . . . millicurie
M&C . . . morphine and cocaine
MCA . . . major coronary artery; megestrol, cyclophosphamide, and Adriamycin (doxorubicin)
MC-Ab . . . monoclonal antibody
MCAD . . . medium chain ACYL CO-A dehydrogenase
MCBP . . . melphalan, cyclophosphamide, BCNU (bischloroethylnitrosourea), and prednisone
MCFA . . . medium-chain fatty acid
mcg . . . microgram
MCH . . . mean corpuscular hemoglobin
MCHC . . . mean cell hemoglobin concentration

mCi . . . . . millicurie
MCI . . . . . mean cardiac index
MCL . . . . . midclavicular line; midcostal line
MCT . . . . . medium chain triglycerides
MCTD . . . . . mixed connective tissue disease
MCV . . . . . mean corpuscular volume
Md . . . . . mendelevium
MD . . . . . medical doctor
MDIs . . . . . metered dose inhalers
MDM . . . . . mid-diastolic murmur; minor determinant mixture
MDP . . . . . mentodextra posterior
MDR . . . . . minimum daily requirement
MDS . . . . . materials distribution system
MDUO . . . . . myocardial disease (of) unknown origin
MDV . . . . . multiple dose vial
MEA . . . . . mercaptoethylamine; multiple endocrine adenomatosis
MeCCNU . . . . . methylchloroethylcyclohexylmitrosourea (semustine)
MeCP . . . . . methyl-CCNU, cyclophosphamide, and prednisone
MECY . . . . . methyltrexate and cyclophosphamide
MED . . . . . minimal erythemal dose
MEET . . . . . multistage exercise electrocardiographics test
MEIA . . . . . microparticle enzyme immunoassay
MEN . . . . . multiple endocrine neoplasia
mEq . . . . . milliequivalent
methyl-CCNU . . . . . methylchloroethylcyclohexylmitrosourea (semustine)
METS . . . . . metastases
MF . . . . . mycosis fungoides
M&F . . . . . male and female; mother and father
M/F . . . . . male to female (ratio)
MFC . . . . . minimum fungicidal concentration
MFR . . . . . mean flow rate
MFU . . . . . medical follow-up
MFVD . . . . . midforceps vaginal delivery
mg . . . . . milligram
mg% . . . . . milligrams per deciliter; milligrams per 100 milliliters; milligrams percent
Mg . . . . . magnesium
MG . . . . . myasthenia gravis
$MgCl_2$ . . . . . magnesium chloride
$MgCO_3$ . . . . . magnesium carbonate
MGP . . . . . methyl green pyronine
$MgSO_4$ . . . . . magnesium sulfate
MH . . . . . malignant hyperthermia; marital history; menstrual history; mental health
M/H . . . . . microcytic hypochromic (anemia)
MHA . . . . . microhemagglutination
MHA-TP . . . . . microhemagglutination *Treponema pallidum*
MHC . . . . . major histocompatibility complex
MHPG . . . . . methoxyhydroxyphenylglycol
MHz . . . . . megahertz
MI . . . . . myocardial infarction; maturation index
MIC . . . . . minimum inhibitory concentration
μ . . . . . micro (10^{-6})
μg . . . . . microgram
μL . . . . . microliter
μm . . . . . micrometer
μm^3 . . . . . cubic micrometer
μmol . . . . . micromole
μmol/L . . . . . micromolar
μOsm . . . . . micro-osmolar
μU . . . . . microunit
MID . . . . . maximum bactericidal dilution
MIE . . . . . medical improvement expected
MIF . . . . . merthiolate-iodine-formalin; migration inhibitory factor
MIT . . . . . migration inhibition test
MITO-C . . . . . mitomycin C
mIU . . . . . milli International unit
mL . . . . . milliliter
MLAP . . . . . mean left atrial pressure
MLC . . . . . mixed leukocyte culture; mixed lymphocyte culture
MLD . . . . . metachromatic leukodystrophy; minimum lethal dose
mL/L . . . . . milliliters per liter
MLR . . . . . mixed lymphocyte reaction
MLT . . . . . medical laboratory technician

MLV .... monitored live voice
mm .... millimeter
mm^2 .... square millimeter
mm^3 .... cubic millimeter
mM .... millimolar; millimole
MMA .... methylmalonic acid
MMC .... minimal medullary concentration
MMD .... myotonic muscular dystrophy
MMEF .... mean midexpiratory flow
MMF .... maximal midexpiratory flow rate
mm Hg .... millimeters of mercury
mmol .... millimole
mmol/L .... millimolar
MMPI .... Minnesota multiple personality inventory
MMR .... mass miniature radiography; mass miniature roentgenography; maternal mortality rate; measles, mumps, rubella
MMT .... manual muscle test
Mn .... manganese
M&N .... morning and night
M/N .... macrocytic/normochronic (anemia); microcytic/normochronic (anemia)
MNS .... MNS blood group
Mo .... molybdenum
MO .... mesio-occlusal
MOA .... mechanism of action
MOA-B .... monoamine oxidase type-B inhibitor
MOAD .. methotrexate, Oncovin (vincristine), L-asparaginase, and dexamethasone
MOB .... mechlorethamine, Oncovin (vincristine), and bleomycin
MOB-PT .... mitomycin C, Oncovin (vincristine), bleomycin, and cisplatin
MOCA .... methotrexate, Oncovin (vincristine), Cytoxan (cyclophosphamide), and Adriamycin (doxorubicin)
MOD .... maturity-onset diabetes
MODM .... maturity-onset diabetes mellitus
MOFS .... multiple-organ failure syndrome
mol .... mole
mol/L .... molar
mol/m^3 .... mole per cubic meter
mol/s .... mole per second
MOMPs .... major outer membrane proteins
MONO .... mononucleosis
MOP-BAP ...... Mustargen (mechlorethamine), Oncovin (vincristine), prednisone, bleomycin, Adriamycin (doxorubicin), and procarbazine
MOPP .... mustargen oncovin procarbazine and prednisone
MOPV .... monovalent oral poliovirus
mOsm .... milliosmole
mOsm/kg .... milliosmoles per kilogram
MPDS .... mandibular pain dysfunction syndrome
mph .... miles per hour
MPH .... Master of Public Health
MPHD .... methoxyhydroxphenolglycerol
MPPT .... methylprednisolone pulse therapy
MPS .... mucopolysaccharidosis
MPV .... mean plasma volume; mean platelet volume
MR .... moderately resistant
MRA .... main renal artery
mrad .... millirad
MRI .... magnetic resonance imaging
MRM .... modified radical mastectomy
MRS .... methicillin-resistant *Staphylococcus aureus*
MRSA .... methicillin-resistant *S. aureus*
MRVP .... mean right ventricular pressure
m/s .... meters per second
MS .... mental status; mitral stenosis; multiple sclerosis
MSAFP .... maternal serum alpha fetoprotein
MSAP .... mean systemic arterial pressure
MSD .... metabolic screening disorders
msec .... millisecond
m/sec .... meters per second
MSH .... melanocyte stimulating hormone
MSL .... midsternal line
MSLT .... multiple sleep latency test
MSOF .... multiple systems organ failure
MSTA .... mumps skin test antigen

MSTI . . . multiple soft tissue injuries
MSUD . . . maple syrup urine disease
mt . . . send of such (mitte talis)
MT . . . medical technologist
MTB . . . mycobacterium tuberculosis
MTC . . . mitomycin-C
MTHF . . . 5-methyl-tetrahydrofolate
MTR . . . mass, tenderness, rebound (abdominal examination)
MTR-O . . . no masses, tenderness, or rebound (abdominal examination)
MTRX . . . methotrexate
MTX . . . methotrexate
MTX's . . . methotrexate
mU . . . milliunit
MUGA . . . multiple gated scan
MUP . . . monitor unit potential
MV . . . minute volume
M-VAC . . . methotrexate, vinblastine, Adriamycin (doxorubicin), and cisplatin
MVB . . . mixed venous blood
MVC . . . maximal vital capacity; maximal voluntary contraction; myocardial vascular capacity
MVE . . . mitral valve echo
MVOA . . . mitral valve orifice area
MVOS . . . mixed venous oxygen saturation
MVP . . . mean venous pressure; mitral valve prolapse
MVPP . . . mustine, vinblastine, procarbazine, and prednisone
MVR . . . mitral valve regurgitation; mitral valve replacement
MVS . . . mitral valve stenosis
MVV . . . maximum voluntary ventilation
MVVPP . . . Mustargen (nitrogen mustard), vincristine, vinblastine, procarbazine, and prednisone
MW . . . mean weight; molecular weight
MWP . . . mean wedge pressure
MyG . . . myasthenia gravis
MyMD . . . myotonic muscular dystrophy
MYO . . . myoglobin
MYOGLB . . . myoglobin
MZ . . . monozygotic
n . . . nano (10^{-9})
N . . . nitrogen; normal
Na . . . sodium
Na_2CO_3 . . . sodium carbonate
NA . . . not applicable; nursing assistant
N&A . . . normal and active
NACI . . . National Advisory Committee on Immunization
NaCl . . . sodium chloride
NAD . . . nicotinamide adenine dinucleotide; no acute distress; no apparent distress
NADH . . . reduced form of NAD
NADP . . . nicotinamide adenine dinucleotide phosphate
NADPH . . . reduced form of NADP
NaF . . . sodium fluoride
NAF . . . nafcillin
Na&K . . . sodium and potassium
NaOH . . . sodium hydroxide
NAPA . . . *N*-acetylprocainamide
NAS . . . no added salt
NATP . . . neonatal autoimmune thrombocytopenic purpura
Nb . . . niobium
NBIL . . . neonatal bilirubin
NBT . . . nitro blue tetrazolium
NC . . . nerve conduction
NCA . . . National Certification Agency; nonspecific cross-reacting antigen
NCCLS . . . National Committee for Clinical Laboratory Standards
NCEP . . . National Cholesterol Education Program
NCI . . . National Cancer Institute
NCPR . . . no cardiopulmonary resuscitation
NCRC . . . nonchild-resistant container
NCS . . . nerve conduction study
NCV . . . nerve conduction velocity
NCVS . . . nerve condition velocity studies
Nd . . . neodymium
N&D . . . nodular and diffuse (lymphoma)
N/D . . . no defects

NDA . . . New Drug Application
NDC . . . National Drug Code Directory
NDD . . . no-dialysis days
Ne . . . neon
NEA . . . neoplasm embryonic antigen
NEC . . . necrotizing enterocolitis
NED . . . no evidence (of) disease
NEMD . . . nonspecific esophageal motility disorder; nonspecific esophageal motor dysfunction
NEOH . . . neonatal/high
NEOM . . . neonatal/medium
NERD . . . no evidence (of) recurrent disease
NETT . . . nasal endotracheal tube
NF . . . normal full-term delivery
ng . . . nanogram
NGT . . . nasogastric tube; normal glucose tolerance
NGU . . . nongonococcal urethritis
NH_4Cl . . . ammonium chloride
NH_4OH . . . ammonium hydroxide
NHD . . . normal hair distribution
NHDL . . . non-high-density lipoprotein
Ni . . . nickel
NICU . . . neonatal intensive care unit
NIH . . . National Institutes of Health
NIS . . . no inflammatory signs
NITD . . . non-insulin-treated disease
NK . . . natural killer
N/K . . . not known
NKA . . . no known allergies
NKDA . . . no known drug allergies
NKFA . . . no known food allergies
NKH . . . nonketotic hyperglycemia; nonketotic hyperosmolar; nonketotic hyperosmotic
NKHA . . . nonketotic hyperosmolar acidosis
NKHG . . . nonketotic hyperglycemia
NKHS . . . nonketotic hyperosmolar syndrome
NKMA . . . no known medication allergies
nL . . . nanoliter
NL . . . normal
NLB . . . needle liver biopsy
NLDL . . . normal low-density lipoprotein
NLE . . . neonatal lupus erythematosus
nm . . . nanometer
NMJ . . . neuromuscular junction disease
nmol . . . nanomole
nmol/L . . . millimicromolar
NMR . . . nuclear magnetic resonance
NMRI . . . nuclear magnetic resonance imaging
NMS . . . neuroleptic malignant syndrome
NND . . . neonatal death
NNE . . . neonatal necrotizing enterocolitis
NNO . . . no new orders
NNS . . . neonatal screen (hematocrit, total bilirubin, and total protein)
NNT . . . neonatally tolerant
No . . . nobelium
NO . . . nasal oxygen
noc . . . in the night (nocturnal)
NOF . . . National Osteoporosis Foundation
NOII . . . nonocclusive intestinal ischemia
NOK . . . next of kin
NOM . . . nonsuppurative otitis media
NONF . . . nonfasting
non rep . . . do not repeat; no refills
NOOB . . . not out of bed
NOR-EPI . . . norepinephrine
NOS . . . no organisms seen
NOT . . . nocturnal oxygen therapy
NOTT . . . nocturnal oxygen therapy trial
Np . . . neptunium
NP . . . nasal prongs; nasopharynx
NPA . . . nasal pharyngeal airway
NPAT . . . nonparoxysmal atrial tachycardia

NPC .... nasopharyngeal cancer; nasopharyngeal carcinoma
NPF .... no predisposing factor
NPO .... nothing by mouth
NPO/HS .... nothing by mouth at bedtime
NPT .... nocturnal penile tumescence
NPTM .... nocturnal penile tumescence monitoring
NPV .... negative pressure ventilation
nr .... do not repeat (non repetatur)
N/R .... not remarkable
NRBCs .... normal red blood cells; nucleated red blood cells
NRC .... National Research Council; Nuclear Regulatory Commission
NREM .... nonrapid eye movement
NRM .... normal range (of) motion
NROM .... normal range of motion
NS .... normal saline; not seen; not significant
N/S .... normal saline
NSA .... normal serum albumin; no salt albumin
NSAID .... nonsteroidal anti-inflammatory drug
NSDA .... nonsteroid-dependent asthmatic
NSE .... neuron specific enolase
NSM .... nonsmoker
NSR .... normal sinus rhythm
NST .... nonstress test
NSU .... nonspecific urethritis
NSV .... nonspecific vaginitis
NSVD .... normal spontaneous vaginal delivery
NSVT .... nonsustained ventricular tachycardia
NT .... nasotracheal
N&T, N+T .... nose and throat
NTA .... natural thymocytotoxic autoantibody
NTG .... nitroglycerine
NTI .... nonthyroidal illness; nonthyroidal index
NTMI .... nontransmural myocardial infarction
NTN .... nephrotoxic nephritis
NTND .... not tender, not distended
NTR .... negative therapeutic reaction
NTS .... nasotracheal suction
NTT .... nasotracheal tube
NTX .... naltrexone
NU .... name unknown
N&V .... nausea and vomiting
NVA .... near visual acuity; normal visual acuity
NVAF .... nonvalvular atrial fibrillation
NVD .... nausea, vomiting, diarrhea; neck vein distention
NYD .... not yet diagnosed; not yet discovered
nyst .... nystagmus
O .... oxygen
O&A .... observation and assessment
OAG .... open-angle glaucoma
OAH .... ovarian androgenic hyperfunction
OAR .... orientation/alertness remediation
OB .... obstetrics; occult blood
O&B .... opium and belladonna
OBS .... organic brain syndrome
OC .... on call; oral contraceptive
O&C, O+C .... onset and course (of disease)
OCAD .... occlusive carotid disease
OCD .... obsessive-compulsive disorder
OCG .... oral cholecystogram
OCs .... oral contraceptives
OCT .... ornithine carbamyl transferase
od .... right eye (oculus dexter)
OD .... overdose
ODAP .... Oncovin (vincristine), dianhydrogalactitol, Adriamycin (doxorubicin), and Platinol (cisplatin)
ODC .... oxygen dissociation curve
ODE .... O-desmethylencainide
ODm .... ophthalmodynamometry
O&E .... observation and examination
O/E .... (ratio of) observed to expected; on examination
OEC .... outer ear canal
OGT .... oral glucose tolerance

OGTT .... oral glucose tolerance test
OH .... hydroxide; hydroxyl
OHCS .... hydroxycorticosteroid
17-OHCS 17-hydroxycorticosteroids
OHG .... oral hypoglycemic
OHL .... oral hairy leukoplakia
OHP .... oxygen under high pressure
O-I .... outer-to-inner
OIF .... oil immersion field
oint .... ointment
OKT .... a group of monoclonal antibodies for typing lymphocytes
OL .... left eye
OLD .... obstructive lung disease
OM .... otitis media
OMAC .... otitis media, acute, catarrhal
OMAD .... Oncovin (vincristine), methotrexate, Adriamycin (doxorubicin), and dactinomycin
OMAS .... otitis media, acute, suppurating
OMC .... open mitral commissurotomy
OMCA .... otitis media, catarrhal, acute
OMCC, OMCCH .... otitis media, catarrhal, chronic
OME .... otitis media (with) effusion
OMN .... oculomotor nerve
OMPA .... otitis media, purulent, acute
OMPC, OMPCh .... otitis media, purulent, chronic
OMSA .... otitis media, suppurative, acute
OMSC, OMSCh .... otitis media, secretory, chronic; otitis media, suppurative, chronic
OMVC .... open mitral valve commissurotomy
ONTG .... oral nitroglycerin
ONTR .... orders not to resuscitate
OO .... oophorectomy
O&O .... off and on
O-O .... outer-to-outer
OOB .... out of bed; out-of-body (experience)
OOBBRP .... out of bed (with) bathroom privileges
OOC .... onset of contractions
OOL .... onset of labor
O&P .... ova and parasites (stool exam)
OPE .... outpatient evaluation
OPG .... ocular plethysmography
OPLL .... ossification (of) posterior longitudinal ligament
OPP .... Oncovin (vincristine), procarbazine, and prednisone; osmotic
OPV .... oral (attenuated) poliovirus vaccine; oral polio vaccine; outpatient visit
OR x1 .... oriented to time
OR x2 .... oriented to time and place
OR x3 .... oriented to time, place, and person
O.R. .... operating room
ORS .... oral rehydration solution
os .... left eye (oculus sinister)
Os .... osmium
OSA .... obstructive sleep apnea
OSAS .... obstructive sleep apnea syndrome
Osm/kg .... osmole per killigram (osmolality)
Osm/L, Osm/l .... osmole per liter (osmolality)
OSM S .... osmolarity serum
OSM U .... osmolarity urine
OT .... objective test; old tuberculin
O/T .... oral temperature
OTA .... open to air
OTC .... ornithine transcarbamylase
OTC Rx .... over-the-counter prescription
OTD .... oral temperature device
OTH .... other
OTT, OT(T) .... orotracheal tube
ou .... each eye (oculus uterque)
OULQ .... outer upper left quadrant
OURQ .... outer upper right quadrant
OUZ .... upper outer zone (quadrant)
ov .... ovarian
o/w .... otherwise
O/W .... oil in water (emulsion)

OWNK ... out of wedlock (and) not keeping (child)
OWR ... ovarian wedge resection
p ... pico (10^{-12})
p_2, P-2 ... pulmonic secod (heart) sound
p24 ... antigen in HIV infection
p50 ... half saturation (oxygen)
P ... peta (10^{15}); phosphorus; pulse
$\bar{P}$ ... [L. *post* after; mean pressure
/P ... partial lower denture
P/ ... partial upper denture
$P_2=A_2$ ... pulmonic second heart sound equal to aortic second heart sounds
$P_2<A_2$ ... pulmonic heart sound less than aortic second heart sound
$P_2>A_2$ ... pulmonic second heart sound greater than aortic second heart sound
^{32}P ... radioisotope of phosphorus
Pa arterial pressure; protactinium; pulmonary arterial (pressure); pulmonary artery (line)
PA ... alveolar pressure; panic attack; partial pressure; passive aggressive; pernicious anemia; phenylalinine; photo-allergy; physical assistance; pituitary-adrenal; platelet associated
P&A ... percussion and auscultation
P-A ... posteroanterior
P/A ... percussion (and) auscultation
PABA ... para-aminobenzoic acid
PAC ... phenacetin (acetophenetidin), aspirin, and caffeine; Platinol (cisplatin), Adriamycin (doxorubicin), and cyclophosphamide); premature atrial contraction
PAC-V ... Platinol (cisplatin), Adriamycin (doxorubicin), and cyclophosphamide
PAd ... pulmonary artery diastolic
PADP ... pulmonary artery diastolic pressure
PAF ... paroxysmal atrial fibrillation
PA&F ... percussion, auscultation, and fremitus
PAF-A ... platelet-activating factor of anaphylaxis
PAFI ... platelet-aggression factor inhibitor
PAFIB ... paroxysmal atrial fibrillation PAF
PAH phenylalanine hydroxylase; pulmonary artery hypertension; pulmonary artery hypotension
PAHA ... *para*-aminohippuric acid
PAHVC ... pulmonary alveolar hypoxic vasoconstriction
PAI ... plasminogen activator inhibitor
PA-LS-ID ... pernicious anemia-like syndrome (and) immunoglobulin deficiency
PAM ... periodic acid-methanamine silver
PAMP ... pulmonary artery mean pressure
PAN ... periarteritis nodosa
P_{ao} ... airway opening pressure
Pao ... ascending aortic pressure
PaO_2 ... partial pressure of arterial oxygen
PAo ... pulmonary artery occlusion (pressure)
PAO ... peak acid output; peripheral airway obstruction
PAO_2 ... partial pressure of oxygen in alveoli
PAO_2-PaO_2 ... alveolar-arterial difference in partial pressure of oxygen
PAOD ... peripheral arterial occlusive disease; peripheral arteriosclerotic occlusive disease
PAOP ... pulmonary artery occlusion pressure
Pap ... Papanicolaou stain
PAP .. peroxidase antiperoxidase; pri. atypical pneum.; prostate acid phosphatase
PA/PS ... pulmonary atresia/pulmonary stenosis
PAR ... pulmonary arteriolar resistance
Para ... paraplegic; parous (having borne one or more children)
para ... number of pregnancies producing viable offspring; paraplegia/paraplegic
para I ... unipara (having borne one child)
para II ... bipara (having borne two children)
para III ... tripara (having borne three children)
para IV ... quadripara (having borne four children)
para O ... nullipara (no child borne)
parasym ... parasympathetic (division of autonomic nervous system)
PARR ... postanesthesia recovery room
PAS .. para-aminosalicylic acid; periodic acid Schiff stain; preadmission screening; pulmonary arterial stenosis; pulmonary artery systolic
Pas Ex ... passive exercise
PAT ... paroxysmal atrial tachycardia; paroxysmal auricular tachycardia; preadmission testing
PATCO ... prednisone, araC, thioguanine, cyclophosphamide, and Oncovin (vincristine)

pat. T .... patellar tenderness
p aur .... behind the ear
PAV .... partial atrioventricular
Paw .... mean airway pressure
PAW .... peak airway pressure; pulmonary artery wedge
PAWP .... pulmonary arterial wedge pressure
Pb .... lead
P&B .... pain and burning; phenobarbital and belladonna
P_{BA} .... brachial arterial pressure
PBA .... percutaneous bladder aspiration
Pb-B .... lead level in blood
PBC ..... peripheral blood cell; pregnancy and birth complications; primary biliary cirrhosis
PBF .... peripheral blood flow; placental blood flow; pulmonary blood flow
PB-Fe .... protein-bound iron
PBG .... porphobilinogen
Pbl .... lead intoxication
PBI .... phenformin; protein-bound iodine
PBL .... peripheral blood leukocytes; peripheral blood lymphocytes
PBLI .... premature birth, live infant
PBLT .... peripheral blood lymphocyte transformation
PBM .... peripheral basement membrane; peripheral blood mononuclear
PBMC .... peripheral blood mononuclear cell
PBMV .... pulmonary blood mixing volume
PBP .... peak blood pressure
PBPs .... penicillin-binding proteins
PBS .... peripheral blood smear
PBZ .... phenoxybenzamine; Pyribenzamine (tripelennanine)
pc .... after meals (post cibum)
PC .... porto-caval; present complaint
pc1 .... platelet count pretransfusion
pc2 .... platelet count post-transfusion
PCA .... parietal cell antibody; percutaneous coronary angioplasty
PCB .... polychlorinated biphenyls
PCD ...... paroxysmal cerebral dysrhythmia; polycystic disease; posterior corneal deposits
PCE .... pseudocholinesterase
PCG .... pneumocardiogram
PCH .... paroxysmal cold hemoglobinuria
PCHE .... pseudocholinesterase
PCI .... prothrombin consumption index
PCK .... polycystic kidney
PCKD .... polycystic kidney disease
PCM .... primary cutaneous melanoma
PCMX .... parachlorometaxylenol
PCN .... penicillin
PCNS .... penicillins
Pco, P_{co} .... carbon monoxide pressure or tension
pCO_2 .... carbon dioxide partial pressure (tension)
PCoA .... posterior communicating artery
PCOD .... polycystic ovarian disease
PCOS .... polycystic ovary syndrome
PCP .... phencyclidine
PCR .... polymerase chain reaction
P c/s .... primary cesarean section
PCT .... postcoital test; prothrombin consumption test
PCTA .... percutaneous coronary transluminal angioplasty
PCU .... patient care unit
p cut .... percutaneous
PCV .... packed cell volume
PCW .... pulmonary capillary wedge (pressure)
PCWP .... pulmonary capillary wedge pressure
PCZ .... procarbazine; prochlorperazine
p/d .... packs per day (cigarettes)
Pd .... palladium
PD ...... patent ductus; percutaneous drain; peritoneal dialysis; postural drainage
PD_{50} .... median paralyzing dose
P(D+) .... probability of having disease
P(D-) .... probability of not having disease
P/D .... packs per day (cigarettes)
PDA .. patent ductus arteriosus; posterior descending (coronary) artery; pulmonary disease anemia

PDB . . . . *para*-dichlorobenzene
PD&C . . . . postural drainage and clapping
PDCB . . . . *para*-dichlorobenzene
PDCD . . . . primary degenerative cerebral disease
PDD . . . . platinum diamminodichloride (cisplatin); pyridoxine-deficient diet
PDE . . . . paroxysmal dyspnea (on) exertion
PDF . . . . peritoneal dialysis fluid
PDFC . . . . premature dead female child
PDH . . . . past dental history
PDI . . . . periodontal disease index
PDL . . . . poorly differentiated lymphocyte
PDLC . . . . poorly differentiated lung cancer
PDLD . . . . poorly differentiated lymphocytic-diffuse
PDLL . . . . poorly differentiated lymphocytic lymphoma
PDLN . . . . poorly differentiated (lymphocytic) lymphoma-nodular
PDM . . . . polymyositis (and) dermatomyositis
PDMC . . . . premature dead male child
PD&P . . . . postural drainage and percussion
PDR . . . . peripheral diabetic retinopathy; *Physician's Desk Reference*
PDS . . . . pain-dysfunction
PDW . . . . platelet distribution width
PE . . . . partial epilepsy; physical examination; physical exercise; pleural effusion; pulmonary edema; pulmonary embolism
PEARLA . . . . pupils equal and react to light and accommodation
PEB . . . . Platinol (cisplatin), etoposide, and bleomycin
PEEP . . . . peak end-expiratory pressure; positive end-expiratory pressure
PEF . . . . peak expiratory flow; pulmonary edema fluid
PEFR . . . . peak expiratory flow rate
PEFT . . . . peak expiratory flow time
PEFV . . . . partial expiratory flow volume
PEG . . . . polyethylene glycol
pen., Pen . . . . penicillin
PEN . . . . parenteral (and) enteral nutrition
PEP . . . . phosphoenolpyruvate
PEPI . . . . pre-ejection period index
PEPP . . . . positive expiratory pressure plateau
PER . . . . peak ejection rate
perf. . . . . perforation
PERF . . . . peak expiratory flow rate
PERK . . . . prospective evaluation (of) radial keratomy
PERL . . . . pupils equal (and) react (to) light (and) accommodation
PERLA . . . . pupils equal, reactive to light and accommodation
PERR . . . . pattern evoked retinal response
PERRLA . . . . pupils equal, round, react (to) light (and) accommodation
PET . . . . peak flow; pericardial fluid; peritoneal fluid; pleural fluid; positron emission tomography; pre-eclamptic toxemia
PeV . . . . peripheral vein
PEWV . . . . pulmonary extravascular water volume
PF . . . . platelet factor; preservative free
PFA . . . . phosphonoformatic acid; profunda femoris artery
PFG . . . . peak-flow gauge
PFK . . . . phosphofructoaldolase
PFM . . . . peak flow meter
PFO . . . . patent foramen ovale
PFR . . . . peak flow rate; pericardial friction rub
PFS . . . . penile flow study; prefilled syringe
PFT . . . . prednisone, fluorouracil, and tomoxifen; pulmonary function test
PFU . . . . plaque forming units
P_G . . . . plasma glucose
pg . . . . picogram
PG . . . . parotid gland; phosphatidyl glycine
PGD . . . . phosphogluconate dehydrogenase
PGE . . . . primary generalized epilepsy; prostaglandin E
pgf . . . . paternal grandfather
PGH . . . . pituitary growth hormone; prostaglandin H
PGI . . . . phosphoglucose isomerase; potassium, glucose, and insulin; prostaglandin I
PGK . . . . phosphoglycerokinase
pgm . . . . paternal grandmother
PGM . . . . paternal grandmother
PGN . . . . proliferative glomerulonephritis
PgR . . . . progesterone receptor
PGs . . . . prostaglandin; pyoderma gangrenosum

PGTR .... plasma glucose tolerance rate
PGTT .... prednisolone glucose tolerance test
PGU .... peripheral glucose uptake; postgonococcal
pH .... measurement of acidity or alkalinity
PH .... past history; persistent hepatitis; personal history
pHa .... arterial blood pH
PHA .... phytohemagglutinin activation
PHCC .... primary hepatocellular carcinoma
PhD .... Doctor of Philosophy
pheo, Pheo .... pheochromocytoma
PHI .... phosphohexoseisomerase
PHIS .... posthead injury syndrome
PHK .... postmortem human kidney
PHP .... persistent hyperphenylalaninemia
pHPT .... primary hyperparathyroidism
PHR .... peak heart rate
PHT .... peroxide hemolysis test; portal hypertension; primary hyperthyroidism; pulmonary hypertension
PHTN .... portal hypertension
PHx .... past history
pi .... platelet count increment
PI .... phosphatidylinositol; protamine insulin; pulmonary infarction
PICC .... peripherally inserted central catheter
PICD .... primary irritant contact dermatitis
PID .... pelvic inflammatory disease
PIE .... postinfectious encephalomyelitis; prosthetic infectious endocarditis
PIF .... peak inspiratory flow
PIH .... pregnancy-induced hypertension
PIHH .... postinfluenza-like hyposmia and hypogeusia
PIIP .... portable insulin infusion pump
PIM .... penicillamine-induced myasthenia
PIMS .... programmable implantable medication system
PIO .... progesterone in oil
PIO_2 .... inspired oxygen tension; partial pressure of inspiratory oxygen
PIV .... parainfluenza virus
PIWT .... partially impacted wisdom teeth
PJS .... Peutz-Jeghers syndrome
PJT .... paroxysmal junctional tachycardia
PJVT .... paroxysmal junctional-ventricular tachycardia
P_K .... plasma potassium
PK .... pyruvate kinase
PKN .... parkinsonism
PKU .... phenylketonuria
PLCC .... primary liver cell cancer
PLL .... peripheral light loss
PLR .... pupillary light reflex
PLS .... primary lateral sclerosis
Plt .... platelet
PLT .... psittacosis-lymphogranuloma venereum-trachoma
PLV .... live poliomyelitis vaccine
Pm .... promethium
PM .... afternoon; pacemaker
PM-1 .... polymorph; postmortem
PMC .... premature mitral closure; pseudomembranous colitis
PMD .... primary myocardial disease; progressive muscular dystrophy
PMEC .... pseudomembranous enterocolitis
PMH .... past medical history
PMI .... past medical illness
PMIS .... postmyocardial infarction syndrome
PM-I .... platelet membrane antigen
pML .... posterior mitral valve leaflet
PMN .... polymorphonuclear neutrophil
PMO .... postmenopausal osteoporosis
pmol .... picomole
PMP .... pain management program; previous menstrual period
PM&R .... physical medicine and rehabilition
PMR .... perinatal morbidity rate; perinatal mortality rate
PMS .... premenstrual syndrome
PMTS .... premenstrual tension syndrome
PN .... parenteral nutrition
P_{N2} .... partial pressure of nitrogen
P_{Na} .... plasma sodium

PNC .... penicillin
PNH .... paroxysmal nocturnal hemoglobinuria
PNP .... nonprotein nitrogen
PNPB .... positive-negative pressure breathing
pNPP .... paranitrophenylphosphate
PNPR .... positive-negative pressure respiration
Pnx .... pneumothorax
po .... by mouth (per os)
pO_2 .... oxygen partial pressure (tension)
Po .... polonium
P&O .... parasites and ova
P-O .... postoperative
POA .... pancreatic oncofetal antigen
PODx .... preoperative diagnosis
POHI .... physically (or) otherwise health-impaired
POHS .... presumed ocular histoplasmosis syndrome
POL .... premature onset (of) labor
POM .... pain on motion
POMP .... prednisone, Oncovin (vincristine), methotrexate, and Purinethol (mercaptopurine)
POMR .... problem oriented medical record
POP .... pain on palpation
POR .... physician of record; problem oriented record
POS .... polycystic ovary syndrome
POVT .... puerperal ovarian vein thrombophlebitis
PP .... paradoxical pulse; pedal pulse; peripheral pulse; postprandial
PPA .... phenylpropanolamine
PPAS .... peripheral pulmonary artery stenosis
PPB .... platelet-poor blood; positive pressure breathing
PPBE .... postpartum breast engorgement
PPBS .... postprandial blood sugar
PPCM .... postpartum cardiomyopathy
PPD .... packs per day (cigarettes); purified protein derivative
P&PD .... percussion and postural drainage
PPF .... plasma protein fraction
PPG .... photoplethysmography
PPH .... persistent pulmonary hypertension; postpartum hemorrhage
PPK .... palmoplantar keratosis
PPL .... penicilloye-polylysine
PPLO .... pleuropneumonia-like organisms
ppm .... parts per million
PPP .... palmoplantar pustulosis; pedal pulse present; peripheral pulse palpable
PPROM .... prolonged premature rupture of membranes
ppt .... precipitate
Pr .... praseodymium; presbyopia
PR .... per rectum
P&R .... pelvic and rectal (examination); pulse and respiration
P-R .. time between P wave and beginning of QRS complex in electrocardiography
P/R .... productivity to respiration (ratio)
PRA .... plasma renin activity; progesterone receptor assay
PRBC .... packed red blood cells
PRBCs .... packed red blood cells
PRED .... prednisone
PRERLA .... pupils round, equal, react to light (and) accommodation
PRF .... progressive renal failure
PRFM .... premature rupture (of) fetal membranes; prolonged rupture (of) fetal membranes
PRG .... phleborheography
PRH .... past relevant history
PRL .... prolactin
PRLA .... pupils react to light and accommodation
prn .... as needed (pro re nata)
PROM .... passive range of motion; premature rupture of membranes; prolonged rupture of membranes
PRP .... polyribophosphate
PRRE .... pupils round, regular, (and) equal
PRSM .... peripheral smear
PS ..... periodic syndrome; phosphatidylserine; population sample; Porter-Silber; pulmonary stenosis; pyloric stenosis
P&S .... pain and suffering
PSA .... prostate specific antigen
PSBO .... partial small bowel obstruction

PSG . . . . polysomnography
PSIS . . . . posterior/superior iliac spine
PSP . . . . phenolsulfonphthalein
PSRBOW . . . . premature spontaneous rupture (of) bag of waters
PSRO . . . . Professional Standards Review Organization
PSS . . . . progressive systemic sclerosis
PS-VER . . . . pattern shift - visual evoked response
PSVT . . . . paroxysmal supraventricular tachycardia
PSW . . . . past sleepwalker
Pt . . . . platinum
PT . . . . pericardial tamponade; physical therapy; prothrombin time
P&T . . . . Pharmacy & Therapeutics
PTA . . . . platelet thromboplastin antecedent; prothrombin activity
PTAH . . . . phosphotungstic acid hematoxylin
PTBA . . . . percutaneous transluminal balloon angioplasty
PTBD . . . . percutaneous transhepatic biliary drainage
PTBD-EF . . . . percutaneous transhepatic biliary drainage-enteric feeding
PTBS . . . . post-traumatic brain syndrome
PTC . . . . phenylthiocarbamide; plasma thromboplastin component
PTCA . . . . percutaneous transluminal coronary angioplasty
PTCR . . . . percutaneous transluminal coronary recanalization
PTD . . . . percutaneous transluminal dilatation
PTED . . . . pulmonary thromboembolic disease
PTH . . . . parathyroid hormone
PTHBD . . . . percutaneous transhepatic biliary drain(age)
PTMDF . . . . pupils, tension, media, disc, fundus
PTP . . . . prothrombin-proconvertin
PTPN . . . . peripheral (vein) total parenteral nutrition
PTR . . . . patella tendon reflex; peripheral total resistance
PTRA . . . . percutaneous transluminal renal angioplasty
PTS . . . . pneumatic tube system
PTT . . . . partial thromboplastin time
PTV . . . . posterior tibial vein
PTWTKG . . . . patient's weight (in) kilograms
Pu . . . . plutonium
PU . . . . peptic ulcer
PUBS . . . . percutaneous umbilical blood sampling
PuD . . . . pulmonary disease
PUD . . . . peptic ulcer disease; pulmonary disease
PUE . . . . pyrexia (of) unknown etiology
pulv . . . . a powder (pulvis)
PUNL . . . . percutaneous ultrasonic nephrolithotripsy
PUO . . . . pyrexia (of) undetermined/unknown origin
PUP . . . . percutaneous ultrasonic pyelolithotomy
PUPPP . . . . pruritic urticarial papules and plaques of pregnancy
PUVA . . . . pulsed ultraviolet actinotherapy
PV . . . . peripheral vein; plasma volume
PVA . . . . polyvinyl alcohol
PVB . . . . Platinol (cisplatin), vinblastine, and bleomycin; premature ventricular beat
PVC . . . . premature ventricular contraction
PVD . . . . peripheral vascular disease
PVE . . . . prosthetic valve endocarditis
PVF . . . . portal venous flow; primary ventricular fibrillation
PVH . . . . pulmonary vascular hypertension
PVI . . . . peripheral vascular insufficiency
PVO . . . . peripheral vascular occlusion; pulmonary venous obstruction; pulmonary venous occlusion
PVOD . . . . peripheral vascular occlusive disease
PVP . . . . penicillin V potassium
PVR . . . . pulse volume recording
PVT . . . . paroxysmal ventricular tachycardia
PWM . . . . pokeweed mitogen
Px . . . . physical
PYP . . . . pyrophosphate
q . . . . every (quaque)
QALE . . . . quality-adjusted life expectancy
QALY . . . . quality-adjusted life years
QBCA . . . . quantitative buffy coat analysis
qd . . . . every day (quaque die)
qh . . . . every hour (quaque hora)
qhr . . . . every hour (quaque hora)
qid . . . . four times a day (quarter in die)

QMI . . . Q-wave myocardial infarction
QNS . . . quantity not sufficient
qod . . . every other day
Qp . . . pulmonary blood
qs . . . sufficient quantity (quantum sufficiat)
qs ad . . . sufficient quantity to make (quantum sufficiat ad)
QTC . . . quantitative tip culture
QUIGS . . . quantitative immune globulins
QUS . . . quantitative ultrasound
qv . . . as much as you will (quam volveris)
R . . . respiration; right
Ra . . . radium
RA . . . rheumatoid arthritis; right atrium
RABG . . . room air blood gas
RAC . . . right atrial catheter
RAD . . . radiation absorbed dose
RADCA . . . right anterior descending coronary artery
RADS . . . reactive airway disease syndrome
RAF . . . rheumatoid arthritis factor
RAI . . . radioactive iodine
RAO . . . right anterior oblique
RAP . . . rheumatoid arthritis precipitins
RAR . . . renal-aortic ratio
RAW . . . airway resistance
Rb . . . rubidium
RBB . . . right breast biopsy; right bundle-branch
RBBB . . . right bundle-branch block
RBBX . . . right breast biopsy examination
RBC . . . red blood cell
RBP . . . resting blood pressure; retinol binding protein
RBS . . . random blood sugar
RC . . . red cell; retrograde cystogram
RC100 . . . red cell; red cell casts
RCM . . . radiographic contrast media; right costal margin
RCMI . . . red cell morphology index
RCS, R/CS . . . repeat cesarean section
rd . . . rutherford
RDOD . . . retinal detachment, oculus dexter (right eye)
RDOS . . . retinal detachment, oculus sinister (left eye)
RDS . . . respiratory distress syndrome
RDVT . . . recurrent deep vein thrombosis
RDW . . . red cell distribution width
Re . . . rhenium
R&E . . . rest and exercise; round and equal
REM . . . rapid eye movement
REMS . . . rapid eye movement sleep
repet . . . to be repeated (repetatur)
Rf . . . rutherfordium
RF . . . renal failure; rheumatoid factor
RFOL . . . results to follow
rGM-CSF . . . granulocyte-macrophage colony stimulating factor
Rh . . . antigen; blood group; rhesus; rhodium
RHA . . . right hepatic artery
RHBV . . . right-heart blood volume
RhIG . . . Rh_o(D) immune globulin
RHL . . . recurrent herpes labialis; right hepatic lobe
Rh_o(D) . . . red cell antigen
RI . . . reticulocyte index
RIA . . . radioimmunoassay
RID . . . radial immunodiffusion
RIPA . . . radioimmunoprecipitation
RISA . . . radioiodinated serum albumin
RK . . . radial keratotomy
RL, R-L, R/L . . . right to left (shunt)
RLL . . . right liver lobe; right lower lobe
RLQ . . . right lower quadrant
RMCA . . . right main coronary artery; right middle cerebral artery
RMSF . . . Rocky Mountain spotted fever
Rn . . . radon
RN . . . registered nurse
RNA . . . ribonucleic acid
RNP . . . ribonucleoprotein

RO . . . . . routine order
R/O . . . . . rule out
ROAD . . . . . reversible obstructive airway disease
RODAC . . . . . replicate organism detection and counting
ROM . . . . . range of motion; range of movement; right otitis media; rupture of membrane
ROS . . . . . review of symptoms; review of systems
ROT . . . . . right occipital transverse
RPBI . . . . . resting penile-brachial index
RPF . . . . . renal plasma flow
RPGN . . . . . rapidly progressive glomerulonephritis
RPI . . . . . reticulocyte production index
rpm . . . . . revolutions per minute
RPO . . . . . right posterior oblique
RPR . . . . . rapid plasma reagin
RQ . . . . . respiratory quotient
RR . . . . . recovery room; respiratory rate
R&R . . . . . rate and rhythm; recent and remote; rest and recuperation
R/R . . . . . rales/ronchi
RRA . . . . . right renal artery
RROM . . . . . resistive range of motion
RSV . . . . . respiratory syncytial virus
RSVC . . . . . right superior vena cava
R/T . . . . . rectal temperature
RTA . . . . . renal tubular acidosis
RTL . . . . . reactive to light (pupils)
RTM . . . . . routine medical care
RTN . . . . . renal tubular necrosis
Ru . . . . . ruthenium
RUG . . . . . right upper quadrant
RUL . . . . . right upper lobe
RUOQ . . . . . right upper outer quadrant
RUQ . . . . . right upper quadrant
RV . . . . . reserve volume
RVA . . . . . right vertebral artery
RVH . . . . . renovascular hypertension; right ventricular hypertrophy
RVHD . . . . . rheumatic valvular heart disease
RVVT . . . . . Russell viper venom test
Rx . . . . . a recipe; drug; medication; prescribe/prescription; prescription drug
s . . . . . without (sine)
S . . . . . sulfur
S_1 . . . . . first heart sound
S_2 . . . . . second heart sound
SA . . . . . sinoatrial; surface area
S-A . . . . . sinoatrial
SAAG . . . . . serum ascites albumin gradient
SACE . . . . . serum angiotensin converting enzyme
SADD . . . . . Standardized Assessment of Depressive Disorders
SADR . . . . . suspected adverse drug reaction
SAH . . . . . subarachnoid hemorrhage
SAL . . . . . suction assisted lipectomy
SAO . . . . . small airway obstruction
SASA . . . . . sulfapyridine and 5-aminosalicylic acid
SAZ . . . . . sulfasalazine
Sb . . . . . antimony
SBB . . . . . small bowel biopsy; specialist in Blood Bank technology
SBE . . . . . subacute bacterial endocarditis
SBL . . . . . serum bactericidal level
SBP . . . . . systemic blood pressure; systolic blood pressure
SBS . . . . . shaken baby syndrome; short bowel syndrome
Sc . . . . . scandium
SC . . . . . sickle cell; subclavian; subcutaneous
S-C . . . . . sickle cell
SCA . . . . . sickle-cell anemia
SCAT . . . . . sheep cell agglutination test
SCC . . . . . squamous cell carcinoma
SCCB . . . . . small cell carcinoma (of) bronchus
SCCHN . . . . . squamous cell carcinoma (of) head (and) neck
SCCL . . . . . small cell carcinoma (of) lung
SCE . . . . . sister chromatid exchange
SCh . . . . . succinylcholine chloride
SCID . . . . . severe combined immunodeficiency

SCIV ..... subclavian intravenous; subcutaneous intravenous
Scl ..... scleroderma; scleroderma antibody
SCL ..... scleroderma
SCPK, S-CPK ..... serum creatine phosphokinase
SCr ..... serum creatinine
SCV ..... squamous cell carcinoma (of) vulva; subclavian vein
SCV-CPR ..... simultaneous compression ventilation-cardiopulmonary resuscitation
SD ..... senile dementia; spontaneous delivery; standard deviation
S&D ..... stomach and duodenum
S-D ..... sickle cell-(hemoglobin) D (disease); strength duration
S/D ..... sharp/dull; systolic/diastolic (ratio)
SDA ..... same day admission
SDAS ..... same day admission for surgery
SDAT ..... senile dementia, Alzheimer type
SDB ..... sleep-disordered breathing
SD&C ..... suction, dilation, and curettage
SDFP ..... single donor frozen plasma
SDHD ..... sudden death heart disease
SDIHD ..... sudden death ischemic heart disease
SDS ..... same day surgery
SD-SK ..... streptodornase-streptokinase
Se ..... selenium
S&E ..... safety and efficiency
SED ..... sedimentation (rate); skin erythema dose
SEM ..... scanning electron microscopy; standard error of the mean
SEP ..... serum electrophoresis; somatosensory evoked potential
SER ..... somatosensory evoked response
SF-EMG ..... single fiber electromyography
SFLE ..... Stress From Life Experience
SG ..... specific gravity
SGA ..... small for gestational age
SGOT ..... serum glutamic oxaloacetic transaminase
SGPT ..... serum glutamic pyruvic transaminase
SGS ..... second generation sulfonylurea
SGTT ..... standard glucose tolerance test
SH ..... serum hepatitis
S&H ..... speech and hearing
S/H ..... sample and hold
SHAA ..... serum hepatitis-associated antigen
SHBG ..... sex hormone binding globulin
Si ..... silicon
SI ..... Système International (SI) units
S&I ..... suction and irrigation
SIADH ..... syndrome of inappropriate antidiuretic hormone
SID ..... sudden infant death; systemic inflammatory disease
SIDS ..... sudden infant death syndrome
Sig ..... mark, write (signa)
SIRF ..... severely impaired renal function
SIS ..... saline infusion sonography
SISI ..... short increment sensitivity index
SK ..... streptokinase
SKAB ..... skeletal antibody
SKSD, SK-SD ..... streptokinase-streptodornase
SL ..... sublingual(ly)
S/L ..... slip lamp (examination)
S:L ..... sucrase to lactase (ratio)
SLCG ..... sulfolithoecholylglycine
SLE ..... systemic lupus erthyematosus
Sm ..... samarium; Smith antigen
SMA ..... sequential/serial multiple analysis; smooth muscle antibody
SMX ..... sulfamethoxazole
SMZ ..... sulfamethoxazole
Sn ..... tin
SND ..... sinus node dysfunction
SNF ..... skilled nursing facility
SO, S&O, S-O ..... salpingo-oophorectomy
SOAP ..... subjective, objective, assessment, and plans
SOAPIE ..... subjective (data), objective (data), assessment, plan, implementation, (and) evaluation (problem-oriented record)
SOB ..... short of breath
SOBOE ..... shortness of breath on exertion
SOD ..... superoxide dismutase

sos .... if there is need (si opus sit)
SPC .... standard plate count
SPCA .... serum prothrombin conversion accelerator
SPE .... septic pulmonary edema
SPECT .... single-photon emission tomography
SPEP .... serum protein electrophoresis
SPI .... selective protein index
SPL .... sound pressure level
SPMI .... status postmyocardial infarction
SPO .... status postoperative
SPOD .... spouse's perception of disease
SPS .... sodium polyanetholsulfonate; sulfite polymyxin sulfadiazine
SQ .... subcutaneous(ly)
SqCCA .... squamous cell carcinoma
sq cell ca .... squamous cell carcinoma
Sr .... strontium
SR .... sedimentation rate; sustained release; systems review
S&R .... seclusion and restraint(s)
SRAW .... specific airway resistance
SRC .... sedimented red cell
SRF .... severe renal failure
SRF-A .... slow-reacting factor of anaphylaxis
SRI .... severe renal insufficiency
SRIF .... somatotropin releasing inhibiting factor
SR/NE .... sinus rhythm, no ectopy
SRNG .... sustained release nitroglycerin
SROM .... spontaneous rupture of membranes
SRSA, SRS-A .... slow-reacting substance (of) anaphylaxis
SRT .... sedimentation rate test; speech reception threshold
SRU .... side rails up
ss .... one-half (semis)
SS .... *Salmonella-Shigella*; saturated solution; subaortic stenosis
S&S .... shower and shampoo; signs and symptoms
S/S .... signs and symptoms
SS-A .... Sjögren syndrome A antibody
SS-B .... Sjögren syndrome B antibody
SSD .... sickle cell disease; silver sulfadiazine
SS-DNA .... single-stranded DNA
SSEP .... somatosensory evoked potential
SSKI .... saturated solution of potassium iodide
SSN .... severely subnormal
SSPE .... subacute sclerosing panencephalitis
S-T .... sickle-cell thalassemia
St AE .... standard above-elbow (cast)
stat .... at once (statim); immediately
STD .... sexually transmitted disease; skin test dose
STDH .... skin test (for) delayed-type hypersensitivity
STH .... somatotropic hormone
STI .... systolic time intervals
STIC .... serum trypsin inhibitory capacity
STLOM .... swelling, tenderness, limitation of motion
STP .... standard temperature and pressure
STS .... serologic test for syphilis
S&U .... supine and upright
supp .... suppository (suppositorium)
SVAS .... subvalvular aortic stenosis
SVBG .... saphenous vein bypass graft
SVC .... slow vital capacity
SVCO .... superior vena cava obstruction
SVC-PA .... superior vena cava-pulmonary artery (shunt)
SVCS .... superior vena cava syndrome
SVD .... single vessel disease
SVPB .... supraventricular premature beat
SVPC .... supraventricular premature contraction
SVR .... systemic vascular resistance
SVT sinoventricular tachyarrhythmia; subclavian vein thrombosis; supraventricular tachyarrhythmia; supraventricular tachycardia
SW .... short wave
SWI .... sterile water injection
Sx .... signs; symptom(s)
syr .... syrup (syrupus)
SYS BP .... systolic blood pressure

T . . . . temperature; tera (10^{12})
T_1 . . . . monoiodotyrosine; tricuspid first heart sound
T+1, T+2, T+3 . . . . first, second, and third stages of increased intraocular tension
T1-T12 . . . . first to twelfth thoracic vertebrae or nerves
T_2 . . . . diiodothyronine
T_3 . . . . triiodothyronine
T_3RU . . . . triiodothyronine redin uptake
T_3UP . . . . triiodothyronine uptake
T_3UR . . . . triiodothyronine uptake ratio
T_4 . . . . levothyroxine; thyroxine
Ta . . . . tantalum
TA . . . . thyroglobulin autoprecipitins
T&A . . . . tonsillectomy and adenoidectomy
TAA . . . . thoracic aortic aneurysm
tab . . . . tablet (tabella)
TAb . . . . therapeutic abortion
TAD . . . . tricyclic antidepressant drug
TAH . . . . total abdominal hysterectomy; transabdominal hysterectomy
tal . . . . such
tal dos . . . . such doses
TAM . . . . tamoxifen
TAT . . . . thematic apperception test; toxin-antitoxin; turnaround time
Tb . . . . terbium
TB . . . . tuberculosis
TBA . . . . to be administered; to be admitted
TBB . . . . transbronchial biopsy
TBC . . . . total body calcium
TBD . . . . total body density
TBE . . . . tick-borne density
TBF . . . . total body fat
TBFB . . . . tracheobronchial foreign body
TBG . . . . thyroxine binding globulin
TBGI . . . . thyroid binding globulin index
TBH . . . . total-body hematocrit
TBI . . . . thyroid binding index; thyroxine binding index; total-body irradiation
TBL . . . . total body load
TBM . . . . tuberculous meningitis
TBN . . . . total body nitrogen
TBNA . . . . transbronchial needle aspiration
TBPA . . . . thyroxine binding prealbumin
TBR . . . . total bed rest
TBSA . . . . total body surface area
TBTT . . . . tuberculin tine test
TBW . . . . total body water
TBWA . . . . total body water
TBX . . . . total-body irradiation
Tc . . . . technetium
^{99m}Tc . . . . radioisotope of technetium Tc 99m
TC . . . . throat culture; total cholesterol
T&C . . . . type and crossmatch
TCA . . . . trichloracetic acid; tricyclic antidepressant
TCABG . . . . triple coronary artery (bypass) graft
TCAD . . . . tricyclic antidepressant
TCAG . . . . triple coronary artery (bypass) graft
TCBS . . . . thiosulfate citrate bile salts sucrose
TCC . . . . transitional cell carcinoma
TCCB . . . . transitional cell carcinoma (of) bladder
TCE . . . . trichloroethanol
TCM . . . . tissue culture medium
TCT . . . . thrombin clotting time
TDK . . . . tardive dyskinesia
TDM . . . . therapeutic drug monitoring
TdT . . . . terminal deoxynucleotidyl transferase
Te . . . . tellurium; tetanus
TE . . . . tetanus
T&E . . . . testing and evaluation
TEA . . . . total elbow arthroplasty
TEAC . . . . tetraethylammonium chloride
TeBG . . . . testosterone-estradiol-binding globulin
TEE . . . . transesophageal echocardiography
TEG . . . . thromboelastogram
TEN . . . . toxic epidermal necrolysis; toxic epidermal necrosis

TENS . . transcutaneous electrical nerve stimulation; transelectrical nerve stimulator
ter . . . terminal
TER . . . total elbow replacement
term. . . . full-term (infant); terminal
tet . . . tetanus
Tet . . . tetralogy of Fallot
TET . . . tetanus; treadmill exercise test
TF . . . tetralogy (of) Fallot
TFEV . . . timed forced expiratory volume
TG . . . triglyceride
TGT . . . thromboplastin generation test
TGV . . . thoracic gas volume
th . . . thoracic
Th . . . thorium
THA . . . transient hemispheric attack
THb . . . total hemoglobin
THC . . . tetrahydrocannabinol
THR . . . targeted heart rate; total hip replacement
Ti . . . titanium
TI . . . total iron
TIA . . . transient ischemic attack
TIBC . . . total iron binding capacity
tid . . . three times a day (ter in die)
TIF . . . tumor-inducing factor; tumor-inhibiting factor
TIT . . . triiodothyronine
TIUV . . . total intrauterine volume
TJA . . . total joint arthroplasty
TJR . . . total joint replacement
TK . . . through (the) knee; transketolase
TKA . . . total knee arthroplasty
TKO . . . to keep open
TKR . . . total knee replacement
TKVO . . . to keep vein open
Tl . . . thallium
TL . . . tubal ligation
TLA . . . translumbar aortogram
TLC . . . tender loving care; thin-layer chromatography; total lung capacity
TLW . . . total lung water
Tm . . . thulium
TM . . . temporomandibular (joint)
t_{max} . . . time of maximal concentration
TMB . . . transient monocular blindness
TMET . . . treadmill exercise test
TMJ . . . temporomandibular joint
TMJ-PDS . . . temporomandibular joint-pain dysfunction syndrome
TMJS . . . temporomandibular joint syndrome
TMP . . . trimethoprim
TMP-SMX . . . trimethoprim-sulfomethoxazole
TMP-SMZ . . . trimethoprim-sulfomethoxazole
TMX . . . tamoxifen
TNS . . . transcutaneous nerve stimulation
TNTC . . . too numerous to count
T&O . . . tubes and ovaries
TOAP . . . thioguanine, Oncovin (vincristine), araC (cytarabine), and prednisone
TOB . . . tobramycin
TOF . . . tetralogy of Fallot
TOGV . . . transposition of great vessels
TOL . . . trial of labor
TOS . . . thoracic outlet syndrome
TP . . . total protein
TPA . . . tissue plasminogen activator; *Treponema pallidum* agglutination
TPC . . . telescoping plugged catheter
TPCV . . . total packed cell volume
TPI . . . *Treponema* immobilization test; triose phosphate isomerase
TPN . . . total parenteral nutrition
TPP . . . thiamine pyrophosphate
TPR . . . temperature, pulse, respiration
TPVR . . . total peripheral vascular resistance
TR . . . turbidity-reducing
TRAP . . . tartrate resistance leukocyte acid phosphatase
TRCV . . . total red cell volume
TRH . . . thyroid releasing hormone

TRIC .... trachoma inclusion conjunctivitis
trig .... triglycerides
TRIS .... tris(hydroxymethyl)aminomethane
trit .... triturate (tritura)
Trml, TRML .... terminal
TRP .... tubular reabsorption of phosphorus
TS .... Tay-Sachs; total solids
TSB .... trypticase soy broth
TSE .... testicular self-examination
TSH .... thyroid stimulating hormone
TSH-RF .... thyroid-stimulating hormone-releasing factor
TSH-RH .... thyroid-stimulating hormone-releasing hormone
TSI .... thyroid stimulating immunoglobulin; total serum iron
tsp .... teaspoon
TSS .... toxic shock syndrome
TSST .... toxic shock syndrome toxin
TT .... tablet triturate; thrombin time
T&T .... time and temperature
TT_4 .... total thyroxine
TTP .... thrombotic thrombocytopenic purpura
TTS .... tarsal tunnel syndrome
TTUTD .... tetanus toxoid up-to-date
TU .... thiouracil; Todd unit; toxic unit; tuberculin unit
TUD .... total urethral discharge
TUN .... total urinary nitrogen
TUPR .... transurethral prostatic resection
TUR .... transurethral resection
TURB .... transurethral resection (of) bladder (tumor)
TURBN .... transurethral resection (of) bladder neck
TURBT .... transurethral resection (of) bladder tumor
TURP .... transurethral prostatectomy; transurethral resection of prostate
TURV .... transurethral resection (of) valves
TV .... tidal volume; total volume
TVC .... triple voiding cystogram
TVU .... total volume (of) urine
TVUS .... transvaginal ultrasound
TWG .... total weight gain
Tx .... therapy; treatment
T&X .... type and crossmatch
TXM .... type and crossmatch
Txn .... transplant
TZ .... transformation zone
U .... uranium
UA, U/A .... uric acid; urinalysis
UAO .... upper airway obstructions
UB12BC .... unsaturated B_{12} binding capacity
UBBC .... unsaturated vitamin B_{12} binding capacity
UBBST .... universal blood and body substance technique
UBC .... unsaturated binding capacity
UBW .... usual body weight
UC .... ulcerative colitis
U&C .... urethral and cervical (cultures)
U/C .... urine culture
UCD .... urine collection device
UCG .... urinary chorionic gonadotropin
UCI .... urethral catheter in; urinary catheter in
UCO .... urethral catheter out; urinary catheter out
UCRE .... urine creatinine
ud .... as directed (ut dictum)
UDP .... uridine diphosphate
UDPG .... uridinediphosphoglucose
U/E .... upper extremity
UE .... under elbow; upper extremity
UEA .... upper extremity arterial
UES .... upper esophageal sphincter
UFC .... urinary free cortisol
UGA .... under general anesthesia
UGI .... upper GI
UIBC .... unbound iron binding capacity
U-I-S .... uroporphyrinogen-I-synthetase
UK .... urokinase
Umax .... maximal urinary osmolality

UMN . . . upper motor neuron
UNa . . . urinary sodium
ung . . . ointment (unguentum)
UO . . . under observation
UOP . . . urinary output
UOQ . . . upper outer quadrant
UOsm . . . urinary osmolality
UP . . . universal precautions
U/P . . . urine-plasma (ratio)
URI . . . upper respiratory illness; upper respiratory infection
URQ . . . upper right quadrant (of abdomen)
URT . . . upper respiratory tract
US . . . ultrasound
U.S. . . . United States
USAN . . . United States Adopted Names
USB . . . upper sternal border
USP . . . United States Pharmacopeia
UTBG . . . unbound thyroxin-binding globulin
ut dict . . . as directed (ut dictum)
UTI . . . urinary tract infection
UTO . . . unable to obtain
UUN . . . urine urea nitrogen
UV . . . ultraviolet; umbilical vein
UVA . . . midrange spectrum; ultraviolet
UVI . . . ultraviolet irradiation
V . . . vanadium
VA . . . visual activity
VAB . . . vincristine, actinomycin D, and bleomycin
VABP . . . ventroarterial bypass pumping
VAD . . . vascular access device; venous admixture
VADA . . . vincristine, Adramycin (doxorubicin), dexamethasone, and actinomycin D
VADR . . . vincristine, Adramycin (doxorubicin), and cyclophosphamide
vas., VAS . . . vasectomy
VB_1 . . . first voided bladder specimen
VB_2 . . . second midstream bladder specimen
VB_3 . . . third midstream bladder specimen
VBAP . . vincristine, BCNU (carmustine), Adriamycin (doxorubicin), and prednisone
VBC . . . vincristine, bleomycin, and cisplatin
VBG . . . venous blood gases
VBL . . . vinblastine
VBM . . . vinblastine, bleomycin, and methotrexate
VBMCP . . . vincristine, BCNU (carmustine), melphalan, cyclophosphamide, and prednisone
VBP . . . vinblastine, bleomycin, and Platinol (cisplatin)
VC . . . vena cava; vital capacity
VCA . . . vancomycin, colistin, and anisomycin; viral capsid antigen
VCA-EB . . . viral capsid antigen, Epstein-Barr
VCAP . . . vincristine, cyclophosphamide, Adriamycin (doxorubicin), and prednisone
VCG . . . vectorcardiogram
VCMP . . . vincristine, cyclophosphamide, melphalan, and prednisone
VCN . . . vancomycin, colistomethane, and nystatin
VCP . . . vincristine, cyclophosphamide, and prednisone
VCR . . . vincristine
VCT . . . venous clotting time
VCU . . . voiding cystourethrogram
VCUG . . . voiding cystourethrogram
VD . . . vascular disease; venereal disease
V&D . . . vomiting and diarrhea
VDAC . . . vaginal delivery after cesarean
VDG, VD-G . . . venereal disease, gonorrhea
VDP . . . vinblastine, decarbazine, and cisplatin; vincristine, daunorubicin, and prednisone
VDRL . . . test for syphilis; Venereal Disease Research Laboratory
VDS . . . vindesine
VE . . . vaginal examination; visual efficiency
VEMP . . vincristine, Endaxan (cyclophosphamide), mercaptopurine, and prednisone
VEP . . . visual evoked potential
VER . . . visual evoked response
VF . . . ventricular fibrillation; vision field
VFAM . . . vincristine, 5-fluorouracil, Adriamycin (doxorubicin), and mitomycin C
V&G . . . vagotomy and gastroenterotomy
VGH . . . very good health

VHD . . . valvular heart disease
VHDL . . . very high density lipoprotein
VIP . . . vasoactive intestinal polypeptide
VLBW . . . very low birth weight
VLD . . . very low density
VLDL . . . very low density lipoprotein
VLDLP . . . very low density lipoprotein
VLDL-TG . . . very low density lipoprotein triglyceride
VLM . . . visceral larva migrans
VMA . . . vanillylmandelic acid
VMO . . . vastus medialis oblique (muscle)
vo . . . verbal order
VP . . . venous pressure
VPA . . . valproic acid
VPCs . . . ventricular premature complexes
VPRBC . . . volume (of) packed red blood cells
VS . . . vital signs
VSD . . . ventricular septal defect
VSS . . . vital signs stable
VSV . . . vesicular stimatitis virus
VT . . . ventricular tachyarrhythmia; ventricular tachycardia
V tach, V-TACH . . . ventricular tachycardia
VTE . . . venous thromboembolism
VTM . . . virus transport media
VU . . . voltage unit
VV . . . varicose vein
V&V . . . vulva and vagina
vW, VW . . . von Willebrand (disease)
vWD . . . von Willebrand disease
vWf, vWF . . . von Willebrand factor
vWS, vWs . . . von Willebrand syndrome
VZ, V-Z . . . varicella-zoster (virus)
VZIG . . . varicella-zoster immune globulin
VZV . . . varicella-zoster virus
W . . . tungsten
wa . . . while awake
WB . . . weight-bearing; whole blood
WBAT . . . weight-bearing as tolerated
WBC . . . white blood cell; white blood cell (count)
WBC/hpf . . . white blood cells per high power field
WBTT . . . weight-bearing to tolerance
WD . . . warm dry; well developed; well differentiated; wet dressing
W/D . . . warm (and) dry
WDF . . . white divorced female
WDHA . . . watery diarrhea-hypokalemia-achlorhydria
WDHH . . . watery diarrhea-hypokalemia-hypochlorhydria
WDLL . . . well-differentiated lymphatic lymphoma
WDM . . . white divorce male
WEE . . . Western equine encephalitis/encephalomyelitis
WF . . . white female
W-F . . . Weil-Felix
WFI . . . water for injection
WFL . . . within functional limits
WIC . . . women, infants, (and) children
WLS . . . wet lung syndrome
WM . . . white male
WN . . . well nourished
WNL . . . within normal limits
WP . . . whirlpool
WPW . . . Wolff-Parkinson-White syndrome
W&S . . . wound and skin
WSF . . . white single female
WSM . . . white single male
WSR . . . Westergren sedimentation rate
w/u, W/U . . . work-up
WWAC . . . walk with aid (of) cane
WWidF . . . white widowed female
WWidM . . . white widowed male
X&D . . . examination and diagnosis
Xe . . . xenon
XKO . . . not knocked out
XN . . . night blindness

XO . . . . gonadal dysgenesis of Turner type
XOM . . . . extraocular movement
X-Prep . . . . bowel evacuation prior to radiography
y . . . . year
Y . . . . yttrium
YAG . . . . yttrium-argon-garnet - a type of laser
Yb . . . . ytterbium
y/o, Y/O . . . . years old
YOB . . . . year of birth
YORA . . . . younger-onset rheumatoid arthritis
Z-E . . . . Zollinger-Ellison
Z/G . . . . zoster (serum) immunoglobulin
ZIg, ZIG . . . . zoster (serum) immunoglobulin
ZIP . . . . zoster immune plasma
Zn . . . . zinc
ZPP . . . . zinc protophorhyrin
Zr . . . . zirconium
ZSR . . . . zeta sedimentation rate

KEY WORD INDEX

The Key Word Index is not intended in any way to suggest patterns of physicians' orders, nor is it complete. Rather, it is the intent of the authors and editors to make the information easier to find and utilize in order to support better patient care.

The Key Word Index provides a reference to the procedure name based on a diagnostic property, disease entity, organ system, or syndrome for which the procedure is useful. It lists descriptions of specific procedures. Some may support possible clinical diagnoses or rule out other diagnostic possibilities.

Each procedure relevant to the indexed diagnosis is listed and weighted. Two symbols (••) indicate that the procedure is diagnostic, that is, it documents the diagnosis if the expected result is found. A single symbol (•) indicates a procedure frequently used in the diagnosis or management of the particular disease. The other listed procedures are useful on a selective basis with consideration of clinical factors and specific aspects of the case.

Diagnoses with *International Classification of Disease—Clinical Modification* (ICD-9-CM) codes are indicated within the [ ] symbol.

(Continued)

(Continued)

(Continued)

(Continued)

(Continued)

(Continued)

(Continued)

(Continued)

(Continued)

(Continued)

BRONCHITIS (ACUTE) [466.0] *(Continued)*

BRONCHITIS (CHRONIC) [491.9]

BRONCHITIS (NOT ACUTE OR CHRONIC) [490]

(Continued)

(Continued)

(Continued)

CARCINOMA [194.3] *(Continued)*

(Continued)

(Continued)

(Continued)

(Continued)

CARCINOMA (SKIN) [173.9]

(Continued)

CARCINOMA (SKIN) [173.9] *(Continued)*

CARCINOMA (SMALL CELL) [M8041/3]

(Continued)

CARDIOMYOPATHY (HYPERTROPHIC) [425.1]

CARDIOMYOPATHY (HYPERTROPHIC OBSTRUCTIVE) [425.1]

(Continued)

(Continued)

(Continued)

CIRCULATORY DISEASE *(Continued)*

CIRRHOSIS [571.5] *see also* ALCOHOLISM; ALPHA$_1$-ANTITRYPSIN DEFICIENCY; ASCITES; CHOLANGITIS (PRIMARY SCLEROSING); CIRRHOSIS (PRIMARY BILIARY); CYSTIC FIBROSIS; ESOPHAGEAL VARICES; GALACTOSEMIA/GALACTOSURIA; GLYCOGEN STORAGE DISEASE; HEMOCHROMATOSIS; HEPATITIS; HEPATITIS (AUTOIMMUNE); JAUNDICE; LIVER; NIEMANN-PICK DISEASE; SYPHILIS; WILSON DISEASE

(Continued)

(Continued)

CONGENITAL BILIARY ECTASIA

CONGENITAL HEART DISEASE [746.9]

(Continued)

COR PULMONALE [416.9]

CORTICOSTEROID (INHALANT)

(Continued)

CORTICOSTEROID (INHALANT) *(Continued)*

CORTICOSTEROID (RECTAL)

CORTICOSTEROID THERAPY

(Continued)

CORTICOSTEROID THERAPY *(Continued)*

(Continued)

CORTICOSTEROID THERAPY *(Continued)*

CORTICOSTEROID (TOPICAL)

COUGH [786.2]

(Continued)

(Continued)

(Continued)

(Continued)

CYSTS *(Continued)*

CYST (SINUS) [478.1]

CYST (THYROID) [246.2]

(Continued)

DIABETES MELLITUS [250.0; 775.1] *(Continued)*

DIALYSIS [V56.0]

DIALYSIS (PERITONEAL) [V56.8]

DIAPHRAGM PARALYSIS [519.4]

DIARRHEA [787.91] *see also* ACQUIRED IMMUNODEFICIENCY SYNDROME (AIDS); ADENOVIRUS INFECTION; AMEBIASIS; CELIAC DISEASE; COLITIS; COLITIS (PSEUDOMEMBRANOUS); COLITIS (ULCERATIVE); CROHN DISEASE; CRYPTOSPORIDIOSIS; CYSTIC FIBROSIS; CYTOMEGALOVIRUS; ENTERIC FEVER; ENTERITIS; ENTEROCOLITIS (NECROTIZING); GASTROENTERITIS; GASTROINTESTINAL TRACT; GIARDIASIS; GLUCAGONOMA; HYPERTHYROIDISM; IGA DEFICIENCY; INFLAMMATORY BOWEL DISEASE; MALABSORPTION/ MALDIGESTIVE DISEASES; MICROSPORIDIOSIS; SMALL INTESTINE; TYPHOID FEVER

Acute diarrhea includes infectious and noninfectious entities. Evaluation of the chronic diarrheal diseases begins with basic testing involving blood and stool.

DISEASES WITH LUNG INVOLVEMENT [517.8] *(Continued)*

(Continued)

DISEASES WITH LUNG INVOLVEMENT [517.8] *(Continued)*

DISSECTION (AORTA) [441.00]

(Continued)

(Continued)

(Continued)

EFFUSIONS/TRANSUDATES/EXUDATES *(Continued)*

ELECTROLYTES *see* ACIDOSIS/ALKALOSIS (ACID-BASE BALANCE); ADDISON DISEASE; BARTTER SYNDROME; CONGESTIVE HEART FAILURE; CUSHING SYNDROME

EMBOLISM [444.9] *see also* ANTICOAGULANT THERAPY; CLAUDICATION; DEEP VEIN THROMBOSIS (DVT); HEMOPTYSIS; RENAL VEIN THROMBOSIS; THROMBOSIS

(Continued)

(Continued)

(Continued)

FARMER'S LUNG DISEASE [495.0] *(Continued)*

FAT EMBOLISM [958.1]

FATIGUE [780.7]

(Continued)

(Continued)

FEVER UNDETERMINED ORIGIN (FUO) [780.6] *(Continued)*

(Continued)

FEVER UNDETERMINED ORIGIN (FUO) [780.6] *(Continued)*

FIBROMUSCULAR DYSPLASIA [447.8]

FIBROMYALGIA [729.1]

FISTULA *(Continued)*

FISTULA (ANAL) [565.1]

FISTULA (ARTERIOVENOUS) [447.0]

FISTULA (BRONCHOPLEURAL) [510.0]

FISTULA (CAROTID-CAVERNOUS) [853.00]

FISTULA (COLON) [569.81]

FLAIL CHEST [807.4]

FLUTTER (ATRIAL) [427.32]

FOLATE DEFICIENCY *see also* ANEMIA (MACROCYTIC/MEGALOBLASTIC)

FOREIGN BODIES

FRACTURE [829.0]

FUNGUS INFECTION [117.9]

(Continued)

(Continued)

GLUCOCORTICOID THERAPY *(Continued)*

(Continued)

GLUCOCORTICOID THERAPY *(Continued)*

(Continued)

(Continued)

GRANULOMATOSIS [686.1] *(Continued)*

GRANULOMATOSIS (EOSINOPHILIC) [277.8]

GRANULOMATOUS DISEASE OF CHILDHOOD [288.1] *see also* CHRONIC GRANULOMATOUS DISEASE; GENETIC COUNSELING; TUBERCULOSIS

(Continued)

HEADACHE [784.0] *(Continued)*

HEADACHE (TENSION) [307.81]

(Continued)

HEART *(Continued)*

(Continued)

HEART *(Continued)*

HEART BLOCK [426.9]

HEART FAILURE [428.9]

(Continued)

HEART FAILURE [428.9] *(Continued)*

(Continued)

(Continued)

HEMORRHAGE [459.0]

(Continued)

(Continued)

(Continued)

HYPERCOAGULABLE STATES *(Continued)*

(Continued)

HYPERCOAGULABLE STATES *(Continued)*

(Continued)

(Continued)

(Continued)

(Continued)

(Continued)

INFILTRATE (PULMONARY) [518.3] *(Continued)*

INFLAMMATION (SPINAL CORD) [720.9]

INFLAMMATION (TESTES) *see* ORCHITIS

INFLAMMATORY BOWEL DISEASE

(Continued)

INFLAMMATORY DISEASES AND STATES *(Continued)*

(Continued)

INFLAMMATORY DISEASES AND STATES *(Continued)*

INTRADUCTAL PAPILLOMA (BREAST) [217]

INTRAPERITONEAL AIR

INTRAPULMONARY HEMORRHAGE

(Continued)

(Continued)

Diabetic ketoacidosis may be defined as hyperglycemia with increased anion gap, metabolic acidosis, and serum or urinary ketones. Other types of ketoacidosis exist as well, including starvation and alcoholism/alcohol withdrawal.

(Continued)

(Continued)

(Continued)

(Continued)

(Continued)

LYMPHOMA [202.8] *(Continued)*

LYMPHOMA (NON-HODGKIN) [202.80]

(Continued)

(Continued)

MALIGNANT NEOPLASM (INTRATHORACIC ORGANS) [194.3]
(Continued)

(Continued)

MALIGNANT NEOPLASM (INTRATHORACIC ORGANS) [194.3]
(Continued)

MALIGNANT NEOPLASM (RESPIRATORY SYSTEM) [165.9]

(Continued)

(Continued)

(Continued)

METASTASIS [199.1] *(Continued)*

(Continued)

METASTASIS [199.1] *(Continued)*

METASTATIC PAIN *(Continued)*

(Continued)

METASTATIC PAIN *(Continued)*

(Continued)

(Continued)

(Continued)

MULTIPLE ENDOCRINE NEOPLASIA (MEN 1, MEN 2) [237.4]
(Continued)

(Continued)

MULTIPLE ENDOCRINE NEOPLASIA (MEN 1, MEN 2) [237.4]
(Continued)

MYCOSIS (SYSTEMIC) [117.9] *(Continued)*

MYELINOSIS (CENTRAL PONTINE) [341.8]

(Continued)

(Continued)

NEOPLASIA *(Continued)*

(Continued)

NEOPLASIA *(Continued)*

NEOPLASM [239.9]

(Continued)

NEOPLASM [239.9] *(Continued)*

(Continued)

NEOPLASM [239.9] *(Continued)*

NEOPLASM (BENIGN) [229.9]

(Continued)

NEOPLASM (BENIGN) [229.9] *(Continued)*

(Continued)

NEOPLASM (BENIGN) [229.9] *(Continued)*

(Continued)

NEOPLASM OF UNCERTAIN BEHAVIOR (RESPIRATORY SYSTEM) [235] *(Continued)*

NEOPLASM (RESPIRATORY SYSTEM) [165.9]

(Continued)

(Continued)

(Continued)

(Continued)

(Continued)

(Continued)

(Continued)

(Continued)

(Continued)

PLEURAL FIBROSIS [511.0] *(Continued)*

PLEURODYNIA [786.52]

PLEURODYNIA (EPIDEMIC) [074.1]

(Continued)

(Continued)

PNEUMONIA [486] *(Continued)*

PNEUMONIA (*ACINETOBACTER*)

PNEUMONIA (ANAEROBIC)

(Continued)

PNEUMONIA (ASPIRATION) [507.0] *(Continued)*

PNEUMONIA (*BACTEROIDES*)

PNEUMONIA (BRONCHO) [485]

(Continued)

(Continued)

PNEUMONIA (INTERSTITIAL) [516.8]

PNEUMONIA (*KLEBSIELLA*) [482.0]

(Continued)

(Continued)

PNEUMONIA (PRIMARY ATYPICAL) [486] *(Continued)*

PNEUMONIA (*PROTEUS*) [482.83]

(Continued)

(Continued)

Manifestations include hirsutism, anovulation, oligomenorrhea or amenorrhea, often with obesity and not infrequently with diabetes mellitus. Total and free serum testosterone concentrations, LH, and insulin are increased.

POLYCYTHEMIA/POLYCYTHEMIA VERA [238.4] *see also* HYPERVISCOSITY; SPLENOMEGALY; TUMOR MARKERS

Hemoglobin >18.5 g/dL for male Caucasians, 17 g/dL for female Caucasians, 17.5 g/dL for male African-Americans, 16.7 g/dL for female African-Americans

POLYDERMATOMYOSITIS

POLYHYDRAMNIOS [657]

POLYMYALGIA RHEUMATICA [725] *see also* ARTERITIS (TEMPORAL); MIXED CONNECTIVE TISSUE DISEASE (MCTD); MUSCLE DISEASE; SCLERODERMA; SYSTEMIC LUPUS ERYTHEMATOSUS (SLE)

(Continued)

(Continued)

PREOPERATIVE EVALUATION

PREOPERATIVE EVALUATION (RESPIRATORY SYSTEM) [V71.8]

PRESYNCOPE [780.2]

(Continued)

PSITTACOSIS [073.9] *see also* LEGIONNAIRES' DISEASE; VASCULITIS

PUBERTY (PRECOCIOUS) [259.1]

PULMONARY ATRESIA [747.3]

PULMONARY BLASTOMYCOSIS [116.0]

(Continued)

(Continued)

PULMONARY FIBROSIS (IDIOPATHIC) [516.3] *(Continued)*

PULMONARY FUNCTION TESTS

PULMONARY HEART DISEASE [416.9]

(Continued)

PULMONARY VASCULAR DISEASE [416.0] *(Continued)*

PYLORIC STENOSIS [537.0] *see also* BARTTER SYNDROME; DEHYDRATION/HYPOVOLEMIA; HYPOKALEMIA; TRISOMY; TURNER SYNDROME; VOMITING

(Continued)

(Continued)

(Continued)

(Continued)

(Continued)

SARCOIDOSIS [135] *(Continued)*

SARCOMA [171.9]

(Continued)

(Continued)

(Continued)

(Continued)

(Continued)

SPUR CELL ANEMIA *see* ANEMIA (SPUR CELL)

SPUTUM INDUCTION

STAPHYLOCOCCUS AUREUS

***STAPHYLOCOCCUS EPIDERMIDIS* (NONPENICILLINASE PRODUCING) [038.1]**

(Continued)

(Continued)

(Continued)

(Continued)

TACHYPNEA [786.09]

(Continued)

THROMBOSIS [453.9] *(Continued)*

(Continued)

(Continued)

(Continued)

TRANSPLANT (HEART) [V42.1] *(Continued)*

TRANSPLANT (LIVER) [V42.7]

TRANSPLANT (LUNG) [V42.6]

(Continued)

(Continued)

(Continued)

(Continued)

(Continued)

(Continued)

WEAKNESS [780.7] *(Continued)*

(Continued)

WEIGHT LOSS [783.2] *(Continued)*

(Continued)

WEIGHT LOSS [783.2] *(Continued)*

WHEEZING [786.09]

ALPHABETICAL INDEX

NOTES

NOTES

NOTES

NOTES

NOTES

NOTES

NOTES

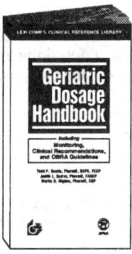

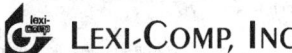

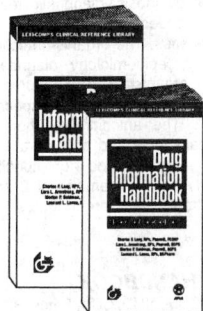

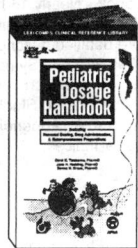

INFECTIOUS DISEASES HANDBOOK

by Carlos M. Isada MD; Bernard L. Kasten Jr. MD; Morton P. Goldman PharmD; Larry D. Gray PhD; and Judith A. Aberg MD

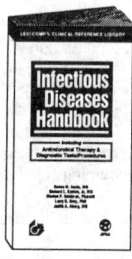

This four-in-one quick reference is concerned with the identification and treatment of infectious diseases. Each of the four sections of the book (175 disease syndromes, 152 organisms, 248 laboratory tests, and 328 antimicrobials) contain related information and cross-referencing to one or more of the other three sections.

The disease syndrome section provides the clinical presentation, differential diagnosis, diagnostic tests, and drug therapy recommended for treatment of more common infectious diseases. The organism section presents the microbiology, epidemiology, diagnosis, and treatment of each organism. The laboratory diagnosis section describes performance of specific tests and procedures. The antimicrobial therapy section presents important facts and considerations regarding each drug recommended for specific diseases of organisms. Also an International Brand Name Index with names from 20 different countries.

DRUG-INDUCED NUTRIENT DEPLETION HANDBOOK

by Ross Pelton, RPh, PhD, CCN; James B. LaValle, RPh, DHM, NMD, CCN; Ernest B. Hawkins, RPh, MS; Daniel L. Krinsky, RPh, MS

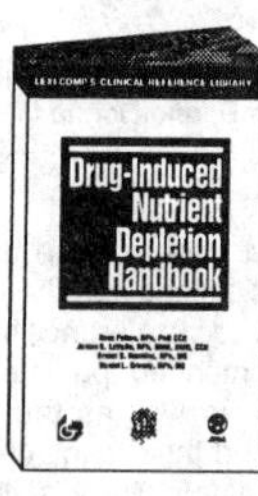

A complete and up-to-date listing of all drugs known to deplete the body of nutritional compounds.

This book is alphabetically organized and provides extensive cross-referencing to related information in the various sections of the book. Nearly 150 generic drugs that cause nutrient depletion are identified and are cross-referenced to more detailed descriptions of the nutrients depleted and their actions. Symptoms of deficiencies, and sources of repletion are also included. This book also contains a Studies and Abstracts section, a valuable Appendix, and Alphabetical & Pharma-cological Indices.

NATURAL THERAPEUTICS POCKET GUIDE

by James B. LaValle, RPh, DHM, NMD, CCN; Daniel L. Krinsky, RPh, MS; Ernest B. Hawkins, RPh, MS; Ross Pelton, RPh, PhD, CCN; Nancy Ashbrook Willis, BA, JD

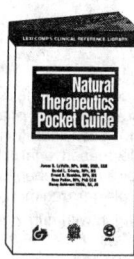

Provides condition-specific information on common uses of natural therapies.

Containing information on over 70 conditions, each including the following: review of condition, decision tree, list of commonly recommended herbals, nutritional supplements, homeopathic remedies, lifestyle modifications, and contraindications & warnings. Provides herbal/nutritional/nutraceutical monographs with over 10 fields including references, reported uses, dosage, pharmacology, toxicity, warnings & interactions, and cautions & contraindications.

Appendix: drug-nutrient depletion, herb-drug interactions, drug-nutrient interaction, herbal medicine use in pediatrics, unsafe herbs, and reference of top herbals.

To order call toll free anywhere in the U.S.: 1-800-837-LEXI (5394)
Outside of the U.S. call: 330-650-6506 or online at www.lexi.com

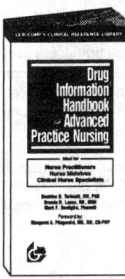

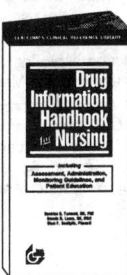

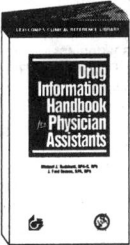

DRUG INFORMATION HANDBOOK for CARDIOLOGY

by Bradley G. Phillips, PharmD; Virend K. Somers, MD, Dphil

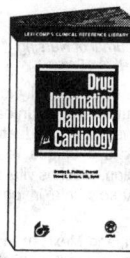

An ideal resource for physicians, pharmacists, nurses, residents, and students. This handbook was designed to provide the most current information on cardio-vascular agents and other ancillary medications.

- Each monograph includes information on Special Cardiovascular Considerations and I.V. to Oral Equivalency
- Alphabetically organized by brand and generic name
- Appendix contains information on Hypertension, Anticoagulation, Cytochrome P-450, Hyperlipidemia, Antiarrhythmia, and Comparative Drug Charts
- Special Topics/Issues include Emerging Risk Factors for Cardiovascular Disease, Treatment of Cardiovascular Disease in the Diabetic, Cardiovascular Stress Testing, and Experimental Cardiovascular Therapeutic Strategies in the New Millenium, and much more . . .

DRUG INFORMATION HANDBOOK for ONCOLOGY

by Dominic A. Solimando, Jr, MA; Linda R. Bressler, PharmD, BCOP; Polly E. Kintzel, PharmD, BCPS, BCOP; Mark C. Geraci, PharmD, BCOP

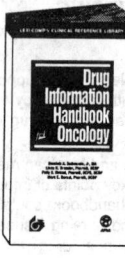

Presented in a concise and uniform format, this book contains the most comprehensive collection of oncology-related drug information available. Organized like a dictionary for ease of use, drugs can be found by looking up the *brand or generic name*!

This book contains 253 monographs, including over 1100 Antineoplastic Agents and Ancillary Medications.

It also contains up to 33 fields of information per monograph including Use, U.S. Investigational, Bone Marrow/Blood Cell Transplantation, Vesicant, Emetic Potential. A Special Topics Section, Appendix, and Therapeutic Category & Key Word Index are valuable features to this book, as well.

ANESTHESIOLOGY & CRITICAL CARE DRUG HANDBOOK

by Andrew J. Donnelly, PharmD; Francesca E. Cunningham, PharmD; and Verna L. Baughman, MD

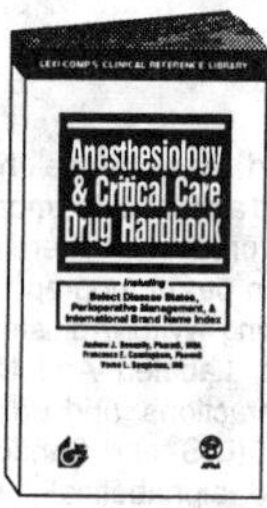

Containing over 2000 medications with up to 25 fields of information presented in each monograph. This handbook also contains the following Special Issues and Topics: Allergic Reaction, Anesthesia for Cardiac Patients in Noncardiac Surgery, Anesthesia for Obstetric Patients in Nonobstetric Surgery, Anesthesia for Patients With Liver Disease, Chronic Pain Management, Chronic Renal Failure, Conscious Sedation, Perioperative Management of Patients on Antiseizure Medication, and Substance Abuse and Anesthesia.

The Appendix includes Abbreviations & Measurements, Anesthesiology Information, Assessment of Liver & Renal Function, Comparative Drug Charts, Infectious Disease-Prophylaxis & Treatment, Laboratory Values, Therapy Recommendations, Toxicology information, *and much more.*

International Brand Name Index with names from over 20 different countries is also included.

To order call toll free anywhere in the U.S.: 1-800-837-LEXI (5394)
Outside of the U.S. call: 330-650-6506 or online at www.lexi.com

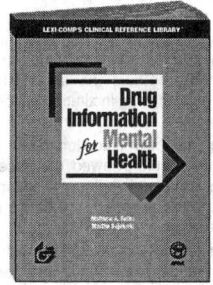

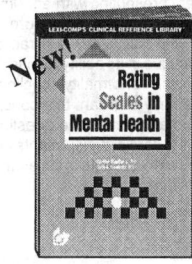

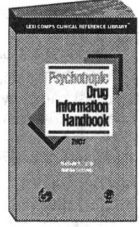

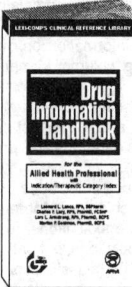

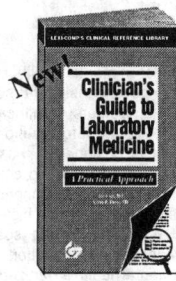

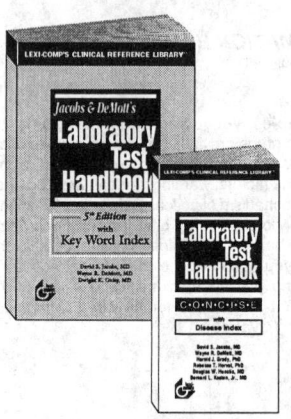

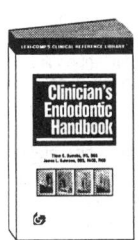

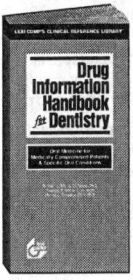

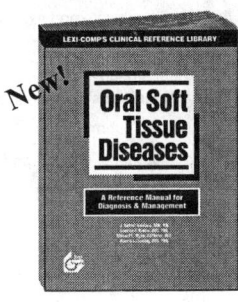

DENTAL OFFICE MEDICAL EMERGENCIES

by Timothy F. Meiller, DDS, PhD; Richard L. Wynn, BSPharm, PhD; Ann Marie McMullin, MD; Cynthia Biron, RDH, EMT, MA; Harold L. Crossley, DDS, PhD

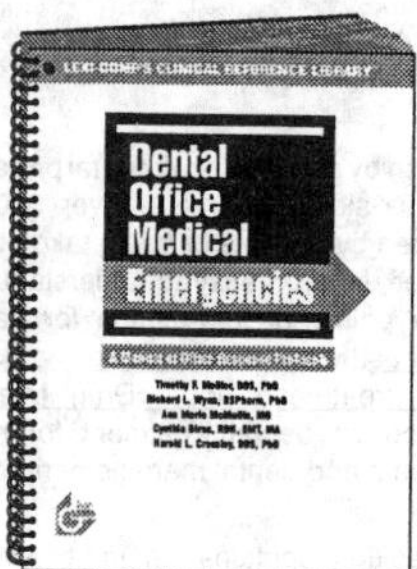

Designed specifically for general dentists during times of emergency. A tabbed paging system allows for quick access to specific crisis events. Created with urgency in mind, it is spiral bound and drilled with a hole for hanging purposes.

- Basic Action Plan for Stabilization
- Allergic / Drug Reactions
- Loss of Consciousness / Respiratory Distress / Chest Pain
- Altered Sensation / Changes in Affect
- Management of Acute Bleeding
- Office Preparedness / Procedures and Protocols
- Automated External Defibrillator (AED)
- Oxygen Delivery

A PATIENT GUIDE TO ROOT THERAPY - Flip Chart

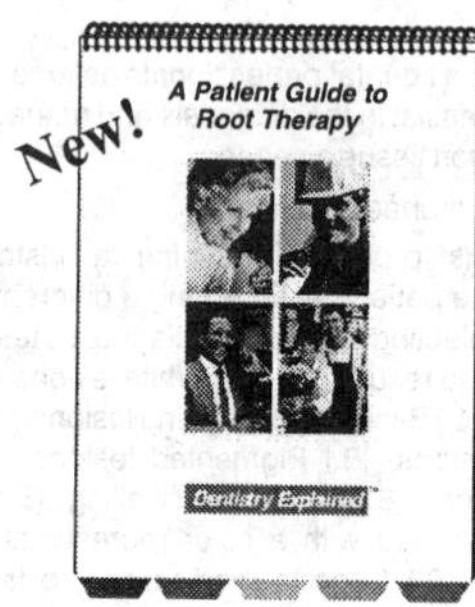

- An ideal tool used to educate and explain to your patients about root canals
- 8 1/2" x 11" colorful tabbed flip chart explaining each of the steps involved in a root canal
- Actual clinical photographs, radiographs, and diagrams

"Take home" patient education pamphlets also included.

A PATIENT GUIDE TO DENTAL IMPLANTS - Flip Chart

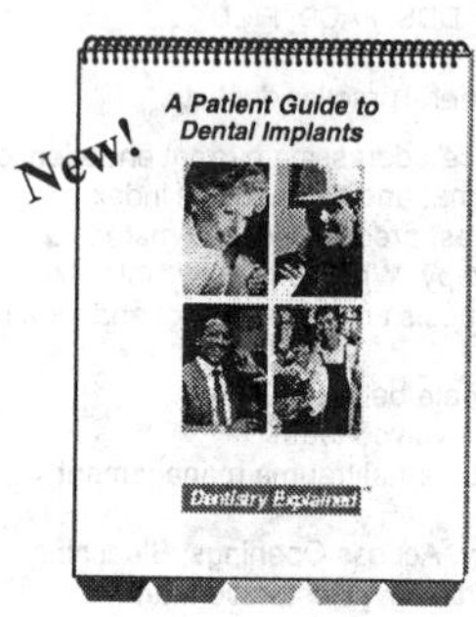

- An ideal tool used to educate and explain to your patients about dental implants
- 8 1/2" x 11" colorful tabbed flip chart explaining each of the steps involved in:
  1.) Single tooth restoration
  2.) Replacement of several teeth
  3.) Implants supported overdenture (4 implants/2 implants)
  4.) Screw-retained denture

"Take home" patient education pamphlets also included.

To order call toll free anywhere in the U.S.: 1-800-837-LEXI (5394)
Outside of the U.S. call: 330-650-6506 or online at www.lexi.com

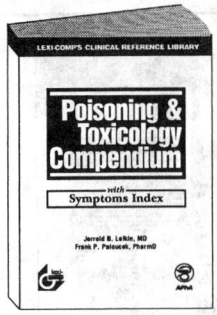

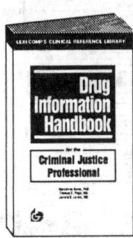

Introducing . . . *Diseases Explained*™

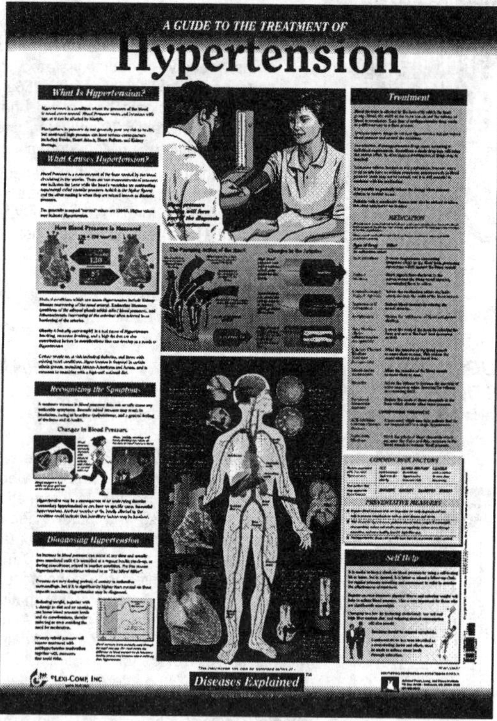

Lexi-Comp is proud to introduce Diseases Explained™, our new series of patient education material. Written in a language a patient can easily understand, each product will help the healthcare professional explain to patients about their specific medical condition.

Available now in a wall chart format and soon to be released as booklets, leaflets, and desk flip charts, this series will help you educate the patient about the cause, symptoms, diagnosis, treatment, and self-help concerning their condition.

Available now:

- Alzheimer's Disease
- Anemia
- Angina
- Asthma
- Anxiety
- Cholesterol
- COPD
- Depression
- Diabetes
- Enlarged Prostate
- Epilepsy
- Essential Tremor
- Glaucoma
- Heart Attack
- Hypertension
- Incontinence
- Insomnia
- Irritable Bowel Syndrome
- Menopause
- Migraine
- Multiple Sclerosis
- Obsessive-Compulsive Disorder
- Osteoporosis
- Otitis
- Panic Disorder
- Parkinson's Disease
- Schizophrenia
- Spasticity
- Stroke
- Thyroid Disease

Visit www.diseases-explained.com/catalog for an updated list of products or for more information call toll free: 1-877-837-5394

Thank you!

for purchasing Lexi-Comp's *Diagnostic Procedures Handbook*, 2nd Edition

Return this postage-paid card so we can keep you up-to-date on all the latest products, promotions and upgrades.

- ☐ Please put me on your **"Mailing List"**.
- ☐ Please put me on your **"Standing Order List"** to automatically receive the new edition each year.

____

Please print the title of the book here that you would like to receive a new edition of automatically each year.

- ☐ Please send me information on **quantity discounts.**

Name (First): ________________ (Last): ________________

Title / Occupation: ________________________

Institution / Company: ________________________

Address: ________________________

City: ________________ State/Province: ____________

Zip/Postal Code: ________________ Country: ____________

Telephone: (_____) ____________ Fax: (_____) ____________

E-Mail Address: ________________________

OTHER AREAS OF INTEREST (listed alphabetically by topic):

- ☐ Advanced Practice Nursing Drug Information
- ☐ Allied Health Professional Drug Information
- ☐ Anesthesiology & Critical Care Drug Information
- ☐ Cardiology Drug Information
- ☐ Criminal Justice Professional Drug Information
- ☐ Dental Office Medical Emergencies
- ☐ Dentistry Drug Information
- ☐ Diagnostic Procedures
- ☐ Drug-Induced Nutrient Depletion
- ☐ Drug Information
- ☐ Endodontic Handbook, Clinician's
- ☐ Geriatric Dosage Information
- ☐ Infectious Diseases
- ☐ Laboratory Tests
- ☐ Lab Medicine, Clinician's Guide to
- ☐ Mental Health Drug Information
- ☐ Natural Therapeutics
- ☐ Nursing Drug Information
- ☐ Oncology Drug Information
- ☐ Pediatric Dosage Information
- ☐ Physician Assistants Drug Information
- ☐ Poisoning & Toxicology
- ☐ Psychotropic Drug Information
- ☐ Rating Scales in Mental Health
  - __ Rating Scales Training Videos

ALSO INTERESTED IN THE FOLLOWING:

- ☐ Formulary or Laboratory Custom Publishing Service
- ☐ Lexi-Comp's CRL™ on CD-ROM __ Academic __ Personal __ Institutional
- ☐ Lexi-Comp database on a hand-held device __ Palm Pilot __ Windows CE™ __ Other

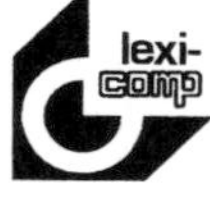

LEXI-COMP, INC

1100 Terex Road • Hudson, OH 44236

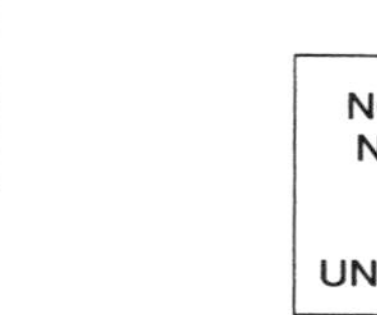

NO POSTAGE
NECESSARY
IF MAILED
IN THE
UNITED STATES

BUSINESS REPLY MAIL

FIRST-CLASS MAIL PERMIT NO 689 HUDSON, OH

POSTAGE WILL BE PAID BY ADDRESSEE

LEXI-COMP, INC.
Diagnostic Procedures Handbook
1100 Terex Road
Hudson, OH 44236-9915